ACADEMIC PRESS LIMITED
24–28 Oval Road
LONDON NW1 7DX

U.S. Edition Published by
ACADEMIC PRESS INC.
San Diego, CA 92101

This book is printed on acid free paper

A catalogue record for this book is available from the British Library

ISBN 0–12–340440–1

Typeset by Fakenham Photosetting, Norfolk
Printed in Great Britain by the University Printing House, Cambridge

Mechanisms and Models in Rheumatoid Arthritis

B. Henderson
Maxillofacial Surgery Research Unit
Eastman Dental Institute and University College London Hospitals
256 Gray's Inn Road
London
WC1X 8LD, UK.

J.C.W. Edwards
Division of Rheumatology
University College London Medical School
Arthur Stanley House
Tottenham Street, London
W1P 9PG, UK.

and

E.R. Pettipher
Department of Immunology and Infectious Diseases
Central Research Division
Pfizer Inc
Groton, CT 06340
USA.

Academic Press
London San Diego New York
Boston Sydney Tokyo Toronto

Mechanisms and Models in Rheumatoid Arthritis

Contents

Introduction

The term rheumatoid arthritis (RA) was coined by Garrod in 1859, but it was only in 1906 that Bannatyne distinguished the pathological changes occurring in RA from those found in the other major arthritic disease of humanity – osteoarthritis.

Research into the aetiology and pathology of RA started in earnest in the 1960s and has accelerated rapidly during the past three decades to the point where RA is now accepted as the prototypic inflammatory disease. We now know a great deal about the cellular and molecular aspects of this disease although it is less clear how much of this vast array of information we understand. The fact that almost all the therapies currently prescribed to treat RA were developed before the 1960s attests to this view of our lack of understanding. However, a number of modalities based on our current understanding of the molecular pathogenesis of RA are currently in clinical trial.

One of the major advances in our understanding of RA has been the development of animal models of this lesion. The first model, adjuvant disease, was developed in the mid 1950s. Since then a slow but steady stream of models have appeared (antigen-induced arthritis, bacterial cell wall arthritis, collagen-induced arthritis, etc) including, in recent years, the use of transgenic animals to determine the effect of gene ablation or supplementation on the arthritic process. Such models have been used in a large number of investigations ranging from fundamental studies of the aetiology and pathogenesis of RA to its response to known or novel drugs.

In this volume we bring together clinicians and basic scientists who are investigating the nature of RA using both clinical material and animal models. It is rare for one volume to encompass both groups of researchers. However, it is important that information from both viewpoints is encompassed to give a modern overview of the mechanisms involved in the aetiology and pathogenesis of RA.

In the first section of this volume the clinical picture of RA is reviewed and current viewpoints of the autoimmune/infectious aetiopathogenesis are discussed followed by a discussion of current and future therapeutic strategies for this condition. The second section describes the general and cellular pathology of RA. This is further expanded in the third section where the role of individual cell populations (synovial cells, chondrocytes, osteoblasts, osteoclasts, lymphocytes, etc), and the process of leukocyte trafficking, in the pathology of RA are discussed in detail. The fourth section contains reviews of the various soluble mediators believed to be involved in the pathogenesis of RA. The fifth and largest section is devoted to animal models of RA and includes reviews on the immunogenetics of experimental arthritis, the discovery of spontaneous models, the development of transgenic models and the use of animal models in drug research.

It is hoped that this book will interest clinical rheumatologists and researchers in various disciplines interested in the study of inflammation and arthritis.

Contributors

M. ALINI, Joint Diseases Laboratory, Shriners Hospital for Crippled Children, Division of Surgical Research, Department of Surgery, McGill University, 1529 Cedar Avenue, Montreal, Quebec H3G 1A6, Canada.

M.E.J. BILLINGHAM, Lilly Research Centre, Erl Wood Manor, Windlesham, Surrey GU20 6PH, UK.

D.R. BLAKE, Professor of Rheumatology and Head of the Bone and Joint Research Unit, The London Hospital, Whitechapel Road, London, UK.

S. BLAKE, Bone and Connective Tissue Research Group, Maxillofacial Surgery Research Unit, Eastman Dental Institute for Oral Health Care Sciences, University of London, 256 Gray's Inn Road, London WC1X 8LD, UK.

M.L. BLIVEN, Department of Immunology and Infectious Diseases, Central Research Division, Pfizer Inc., Groton, CT 06340, USA.

T.E. CAWSTON, Rheumatology Research Unit, Addenbrookes Hospital, Hill's Road, Cambridge, CB2 2QQ, UK.

C.Q. CHU, Division of Clinical Immunology, The Mathilda and Terence Kennedy Institute of Rheumatology (incorporating the Charing Cross Sunley Research Centre Trust), 6 Bute Gardens, Hammersmith, London W6 7DW, UK.

B.C. COLE, Professor of Medicine, Division of Rheumatology, University of Utah School of Medicine, 50 North Medical Drive, Salt Lake City, Utah 84132, USA.

R. DYNESIUS-TRENTHAM, Division of Rheumatology and Department of Medicine, Beth Israel Hospital and Harvard Medical School, 330 Brookline Avenue, Boston MA 02215, USA.

J.C.W. EDWARDS, Senior Lecturer and Consultant in Rheumatology, Synovial Biology Unit, Division of Rheumatology, University College London Medical School, Arthur Stanley House, Tottenham Street, London W1P 9PG, UK.

M. FELDMANN, Professor of Immunology, The Mathilda and Terence Kennedy Institute of Rheumatology (Incorporating the Charing Cross Sunley Research Centre Trust), 6 Bute Gardens, Hammersmith, London W6 7DW, UK.

G.S. FIRESTEIN, Director of Immunology, Gensia Pharmaceuticals, 11025 Roselle St., San Diego, CA 92121, USA.

A.J. FREEMONT, Senior Lecturer in Osteo-articular Pathology, Department of Rheumatology, University of Manchester, Stopford Building, Oxford Road, Manchester M13 9PT, UK.

S.J. FOSTER, Vascular Inflammatory and Musculo-skeletal Research Department, ZENECA Pharmaceuticals, Mereside, Alderley Park, Macclesfield, Cheshire SK10 4TG, UK.

R.E. GAY, Research Associate Professor of Medicine, The University of Alabama at Birmingham, Division of Clinical Immunology and Rheumatology, UAB Station/ THT 433, Birmingham, AL 25294, USA.

S. GAY, Professor of Medicine, The University of Alabama at Birmingham, Division of Clinical Immunology and Rheumatology, UAB Station/THT 433, Birmingham, AL 35294, USA.

M. GOWEN, Department of Cellular Biochemistry, Units of Bone Biology and Immunology, SmithKline Beecham, 709 Swedeland Road, King of Prussia, PA 19406, USA.

M.M. GRIFFITHS, Research Service, Veteran's Affairs Medical Center and Division of Rheumatology, University of Utah Medical School, Salt Lake City, Utah 84132, USA.

R.J. GRIFFITHS, Department of Immunology and Infectious Diseases, Central Research Division, Pfizer Inc., Groton, CT 06340, USA.

B. HALLIWELL, Professor of Biochemistry, Pharmacology Group, King's College, University of London, Manresa Road, London SW3 6LX, UK and Pulmonary Medicine, UC Davis Medical Center, 4301 X St., Sacramento, CA 95817, USA.

S. HARRIS, Group Leader, Biochemical Targets, Glaxo Group Research Ltd., Greenford Road, Greenford, Middlesex UB6 0HE, UK.

B. HENDERSON, Boissard Professor of Biochemistry, Chairman of Division, Eastman Dental Institute for Oral Health Care Sciences and University College London Hospitals, University of London, 256 Gray's Inn Road, London WC1X 8LD, UK.

A.P. HOLLANDER, Shriners Hospital for Crippled Children, Division of Surgical Research, Department of Surgery, McGill University, 1529 Cedar Avenue, Montreal, Quebec H3G 1A6, Canada. *Current address:* Department of Human Metabolism and Clinical Biochemistry, University of Sheffield Medical School, Beech Hill Road, Sheffield S10 2RX, UK.

A.J. LEWIS, Vice President, Wyeth-Ayerst Research, Princeton, NJ 08534, USA.

P.E. LIPSKY, The Harold C. Simmons Arthritis Research Center, The University of Texas Southwestern Medical Center, 5323 Harry Hines Boulevard, Dallas, TX 75235, USA.

R.N. MAINI, Director, The Mathilda and Terence Kennedy Institute of Rheumatology (Incorporating the Charing Cross Sunley Research Centre Trust), 6 Bute Gardens, Hammersmith, London W6 7DW, UK.

P.I. MAPP, ARC Bone and Joint Research Unit, The London Hospital, Whitechapel Road, London, UK.

I.B. McINNES, Wellcome Trust Clinical Fellow, Centre for Rheumatic Diseases, University Department of Medicine, Glasgow Royal Infirmary, Glasgow G31 2ER, UK.

R.M. McMILLAN, Vascular, Inflammatory and Musculo-skeletal Research Department, ZENECA Pharmaceuticals, Mereside, Alderley Park, Macclesfield, Cheshire SK10 4TG, UK.

N. OPPENHEIMER-MARKS, The Harold C. Simmons Arthritis Research Center, The University of Texas Southwestern Medical Center, 5323 Harry Hines Boulevard, Dallas, TX 75235, USA.

F.X. O'SULLIVAN, Associate Professor of Internal Medicine, University of Missouri-Columbia, Columbia, MO 65212, USA.

I.G. OTTERNESS, Research Advisor, Department of Immunology and Infectious Diseases, Central Research Division, Pfizer Inc., Groton, CT 06340, USA.

G.S. PANAYI, ARC Professor of Rheumatology, United Medical and Dental Schools of Guy's and St Thomas's Hospitals, Guys Hospital, 4th Floor Hunt's House, London SE1 9RT, UK.

E.R. PETTIPHER, Senior Scientist, Department of Immunology and Infectious Diseases, Central Research Division, Pfizer Inc., Groton, CT 06340, USA.

A.R. POOLE, Director, Joint Diseases Laboratory, Shriners Hospital for Crippled Children, Division of Surgical Research, Department of Surgery, McGill University, 1529 Cedar Avenue, Montreal, Quebec H3G 1A6, Canada.

A. SAWITZKE, Assistant Professor of Medicine, Division of Rheumatology, University of Utah School of Medicine, 50 North Medical Drive, Salt Lake City, Utah 84132, USA.

J.H. SCHWAB, Department of Microbiology and Immunology, University of North Carolina School of Medicine, CB 7290, Chapel Hill, NC 27599, USA.

J.S. SHAW, Vascular, Inflammatory and Musculo-skeletal Research Department, ZENECA Pharmaceuticals, Mereside, Alderley Park, Macclesfield, Cheshire SK10 4TG, UK.

T. SKERRY, Department of Anatomy, School of Veterinary Science, University of Bristol, Southwell Street, Bristol BS2 8EJ, UK.

R.D. STURROCK, McCleod/ARC Professor of Rheumatology, Centre for Rheumatic Diseases, University Department of Medicine, Glasgow Royal Infirmary, Glasgow G31 2ER, UK.

D.E. TRENTHAM, Chief, Division of Rheumatology and Associate Professor of Medicine, Beth Israel Hospital and Harvard Medical School, 330 Brookline Avenue, Boston MA 02215, USA.

F.A.J. VAN DE LOO, Department of Rheumatology, University Hospital, Nijmegen, The Netherlands.

S.M. WAHL, Cellular Immunology, NIDR, NIH, Building 30, Room 326, 9000 Rockville Pike, Bethesda, MD 20892, USA.

B.M. WEICHMAN, Wyeth-Ayerst Research, Princeton, NJ 08543, USA.

L.S. WILKINSON, Division of Rheumatology, University College London Medical School, Arthur Stanley House, Tottenham Street, London W1P 9PG, UK.

P.H. WOOLEY, Associate Professor of Internal Medicine, Immunology and Microbiology, Division of Rheumatology, Department of Internal Medicine, Wayne State University Medical School, Hutzet Hospital 2E, 4707 St Antoine Blvd, Detroit, MI 48201, USA.

D.E. WOOLLEY, Reader in Biochemistry, Department of Medicine, University Hospital of South Manchester, Nell Lane, West Didsbury, Manchester M20 8LR, UK.

J. ZAGORSKI, Cellular Immunology, NIDR, NIH, Building 30, Room 326, 9000 Rockville Pike, Bethesda, MD 20892, USA.

J. ZHANG, Wyeth-Ayerst Research, Princeton, NJ 08543, USA.

Introduction to
Rheumatoid Arthritis

1 Clinical Aspects of Rheumatoid Arthritis

I.B. McInnes and R.D. Sturrock

HISTORY

The antiquity of rheumatoid arthritis (RA) is a disputed subject as there are no convincing records documenting the existence of RA in ancient and mediaeval literature. Anecdotal case descriptions exist in the ancient Hindu and Greek medical writings (Sturrock *et al.*, 1977) which are suggestive of the existence of RA but frequently chronic rheumatic disease is described as 'gout' in mediaeval writings and in references occurring in the literature up to the nineteenth century. The evidence from paleopathology suggests that osteoarthritis was common in ancient and mediaeval times (Thould and Thould, 1983) but, unfortunately, the small bones of the hands and feet are invariably missing from ancient skeletal remains so that the characteristic bony erosions of RA cannot be looked for.

The earliest clear description of RA is to be found in the French literature with a description by Landre-Beauvais who used the term 'gout asthenique primitife' to describe a case (Snorrason, 1952). Subsequent descriptions followed but the term 'rheumatoid arthritis' was first used by A.B. Garrod in 1859 (Garrod, 1859).

EPIDEMIOLOGY

RA has a worldwide distribution but it lacks a precise definition and several sets of criteria have been developed to facilitate diagnosis. Most epidemiological surveys have used the criteria defined by Ropes *et al.* in 1958 and Table 1 lists these criteria alongside the most recent revision proposed by the American Rheumatism Association (Arnett *et al.*, 1987). Using the Ropes criteria the overall prevalence rate for definite RA in western Europe is about 1% with a female to male ratio of 3:1 and a peak age of onset between the fifth and sixth decades of life. Annual incidence rates vary from 90 to 300 new cases per 100 000 (Hazes and Silman, 1990). There are variations in prevalence rates between different ethnic groups with low rates in the rural African population and in the Chinese.

Genetic factors are important with a strong association between RA and HLA-DR4 which is now increasingly recognized to be a disease severity risk factor rather than a disease marker (Thomson *et al.*, 1993, reviewed in more detail in Chapter 2, this volume). Concordance rates for the disease in monozygotic twins is surprisingly low at approximately 11% (Silman *et al.*, 1993).

CLINICAL FEATURES

RA is a disease with a wide clinical spectrum and is often difficult to diagnose in the early stages of onset. Many patients may present with non-specific systemic features

Mechanisms and Models in Rheumatoid Arthritis
ISBN 0–12–340440–1

Table 1a. ARA criteria for rheumatoid arthritis of 1958 (Ropes *et al.*, 1958).

Morning stiffness
Pain on motion or tenderness in at least one joint
Swelling of one joint, representing soft tissue or fluid
Swelling of at least one other joint
Symmetrical joint swelling
Subcutaneous nodules
Typical radiological arthritic changes
Positive test for rheumatoid factor in serum
Poor mucin precipitate from synovial fluid
Characteristic histological changes in synovial membrane
Characteristic histiopathology of rheumatoid nodules

Exclusions
The typical rash of lupus
High concentrations of lupus erythematosus cells
Histological evidence of polyarteritis nodosa
Weakness of neck, trunk, and pharyngeal muscles or persistent muscle swelling or dermatomyositis
Definite scleroderma
Clinical picture characteristic of rheumatic fever
Clinical picture characteristic of gouty arthritis
Tophi
A clinical picture of acute infectious arthritis
Tubercle bacilli in the joints or histological evidence of joint tuberculosis
Clinical picture characteristic of Reiter's syndrome
Clinical picture characteristic of shoulder–hand syndrome
Clinical picture characteristic of hypertrophic pulmonary osteoarthropathy
Clinical picture characteristic of neuroarthropathy
Homogentisic acid in the urine, detectable grossly with alkalinization
Histological evidence of sarcoid or positive Kveim test
Multiple myeloma
Characteristic skin lesions of erythema nodosum
Leukaemia or lymphoma
Agammaglobulinaemia

Table 1b. The revised criteria of 1987 (ARA/ACR) Arnett *et al.* (1988).

Criterion	Comment
Morning stiffness	Duration >1 h lasting >6 weeks
Arthritis of at least 3 areas	Soft tissue swelling or exudation lasting >6 weeks
Arthritis of hand joints	Wrist, metacarpophalangeal joints or proximal interphalangeal joints lasting >6 weeks
Symmetrical arthritis	At least one area, last >6 weeks
Rheumatoid nodules	As observed by a physician
Serum rheumatoid factor	As assessed by a method positive in less than 5% of control subjects
Radiographic changes	As seen on anteroposterior films of wrists and hands

such as malaise, weight loss and a low grade fever associated with the onset of pain, stiffness and swelling of one or more joints.

JOINT ABNORMALITIES

Characteristically the small joints of the hands, wrists and feet are affected first in a symmetrical fashion but any synovial joint can be involved (Table 2). There are three forms of clinical presentation into which most cases of RA can broadly be recognized (Fig. 1):

Table 2.

| | % joints initially involved | | | % finally involved |
	Right	Left	Bilateral	
MCP	65	58	52	87
Wrist	60	57	48	82
PIP	63	53	45	63
MTP	48	47	43	48
Shoulder	37	42	30	47
Knee	35	30	24	56
Ankle	25	23	18	53
Elbow	20	15	14	21

PIP, proximal interphalyngeal joint; MCP, metacarpophalyngeal joint; MTP, metatarsophalyngeal joint.

● A chronic progressive form in which the disease begins with minimal joint involvement and then progresses slowly over a period of years to multiple joint disease with severe functional limitation. This is the most common pattern of arthritis seen.
● An intermittent course punctuated by acute episodes of arthritis with periods of remission in between.
● An explosive onset with multiple joint involvement and acute synovitis which may go into partial remission after 3 years or so. This pattern of RA is more commonly seen when RA begins in the elderly patient.

The typical joint deformities of the hands and feet are shown in Figs 2 and 3. Soft tissue swelling, ulna deviation of the fingers and tenderness over the proximal interphalyngeal and metacarpophalyngeal joints are characteristic of hand involvement whilst clawing and crowding of the toes with subluxation of the metatarsal heads, underneath which callosities often develop, are the hallmarks of foot disease. Large joints such as the knee and hip are often affected (Figs 4 and 5) with resulting deformity and pain which necessitates joint replacement surgery.

The proliferating synovial tissue at the wrist may involve muscle flexor and extensor tendons resulting in tendon rupture.

Of particular importance is the degree of arthritis occurring in the cervical spine which may result in atlantoaxial subluxation and compression of the cervical cord causing a cervical myelopathy (Fig. 6).

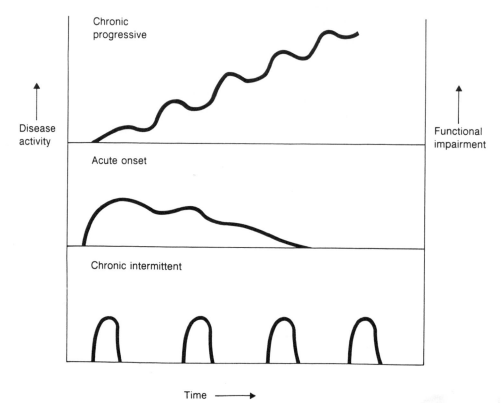

Figure 1. Three patterns of the clinical progress of rheumatoid arthritis are demonstrated. The most common pattern is of chronic progressive disease.

EXTRA ARTICULAR FEATURES

Rheumatoid arthritis is not confined to the joints alone and may involve many other body systems. Some clinicians have used the term 'rheumatoid disease' to emphasize the multisystem aspects of RA. The most common extra-articular features are shown in Fig. 7.

ANAEMIA

This is the most common extra-articular feature of RA and is associated with active disease (Smith *et al.*, 1992). Characteristically it is described as being normocytic and normochromic but in practice this classical presentation is uncommon and the more usual presentation is of a microcytosis with normal iron stores. The precise mechanism for the anaemia is not known but involves a block in utilization of iron for haemopoiesis.

NODULES

Nodules are subcutaneous, rounded, rubbery lesions which characteristically occur over bony prominences and are seen in patients with seropositive RA. They are often

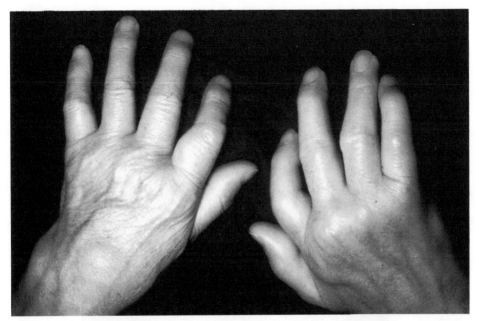

Figure 2. Typical hand deformities of rheumatoid arthritis showing ulnar deviation of the fingers and swelling of the metacarpophalangeal and proximal interphalangeal joints.

observed and felt around the elbow (Fig. 8) but may cause pressure effects when forming over the sacral area with resultant skin breakdown and the development of a vasculitic ulcer (Fig. 9). Rheumatoid nodules can occur in the lungs and heart and in the former site are sometimes confused with a lung tumour. The histology of a nodule consists of a central core of fibrinoid necrosis around a small blood vessel with a chronic inflammatory infiltrate of macrophages and an outer layer of fibroblasts arranged in a 'palisade' (Fig. 10).

EYE DISEASE

The eye may be involved in RA in a variety of ways. The most common form of eye disease is episcleritis which consists of an area of focal inflammation of the superficial layers of the sclera and is associated with discomfort, 'a feeling of sand in the eyes', but not much pain. Scleritis is an extension of this with involvement of the deeper layers of the sclera and widespread inflammation associated with severe pain (Fig. 11). A more indolent form of scleritis results in a slate grey or blue discoloration due to the underlying choroid becoming visible.

Patients who develop scleritis have a poorer overall prognosis and are more likely to develop vasculitis.

VASCULITIS

Inflammation of the vessel wall of small arterioles and venules in RA patients is usually a complication of seropositive disease and the most common manifestation is

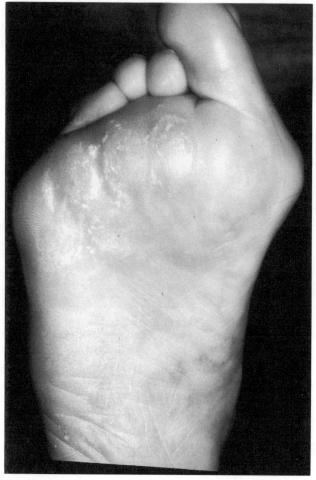

Figure 3. Foot deformity in rheumatoid arthritis showing clawing of the toes, subluxation of the metatarsal heads and callosities forming over bony prominences.

of nail fold infarcts and 'splinter' haemorrhages underneath the nails (Fig. 12). Vasculitis of the skin vessels may result in ulcer formation and extensive skin necrosis whilst digital artery vasculitis leads to florid gangrene (Fig. 13). Severe rheumatoid vasculitis is a life-threatening condition with multi-organ disease of the heart, lungs, nerves and bowel. There an associated immune disturbance with high levels of circulating immune complexes and usually low C4 levels and evidence of complement activation.

SJÖGREN'S SYNDROME

Chronic inflammation of the lacrimal and salivary glands characterized by a reduction in tear (Fig. 14) and saliva production results in the symptoms of dry eyes and a dry mouth. An increased frequency of dental caries and eye infections is seen in these

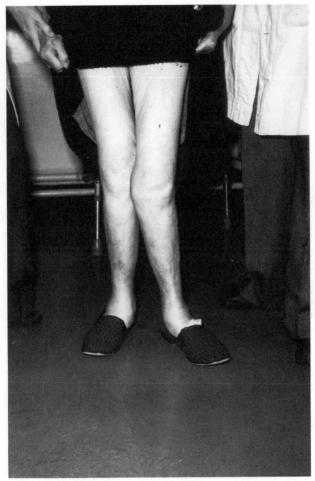

Figure 4. Swelling and instability of the left knee with a typical valgus deformity of rheumatoid arthritis.

patients and there is also an increased risk of the occurrence of a non-Hodgkin's lymphoma (Porter, 1993).

FELTY'S SYNDROME

This is a syndrome occurring in a small subset of RA patients with a DR4 positivity frequency of 90% or more (Campion *et al.*, 1990). The clinical features consist of splenomegaly, lymphadenopathy and a pancytopenia. Leg ulceration may also be a complication and the patients are prone to recurrent infections with staphylococci and Gram-negative bacteria. The precise aetiology is unknown but these patients exhibit high titre rheumatoid factors and antinuclear antibodies and granulocyte function is impaired. Some patients may respond to splenectomy with a rise in the white cell and platelet counts but the results of this procedure are variable and improvement of the

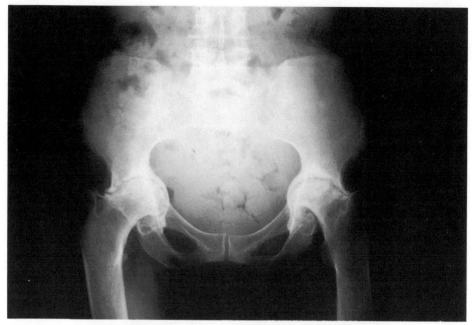

Figure 5. X-ray of the hips showing gross rheumatoid arthritis with protrusio acetabulli.

haematological features can occur following the use of slow-acting antirheumatic drugs such as azathioprine and methotrexate.

IMAGING IN RA

The contribution of plain X-ray films in management of RA has been complimented in recent years by the increased availability of computerized tomography (CT) and, subsequently, of magnetic resonance imaging (MRI). Related procedures including arthrography and conventional tomography are less frequently carried out as a result. In this section, the cardinal plain radiologic signs of RA will be described and thereafter the role of CT and, particularly, MRI will be discussed. Plain radiography allows diagnosis and thereafter therapeutic monitoring, and remains the gold standard in evaluating disease progression in RA. The characteristic symmetrical pattern of synovial joint involvement has been described and assists in radiologic diagnosis.

Classical features recognized reflect the inflammatory pathogenesis underlying joint damage. Thus, osteoporosis is an early feature and, initially, is of periarticular distribution, although it may become generalized, particularly in the axial skeleton. Narrowing of the joint space secondary to articular cartilage loss is usually diffuse and characteristically pancompartmental within joints (Fig. 15). Erosions, which represent bony destruction, are initially evident on bone unprotected by cartilage and therefore exposed directly to cytokine and enzyme mediators in synovial tissue. Early changes are found in the dorsoradial aspect of the head of the second metacarpophalyngeal (MCP) joint, third MCP and proximal interphalangeal (PIP) joint, and in the first and fifth metatarsophalangeal (MTP) joint heads in the feet. Severe erosive appearances

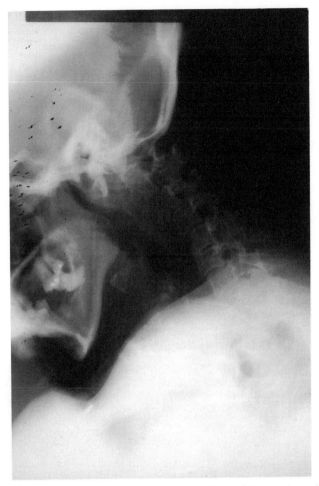

Figure 6. Lateral view of the cervical spine in rheumatoid arthritis showing atlanto-axial subluxation and multiple subaxial dislocation of the cervical vertebrae.

may reflect collapse of underlying osteoporotic bone and often are accompanied by secondary osteoarthritic changes including osteophyte formation. Such compressive events account for acetabular protrusion at the hip representing migration of the acetabular margin medial to the ilioischial line. Bony cysts in the subchondral area are common and rarely, if predominant, may be described as pseudocystic RA. Soft tissue examination is important and may demonstrate fusiform peri-articular swelling early in the disease process or the presence of intra-articular effusions. Ultimately, bony ankylosis may occur but in RA is rarely seen outwith the wrist and tarsal bones.

The dynamic evolution of these changes seems to be that of rapid initial progression which slows thereafter. Several scoring systems using standard films have been devised to standardize assessment of these changes to facilitate therapeutic monitoring and drug comparison. Thus, Larsen's method uses standard radiographs against which samples are compared (Larsen and Thoen, 1987). Other methods, such as that of Sharp *et al.* (1985) derive joint space narrowing and erosive scores allowing statisti-

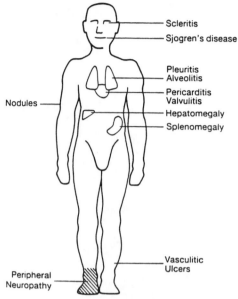

Figure 7. Diagram showing the common extra-articular features of rheumatoid arthritis.

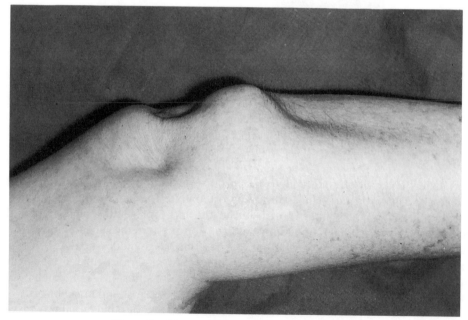

Figure 8. Rheumatoid nodules over the elbow.

cal analysis. Although the latter may be more sensitive to changes over time, the former approach is quicker and no universally accepted standard yet exists (Cuchacovich *et al.*, 1992). An alternative approach is the use of quantitative micro-

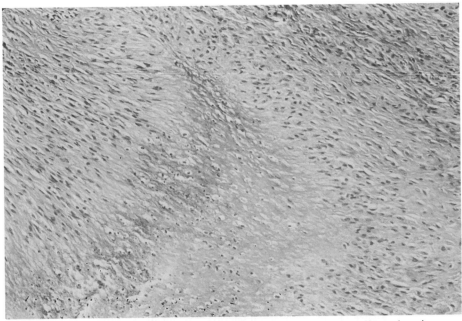

Figure 9. Histology of a rheumatoid nodule showing fibrinoid necrosis, a chronic inflammatory cell infiltrate and 'palisading' of fibroblasts.

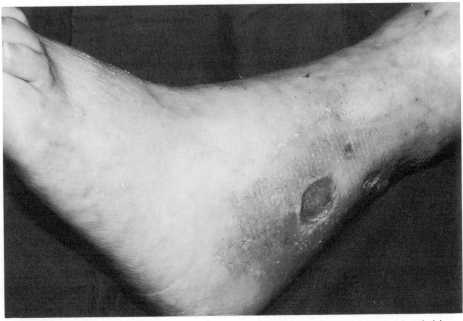

Figure 10. A vasculitic ulcer on the lateral aspect of the ankle in rheumatoid arthritis.

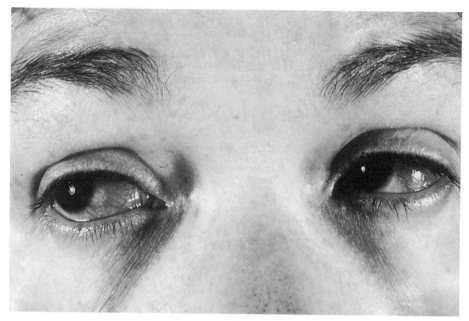

Figure 11. Severe bilateral scleritis in rheumatoid arthritis.

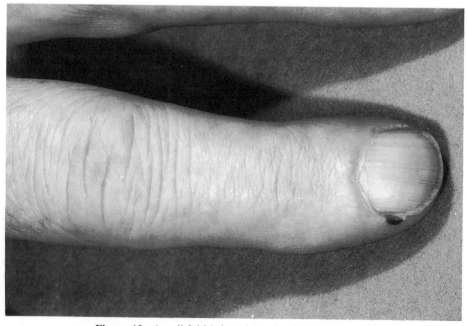

Figure 12. A nail fold infarct in early digital vasculitis.

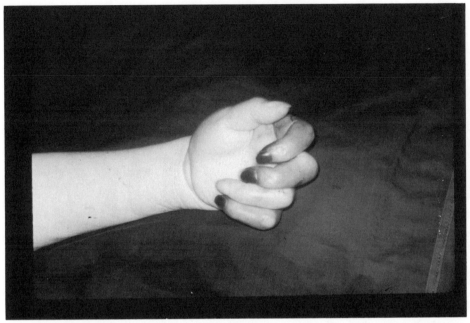

Figure 13. Severe digital vasculitis with early gangrene in rheumatoid arthritis.

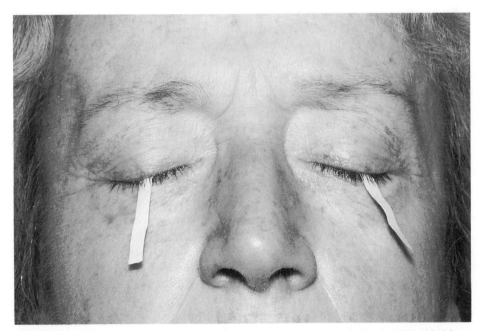

Figure 14. A photograph showing a Schirmer's test in a patient with rheumatoid arthritis in Sjogren's syndrome. Dryness of the eyes is illustrated by the lack of wetting of the blotting paper strip placed underneath the lower eye-lid.

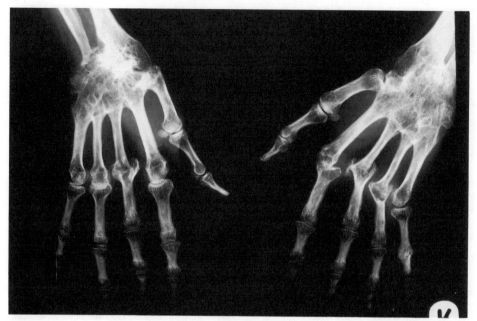

Figure 15. X-rays of the hands of the patient with rheumatoid arthritis showing erosions and subluxations of the metatarsophalangeal joints with ankylosis of the carpal bones of both wrists.

focal radiography which employs a smaller X-ray source to create macroradiographs which provide high magnification and spatial resolution (Buckland-Wright *et al.*, 1993). This allows quantification of disease progression and of erosion repair and has been used to assess the impact of disease modifying antirheumatic drug (DMARD) therapy.

CT scanning allows resolution of complex joints with their related soft tissue structures and has provided useful imaging for preoperative assessment particularly at the hip, shoulder and temporomandibular joint. In combination with MRI of the cervical spine area, CT with contrast enhancement remains valuable in planning neurosurgical stabilization in cases of spinal cord and nerve root compression. In other systems, CT is the investigation of choice to diagnose pulmonary fibrosis complicating RA.

MRI offers superior soft tissue contrast and a high level of spatial resolution as compared to CT and has increasing use in RA for early diagnosis and in management of disease complications, particularly of the neck. Plain X-rays are poor early discriminators of joint erosion and synovial tissue changes, although early detection of inflammatory changes may be therapeutically important. Several studies have shown MRI with gadolinium enhancement of wrist and hand to be superior to conventional X-rays in detecting bone erosions (Jorgensen *et al.*, 1993). Moreover, the precise location within joints of synovitic changes may be established and characterized. Contrast injection allows discrimination of synovitis from effusions, hypervascular from fibrotic synovial thickening and subchondral pannus from subchondral sclerosis. Many other soft tissue abnormalities are revealed including avascular necrosis, bone marrow oedema, tendon inflammation and rupture, muscle atrophy and tears (e.g. rotator cuff lesions) (Heron, 1992). MRI is also useful in clarifying causes of carpal tunnel syndrome, a common complication in RA (Reichner and Kellerhouse, 1990). Thus, MRI has superseded arthrography and stands comparison with arthroscopy in diagnostic value in many arthropathies, although naturally no histological diagnosis is obtained.

MRI is the preferred investigation of rheumatoid cervical myelopathy (Fig. 16).

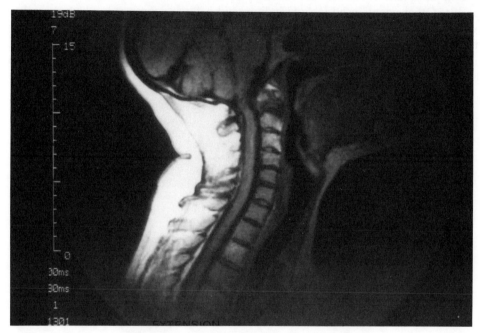

Figure 16. An MRI scan of the cervical spine.

Atlanto-axial subluxation and impaction (vertical) and cervical spine subluxations are well demonstrated, as are the effects of flexion and extension on spinal cord integrity (Ginig *et al.*, 1990). In addition to revealing instability, the presence and effects of local pannus formation may be revealed. Although less common in RA, lumbar disc lesions may be similarly delineated in combination with CT scanning. Thus, MRI offers a sensitive image of synovial destruction and sequential studies following DMARD therapy will provide an important measure of drug efficacy.

Infrared thermography has been used to detect increased heat loss from the skin surface over an inflamed joint. The intensity of the infrared radiation measured is a reflection of increased blood flow in tissues near to the skin surface with heat being conducted to the skin surface and subsequently being detected as radiant heat. This is an indirect assessment of the inflammatory response. It is possible to scan over an area of interest and to produce an image (Plate I) which can be quantified by computer analysis to generate a thermographic index. Some centres using this technique have demonstrated changes in heat radiation which mirror clinical changes occurring during therapy with second line drugs for RA such as methotrexate and D-penicillamine (Devereaux *et al.*, 1985). Infrared thermography is also capable of detecting abnormal heat patterns in soft tissue conditions such as tennis elbow and algodystrophy

(Thomas *et al.*, 1992). The major disadvantage of this technique is the need for a temperature controlled environment – a problem which may be overcome by microwave thermography in the future (Fraser *et al.*, 1987).

Radionuclide scanning offers an alternative diagnostic approach which takes advantage of the hypervascular inflamed synovium and hyperaemia of adjacent bone. Tc-99m phosphate complexes are taken up by actively inflamed joints but this is non-specific. Other agents used include indium and gallium compounds which are selectively taken up as a function of their affinity for iron-binding proteins found in inflamed synovium. There is some evidence that the site of maximal persistent uptake may predict erosive disease, if scanning is carried out early in the course of RA (Rosenthal, 1991) (Fig. 17). Recently Tc-99m polyclonal human immunoglobulin has

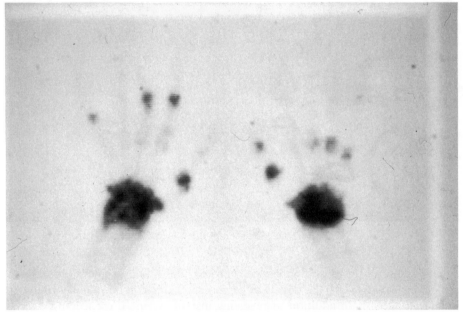

Figure 17. Isotope scan using a bone-seeking isotope in a patient with active rheumatoid arthritis showing uptake over the wrists and small joints of the fingers.

been found to detect active synovitis and may derive some quantitative results (Pons *et al.*, 1993). This technique may allow determination of active disease in the context of chronic inflammation, which is poorly defined by conventional Tc^m scanning. Finally, labelled leucocytes (Tc, gallium, indium) accumulate at sites of leucocyte migration and may be useful in detection of septic foci, especially after joint arthroplasty.

MEDICAL MANAGEMENT

The rheumatologist has a relatively wide range of drugs at his disposal to attempt to treat rheumatoid arthritis. These include non-steroidal anti-inflammatory drugs (NSAIDs), steroids, DMARDs including gold compounds, penicillamine, (hydroxy)-chloroquine, methotrexate and immunosuppressive agents such as azathioprine and cyclophosphamide. While these various drugs can offer symptomatic relief they appear to have limited effect on the processes which result in the destruction of articular cartilage and bone.

It is to be hoped that experimental therapies currently under investigation will begin to provide rational treatment for the pathology of RA. The clinical application of currently used therapies and the future therapies for rheumatoid arthritis are reviewed by Panayi in Chapter 3, this volume. Additional reviews of the use of experimental therapies in the treatment of RA can be found in Chapters 14 (Firestein), 15 (McMillan *et al.*) and 29 (Griffiths), this volume.

SURGICAL MANAGEMENT

The outcome of inflammatory synovitis is mechanical disruption which may be amenable to surgical management. Some 70% of RA patients will undergo orthopaedic intervention within 10 years of commencing DMARD therapy (Capell and Kelly, 1990). Options available include synovectomy, arthrodesis, arthroplasty, osteotomy and tendon transfer. 'Surgical' remit may also include radioactive synovectomy. Indications for surgery may be pain, nocturnal disturbance, deformity or progressive loss of function which is not responsive to medical approaches. Multidisciplinary consideration is required, at least by orthopaedic surgeons and rheumatologists, and also must involve the patient so that realistic expectations are achieved. Problem joints should not be considered in isolation, but rather a co-ordinated approach should be formulated. Thus, upper limb procedures may precede knee replacement to facilitate mobilization following the latter. Similarly, cervical spine disease may require stabilization prior to other surgical procedures being undertaken. General medical considerations including anaemia, intercurrent cardiac disease and other extra-articular manifestations of RA, and even RA activity itself, should be optimized. Postoperative recovery is dependent largely on dedicated paramedical staff, particularly physiotherapists.

Synovectomy is possible at a number of joints, but has recently declined in popularity with increasing reliance on arthroplasty. Procedures at the knee and wrist, however, are popular in some centres and may provide transient relief from symptoms. First introduced in the nineteenth century (Swett, 1973), synovectomy may exert beneficial effect by removal of aggressive inflammatory tissue (debulking effect) or, more simply, by mechanical reduction of hypertrophied synovium with improved biomechanics. Thus, 85% clearance is achieved at knee synovectomy, and although experimental models suggest that reformation of synovial tissue occurs within 8 weeks, some 80% of patients report benefit (Mitchel and Shepherd, 1972). Beneficial effect beyond 5 years is difficult to demonstrate but several studies suggest less swelling at the treated joint even at 10 years when compared to the opposite joint. However, there is no effect on general disease progression nor on long-term radiological damage sustained by the operated joint (Brattstrom *et al.*, 1985).

Arthroplasty now dominates the surgical management of RA. Replacement of hip, knee, MCP, elbow and shoulder joints is routinely undertaken and outcome continues to improve as materials, surgical technique and understanding of the biology of failed arthroplasty improves (Figs 18 and 19). This has allowed consideration of joint replacement in younger patients, with different demands on the prosthesis and surgeon, and

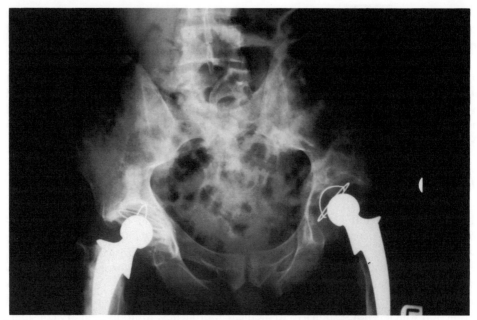

Figure 18. X-ray of the pelvis showing bilateral total hip arthroplasty in rheumatoid arthritis.

also has required the development of revision techniques with acceptable outcome. Moreover, allograft bone grafting has increased the therapeutic options in revision surgery and in primary management of advanced disease.

Most reports of results following hip and knee replacement claim satisfactory pain relief in around 90% of cases (Stuart and Ranel, 1988), with corresponding improvements in function. Prosthesis survival is usually greater than 10 years, with many patients now reaching 15 years survival after large joint arthroplasty. Results for shoulder and elbow replacement are less satisfactory than those for hip and knee (Saver and Kelly, 1990). Complications are principally those of infection, venous thrombosis and mechanical considerations. Infection may occur early, where operative contamination is suspected, and late, in which haematogenous inoculation is most probable.

Early infection varies between 1.5 and 4% of primary arthroplasties, with implicated organisms including *S. aureus*, *S. epidermidis* and Gram-negative species. Susceptibility is increased by concomitant diabetes, psoriasis, urinary infection, immunosuppression and indeed by RA itself. Staged revision in such cases is necessary, whereby prosthetic removal is followed by 'sensitivity directed' antibiotic therapy and later by re-implantation with antibiotic-impregnated cement. Arthrodesis remains as a less satisfactory alternative, although this may offer symptomatic relief. Aseptic loosening may occur in up to 57% of hip arthroplasties at 5 years. This may have mechanical origin, but is hastened by free cement particles which activate macrophages and can be shown *in vitro* to stimulate TNFα and other osteocytoclastic cytokine synthesis. The role of such mechanisms *in vivo* remains subject to intense investigation. Loosening may involve the socket of a hip prosthesis or may lead to endosteolysis of the femoral component, a feature occasionally seen also in knee

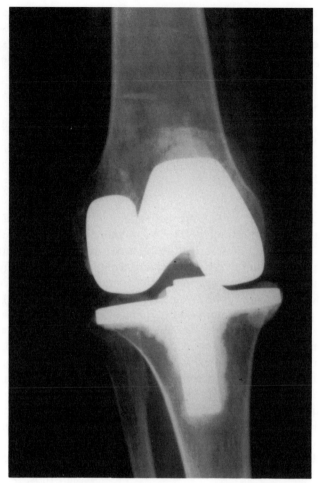

Figure 19. X-ray of the knee showing a semi-constrained knee arthroplasty in rheumatoid arthritis.

replacement. The induction of experimental arthritis by infectious agents is reviewed in Chapters 3 and 22.

Deep venous thrombosis is found in more than 50% of patients postarthroplasty, with incidence of pulmonary embolus, variably reported at 1.5–6% (Stringer *et al.*, 1989). Peri-operative anticoagulation regimes vary considerably in different centres and no consensus exists on an optimal approach. Reduced incidence of venous thrombosis has been reported for RA patients compared to those with osteoarthritis (OA) (Sikorski *et al.*, 1981). Specific complications occur related to individual joints, for example peroneal nerve palsy and femoral neck fracture can follow knee replacement.

Tendon transfer is particularly important in surgery of RA hands and also of feet. Silastic MCP replacement is commonly carried out with some success, although the aim in such procedures must always be improved function rather than purely cosmetic correction of deformity. Wrist synovectomy is a useful procedure for carpal tunnel syndrome.

Specialist orthopaedic and neurosurgical expertise is paramount in the management of cervical spine disease. Imaging with MRI and CT myelogram (discussed elsewhere) has greatly altered the potential for prophylactic stabilization of the spine, although the choice of procedure remains subject to investigation. More advanced spinal disease is associated with increased mortality, and earlier assessment is encouraged. However, the long-term outcome of early prophylactic surgery is not established and awaits large, multicentre trials addressed at this problem.

In summary, surgery offers much to complement the medical management of RA, and is delivered optimally by a team approach to care.

PROGNOSIS IN RA

Efforts to predict outcome in RA are dependent on the stage of disease at which assessment is attempted (Kirwan, 1992). The fundamental antigenic stimulus, and its timing, remain elusive and therefore difficulty arises in interpreting indices of disease activity at a single point in time. Erosive changes may be detectable by MRI within 3 months of clinical onset of disease, and 90% of patients who develop erosive disease will show evidence of this within 2 years (Brook and Corbett, 1977). Thus, it is of importance to predict such patients and perhaps offer more aggressive therapy at an earlier stage. Although laboratory variables have provided a focus for prospective study, there has been a realization recently that clinical staging, analogous to that for Hodgkin's lymphoma, may offer valuable prognostic information (Pincus and Callahan, 1990). Prognosis is best considered separately in terms of mortality and of morbidity.

Life expectancy is reduced in RA by 8–15 years, and this is particularly so for males and those of older age at onset. This increased mortality in comparison to population controls is accounted for mainly by infection, cardiovascular disease, renal disease, including amyloid, gastrointestinal disease (often drug related) and complications directly attributable to RA (Prior et al., 1984). Many studies, both case controlled and prospective, have now identified factors which appear to predict increased risk of mortality (Erhardt et al., 1989). Rheumatoid factor positivity (IgA, IgM particularly), extra-articular disease, including vasculitis and cryoglobulinaemia, persistent acute phase response, number of involved joints and, interestingly, poor functional scores have been implicated in this respect. However, some of these series are subject to case acquisition bias, as they have been done in referral centres. Those studies centred more firmly on community-based diagnosis do identify increased mortality, but may predict subgroups who are 'predisposed' to fare worse (Abruzzo, 1982). The association of HLA status, particularly HLA-DR1, DR4, DR6 and DR10, with susceptibility to and severity of RA has shed interesting light on this debate. Certain alleles at the HLA-DRB1 locus (corresponding to HLA-DR4), appear to predict more aggressive disease, as do other loci coding for the 'shared epitope', in addition to predicting disease susceptibility (Weyand et al., 1992). Clinical trials evaluating these markers prospectively are underway which may provide genetic explanations for the clinically heterogeneous subgroups which emerge on analysis of large patient populations (see Chapters 2 and 4). Finally, the literature is divided on the incidence of neoplasia in RA, with associated increased mortality. Recent population-based data from Finland would suggest a significant increase in lymphoid tumours (Gridley *et al.*, 1993), although several other studies have previously failed to report this association.

Prediction of disability provides peculiar problems in study design, primarily because the time of disease onset is unknown. Clearly, seropositive DR4 positive females carry a poorer prognosis for disability. However, early onset of nodules, Raynaud's phenomenon, acute phase response and erosions all suggest increased morbidity, but may not be evident on first assessment, and are therefore of reduced value in selecting those requiring aggressive therapy. Rheumatoid factors and HLA status may be of some benefit as already discussed. However, functional scores appear to be of considerable value in prediction of disability. Many methods are described, including walking time, button test, grip strength and health assessment question-naires. Using this approach, early loss of function in RA may be demonstrated, which is often progressive, despite subjective clinical improvement (Pincus and Callahan, 1992). Thus, around 80% of patients will deteriorate significantly and of these some 10–20% will be seriously disabled after 10 years (Scott *et al.*, 1987). Poor education and by association, lower social class, predict greater disability in RA and there is some evidence that increased number of work hours may reduce the rate of deterioration, although, more disabled RA patients may not be able to work *a priori*.

Despite 'disease modifying' therapy, outcome in terms of function or mortality in treated patients does not appear to be altered. For this reason, earlier aggressive therapy, perhaps during a therapeutic window of opportunity, has been suggested (Fries, 1990). Firm prognostic indicators are required to identify those who are most at risk and have, accordingly, most potential to benefit from early intervention.

REFERENCES

Abruzzo JL (1982) Rheumatoid arthritis and mortality. *Arthritis Rheum* **25**: 1020–1023.

Arnett FC, Edworthy SM & Block DA (1988) The American Rheumatism Association 1987 revised criteria for the classification of rheumatoid arthritis. *Arthritis Rheum* **31**: 315–324.

Brattstrom H, Czurda, Gschwend et al. (1985) Longterm results of knee synovectomy in early cases of RA. *Clin Rheumatol* **4**: 19.

Brook A & Corbett M (1977) Radiographic changes in early rheumatoid disease. *Ann Rheum Dis* **36**: 71–73.

Buckland-Wright JC, Clarke GS, Chikanza IC & Grahame R (1993) Quantitative microfocal radiography detects changes in erosion area in patients with early RA treated with Myocrisin. *J Rheumatol* **20**: 243–247.

Campion G, Maddison PJ, Goulding N et al. (1990) The Felty syndrome: a case-matched study of clinical manifestations and outcome, serologic features and immunogenetic associations. *Medicine Baltimore* **69**(2): 69–80.

Capell HA & Kelly IG (1990) Surgical management of rheumatic diseases. *Ann Rheum Dis* **49**: 823–882.

Cuchacovich M, Couret M, Peray P et al. (1992) Precision of the Larsden and the Sharp methods of assessing radiologic changes in patients with RA. *Arthritis Rheum* **35**: 736–739.

Deavereaux MD, Parr GR, Thomas DPP & Hazleman BL (1985) Disease activity indexes in rheumatoid arthritis – a prospective, comparative study with thermography. *Ann Rheum Dis* **44**: 434–437.

Erhardt CC, Mumford RA, Venables PJW & Maini RN (1989) Factors predicting a poor life prognosis in RA: an eight year prospective study. *Ann Rheum Dis* **48**: 7–13.

Fraser S, Land D & Sturrock RD (1987) Microwave thermography – an index of inflammatory joint disease. *Br J Rheumatol* **26**: 37–39.

Fries JF (1990) Re-evaluating the therapeutic approach to rheumatoid arthritis. *J Rheumatol* (**supplement 17**): 14–18.

Garrod AB (1859) *Nature and Treatment of Gout and Rheumatoid Gout*. London: Walton and Maberly.

Ginig M, Higer HP, Meairs S, Faust-Tinnefeldt G & Kapp H (1990) MRI of the craniocervical junction in RA: value, limitations, indications. *Skeletal Radiol* **19**: 341–346.

Gridley G, McLaughlin JK, Ekbom A et al. (1993) Incidence of cancer among patients with rheumatoid arthritis. *J Nat Cancer Inst* **85**: 307–311.

Hazes JM & Silman AJ (1990) Review of UK data on the rheumatic diseases – 2 Rheumatoid arthritis. *Br J Rheumatol* **29**: 161–165.

Heron CW (1992) Magnetic resonance imaging in rheumatology. *Ann Rheum Dis* **51**: 1287–1291.

Jacoby RK, Jayson MI & Cosh JA (1973) Onset, early stages, and prognosis of rheumatoid arthritis: a clinical study of 100 patients with 11 year follow-up. *Br Med J* **2**: 96–100.

Jorgensen C, Cyreval C, Araya JM et al. (1993) Sensitivity of MRI of the wrist in very early RA. *Clin Exp Rheumatol* **11**: 163–168.

Kirwan JR (1992) A theoretical framework for process, outcome and prognosis in RA. *J Rheumatol* **19**: 333–336.

Larsen A, Thoen J (1987) Hand radiography of 200 patients with rheumatoid arthritis repeated after an interval of 1 year. *Scand J Rheumatol* **16**: 395–401.

Mitchel N & Shepard N (1972) Effect of synovectomy on synovium and cartilage in early RA. *Clin Orthop* **89**: 178–196.

Pincus T & Callahan LF (1990) Remodelling the pyramid or remodelling the paradigms concerning RA – Lessons from Hodgkin's disease and coronary artery disease. *J Rheumatol* **17**: 1582–1585.

Pincus T & Callahan LF (1992) Rheumatology function tests: grip strength, walking time, button test and questionnaires document can predict longterm morbidity and mortality in RA. *J Rheumatol* **19**: 1051–1057.

Pons F, Moya F, Herranz R et al. (1993) Detection and quantitative analysis of joint activity inflammation with 99Tcm polyclonal human immunoglobulin G. *Nucl Med Commun* **14**: 225–231.

Porter DR (1993) Lymphadenopathy in rheumatoid arthritis. *Rheumatol Review* **2**: 159–162.

Prior P, Symmonds DPM, Scott DL et al. (1984) Cause of death in RA. *Br J Rheumatol* **23**: 92–99.

Reichner MA & Kellerhouse LT (1990) *MRI of the Wrist and Hand*. New York: Raven Press.

Ropes MW, Bennett GA, Cobb S et al. (1958) 1958 revision of diagnostic criteria for rheumatoid arthritis. *Bull Rheum Dis* **9**: 175–176.

Rosenthall L (1991) Nuclear medicine techniques in arthritis. *Rheum Dis Clin of N America* **17**: 585–597.

Saver WA & Kelly IK (1990) Surgery of the rheumatoid elbow and surgery of the rheumatoid shoulder. *Ann Rheum Dis* **49**: 823–882.

Scott DL, Symmons DPM, Coulton BL & Popert AJ (1987) Longterm outcome of treating RA: results after 20 years. *Lancet* **1**: 1108–1111.

Sharp JT, Young DY, Bluhm GB et al. (1985) How many joints in the hands and wrists should be included in a score of radiological abnormalities used to assess RA? *Arthritis Rheum* **28**: 1326–1335.

Sikorski JM, Hampson WG & Staddon GT (1981) The natural history and aetiology of deep vein thrombosis after total hip replacement. *J Bone Joint Surg* **63**: 171–177.

Silman AJ, MacGregor AJ, Thomson W et al. (1993) Twin concordance rates for rheumatoid arthritis: results from a nationwide study. *Br J Rheumatol* **32**: 903–907.

Smith MA, Knight SM, Maddison PJ & Smith JG (1992) Anaemia of chronic disease in rheumatoid arthritis: effect of the blunted response to erythropoietin and of interleukin-1 production by marrow macrophages. *Ann Rheum Dis* **51**: 753–757.

Snorrason E (1952) Landre-Beauvis and his Goutte Asthenique Primitive. *Acta Med Scand* **142**: 115.

Stringer MD, Steadman CA, Hedges AR et al. (1989) Deep vein thrombosis after elective knee surgery. An incidence study in 312 patients. *J Bone Joint Surg* **71B**: 492–497.

Stuart MT & Ranel JA (1988) Total knee arthroplasty in young adults who have RA. *J Bone Joint Surg* **70A**: 84–87.

Sturrock RD, Sharma JN & Buchanan WW (1977) Evidence of rheumatoid arthritis in ancient India. *Arthritis Rheum* **20**: 42.

Swett P (1973) Synovectomy in chronic infectious arthritis. *J Bone Joint Surg* **5**: 110.

Thomas D, Siahamis G, Marion M & Boyle C (1992) Computerized infrared thermography and isotopic bone scanning in tennis elbow. *Ann Rheum Dis* **51**: 103–107.

Thomson W, Pepper L, Payton A et al. (1993) Absence of an association between HLA-DRB1*04 and rheumatoid arthritis in newly diagnosed cases from the community. *Ann Rheum Dis* **52**: 539–541.

Thould AK & Thould BT (1983) Arthritis in Roman Britain. *Br Med J* **287**: 1909–1911.

Weyand CM, Hicok KC, Conn DL & Goronzy JJ (1992) The influence of HLA-DRb1 genes on disease severity in RA. *Ann Int Med* **117**: 801–806.

2 Aetiopathogenesis of Rheumatoid Arthritis

R.N. Maini, C.Q. Chu and M. Feldmann

INTRODUCTION

The cause of rheumatoid arthritis (RA) still remains unknown in spite of many years of intensive investigation, but current thinking favours the concept that it is a multi-factorial disease. It is envisaged that in genetically susceptible individuals an environmental agent(s) initiates an autoimmune disease process which culminates in inflammatory and destructive features. However, our understanding of the pathogenesis of RA at the molecular level has progressed rapidly in recent years and this has resulted in the evolution of new models of therapy, targeting specific molecules. The purpose of this chapter is to review the recent advances in studies on aetiology and pathogenesis of RA with a focus on immunological aspects.

AETIOLOGY

GENETIC FACTORS

Over the past two decades there has been considerable progress in our understanding of the genetic factors contributing to susceptibility to RA. This was marked by the discovery of the association of this disorder with human leukocyte antigen (HLA) class II genes, but it is still not entirely clear whether the HLA genes determine susceptibility to RA or merely identify patients with the worst outcome of the disease.

Contribution of genetic factors to susceptibility to RA was first hinted by familial aggregation and disease concordance in twins. Earlier familial studies showed a slight increase in the frequency of RA in first-degree relatives of patients with rheumatoid arthritis, especially if the probands were seropositive for rheumatoid factor (Lawrence, 1970). Hospital-based twin studies showed that the prevalence of RA in monozygotic twins was as high as 30%, compared with 5% in dizygotic twins. More recent studies have attempted to assess the prevalence of RA in monozygotic twins in the general population, and have arrived at concordance rates between 10 and 20% (Silman *et al.*, 1989). Clearly RA is not a dominant single gene disorder, but results from polygenic influences.

In the 1970s, Stastny (1974, 1978) first described the association of RA with HLA-Dw4 in Caucasian patients. Subsequent work has repeatedly confirmed this finding in Caucasians, and it is estimated that 60–70% of patients with RA are HLA-DR4 positive, compared with 20–25% of control populations (Panayi *et al.*, 1979; Jaraquemada *et al.*, 1979; Karr *et al.*, 1980). A similar increased frequency of HLA-DR4 has been found in many other races and ethnic groups (reviewed by Ollier and Thomson, 1992). However, as a greater range of populations was studied it was

Mechanisms and Models in Rheumatoid Arthritis
ISBN 0–12–340440–1

realized that RA is not always associated with DR4. For example, in Israeli Jews and an Indian immigrant community in the United Kingdom, and in DR4-negative Caucasian patients, an increased frequency of HLA-DR1 has been found. Moreover, DR10 is the associated phenotype in Spanish (Sanchez *et al.*, 1990), DR6 in Yakima American Indians (Willkens *et al.*, 1982), and DR9 in Chilean patients (Massardo *et al.*, 1990). Both DR1 and DR10 have recently been found at an increased frequency in Greek patients although no apparent association with HLA was demonstrated in earlier studies (reviewed by Ollier and Thomson, 1992). In addition, not all of the DR4 subsets are associated with RA. Dw4 and Dw14 are associated with RA in several studies, Dw15 is only associated with RA in Japanese and Chinese (Ohta *et al.*, 1982; Seglias *et al.*, 1992), while Dw10 and Dw13 are not associated with RA in any ethnic group (Ollier and Thompson, 1992).

The mechanism of the association between HLA-DR and RA is not clear. However, attempts to understand the apparent discrepancy of associations and understanding of the structure of MHC molecules have led to the development of 'shared epitope' hypothesis (Gregersen *et al.*, 1987). The importance of HLA class II molecules lies in their participation in a trimolecular model of reaction that involves the HLA antigen-binding cleft formed by the α and β chains of antigen-presenting cell binding to a processed linear peptide antigen of at least nine amino acids, with the HLA–antigen complex in turn binding to the variable portion of the T-cell receptor (Brown *et al.*, 1993). Comparison of the amino acid sequences of HLA-DR4 subtype molecules has revealed the important differences between RA-associated (Dw4, Dw14, Dw15) and non-associated (Dw10, Dw13) in their third hypervariable region of the β chain, especially at amino acid residues 70–74 (Table 1). The shared sequence

Table 1. HLA-DR associations with rheumatoid arthritis defined by DRβ1 third hypervariable region sequence 70–74

DR Type	Sequence 70	71	72	73	74	Association
DR4-Dw4	Q	K	R	A	A	Positive
-Dw14	Q	R	R	A	A	Positive
-Dw15	Q	R	R	A	A	Positive
DR1	Q	R	R	A	A	Positive
DR6-Dw16	Q	R	R	A	A	Positive
DR4-Dw10	D	E	R	A	A	Negative
-Dw13	Q	R	R	A	E	Negative

is also carried by DR1 and by DR6/Dw16, which is also associated with RA. Dw4, Dw14 and Dw15 share similarities with each other (with a conservative substitution of glutamine by lysine at position 71 in Dw4) (Winchester and Gregersen, 1988; Salmon, 1992). This sequence predicts susceptibility to RA and, for example, is associated with RA in 83% of Caucasians in Britain (Wordsworth *et al.*, 1989). In contrast, in non-RA associated DR4–Dw10, the charged basic amino acids glutamine and arginine in positions 70 and 71 are replaced by the acidic amino acids aspartic and glutamic acid. In DR4-Dw13, alanine is substituted for glutamic acid in position 74. Molecular modelling suggests that amino acid residues 70–74 are located in the α helix forming one side of the peptide-binding cleft, and are likely to be involved in antigen binding.

Acidic substitutions at positions 71 and 74, where the side chains of amino acids are probably oriented toward the antigen-binding site, could profoundly alter protein structure and thereby alter affinity for peptide binding (Rudensky et al., 1991).

Interestingly, in the experimental animal arthritis model, mouse class II region genes have been shown to be associated with susceptibility of the development of collagen induced arthritis (see Chapters 19 and 23, this volume). Mouse strains of H-2q or H-2r are susceptible, but those of H-2p are resistant. Structure analysis of class II molecules showed that I-Aq and I-Ar share considerable homology, but I-Aq and I-Ap differ, although only by four amino acids.

Predictions that protein structures on the HLA molecule are important in susceptibility to RA are supported by the outcome of serotyping with alloantisera and monoclonal antibodies, as well as of reactivity with homozygous T cells and T-cell clones (Goronzy et al., 1986; Winchester and Gregersen, 1988).

It has been thought that the disease-associated MHC class II molecules may affect T-cell receptor selection influencing the formation of the T cell repertoire. In a T-cell receptor transgenic mouse model, the positive selection of T-cell receptors in the thymus is highly dependent on the MHC density expressed on the cell surface (Berg et al., 1990). Several groups have observed that RA patients with severe disease tend to be more frequently associated with DR4 (Lanchbury et al., 1991; van Zeben et al., 1991; Wordsworth et al., 1992; Weyand et al., 1992). For example, Felty's syndrome has an amost complete association with DR4–Dw4, and severe forms of RA are significantly associated with genotypes that contain the Dw4/Dw14 and Dw4/DR1 alleles. However, milder forms of RA have little or no association with HLA (van Zeben et al., 1991). Weyand and colleagues (1992) have hypothesized that the density of disease-associated major histocompatibility complex (MHC) molecules is of critical importance in the pathogenesis of RA, possibly via influence on the shape of T-cell repertoire (Weyand et al., 1992; Goronzy and Weyand, 1993).

He et al. (1992) showed that Dw4 or Dw14 allospecific T-cell clones are capable of inducing rheumatoid factor production from B cells crosslinked with staphylococcal endotoxin-D, suggesting a role of T cells and possibly superantigens in the selective production of rheumatoid factor.

As mentioned earlier, RA is a polygenic disease; the contribution of HLA has been calculated from studies of HLA in multicase families to possibly only account for 37% of the genetic factors involved (Deighton et al., 1989). Other susceptible genes have been sought, and associations with T-cell receptors in gene polymorphisms and deletions of immunoglobulin genes have been observed (Olee et al., 1991). The picture is currently incomplete and the relative importance of its components has not been documented.

INFECTIOUS FACTORS

Infectious agents have long been thought to contribute to the aetiology of RA (reviewed in Chapters 3 and 21, this volume). Many bacteria and viruses are known to be arthritogenic in animal models and in humans, but none of the micro-organisms has been identified to be the causative pathogen of RA. In attempts in earlier studies to demonstrate microbial organisms directly from joints, positive findings of mycoplasma, diphtheroids and viruses have either been attributed to laboratory contamination or have been refuted on grounds of a lack of reproducibility.

With the thought that infectious agents may trigger autoimmunity, many studies have sought to implicate microbes in the aetiology of RA by seeking evidence of hyperimmune reactivity to microbial antigens. Epstein–Barr virus (EBV), a ubiquitous virus, has been linked with RA largely because of the detection of increased antibody titres to EBV antigens in RA patients and an induced RA nuclear antigen (Venables *et al.*, 1981; Venables, 1988). Roudier *et al.* (1989) and Albani *et al.* (1992) observed a remarkable similarity in the sequence of the third hypervariable region of HLA-DR4-Dw4 and sequences present in an EBV-encoded protein gp110 and a bacterial heat-shock protein dnaJ. T cells and antibodies reactive with these exogenous peptides are crossreactive with the native Dw4 third hypervariable region peptide. The shared epitope between EBV and HLA-DR1 has led to several proposals regarding the aetiological role of EBV in RA. One suggestion is that deletion of T cells in HLA-DR4-susceptible individuals could result in impaired T-cell mediated killing of cells productively infected with the virus. The persistence of EBV in B lymphocytes of patients with RA in greater than normal amounts could thus lead to the hyperreactivity of B cells and autoantibody production typical of the disease. Other described crossreactivities of EBV nuclear antigens with the autoantigens collagen, actin, and cytokeratin, and to an antigen in the synovial membrane, have suggested mechanisms for the induction of autoimmunity and for localization of immune cells to joints (Baboonian *et al.*, 1991). However, so far, there is no evidence suggesting a primary causative role for EBV, and current data can not explain why only a small proportion of individuals infected with EBV might develop RA, and conversely, that there are well-documented patients with RA with no evidence of EBV infection (Venables *et al.*, 1981).

A high incidence of arthritis in patients infected with retroviruses in Japan has suggested their involvement in the pathogenesis of RA (reviewed in Iwakura *et al.*, 1991). Transgenic mice carrying the human T-cell leukaemia virus-1 (HTLV-1) genome provided direct evidence that this virus can cause arthritis (Iwakura *et al.*, 1991). In this model, approximately one-third of the mice highly expressing the transgene developed chronic, erosive arthritis, with synovial inflammation and cartilage destruction, closely resembling pannus seen in RA. Low levels of rheumatoid factor were also occasionally detected. The mechanisms of the arthritis development in these mice are not known, but it was of particular interest that the mRNA for tax, a transacting transcriptional activator, was highly expressed by cells in the joints. Thus it is likely that the arthritis in this model is due to increased expression of cytokines in the joints. Supporting this hypothesis is the preliminary observation that interleukin (IL)-1α mRNA is expressed in the joints of these mice, as it is in RA.

Involvement of *Mycobacterium tuberculosis* in the aetiology of RA has attracted much attention in recent years. In an animal model of adjuvant arthritis (see Chapter 20), mycobacterial protein showed immunological crossreactivity and sequence similarity to a cartilage link protein, a finding that suggested a possible reason for the localization of the immune response to joints (van Eden *et al.*, 1985). The link with human RA was suggested by the demonstration of reactivity of synovial T cells to mycobacterial antigens in RA (Holoshitz *et al.*, 1986). The mycobacterial 65 kDa protein was subsequently shown to belong to the family of heat-shock protein (hsp)

65, which are expressed in a variety of bacteria and also in the inflamed synovium of RA (van Eden *et al.*, 1988; de Graeff-Meeder *et al.*, 1990). Whether human hsp is a major target of T-cell autoreactivity in RA, however, is unproven, as there are significant differences in sequence and epitopes expressed by bacterial and human hsp. Arguing against a role is the fact that identical responses to hsp65 are also found in other inflammatory sites, for example, pleural effusions (Res *et al.*, 1990). Attempts to suppress RA by vaccination with T cells derived from joints, in a protocol similar to that successfully used in adjuvant arthritis, could have provided support for the importance of mycobacterial immunity, but preliminary attempts have not been successful (van Laar *et al.*, 1991).

Ebringer *et al.* (1985) detected the elevated levels of IgG antibody to *Proteus mirabilis* in serum of patients with RA but not in ankylosing spondylitis or control subjects. This has been interpreted as showing the aetiological importance of this micro-organism in RA (Ebringer *et al.*, 1985). It has been proposed that persistence of the organism in the urinary tract, especially of women, may provide the nidus of infection that triggers a deleterious immune response culminating in RA. The possible role of infectious agents in RA aetiology and pathogenesis is fully reviewed in Chapters 3 and 21.

OTHER AETIOLOGICAL FACTORS

Aside from the possible part that infectious agents may play, the predominance of RA in females, in the premenopausal period, compared to males and the protective effect of the contraceptive pill, presumably due to its progesterone content, have suggested that sex hormones may accelerate or retard its onset (Lahita, 1990). Other aetiological factors that have been considered include diet and stress, but their role in initiating disease is debatable, and may be more significant in altering disease expression and outcome.

Chikanza *et al.* (1992) recently reported that a group of patients with RA had a disturbed pattern of diurnal secretion of cortisol and a deficient response to surgery, suggesting a defect in hypothalamic function. A defective hypothalamic–pituitary–adrenal response has been observed in female Lewis rats which are susceptible to streptococcal cell-wall induced arthritis (Sternberg *et al.*, 1989a,b). That these neuro-endocrine responses are important in the pathogenesis of disease is suggested by the observation that giving corticosteroid in small doses simultaneously with streptococcal cell wall improves the course of the induced arthritis and, conversely, blockade of the glucocorticoid receptor accelerates disease in resistant Fisher rats (Sternberg *et al.*, 1989b). Neuroendocrine involvement in the pathology of RA is discussed by Mapp and Blake in Chapter 16, this volume.

PATHOGENESIS

INITIATION OF THE DISEASE

Without knowing the causative agent, it is impossible to describe accurately how RA is initiated. Various hypotheses have been proposed to explain how an environmental agent might induce autoimmunity leading to an autoimmune disorder. As in the context of autoimmune diseases in general, environmental agents are considered to trigger rather than directly involve the disease process. An old but still popular hypothesis is the induction of autoimmunity by 'antigenic mimicry' or 'molecular mimicry'. This theory implies that an immune response to an extrinsic antigen (usually microbial), closely resembling a self antigen or molecule, crossreacts with the auto-antigen. Then the autoantigen perpetuates the immune response and this results in injury to host tissues. Despite the popularity of this concept, there is as yet no proven role for this mechanism in RA.

Feldmann and colleagues (reviewed by Feldmann, 1989) have proposed that ab-errant and up-regulated expression of HLA class II molecules can induce auto-immunity. A local immune response to any environmental reagents may cause a release of enough cytokines into the environment to up-regulate local antigen-presenting capacity, so allowing autoantigens otherwise 'hidden' from the immune system due to lack of HLA class II expression to be presented to autoreactive T cells that have escaped elimination or tolerance induction. This hypothesis was first pro-posed for endocrine autoimmune diseases, with the suggestion that the endocrine epithelium becomes the critical source of (atypical) autoantigen presentation. Sub-stantial evidence has since accumulated that this scheme may apply in both experi-mental models and human diseases. Transgenic mice producing interferon (IFN)-γ in their islets of Langerhans under the control of the insulin promoter develop an immune, T-cell dependent diabetes, with autoreactive T cells lysing islets and reject-ing transplanted islets (Sarvetnick et al., 1990). In human Graves' thyroiditis, the antigen-presenting capacity of thyrocytes has been documented, as well as the presence of activated autoantigen-reactive T cells, and of local cytokines needed to maintain both antigen-presenting function and T-cell activation (reviewed by Feldmann et al., 1991). In RA synovial membrane, abundant antigen-presenting function resides in macrophages, dendritic cells, B cells, endothelium, and possibly activated T cells, although which of these is most deeply involved in antigen presen-tation is not known. The presence of CD5$^+$ B cells and their descendants may con-tribute significantly to local antigen-presenting function by binding to autoantibody containing immune complexes in their immunoglobulin receptor (Andrew et al., 1991).

It is probable that a localized autoimmune response is determined by the restricted distribution of critical autoantigens. For example, in Graves' disease, antigens syn-thesized by thyroid epithelial cells – thyroglobulin, thyroid peroxidase, and thyroid-stimulating hormone receptor – are the targets which can be recognized by both T and B cells. In RA the important autoantigens that drive pathogenic T cells are not known. Several candidate antigens present in cartilage such as collagen type II, IX, and XI recognized by T and B cells could fulfil this role. Londei et al. (1989) have shown that type II collagen-specific T cells, expressing IL-2 receptor (IL-2R) and hence activated in vivo persisted in the same joint of a patient with RA over 4 years of active disease. These antigens, as well as other cartilage- or chondrocyte-specific antigens, could be of importance in the initial localization of immune response to synovial joints. Other autoantigens recognized by T cells in RA, such as hsp 65 antigen, or the antigen implicated in the autologous mixed lymphocyte reaction, are unlikely to be candidates because they are ubiquitous in cell types in most tissues.

However, it has to be acknowledged that such T cells could be of importance in maintaining the disease process and its extra-articular manifestations.

It is still debatable whether RA should be considered as a single disease, with all cases having the same aetiology, or whether it should be viewed as a syndrome, with a range of aetiological factors initiating the same pathogenetic mechanism and so producing a similar constellation of clinical features.

CELL RECRUITMENT

A hallmark of RA pathology is the remarkable increase of cellularity accompanied by angiogenesis in the synovial membrane. As shown by immunostaining techniques, the vast majority of the increased number of cells in the rheumatoid joint are of lympho-haematopoietic origin. This reflects the increase of cellular recruitment from the circulation, and probably also an increased retention of cells in the synovial membrane. Expression of cell adhesion molecules on endothelial cells and their complementary ligands on the surface of leukocytes appears to be critical in determining the site of leukocyte emigration and the nature of the leukocytes migrating into an inflammatory lesion. Isolated rheumatoid synovial endothelial cells constitutively express endothelial leukocyte adhesion molecule (ELAM)-1 (now known as E-selectin), and intercellular adhesion molecule (ICAM)-1 and their expression can be up-regulated by IL-1 and tumour necrosis factor (TNF) (Abbot et al., 1992). Several immunohistochemical staining studies have shown that ICAM-1, vascular cell adhesion molecule (VCAM)-1 and ELAM-1 are all highly expressed by rheumatoid synovial vascular endothelial cells and cells in the lining layer (Koch et al., 1991, Morales-Ducret et al., 1992; Wilkinson et al., 1993; Chu, unpublished observation). It has recently been shown that VCAM-1 and very late activation antigen (VLA)-4 interactions are important in mediating binding of T cells to endothelial cells, and lymphocyte function-associated molecule (LFA)/ICAM-1 interactions are crucial to subsequent transendothelial migration of T cells (Oppenheimer-Marks et al., 1991; see Chapter 11, this volume).

In RA, VLA-4 may bind to alternatively spliced sequence of fibronectin. The predominance of T cells in RA synovial membrane with the phenotype of memory cells (CD45RO$^+$, CD29$^+$) has suggested local differentiation of T cells. However, increased expression of VLA-4 on CD45RO$^+$ T cells may suggest a selective migration of memory T cells into the inflamed synovial membrane. In fact, CD45RO$^+$ T cells showed a better adherence to endothelial cell as compared with CD45RO$^-$ T cells (Pitzalis et al., 1987). RA synovial T cells have a significantly greater capacity to migrate transendothelially, compared with those in normal and RA peripheral blood (Cush et al., 1992). The binding of VLA-4 to fibronectin and to VCAM-1 expressed by lining cells may result in an enhanced retention of T cells in RA synovial membrane.

Equally important in cell recruitment is the action of chemotactic factors, which promote the migration of cells into a site. Some of these mediators have been identified within rheumatoid joints. Thus, IL-8, which is chemotactic for neutrophils and T cells, is abundant in such joints (Brennan et al., 1990a; Endo et al., 1991); RANTES, a cytokine produced by T cells and related to the IL-8 or chemokine family, and which is chemotactic for CD4-CD45RO$^+$ cells and monocytes (Schall et al., 1990), is also present. As RANTES is chemotactic for the cells most abundant in the membrane it may be of major importance in determining the cell composition of the rhematoid joint. In addition, other cytokines such as IL-1, TNF, and transforming growth factor (TGF)-β have also been shown to be chemotactic for monocytes and T cells (reviewed in Ziff, 1989). Split complement components C3a and C5a, present in RA joints (Jose et al., 1990; Abbink et al., 1992) are chemotactic for neutrophils. The recruitment of leukocytes to arthritic joints is reviewed in detail in Chapter 11, this volume.

T CELLS IN RA

Central to our discussion is the assumption that T cells play a critical role in the pathogenesis of RA. However, Firestein and Zvaifler (1990) have questioned this supposition on the grounds that in chronic phases of RA, T cells produce little IL-2, IFNγ, lymphotoxin (LT), or IL-4, and express little IL-2 receptor, compared to phytohaemagglutinin-activated cells. However, in our view, other lines of evidence indicate that T cells are important in both the initiation and maintenance of RA. Firstly, there is an abundance of T cells in rheumatoid joints in contrast to their absence in normal and paucity in osteoarthritic joints. T lymphocytes are a large population of cells in rheumatoid joints, comprising 20–50% of the cells extracted from synovial membrane, with a predominance of CD4$^+$ cells. Secondly, T cells in rheumatoid joints exhibit activation markers. Of the total T cells, about 50% express HLA class II, and some (2–12%) express p55 IL-2Rs (Brennan et al., 1988a, Londei et al., 1989). Almost all of the CD4$^+$ T cells in rheumatoid joints express CD45RO indicating a primed or memory state (Pitzalis et al., 1987, 1991). Other surface markers indicating activation include up-regulated expression of VLA-1/4, CD69, and CDw60 (Hemler et al., 1986; Fox et al., 1990; Laffon et al., 1991; Afeltra et al., 1993).

Thirdly is the fact that the proportions of different types of T cells in rheumatoid joints are not the same as in peripheral blood. As mentioned above, CD45RO predominate in joints, in contrast to the findings in blood, where 50% are CD45RO$^+$, indicating a virgin state. Selective enrichment of γ/δ T cells in active rheumatoid joints has been described, and some of the γ/δ T cells recognize mycobacterial antigens (Holoshitz et al., 1989). In our studies, some patients have increased numbers of γ/δ T cells in their blood; this patient population also showed an increase in circulating CD5$^+$ B cells (Brennan et al., 1988b, 1989a). Such findings indicate that T cells are not passively trafficking in an inflammatory response.

Fourth is the observation that antigen-specific activated T cells persist in rheumatoid joints. For example, we found that collagen type II-specific T cells expressing IL-2R were present in three operative specimens in a patient with RA over a period of more than 4 years (Londei et al., 1989).

Fifth is the apparent efficacy of T-cell directed treatment in patients with RA, such as cyclosporin, monoclonal antibodies to CD4 (Herzog et al., 1989; Horneff et al., 1991; Reiter et al., 1991), and the resolution of RA in patients developing AIDS (Calabrese et al., 1989). In addition, data from experimental models of arthritis have clearly demonstrated that the development of arthritis is T cell-dependent (see Section 5).

Attempts have been made to define a restricted pattern of Vβ chains of the T cell receptors in RA. Paliard and colleagues (1991) observed expansion of Vβ14$^+$ T cells in the synovial fluid of RA patients compared with low expression of Vβ14 in peripheral blood of the same patients, suggesting the possibility that activation of T cells was mediated by superantigens. However, this overrepresentation of Vβ14 was not confirmed by other investigators, in that use of multiple Vβ gene families by rheumatoid synovial T cells was reported (Uematsu *et al.*, 1991). Thus, Howell *et al.* (1991) analysed the activated T cells (IL-2R-positive) isolated from RA synovial fluids and found predominant expression of Vβ3, Vβ14 and Vβ17. This finding is interesting, as this may reflect the dominant influence of superantigens. Distinct patterns of selection of Vβ family have been shown for different streptococcal and staphylococcal enterotoxin superantigens. Of particular interest is the considerable sequence homology between Vβ3, 14 and 17 families in the third complementarity-determining region, where the Vβ binding site for several superantigens is found (Baccala *et al.*, 1992). Clearly, no definite conclusion can be drawn at the present, as much more work is needed in this area; synovial T cells from a larger population of RA patients need to be examined for their antigen receptor usage and the specificity of these T cells needs to be defined. The role of specific Vβ families in experimental models of arthritis is discussed in detail in this volume by Wooley (Chapter 19) and by Trentham and Dynesius-Trentham (Chapter 23).

B-CELL LINEAGE

There are abundant plasma cells in rheumatoid synovial membrane, although B cells are in small numbers. They have been shown to produce autoantibodies such as anticollagen antibodies and rheumatoid factors. Immune complexes containing rheumatoid factor isolated from RA patients can induce monocytes to produce cytokines such as IL-1 and TNF (Chantry *et al.*, 1989), reflecting one of the mechanisms that rheumatoid factors contribute to the pathogenesis of this disease.

The specificity of the antibodies produced in rheumatoid joints has been investigated by cell fusion techniques. Large numbers of hybridomas producing IgM and IgG were detected (Maini, 1989). While a few of these were polyreactive, and some produced rheumatoid factor, the majority did not bind to a battery of autoantigens tested. However, it has been claimed that the majority of rheumatoid joints containing B cells produce antibody to collagen type II and IgG Fc (Tarkowski *et al.*, 1989).

In examining the B-cell repertoire activated in rheumatoid joints, attempts are being made to ascertain whether there is any evidence of a restricted use of certain genes selected from among the multiple heavy-chain V genes available in the genome. Analysis by Northern blotting of B-cell hybridomas generated from an RA patient's synovium revealed a predominance of Vh4 gene family (Brown *et al.*, 1992). Such overpresentation may result from selection pressures created by specific antigens or superantigens. Alternatively, regulatory elements in flanking regions active in RA may favour recombination of particular individual gene elements and so skew the activated B-cell repertoire. As primed B cells present antigen to T cells more efficiently than do macrophages (Lanzavecchia, 1985) and are probably important in the development and maintenance of the immune network in neonatal and adult life (reviewed by Plater-Zyberk *et al.*, 1992), a greater understanding of the role of B cells should illuminate the pathogenesis of RA.

ANTIGEN-PRESENTING CELLS

Various cell types in rheumatoid synovial joints with antigen-presenting capacity could serve as antigen-presenting cells in immune responses. It is not clear which of these are of major importance in different stages of disease. Macrophages and monocytes comprising some 30–50% of the cell pool in rheumatoid synovial membrane are professional antigen-presenting cells. In view of their persistent presence in large quantities, activated status, and distribution throughout the synovial tissue in close apposition with T cells, these cells could be of importance in the perpetuation of the immune response in the joints.

Chondrocytes have been thought to play an important role in initiating immune responses toward cartilage in inflammatory arthritis, including RA, by presenting cartilage-specific antigens to T cells. Activated chondrocytes can secrete cytokines and express HLA class II and ICAM-1 which facilitates antigen-presenting cell function. Rabbit chondrocytes constitutively expressing Ia antigens have been shown to be potent antigen-presenting cells. Alsalameh et al. (1991) reported that human articular chondrocytes upon activation express class II and can present tetanus toxoid to allogeneic or autologous T cells, although the antigen-presenting function is not so potent as that of blood monocytes.

Dendritic cells which are absent in normal synovial membrane are present in large numbers in rheumatoid synovial fluid (March, 1987; Tsai et al., 1989), and are also demonstrated in rheumatoid synovial membrane (van Dinther-Janssen et al., 1990). These cells express class II (Klareskog et al., 1981; Poulter et al., 1981) and produce cytokines such as IL-1 (Duff et al., 1985). The dendritic cells from rheumatoid synovial fluid are potent antigen-presenting cells (Tsai et al., 1989). Bhardwaj et al. (1992) have recently shown that normal blood dendritic cells are 10–50-fold more potent than monocytes or B cells in presenting a range of microbial superantigens to T cells as has previously been shown for antigens (Katz et al., 1986). Furthermore, these dendritic cells are capable of presenting superantigens to T cells even at femtomolar concentrations and thus may function at low numbers at which monocytes and B cells are inactive.

We have shown that murine splenic CD5[+] B cells are more potent than CD5[−] B cells in presenting goat IgG to T cells (Plater-Zyberk et al., 1992). It is interesting to speculate that CD5[+] B cells in rheumatoid joints which produce rheumatoid factors may take up immune complexes and present the relevant antigens (Maini, 1989).

EXPRESSION OF CYTOKINES AND THEIR RECEPTORS

Over the past decade, production of cytokines in rheumatoid joints has been extensively studied and a profile of cytokines has been outlined. As shown in Table 2, it appears that monocyte/macrophage-derived cytokines, such as IL-1, TNFα, IL-6, and IL-8 are readily detected in abundance, whereas cytokines produced by T cells such as IL-2, IL-4, IFNγ are difficult to detect or expressed sparsely at the protein level (Feldmann et al., 1991; Firestein, 1991). Others, such as LT, are detectable at the mRNA level, but barely detectable at the protein level (Feldmann et al., 1991). Several possibilities have been considered for the dearth of T-cell cytokines; for example, local consumption by target cells, binding to inhibitors or down-regulated by

Table 2. Expression of cytokines in rheumatoid joints

Cytokine	mRNA	Protein level	Cellular source
T-cell cytokine			
IL-2	+	Low	T cells
IL-4	?	Not detectable	
IL-10	+	Medium	Monocytes, T cells?
IFN-γ	+	Low	T cells
TNFβ (LT)	+	Not detectable	T cells?
Macrophage cytokine			
IL-1α	+	High	Macrophages, T cells, fibroblasts, endothelial cells, chondrocytes
IL-1β	+	High	Macrophages, T cells, fibroblasts, chondrocytes
IL-6	+	High	Macrophages, T, B cells, chondrocytes, fibroblasts
IL-8	+	High	Macrophages, endothelial cells, chondrocytes
TNFα	+	High	Macrophages, T cells, endothelial cells, fibroblasts, chondrocytes
GM-CSF	+	High	Endothelial cells, macrophages, chondrocytes
TGF-β	+	High	Macrophage, fibroblasts, chondrocytes, T cells
LIF	+	High	Macrophages, chondrocytes
PDGF-A	+	High	Macrophages, fibroblasts
PDGF-B	+	High	Macrophages, fibroblasts
FGF-1 (acidic FGF)	+	High	Macrophages, fibroblasts, endothelial cells, lymphocytes
FGF-2 (basic FGF)	+	High	Macrophages, endothelial cells, fibroblasts

inhibitory cytokines such as IL-10 or TGFβ. Concentrations that are not detectable in supernatant assays may still be biologically sufficient in a microcellular environment by direct contact, for example (Feldmann *et al.*, 1991). This possibility is reinforced by the increasing list of cytokines expressed on cell membranes, for example IL-1α, TNFα, macrophage colony stimulating factor (M-CSF), etc.

The pattern of cytokine production in rheumatoid joints established thus far has been based almost exclusively on synovium from patients with well-established disease. This pattern may not represent the changes occurring in the initial or early stages of the disease, where T-cell cytokines may be produced in large amounts, but are down-regulated rapidly with disease progression. In mice with experimental allergic encephalomyelitis, mRNAs for IFNγ, IL-2, IL-4 and IL-6 in the central nervous system were all highly expressed at the onset, but declined rapidly with the progression of the disease and a concomitant rise of IL-10 (Kennedy *et al.*, 1992). However, IL-1α tends to persist at higher levels throughout the disease process (Kennedy *et al.*, 1992). We have observed the transient kinetics of IFNγ production, and relative persistence of IL-1 and TNFα in tuberculin-induced delayed type hypersensitivity in human skin biopsies (Chu *et al.*, 1992a). This type of cytokine kinetics may occur during the early stages of RA but it is obviously difficult to monitor in humans. Following the kinetics of cytokine expression in animal models of arthritis such as collagen-induced arthritis would be helpful in clarifying this issue and also in understanding the role of T cells in the initiation of the disease.

Cytokines act on target cells via binding to their receptors expressed by these cells. We have shown that both p55 and p75 TNF receptors (TNF-R) are highly expressed by rheumatoid synovial cells which are situated in the region of TNFα production, and some TNFα-producing cells also express its receptors (Brennan *et al.*, 1992a; Deleuran *et al.*, 1992a). Similarly, type I IL-1 receptor is also widely expressed by rheumatoid synovial cells (Deleuran *et al.*, 1992b). Both TNF-R and type I IL-1 receptor are expressed by pannus cells and chondrocytes (Deleuran *et al.*, 1992a,b), suggesting that TNFα and IL-1 may induce tissue destruction via pannus cells, and also by acting directly on chondrocytes.

ROLE OF CYTOKINES IN RA PATHOLOGY

It is generally accepted that regardless of the actual cause (aetiology) of RA, cytokines are important mediators which are essential for many processes in the pathogenesis of RA. A critical step in the generation of an immune or inflammatory reaction is activation of macrophages and induction of HLA class II expression. IFNγ is potentially the most potent cytokine at inducing such expression in the absence of other factors (Portillo *et al.*, 1989). However, negligible amounts of IFNγ (Firestein and Zvaifler, 1987) are detected in rheumatoid joints, suggesting that other factors alone or in combination with IFNγ are involved. Granulocyte-monocyte colony-stimulating factor (GM-CSF), capable of inducing HLA-DR expression on human monocytes (Chantry *et al.*, 1990) and present in abundance in rheumatoid joints (Xu *et al.*, 1989; Haworth *et al.*, 1991), could be an important macrophage activator and induce HLA class II expression in monocytes in rheumatoid joints (Alvaro-Garcia *et al.*, 1989). However, the most significant inhibition of the expression of class II which we have observed in the rheumatoid synovial cell cultures was with anti-TNFα antibody and exceeded that observed with antibodies to IFNγ or GM-CSF (Brennan, F., Haworth, C., and Feldmann, M., unpublished observation). The effect of anti-TNFα is unlikely to be direct, since TNFα by itself does not induce the expression of HLA class II (Pujol-Borrell *et al.*, 1987). This suggests that many different cytokines may work together to induce this expression, or that as-yet-undefined molecules may be involved. Alternatively (or in addition), cell–cell interactions through cell adhesion molecules may be necessary to maintain HLA-Class II expression. Of interest is the observation that TNFα is a potent inducer of many adhesion molecules including ICAM-1 and VCAM-1 (Pober *et al.*, 1986; Rice and Bevilacqua, 1989).

Angiogenesis is a characteristic feature of RA synovial membrane. From studies of modulation of angiogenesis in tumour tissues, many factors have been shown to be involved in new vessel formation (reviewed by Colville-Nash and Scott, 1992). A number of these factors have been found in RA synovial membrane including TNFα, IL-1 (Buchan *et al.*, 1988a,b), and basic and acidic fibroblast growth factors (FGF) (Sano *et al.*, 1990, 1993; Remmers *et al.*, 1991; Sano *et al.*, 1993). It is not clear which is of particular importance in the angiogenesis noted in RA synovial inflammation.

The activation and differentiation of T and B lymphocytes are finely controlled by cytokines. For B cells, IL-4 and IL-6 are most important. IL-4 is a potent B-cell growth factor, but is detected in negligible amounts in rheumatoid joints, so its role in B-cell activation in RA is questionable. In contrast, high levels of IL-6 produced by RA synovial cells (Hirano et al., 1988; Field et al., 1991) may be responsible for production of high levels of autoantibodies including rheumatoid factors. The latter may further contribute to the pathogenesis of RA by forming immune complexes which can induce IL-1 production (Chantry et al., 1989). TNFα and TNFβ (LT) can also act as B-cell growth factors (Kehrl et al., 1986, 1987). In addition, IL-10, also detected in RA joints (Katsikis et al., 1993), is also a potent B-cell stimulator (Moore et al., 1990). IL-7 has recently been shown to be a T-cell growth factor (Londei et al., 1990) and could be another important candidate for T-cell growth regulation in RA, but it is currently not known whether IL-7 is expressed in RA joints.

Cytokines produced by monocytes/macrophages are proinflammatory and induce tissue destruction. For example, TNFα, IL-1 and IL-8 have all been shown to cause synovitis directly (Pettipher et al., 1986; Henderson and Pettipher, 1989; O'Byrne et al., 1990; Endo et al., 1991) and TNFα and IL-1 can also cause cartilage degradation when injected intra-articularly in rabbit knee joints. Transgenic mice bearing a human TNFα transgene modified in the 3'-region express higher levels of TNFα and develop a chronic arthritis resembling RA which is prevented by anti-TNFα treatment (Keffer et al., 1991). In human RA, TNFα and IL-1 are likely to be important cytokines that are responsible for cartilage destruction. Both TNFα and IL-1 can stimulate synovial cells and chondrocytes to produce metalloproteinases which destroy the extracellular matrix components such as collagen and proteoglycan (reviewed by Firestein, 1992; Dinarello, 1992). They also inhibit matrix synthesis. These cytokines have been found in the cartilage/pannus junction (Chu et al., 1991a, 1992b) where cartilage damage takes place and chondrocytes express receptors for them (Deleuran et al., 1992a,b), suggesting their direct involvement in cartilage destruction. Lotz et al. (1992) recently found that high levels of leukaemia inhibitory factor (LIF) are produced by RA synovial cells and chondrocytes. LIF may be an important mediator for bone resorption in addition to TNF and IL-1.

We have postulated that TNFα is a pivotal cytokine in the pathogenesis of RA (Feldman et al., 1991; Brennan et al., 1992b), based on the fact that TNFα is a proinflammatory cytokine causing arthritis and it is required for other inflammatory cytokine (e.g. IL-1 and GM-CSF) production by RA synovial cells (Brennan et al., 1989b) and present in abundance in rheumatoid joints (di Giovine et al., 1988). This hypothesis has been tested in vivo in collagen-induced arthritis. Treatment of collagen type-II induced arthritis in DBA/1 mice with anti-TNFα antibodies considerably reduced the severity, both clinically and histologically, of the arthritis (Williams et al., 1992). Highly relevant to human disease was the capacity of the treatment to reduce the clinical and histological severity of the disease when the antibodies were administered after the onset of clinical arthritis. These results not only confirm the importance of TNFα in the pathogenesis in arthritis, but also have implications for possible models of therapy in human arthritis. Using a similar protocol with a human–mouse chimeric anti-human TNFα antibody, a trial of blockade of TNFα in RA patients is in progress. Results from phase I of the open trial show that all 20 patients with chronic RA who had failed conventional treatment clinically improved with anti-TNFα treatment, and had reduction of the acute phase response (Elliott et al., 1993). Similar results have been obtained in a randomised double-blind placebo controlled trial (Elliott *et al.*, 1994).

In chronic RA, tissue repair occurs concomitantly with the inflammatory and destructive process. Fibrosis is an important component and complication of RA. It is implicated in deformation of joints, and also in systemic complications such as pulmonary fibrosis. TGFβ-induced collagen synthesis by synovial fibroblasts and proteoglycan synthesis by chondrocytes, and inhibition of protease release from these cells could be important in promoting fibrosis and reducing cartilage destruction in RA (reviewed in Chu *et al.*, 1991b). The presence of high levels of TGFβ in RA (Brennan *et al.*, 1990b), especially in the invasive cartilage/pannus junction (Chu *et al.*, 1992b), suggests it may partly counteract the effects of TNFα and IL-1 in cartilage destruction. The presence of TGFβ in the transitional fibroblastic zone of diffuse fibroblastic junction is compatible with the proposal that such tissue is in an anabolic state of healing or differentiation (Allard *et al.*, 1987; Chu *et al.*, 1992b). Platelet-derived growth factors (PDGF) are potent fibroblast growth factors and can stimulate synovial fibroblast-like cell proliferation. High levels of PDGF and their receptors have been demonstrated in RA synovial membrane, suggesting a role for PDGF fibrosis in RA joints (Remmers *et al.*, 1991; Sano *et al.*, 1993). IL-1 and TNFα have been shown to induce fibrosis, but this may act indirectly via induction of PDGF (Raines *et al.*, 1989).

CYTOKINE REGULATION

Expression of cytokine mRNA by *in vitro*-activated normal peripheral blood mononuclear cells is transient (24–48 h). This is in contrast to that of RA synovial membrane cells, which is relatively persistent. In a chronic disease only persistent features can be relevant to the maintenance of the disease process, so the consistence and persistence of cytokine production suggested that it was of importance in the pathogenesis (Buchan *et al.*, 1988a,b). Initial studies of the expression of IL-1 in rheumatoid joints revealed that all samples contained IL-1 mRNA, suggesting that cytokine production in the rheumatoid joint may be relatively stable and persistent. Further evidence showing persistent production of cytokines came from *in vitro* culturing of isolated synovial cells from rheumatoid joints, where both IL-1α and IL-1β mRNA survived for up to the 5-day culture period in the absence of exogenous stimulus (Buchan *et al.*, 1988a). This indicates that the signals necessary to regulate cytokine production are present in the rheumatoid joints.

Cytokines in *in vitro* experiments can induce other cytokine production in many cell types. We have shown that TNFα and β (LT) are the strongest non-microbial signals for the regulation of IL-1 production. For this reason, neutralizing antibodies to these two cytokines were chosen to investigate the regulation of IL-1 production by rheumatoid synovial cells. The results were striking, in that anti-TNFα completely abolished IL-1 production after the first day of culture, but anti-TNFβ did not show any effect; neither did normal rabbit IgG (Brennan *et al.*, 1989c). Reduction of mRNA for IL-1 showed even more rapid kinetics, and lack of an early effect on the amount of protein indicates that already ongoing synthesis of IL-1 was not affected, but the subsequent activation was inhibited. In comparison, no effect of anti-TNFα antibody on IL-1 production was observed in osteoarthritic synovial cells, although there is immunoreactive TNFα. This is because most TNFα in osteoarthritis is not biologically active. In addition, anti-TNFα antibody also markedly inhibited the production of GM-CSF by RA synovial cells in culture, although the effect is slower (Haworth *et al.*, 1991), and partially inhibited class II expression and the aggregation of cells normally observed in these cultures. This clearly indicates that TNFα is an important cytokine which is required for other cytokine production in rheumatoid joint cells.

However, what regulates TNFα production in rheumatoid synovial cells remains unknown. Preliminary results from our laboratory showed that IL-10 may be a potent down-regulator of TNFα production, that exogenous IL-10 strongly inhibits TNFα gene expression in cultured rheumatoid synovial cells, and that anti-IL-10 causes the increase of TNFα level (Katsikis *et al.*, 1994). This may provide a further clue for the new approaches to the treatment of RA. The effect of manipulating cytokines in experimental models of arthritis is reviewed in Chapter 26, this volume.

CYTOKINE ANTAGONISTS

It has been found recently that many cytokine receptors exist in soluble forms which probably derive from the cleavage of the extracellular part of the transmembrane receptors. Most of the soluble cytokine receptors are able to bind to their complementary ligands competing with the cell-membrane bound forms and act as cytokine inhibitors, for example, soluble IL-1, -2 (p55), -4, -6 and -7 receptors and soluble interferon receptor and soluble TNF-R, which may act as regulators for cytokine network. Both p55 and p75 TNF-R have a soluble form capable of binding to TNF in high affinity and thereby inhibiting TNF activities (Olsson *et al.*, 1989; Seckinger *et al.*, 1989; Engelmann *et al.*, 1990). They are present in elevated levels in serum and in the synovial fluids of patients with RA (Cope *et al.*, 1992; Roux-Lombard *et al.*, 1993), suggesting an augmentation of the TNF inhibitory system. However, these up-regulated levels of soluble TNF receptors do not fully neutralize the TNFα produced by cells from RA joints in culture, whereas they generally appear to be sufficient to neutralize TNFα produced by cells from osteoarthritic joints in culture (Brennan *et al.*, unpublished observations). Thus, in the cartilage-destructive disease of RA there appears to be an attempt at homeostasis, which, however, is inadequate.

Interleukin-1 receptor antagonist (IL-1ra) is the only one cytokine receptor antagonist described so far. IL-1ra belongs to the IL-1 family and has 30% homology with IL-1β. It competes with approximately equal affinity with IL-1 to bind to both IL-1 receptors but does not transduce any signal, thereby acting as a receptor blocking agent (reviewed by Arend, 1991). It is also present in rheumatoid joints (Deleuran *et al.*, 1992b; Firestein *et al.*, 1992a) in relatively larger amounts than IL-1 (IL-1ra : IL-1 = 1.25) (Firestein *et al.*, 1994), but is seems it is not sufficient to block IL-1 activities, as quantities greatly in excess of those of IL-1 (i.e. 1000/1) are necessary to exert inhibitory effects (Arend, 1991). Although the physiological role of these natural inhibitors is not entirely clear, they are potentially useful as therapeutic agents in RA therapy. Indeed, these soluble TNF-R (dimeric fusion protein) and IL-1ra have been used in animal models of arthritis and proved effective (Wooley *et al.*, 1993a; Wooley *et al.*, 1993b). Further discussion of cytokine antagonists and their therapeutic role is to be found in Chapters 13 and 26, this volume.

CONCLUDING REMARKS

The aetiology of RA still remains unsolved, and will continue to attract intensive interest in the next decade. Identification of non-HLA genes contributing to susceptibility to RA will be defined in the foreseeable future, and will provide further clues concerning the pathogenesis.

Therapeutic trials involving blockade of cytokines such as TNFα and IL-1 using neutralizing antibodies in RA patients and IL-1ra are in progress. Our clinical trials with a human–mouse chimeric anti-TNFα antibody has been shown to benefit patients. Use of soluble cytokine receptors (e.g. soluble TNF-R) is envisaged, and will be tried shortly. Gene therapy leading to blockade of inflammatory cytokine activities, for example, by the introduction of IL-1ra gene into rheumatoid joints, has been proposed.

These (and other) therapeutic trials directed at specific molecules will contribute greatly to our understanding of the pathogenesis of RA. The consequent refinement of our concepts of the pathogenesis of RA will motivate the development of more effective therapies and preventive measures.

REFERENCES

Abbink JJ, Kamp AM, Nuijens JS, Erenberg AJ, Swaak AJ & Hack CE (1992) Relative contribution of contact and complement activation to inflammatory reactions in arthritic joints. *Ann Rheum Dis* **51**: 1123–1128.

Abbot SE, Kaul A, Stevens CR & Blake DR (1992) Isolation and culture of synovial microvascular endothelial cells: characterization and assessment of adhesion molecule expression. *Arthritis Rheum* **35**: 401–406.

Afeltra A, Galeazzi M, Ferri GM, Amoroso A, De pita' O, Porzio F et al. (1993) Expression of CD69 antigen on synovial fluid T cells in patients with rheumatoid arthritis and other chronic synovitis. *Ann Rheum Dis* **52**: 457–460.

Albani S, Tuckwell JE, Esparza L, Carson DA & Roudier J (1992) The susceptibility sequence to rheumatoid arthritis is a cross-reactive B cell epitope shared by the *Escherichia coli* heat shock protein dnaJ and the histocompatibility leukocytes antigen DRB10401 molecule. *J Clin Invest* **89**: 327–331.

Allard SA, Muirden KD, Camplejohn KL & Maini RN (1987) Chondrocyte-derived cells at the rheumatoid cartilage-pannus junction identified with monocloncal antibodies. *Rheum Int* **7**: 153–159.

Alsalameh S, Jahn B, Krause A, Kalden JR & Burmester GR (1991) Antigenicity and accessory cell function of human articular chondrocytes. *J Rheumatol* **18**: 414–421.

Alvaro-Garcia JM, Zvaifler NJ & Firestein GS (1989) Cytokines in chronic inflammatory arthritis. IV. Granulocyte/macrophage colony stimulating factor-mediated induction of class II MHC antigen on human monocytes: a possible role in rheumatoid arthritis. *J Exp Med* **170**: 865–875.

Andrew EM, Plater-Zyberk C, Brown CMS, Williams DG & Maini RN (1991) The potential role of B lymphocytes in the pathogenesis of RA. *Br J Rheumatol* **30** (**supplement 1**): 47–52.

Arend WF (1991) Interleukin-1 receptor antagonist – a new member of the IL-1 family. *J Clin Invest* **88**: 1445–1451.

Baboonian C, Venables PJW, Williams DG, Williams RO & Maini RN (1991) Cross-reaction of antibodies to a glycine-alanine repeat sequence of Epstein-Barr virus nuclear antigen-1 with collagen, cytokeratin, and actin. *Ann Rheum Dis* **50**: 772–775.

Baccala R, Smith LR, Vestberg M, Peterson PA, Cole BC & Theofilopoulos AN (1992) Mycoplasma arthritis mitogen: Vβ engaged in mice, rats and humans, and requirements of HLA-DRα for presentation. *Arthritis Rheum* **35**: 434–442.

Berg LJ, Frank CD & Davis MM (1990) The effects of MHC gene dosage and allelic variations on T cell receptor selection. *Cell* **60**: 1043–1053.

Bhardwaj N, Friedman SM, Cole BC & Nisanian AJ (1992) Dendritic cells are potent antigen-presenting cells for microbial superantigens. *J Exp Med* **175**: 267–273.

Brennan FM, Allard S, Londei M, Savill C, Boylston A, Carrel S et al. (1988a) Heterogeneity of T cell receptor idiotypes in rheumatoid arthritis. *Clin Exp Immunol* **73**: 417–423.

Brennan FM, Londei M, Jackson A, Hercend T, Brenner MB, Maini RN & Feldmann M (1988b) T cells expressing γδ chain receptors in rheumatoid arthritis. *J Autoimmunity* **1**: 319–326.

Brennan FM, Plater Zyberk C, Maini RN & Feldmann M (1989a) Co-ordinate expansion of 'foetal type' lymphocytes (TCR $\gamma\delta^+$ T and CD5$^+$ B) in rheumatoid arthritis and primary Sjögren's syndrome. *Clin Exp Immunol* **77**: 175–178.

Brennan FM, Chantry D, Jackson AM, Maini RN & Feldmann M (1989b) Cytokine production in culture by cells isolated from the synovial membrane. *J Autoimmunity* **2 (supplement)**: 177–186.

Brennan FM, Chantry D, Jackson A, Maini RN & Feldmann M (1989c) Inhibitory effect of TNFα antibodies on synovial cell interleukin-1 production in rheumatoid arthritis. *Lancet* **ii**: 244–247.

Brennan FM, Zachariae COC, Chantry D, Larsen CG, Turner M, Maini RN & Feldmann M (1990a) Detection of interleukin-8 (IL-8) biological activity in synovial fluids from patients with rheumatoid arthritis and production of IL-8 mRNA by isolated synovial cells. *Eur J Immunol* **20**: 2141–2144.

Brennan FM, Chantry D, Turner M, Foxwell B, Maini RN & Feldmann M (1990b) Detection of transforming growth factor β in rheumatoid arthritis synovial tissue: lack of effect on spontaneous cytokine production in joint cell cultures. *Clin Exp Immunol* **81**: 278–285.

Brennan FM, Gibbons DL, Mitchell T, Cope AP, Maini RN & Feldmann M (1992a) Enhanced expression of TNF receptor mRNA and protein in mononuclear cells isolated from rheumatoid arthritis synovial joints. *Eur J Immunol* **22**: 1907–1912.

Brennan FM, Maini RN & Feldmann M (1992b) TNFα – A pivotal role in rheumatoid arthritis? *Br J Rheumatol* **31**: 293–298.

Brown JH, Jardetzky TS, Gorga JC, Stern LJ, Urban RG, Strominger JL et al. (1993) Three-dimensional structure of the human class II histocompatibility antigen HLA-DR1. *Nature* **364**: 33–39.

Brown CMS, Longhurst C, Haynes G, Plater-Zyberk C, Malcolm A & Maini RN (1992) Immunoglobulin heavy chain variable region gene utilization by B cell hybridomas derived from rheumatoid synovial tissue. *Clin Exp Immunol* **89**: 230–238.

Buchan G, Barrett K, Turner M, Chantry D, Maini RN & Feldmann M (1988a) Interleukin-1 and tumour necrosis factor mRNA expression in rheumatoid arthritis: prolonged production of IL-1α. *Clin Exp Immunol* **73**: 449–455.

Buchan G, Barrett K, Fujita T, Taniguchi T, Maini RN & Feldman M (1988b) Detection of activated T cell products in the rheumatoid joint using cDNA probes to interleukin 2, IL-2 receptor and interferon γ. *Clin Exp Immunol* **71**: 295–301.

Calabrese LH, Wilke WS, Perkins AD and Tubbs RR (1989) Rheumatoid arthritis complicated by infection with human immunodeficiency virus and the development of Sjogren's syndrome. *Arthritis Rheum* **32**: 1453–1457.

Chantry D, Winearls CG, Maini RN and Feldmann M (1989) Mechanism of immune complex mediated damage: induction of interleukin 1 by immune complexes and synergy with interferon g and tumour necrosis factor α. *Eur J Immunol* **19**: 189–192.

Chantry D, Turner M, Brennan F, Kingsbury A & Feldmann M (1990) Granulocyte-macrophage colony stimulating factor induces both HLA-DR expression and cytokine production by human monocytes. *Cytokine* **2**: 60–67.

Chikanza IC, Petrou P, Kingsley G, Chrousos G & Panayi GS (1992) Defect hypothalamic response to immune and inflammatory stimuli in patients with rheumatoid arthritis. *Arthritis Rheum* **35**: 1281–1288.

Chu CQ, Field M, Feldmann M and Maini RN (1991a) Localization of tumor necrosis factor α in synovial tissues and at the cartilage-pannus junction in patients with rheumatoid arthritis. *Arthritis Rheum* **34**: 1125–1132.

Chu CQ, Field M, Abney E, Zheng RQH, Allard S, Feldman M et al. (1991b) Transforming growth factor β1 in rheumatoid synovial membrane and cartilage/pannus junction. *Clin Exp Immunol* **86**: 380–386.

Chu CQ, Field M, Andrew E, Haskard D, Feldmann M & Maini RN (1992a) Detection of cytokines at the site of tuberculin-induced delayed-type hypersensitivity in man. *Clin Exp Immunol* **90**: 522–529.

Chu CQ, Field M, Allard S, Abney E, Feldman M & Maini RN (1992b) Detection of cytokines at the cartilage/pannus junction in patients with rheumatoid arthritis: implications for the role of cytokines in cartilage destruction and repair. *Br J Rheumatol* **31**: 653–661.

Colville-Nash PR & Scott DL (1992) Angiogenesis and rheumatoid arthritis: pathogenic and therapeutic implications. *Ann Rheum Dis* **51**: 919–925.

Cope A, Adeka D, Doherty M, Engelmann H, Gibbons DL, Jones AC et al. (1992) Soluble tumour necrosis factor (TNF) receptors are increased in the sera and synovial fluids of patients with rheumatic disease. *Arthritis Rheum* **35**: 1160–1169.

Cush JJ, Pietschmann P, Oppenheimer-Marks N & Lipsky PE (1992) The intrinsic migratory capacity of memory T cells contribute to their accumulation in rheumatoid synovium. *Arthritis Rheum* **35**: 1434–1444.

de Graeff-Meeder ER, Voorhorst V, van Eden W, Schuurman HJ, Huber J, Barkley D et al. (1990) Antibodies to the mycobacterium-65 kD heat-shock protein are reactive with synovial tissue of adjuvant arthritic rats and patients with rheumatoid arthritis and osteoarthritis. *Am J Pathol* **137**: 1013–1017.

Deighton CM, Walker DJ, Griffiths ID & Roberts DF (1989) The contribution of HLA to rheumatoid arthritis. *Clinical Genetics* **36**: 178–182.

Deleuran BW, Chu CQ, Field M, Brennan FM, Mitchell T, Feldman M et al. (1992a) Localization of tumour necrosis factor receptors in the synovial tissue and cartilage/pannus junction in rheumatoid arthritis: implications for local actions of tumour necrosis factor α. *Arthritis Rheum* **35**: 1170–1178.

Deleuran BW, Chu CQ, Field M, Brennan FM, Katsikis P, Feldmann M et al. (1992b) Localization of interleukin-1α, type 1 interleukin-1 receptor and interleukin-1 receptor antagonist in the synovial membrane and cartilage/pannus junction in rheumatoid arthritis. *Br J Rheumatol* **21**: 801–809.

di Giovine FS, Nuki G & Duff GW (1988) Tumour necrosis factor in synovial exudates. *Ann Rheum Dis* **47**: 768–772.

Dinarello CA (1992) Interleukin-1 and tumour necrosis factor: effector cytokines in autoimmune diseases. *Semin Immunol* **4**: 133–145.

Duff GW, Forre O, Waalen K, Dickens E & Nuki G (1985) Rheumatoid arthritis synovial dendritic cells produce interleukin-1. *Br J Rheumatol* **24** (**supplement 1**): 94–97.

Ebringer A, Ptaszynska T, Corbett M, Wilson C, Macafee Y, Avakian H et al. (1985) Antibodies to proteus in RA. *Lancet* **ii**: 305–307.

Elliott MJ, Maini RN, Feldmann M, Long-Fox A, Charles P, Katsikis P et al. (1993) Treatment of rheumatoid arthritis with chimeric monoclonal antibodies to TNFα. *Arthritis Rheum* **36**: 1681–1690.

Endo H, Akahoshi T, Takagishi K, Kashiwazaki S & Matsushima K (1991) Elevation of interleukin-8 (IL-8) levels in joint fluids of patients with rheumatoid arthritis and the induction by IL-8 of leukocyte infiltration and synovitis in rabbit joints. *Lymphokine Cytokine Res* **10**: 245–252.

Engelmann H, Novick D & Wallach D (1990) Two tumour necrosis factor-binding proteins purified from human urine. *J Biol Chem* **265**: 1531–1536.

Feldmann M (1989) Molecular mechanisms involved in human autoimmune diseases: relevance of chronic antigen presentation, Class II expression and cytokine production. *Immunology* (**supplement 2**): 66–71.

Feldmann M, Brennan FM, Chantry D, Haworth C, Turner M, Katsikis P et al. (1991) Cytokine assays: role in evaluation of the pathogenesis of autoimmunity. *Immunol Rev* **119**: 105–123.

Field M, Chu C, Feldmann M & Maini RN (1991) Interleukin-6 in the synovial membrane in rheumatoid arthritis. *Rheumatol Int* **11**: 45–50.

Firestein GS (1991) Immunopathogenesis of rheumatoid arthritis. *Cur Opin Immunol* **31**: 398–406.

Firestein GS (1992) Mechanisms of tissue destruction and cellular activation in rheumatoid arthritis. *Cur Opin Rheum* **4**: 348–353.

Firestein GS & Zvaifler NJ (1987) Peripheral blood and synovial fluid monocyte activation in inflammatory arthritis. II. Low levels of synovial fluid and synovial tissue interferon suggest that γ-interferon is not the primary macrophage activating factor. *Arthritis Rheum* **30**: 864–871.

Firestein GS, Zvaifler NJ (1990) How important are T cells in chronic rheumatoid synovitis? *Arthritis Rheum* **33**: 768–773.

Firestein GS, Berger AE, Tracey DE, Chosay JG, Chapman DL, Paine MM et al. (1992a) IL-1 receptor antagonist protein production and gene expression in rheumatoid arthritis and osteoarthritis synovium. *J Immunol* **149**: 1054–1062.

Firestein GS, Paine MM, Boyle DL, Yu C, Zvaifler NJ & Arend WP (1992b) IL-1ra:IL-1 balance in rheumatoid arthritis (RA) and osteoarthritis (OA) synovial cells. *Arthritis Rheum* **35**: s143.

Firestein GS, Boyle DL, Yu C, Paine MM, Whisenand TD, Zvaifler NJ & Arend WP (1994) Synovial interleukin-1 receptor antagonist and interleukin-1 balance in rheumatoid arthritis. *Arthritis Rheum* **37**: 644–652.

Fox DA, Millard JA, Kan L, Zedes WS, Davies W, Higgs J et al. (1990) Activation pathways of synovial T lymphocytes: expression and function of the UM4D4/CDw60 antigen. *J Clin Invest* **86**: 1124–1136.

Goronzy JJ & Weyand CM (1993) Interplay of T lymphocytes and HLA-DR molecules in rheumatoid arthritis. *Cur Opin Rheumatol* **5**: 169–177.

Goronzy J, Weyand PM & Fathman CG (1986) Shared T cell recognition sites on human histocompatibility leukocyte antigen class II molecules of patients with seropositive rheumatoid arthritis. *J Clin Invest* **77**: 1042–1049.

Gregersen PK, Silver J & Winchester RJ (1987) The shared epitope hypothesis. An approach to understanding the molecular genetics of susceptibility to rheumatoid arthritis. *Arthritis Rheum* **30**: 1205–1213.

Haworth C, Brennan FM, Chantry D, Turner M, Maini RN & Feldmann M (1991) Expression of granulocyte-macrophage colony-stimulating factor in rheumatoid arthritis: regulation by tumour necrosis factor α. *Eur J Immunol* **21**: 2575–2579.

He X, Goronzy J and Weyand C (1991) Selective induction of rheumatoid factors by superantigens and human helper T cells. *J Clin Invest* **89**: 673–680.

Hemler ME, Glass D, Coblyn JS and Jacobson JG (1986) Very late activation antigens on rheumatoid synovial fluid T lymphocytes: association with stages of T cell activation. *J Clin Invest* **78**: 696–702.

Henderson B & Pettipher ER (1989) Arthritogenic actions of recombinant IL-1 and tumour necrosis factor alpha in the rabbit: evidence for synergistic interactions between cytokines *in vivo*. *Clin Exp Immunol* **75**: 306–310.

Herzog C, Walker C, Müller W, Rieber P, Reiter C, Riethmüller G et al. (1989) Anti CD4 antibody treatment of patients with RA: effect on clinical course and circulating T cells *J Autoimmunity* **2**: 627–642.

Hirano T, Matsuda T, Turner M, Miyasaka N, Buchan G, Tang B et al. (1988) Excessive production of interleukin 6/B cell stimulatory factor-2 in rheumatoid arthritis. *Eur J Immunol* **18**: 1797–1801.

Holoshitz J, Klajman A, Druker I, Lapidot Z, Yaretzky A, Frenkel A et al. (1986) T lymphocytes of rheumatoid arthritis patients show augmented reactivity to a fraction of mycobacteria cross-reactive with cartilage. *Lancet* **ii**: 305–309.

Holoshitz J, Koning F, Coligan JE, De Bruyn J & Strober S (1989) Isolation of CD4-CD8- mycobacteria-reactive T lymphocyte clones from rheumatoid arthritis synovial fluid. *Nature* **339**: 226–229.

Horneff G, Burmester GR, Emmrich F and Kalden JR (1991) Treatment of rheumatoid arthritis with an anti-CD4 monoclonal antibody. *Arthritis Rheum* **34**: 129–140.

Howell MD, Diveley JP, Lundeen KA, Esty A, Winters ST, Carlo DJ et al. (1991) Limited T-cell receptor beta-chain heterogeneity among interleukin-2 receptor-positive synovial T cells suggests a role for super-antigen in rheumatoid arthritis. *Proc Natl Acad Sci USA* **88**: 10921–10925.

Iwakura Y, Yosu M, Yoshida E, Takiguchi M, Sato K, Kitajima I et al. (1991) Induction of inflammatory arthropathy resembling rheumatoid arthritis in mice transgenic for HTLV. *Science* **253**: 1026–1028.

Jaraquemada D, Pachoula-Papasteriadis C, Festenstein H, Sachs JA, Roitt IM, Corbett M et al. (1979) HLA-D and DR determinants in rheumatoid arthritis. *Transplant Proc* **11**: 1306.

Jose PJ, Moss IK, Maini RN and Williams TJ (1990) Measurement of the chemotactic complement fragment C5a in rheumatoid synovial fluids by radioimmunoassay: role of C5a in the acute inflammatory phase. *Ann Rheum Dis* **49**: 747–752.

Karr RW, Rody JE, Lee T & Schwartz BD (1980) Association of HLA-DRw4 with rheumatoid arthritis in black and white patients. *Arthritis Rheum* **23**: 1241–1245.

Katsikis P, Chu CQ, Maini RN & Feldmann M (1994) Immunoregulatory role of interleukin 10 in rheumatoid arthritis. *J Exp Med* **179**: 1517–1527.

Katz DR, Feldmann M, Tees R & Schreier MH (1986) Heterogeneity of accessory cells interacting with T-helper clones. *J Immunol* **58**: 167–172.

Keffer J, Lesley P, Cazlaris H, Geogopoulos S, Kaslaris E, Kioussis D et al. (1991) Transgenic mice expressing human tumour necrosis factor: a predictive gene model of arthritis. *EMBO J* **10**: 4025–4031.

Kehrl JH, Roberts AB, Wakefield LM, Jakowlew S, Sporn MB & Fauci AS (1986) Transforming growth factor β is an important immunomodulatory protein for human B lymphocytes. *J Immunol* **137**, 3855–3860.

Kehrl JH, Miller A & Fauci AS (1987) Effect of tumor necrosis factor-α on mitogen-activated human B cells. *J Exp Med* **166**: 786–791.

Kennedy MK, Torrance DS, Picha KS & Mohler KM (1992) Analysis of cytokine mRNA expression in the central nervous system of mice with experimental autoimmune encephalomyelitis reveals that IL-10 mRNA expression correlates with recovery. *J Immunol* **149**: 2496–2505.

Klareskog L, Forsum U, Tjernlund UM, Kabelitz D & Wigren A (1981) Appearance of anti-HLA-DR reactive cells in normal and rheumatoid synovial tissue. *Scand J Immunol* **14**: 183–192.

Koch AE, Burrows JC, Haines GK, Carlow TM & Harlan JM (1991) Immunolocalization of endothelial and leukocyte adhesion molecules in human rheumatoid and osteoarthritic synovial tissues. *Lab Invest* **64**: 313–320.

Laffon A, Garcia-Vicuna R, Humbria A, Postigo AA, Corbi AL, de Landazuri MO et al. (1991) Upregulated expression and function of VLA-4 fibronectin receptors on human activated T cells in rheumatoid arthritis. *J Clin Invest* **88**: 546–552.

Lahita RG (1990) Sex hormones and the immune system. Part 1: Human data. *Bailliere's Clin Rheumatol* **4**: 1–12.

Lanchbury JSS, Jaeger EEM, Sansom DM, Hall MA, Wordsworth P, Stedeford J et al. (1991) Strong primary selection for the Dw4 subtype of DR4 accounts for the HLA-DQw7 association with Felty's Syndrome. *Hum Immunol* **32**: 56–64.

Lanzavecchia A (1985) Antigen-specific interaction between T and B cells. *Nature* **314**: 537–539.

Lawrence JS (1970) Rheumatoid arthritis: nature or nurture? *Ann Rheum Dis* **29**: 357–369.

Londei M, Savill C, Verhoef A, Brennan F, Leech ZA, Duance V et al. (1989) Persistence of collagen type II specific T cell clones in the synovial membrane of a patient with RA. *Proc Natl Acad Sci USA* **86**: 636–640.

Londei M, Verhoef A, Hawrylowicz C, Groves J, De Berardinis P & Feldmann M (1990) Interleukin 7 is a growth factor for mature human T cells. *Eur J Immunol* **20**: 425–428.

Lotz M, Moats T & Villiger PM (1992) Leukemia inhibitory factor is expressed in cartilage and synovium and can contribute to the pathogenesis of arthritis. *J Clin Invest* **90**: 888–896.

Maini RN (1989) Exploring immune pathways in rheumatoid arthritis. *Br J Rheumatol* **28**: 466–479.

March LM (1987) Dendritic cells in the pathogenesis of rheumatoid arthritis. *Rheumatol Int* **7**: 93–100.

Massardo L, Jacobelli S, Rodriguez L, Rivero S, Gonzalez A & Marchetti R (1990) Weak association between HLA-DR4 and rheumatoid arthritis in Chilean patients. *Ann Rheum Dis* **49**: 290–292.

Moore KW, Vieiva P, Fiorentino DF, Trounstine ML, Khan TA & Mosmann TR (1990) Homology of cytokine synthesis inhibitory factor (IL-10) to the Epstein-Barr virus gene BCRF 1. *Science* **248**: 1230–1234.

Morales-Ducret J, Wayner E, Elices MJ, Alvaro-Gracia JM, Zvaifler NJ & Firestein GS (1992) α4/β1 integrin (VLA-4) ligands in arthritis. Vascular cell adhesion molecule-1 expression in synovium and on fibroblast-like synoviocytes. *J Immunol* **149**: 1424–1431.

O'Byrne EM, Blancuzzi V, Wilson DE, Wong M & Jeng AY (1990) Elevated substance P and accelerate cartilage degradation in rabbit knee injected with interleukin-1α and tumour necrosis factor. *Arthritis Rheum* **33**: 1023–1028.

Ohta N, Nishimura YK, Tanimoto K, Horiuchi Y, Abe C, Shiokawa Y et al. (1982) Association between HLA and Japanese patients with rheumatoid arthritis. *Hum Immunol* **5**: 123–132.

Olee T, Yang PPM, Siminovitch KA, Olsen NJ, Hillson J, Wu J et al. (1991) Molecular basis of an autoantibody-associated restriction fragment length polymorphism that confers susceptibility to autoimmune diseases. *J Clin Invest* **88**: 193–203.

Ollier W & Thomson W (1992) Population genetics of rheumatoid arthritis. *Rheum Dis Clin N Am* **18**: 741–759.

Olsson I, Lantz M & Nilsson E (1989) Isolation and characterization of a tumour necrosis factor binding protein from urine. *Eur J Haematol* **42**: 270–275.

Oppenheimer-Marks N, Davies LS, Bogue DT, Ramberg J & Lipsky PE (1991) Differential utilization of ICAM-1 and VCAM-1 during the adhesion and transendothelial migration of human T lymphocytes. *J Immunol* **147**: 2913–2921.

Paliard X, West SG, Lafferty JA, Clements JR, Kappler JW, Marrack P et al. (1991) Evidence for the effects of a superantigen in rheumatoid arthritis. *Science* **253**: 325–329.

Panayi GS, Woolley PH and Batchelor JH (1979) HLA-DRW4 and rheumatoid arthritis. *Lancet* **i**: 730–734.

Pettipher ER, Higgs GA & Henderson B (1986) Interleukin 1 induces leukocyte infiltration and cartilage proteoglycan degradation in the synovial joint. *Proc Natl Acad Sci USA* **83**: 8749–8753.

Pitzalis C, Kingsley G, Murphy J & Panayi G (1987) Abnormal distribution of the helper-inducer and suppressor-inducer T lymphocyte subsets in the rheumatoid joint. *Clin Immunol Immunopathol* **45**: 252–258.

Pitzalis C, Kingsley GH, Covelli M, Meliconi R, Markey A & Panayi GS (1991) Selective migration of the human helper-inducer memory T cell subset: confirmation by *in vivo* cellular kinetic studies. *Eur J Immunol* **21**: 369–376.

Plater-Zyberk C, Brown CMS, Andrew EM & Maini RN (1992) CD5$^+$ B in rheumatoid arthritis. *Ann NY Acad Sci* **651**: 540–550.

Pober JS, Gimbrone MA, Jr, Lapierre LA, Mendrick DL, Fiers W, Rothlein R et al. (1986) Overlapping patterns of activation of human endothelial cells by interleukin 1, tumour necrosis factor, and immune interferon. *J Immunol* **137**: 1893–1896.

Portillo G, Turner M, Chantry D & Feldmann M (1989) Effect of cytokines on HLA-DR and IL-1 production by a monocytic tumour, THP-1. *Immunology* **66**: 170–175.

Poulter LW, Duke O, Hobbs S, Janossy G & Panayi G (1981) Histochemical discrimination of HLA-DR positive cell populations in the normal and arthritic synovial lining. *Clin Exp Immunol* **48**: 381–388.

Pujol-Borrell R, Todd I, Doshi M, Bottazzo GF, Sutton R, Gray D et al. (1987) HLA class II induction in human islet cells by interferon-g plus tumour necrosis factor of lymphotoxin. *Nature* **326**: 304–306.

Raines EW, Dower SK & Ross R (1989) Interleukin 1 mitogenic activity for fibroblasts and smooth muscle cells is due to PDGF-AA. *Science* **243**: 393–397.

Reiter C, Kaavand B, Rieber EP, Schattenkirchner M, Riethmuler G and Kruger K (1991) Treatment of rheumatoid arthritis with monoclonal CD4 antibody M-T151. Clinical results and immunopharmacologic effects in an open study, including repeated administration. *Arthritis Rheum* **34**: 525–536.

Remmers EF, Sano H & Wilder RL (1991) Platelet-derived growth factors and heparin-binding (fibroblast) growth factors in the synovial tissue pathology of rheumatoid arthritis. *Semin Arthritis Rheum* **21**: 191–199.

Res PC, Telgt D, van Laar JM, Pool MO, Breedveld FC & De Vries RR (1990) High antigen reactivity in mononuclear cells from sites of chronic inflammation. *Lancet* **336**: 1406–1408.

Rice GE & Bevilacqua MP (1989) An inducible endothelial cell surface glycoprotein mediates melanoma adhesion. *Science* **246**: 1303–1306.

Roudier J, Petersen J, Rhodes G, Luka J & Carson DA (1989) Susceptibility to rheumatoid arthritis maps to a T cell epitope shared by the HLA Dw4 DR beta 1 chain and the Epstein Barr virus glycoprotein gp110. *Proc Natl Acad Sci USA* **86**: 5104–5108.

Roux-Lombard P, Punzi L, Hasler F, Bas S, Todesco S, Gallati H et al. (1993) Soluble tumour necrosis factor receptors in human inflammatory synovial fluids. *Arthritis Rheum* **36**: 485–489.

Rudensky AY, Preston-Hurlburt P, Hong S-C, Barlow A & Janeway CA (1991) Sequence analysis of peptides bound to class II molecules. *Nature* **353**: 622–627.

Salmon M (1992) The immunogenetic component of susceptibility to rheumatoid arthritis. *Cur Opin Rheum* **4**: 342–347.

Sanchez B, Moreno I, Magarino R, Garzon M, Gonzalez MF, Garcia A et al. (1990) HLA-DRw10 confers the highest susceptibility to rheumatoid arthritis in a Spanish population. *Tissue Antigens* **36**: 174–176.

Sano H, Forough R, Maier JA, Case JP, Jackson A, Engleka K et al. (1990) Detection of high levels of heparin binding growth factor-1 (acidic fibroblast growth factor) in inflammatory arthritis joints. *J Cell Biol* **110**: 1417–1426.

Sano H, Engleka K, Mathern P, Hla T, Crofford LJ, Remmers EF et al. (1993) Coexpression of phospho-tyrosine-containing proteins, platelate-derived growth factor-B, and fibroblast growth factor-1 in situ in synovial tissues of patients with rheumatoid arthritis and Lewis rats with adjuvant or streptococcal cell wall arthritis. *J Clin Invest* **91**: 553–565.

Sarvetnick N, Shizuru J, Liggitt D, Martin L, McIntyre B, Gregory A et al. (1990) Loss of pancreatic islet tolerance induced by B cell expression of interferon-γ. *Nature* **346**: 844–847.

Schall TJ, Bacon K, Toy KJ & Goeddel DV (1990) Selective attraction of monocytes and T lymphocytes of the memory phenotype by cytokine RANTES. *Nature* **347**: 669–671.

Seckinger P, Isaaz S & Dayer J-M (1989) Purification and biologic characterization of a specific tumor necrosis factor inhibitor. *J Biol Chem* **264**: 11966–11973.

Seglias J, Li EK, Cohen MG, Wong RWS, Potter PK & So AK (1992) Linkage between rheumatoid arthritis susceptibility and the presence of HLA-DR4 and DRβ allelic third hypervariable sequences in Southern Chinese persons. *Arthritis Rheum* **35**: 163–167.

Silman AJ, Ollier W, Hayton RM, Holligan S & Smith K (1989) Twin concordance rates for rheumatoid arthritis: preliminary results from a nationwide study. *Br J Rheumatol* **28** (**supplement 2**): 95.

Stastny P (1974) Mixed lymphocyte culture typing cells from patients with rheumatoid arthritis. *Tissue Antigens* **4**: 571–579.

Stastny P (1978) Association of the B cell alloantigen DRw4 with rheumatoid arthritis. *N Engl J Med* **97**: 664–761.

Sternberg EM, Hill JM, Chrousos GP, Kamilaris T, Listwak SJ, Gold PW et al. (1989a) Inflammatory mediator-induced hypothalamic-pituitary-adrenal axis activation is defective in streptococcal cell wall arthritis-susceptible Lewis rats. *Proc Natl Acad Sci USA* **86**: 2374–2378.

Sternberg EM, Young WS, Bernardini R, Calogero AE, Chrousos GP, Gold PW et al. (1989b) A central nervous system defect in biosynthesis of corticotropin-releasing hormone is associated with susceptibility to streptococcal cell-wall induced arthritis in Lewis rats. *Proc Natl Acad Sci USA* **86**: 4771–4775.

Tarkowski A, Klareskog L, Carlsten H, Herberts P & Koopman WJ (1989) Secretion of antibodies to types I and II collagen by synovial tissue cells in patients with rheumatoid arthritis. *Arthritis Rheum* **32**: 1087–1096.

Tsai V, Bergroth V & Zvaifler NJ (1989) Dendritic cells in health and disease. In Feldmann M, Maini RN & Woody JN (eds) *T Cell Activation in Health and Disease*, pp 33–44. London: Academic Press.

Uematsu Y, Wege H, Straus A, Ott M, Bannwarth W, Lanchbury J et al. (1991) The T-cell receptor repertoire in the synovial fluid of a patient with rheumatoid arthritis is polyclonal. *Proc Natl Acad Sci USA* **88**: 8534–8538.

van Dinther-Janssen ACHM, Pals ST, Scheper PR, Breedveld F & Meijer CJLM (1990) Dendritic cells and high endothelial venules in the rheumatoid synovial membrane. *J Rheumatol* **17**: 11–17.

van Eden W, Holoshitz J, Nevo Z, Frenkel A, Klajman A & Cohen IR (1985) Arthritis induced by a T lymphocyte clone that responds to mycobacterium tuberculosis and to cartilage proteoglycans. *Proc Natl Acad Sci USA* **82**: 5117–5120.

van Eden W, Thole JER, van der Zee R, Noordzig A, van Embden JDA, Hensen EJ et al. (1988) Cloning of the mycobacterial epitope recognised by thymocytes in adjuvant arthritis. *Nature* **331**: 171–173.

van Laar JM, Miltenburg AM, Verdonk MJ, Daha MR, de Vries RR & Breedveld FC (1991) T cell vaccination in rheumatoid arthritis. *Br J Rheumatol* **30** (**supplement 2**): 28–29.

van Zeben D, Hazes JMW, Zwinderman AH, Cats A, Schreuder GMT, D'Amaro J et al. (1991) Association of HLA-DR4 with a more progressive disease course in patients with rheumatoid arthritis. *Arthritis Rheum* **43**: 822–830.

Venables PJW (1988) Epstein-Barr virus infection and autoimmunity in rheumatoid arthritis. *Ann Rheum Dis* **47**: 265–269.

Venables PJW, Roffe LM, Erhardt CC, Maini RN, Edwards JMB & Porter AD (1981) Titers of antibodies to RANA in rheumatoid arthritis and normal sera. *Arthritis Rheum* **24**: 1459–1469.

Weyand CM, Xie C & Goronzy JJ (1992) Homozygosity for the HLA-DRB1 allele selects for extra-articular manifestations in rheumatoid arthritis. *J Clin Invest* **89**: 2033–2039.

Wilkinson LS, Edwards JCW, Poston RN & Haskard DO (1993) Expression of vascular cell adhesion molecule-1 in normal and inflamed synovium. *Lab Invest* **68**: 82–88.

Williams RO, Feldmann M & Maini RN (1992) Anti-tumour necrosis factor ameliorates joint disease in murine collagen-induced arthritis. *Proc Natl Acad Sci USA* **89**: 9784–9788.

Willkens RF, Hansen JA, Malmgren JA, Nisperos B, Mickelson EM & Watson MA (1982) HLA antigens in Yakima Indians with rheumatoid arthritis. *Arthritis Rheum* **25**: 1435–1439.

Winchester RJ & Gregersen PK (1988) The molecular basis of susceptibility to rheumatoid arthritis: the conformational equivalence hypothesis. *Spring Semin Immunopathol* **10**: 119–139.

Wooley PH, Dutcher J, Widmer MB & Gillis S (1993a) Influence of a recombinant human soluble tumor necrosis factor receptor Fc fusion protein on type II collagen-induced arthritis in mice. *J Immunol* **151**: 6602–6607.

Wooley PH, Whalen JD, Chapman DL, Berger AE, Richard KA, Aspar DG & Staite ND (1993b) The effects of an interleukin-1 receptor antagonist protein on type II collagen-induced arthritis and antigen-induced arthritis in mice. *Arthritis Rheum* **36**: 1305–1314.

Wordsworth BP, Lanchbury JSS, Sakkas LI, Welsh KI, Panayi GS & Bell JI (1989) HLA-DR4 subtype frequencies in rheumatoid arthritis indicate that DRβ1 is the major susceptibility locus within the HLA class II region. *Proc Natl Acad Sci USA* **86**: 10049–10053.

Wordsworth BP, Pile KD, Buckley JD, Lanchbury JSS, Ollier B, Lathrop M et al. (1992) HLA hetero-zygosity contributes to susceptibility to rheumatoid arthritis. *Am J Hum Genet* **51**: 585–591.

Xu WD, Firestein GS, Taetle R, Kaushansky K & Zvaifler NJ (1989) Cytokines in chronic inflammatory arthritis. II. Granulocyte-macrophage colony-stimulating factor in rheumatoid synovial effusions. *J Clin Invest* **83**: 876–882.

Ziff M (1989) Role of endothelium in chronic inflammation. *Spring Semin Immunopathol* **11**: 199–214.

3 Mycoplasmas, Superantigens and Autoimmune Arthritis

Barry C. Cole and Allen Sawitzke

INTRODUCTION

Infectious agents including viruses, bacteria and mycoplasmas have long been considered as prime candidates for the etiology of the human rheumatic autoimmune diseases. Proposed mechanisms of induction of disease have included chronic infection, deposition of immune complexes, and breakdown of self tolerance mediated by modification of host proteins or by molecular mimicry of cartilage or other self components. Recently, new hypotheses for induction of autoimmunity have been forthcoming based upon the interaction of lymphoid cells with superantigens (SAgs), a new class of immunostimulants that are produced by viruses, bacteria and mycoplasmas. We shall begin by summarizing current ideas on the aetiopathogenesis of human rheumatoid arthritis (RA). Then, using the SAg *Mycoplasma arthritidis* mitogen (MAM) as a model, we will show how SAgs can trigger or enhance RA.

AETIOPATHOGENESIS OF RHEUMATOID ARTHRITIS

PATHOGENETIC FEATURES

The major pathological features of RA within the synovium are: infiltration by mononuclear phagocytes, lymphocytes and polymorphonuclear cells; clusters of $CD4^+$ T cells; scattered $CD8^+$ T cells; increased HLA-DR expression; secretion of rheumatoid factor (RF); immune complex formation; complement activation; late T-cell activation markers (VLA-1) with a detectable but smaller representation of early activation factors including IL-2 (Harris, 1993; see also Chapters 2 and 11, this volume). Several theories of pathogenesis are undergoing active investigation in an effort to elucidate the aetiology of this disease. Most are based upon one of three premises: (a) autoreactive T-cell proliferation; (b) an autocrine/paracrine regulatory defect affecting primarily macrophages, dendritic cells and fibroblast-like cells; or (c) an antigen driven T-cell response that is environmentally triggered (Firestein and Zvaifler, 1992).

T-CELL INVOLVEMENT

Evidence for involvement of T cells in the RA disease process includes the detection of T-cell infiltrates within rheumatoid synovium, oligoclonality of the T-cell receptors (TCR) present on synovial T cells (Howell *et al.*, 1991), prolonged remissions in patients with AIDS (Harris, 1993), and the positive response of patients to therapies that are principally directed against T cells (thoracic duct drainage, Cyclosporin-A, total lymph node irradiation (TLI), and antibodies against T-cell surface markers (CD4, CDw52)) (Harris, 1993). Additionally, both the collagen-induced arthritis (CIA) (Trentham, 1993; Trentham and Dynesius-Trentham, Chapter 23, this volume) and adjuvant arthritis (AA) (Taurog *et al.*, 1983; Billingham, Chapter 20, this volume) models of RA are at least partially transferable by passive T-cell transfer. When these observations are combined with the pivotal role played by T cells in the normal immune response, aberrant T-cell behaviour becomes a very appealing theory for explaining many of the pathologic features of RA.

AUTOCRINE/PARACRINE FACTORS

Mononuclear cells (dendritic cells, macrophages, synovial cells) may play an important role in the pathogenesis of RA as based upon the observation of high levels of activation markers including HLA-DR and/or the characteristic morphologic changes of mononuclear cells within the RA synovium (Firestein and Zvaifler, 1992). Cytokine profiles present within the joint as detected by *in situ* hybridization or synovial fluid analysis (Firestein *et al.*, 1988; Miossec *et al.*, 1990) also favour their activation. High levels of IL-1, IL-6, GM-CSF and TGFβ are observed, while lymphocyte products including IL-2, IL-4 and γ-interferon are low. These cytokine patterns suggest a stage of late activation and imply that the T cells could have accumulated in the joint as a consequence of their increased adhesion molecules present rather than as an initiating event (Firestein and Zvaifler, 1992). Further discussion of cytokines is found in Chapters 2, 4, 9, 10, 12, 13 and 26, this volume.

ENVIRONMENTAL TRIGGERS

Infectious agents have been considered capable of triggering the disease process in genetically susceptible individuals as supported by the association of streptococcus with rheumatic fever (Bisno, 1993) and *Borrelia burgdorferi* with Lyme disease (Stere, 1989). Many other infectious agents have been claimed to have qualities that would make them strong candidates for RA disease triggers. Most studied among them are Epstein-Barr virus (Roudier *et al.*, 1988; Deacon *et al.*, 1991), parvovirus (Smith and Ryan, 1988), retrovirus (Krapf *et al.*, 1989; Ranki *et al.*, 1992) and mycoplasma (Cole *et al.*, 1985c; Barile *et al.*, 1991). Proposed mechanisms of tolerance breakdown include simple infection complicated by crossreactive epitopes to host products (mimicry), production of neoantigens (altered-self), and uncovering of sequestered self-antigens (Rose and Mackay, 1992). None of these mechanisms necessarily requires that the infectious trigger remains throughout the disease course, but only that it initiates the process. The role of bacterial and viral factors in the pathogenesis or experimental arthritis is detailed in Chapter 21, this volume.

ARTHRITIS CAUSED BY MYCOPLASMAS

The most common infectious agents of naturally occurring animal arthritides are the mycoplasmas, as reviewed in detail elsewhere (Cole *et al.*, 1985c). Although evidence for the involvement of mycoplasmas in human RA is inconclusive, the characteristics of the animal diseases are remarkably similar to the human disease. Some mycoplasma species produce a triad of symptoms that includes respiratory, genitourinary and joint disease. Many domestic hosts such as cattle, sheep, goats, swine and chickens are susceptible to more than one relatively host-specific mycoplasma species. Perhaps the most convenient experimental model of arthritis is that caused in rats, mice and rabbits by *Mycoplasma arthritidis*. Murine disease begins as live organisms migrate into the joint and establish a local infection possibly by possessing site-specific adhesion molecules (Washburn *et al.*, 1993). At this stage of acute inflammation, organisms can readily be cultured from the joints, but later they become increasingly difficult to recover. The chronic phase of mycoplasmal arthritis exhibits all of the features of the human rheumatoid joint including infiltration of the synovium with lymphocytes, plasma cells and macrophages; formation of lymphoid follicles; neovascularization with villous and synovial lining hypertrophy, pannus formation and destruction of cartilage and bone (Fig. 1). Periods of remission and exacerbation have been observed and disease activity can persist for the life of the animal (Cole *et al.*, 1985c).

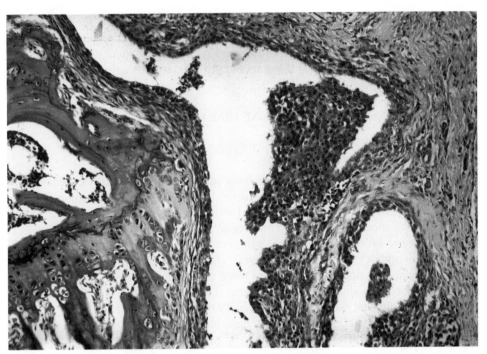

Figure 1. Section of a mouse ankle joint 76 days after i.v. injection of *M. arthritidis*, haematoxylin and eosin ×450. Synovial villus with heavy infiltration by mononuclear cells. Pannus erosion of articular cartilage and bone destruction with dense areas of collagen deposition are also seen. From Cole *et al.* (1971), with permission.

There is clear evidence that host responses are suppressed or bypassed during the early stages of infection with *M. arthritidis* since neutralizing and opsonizing antibodies against the organisms fail to develop and organisms persist in the peripheral circulation. Mimicry has been proposed as one mechanism by which the organisms evade immune recognition (Cahill *et al.*, 1971). The inflammatory response within the joint is believed to be due to activation of both T and B cells as well as to activation of macrophages by the organisms or their products (Cole *et al.*, 1985a). The mechanisms of disease chronicity in *M. arthritidis* infections remain to be established. Deposition of immune complexes in the cartilage or arthritic rabbit joints has been demonstrated although the nature of the complexes is not known (Washburn *et al.*, 1980). Low levels of infection may be sufficient to drive a continued immune response to sequestered antigens (Cole *et al.*, 1985c) or to self antigens as recently proposed by Busche and coworkers (Busche *et al.*, 1990). As we shall discuss later, SAgs may play a key role in the chronicity and flares seen in human disease.

SUMMARY

It remains to be determined which of the above theories for the aetiopathogenesis of RA is correct. However, it is evident that RA is a complex disease process and that control of disease expression is dependent upon multiple factors. When this observation is combined with the known role of MHC class II alleles in RA, the obvious importance of any factor that can alter the interaction of the *class II–TCR–antigen* complex (ternary complex) is readily apparent. SAgs are able to interact with the components of the ternary complex in unique ways that result in activation of T and B cells, thereby potentially uniting these seemingly unrelated theories of disease pathogenesis.

SUPERANTIGENS AND AUTOIMMUNE DISEASE

CHARACTERISTICS OF SUPERANTIGENS

SAgs in the form of soluble toxins have been identified in staphylococci (Choi *et al.*, 1989; Marrack *et al.*, 1990), streptococci (Imanishi *et al.*, 1990), pseudomonas (Legaard *et al.*, 1992) and mycoplasmas (Cole *et al.*, 1989). Cell-associated SAgs have also been found in streptococcal M proteins (Tomai *et al.*, 1991) and *Yersinia enterocolitica* cell walls (Stuart and Woodward, 1992). A group of endogenous SAgs previously referred to as minor lymphocyte stimulating antigens (Mls) are now known to be products of murine retroviral tumor viruses (Acha-Orbea and Palmer, 1991). In addition, SAg activity has also been identified in rabies virus (Lafon *et al.*, 1992) and also in the virus responsible for murine AIDS (Hugin *et al.*, 1991). Indirect evidence that a SAg may play a role in human AIDS has also been presented (Laurence *et al.*, 1992).

What are the characteristic properties of SAgs? Firstly, they are potent T-cell mitogens. A diagrammatic representation of T_H-cell and B-cell activation by MAM-like molecules is shown in Fig. 2. Unlike classic antigens, SAgs directly bind to MHC molecules outside of the antigen groove (Dellabona *et al.*, 1990) and without the need for processing (Cole *et al.*, 1986a) by antigen presenting cells (APC). Furthermore, they are recognized by the β chains of the variable region (Vβ) of the T-cell receptor for antigen (TCR) largely irrespective of other restriction elements such as Vα, Dβ or Jβ (White *et al.*, 1989). As a result, all T cells bearing the Vβ chains with which that SAg interacts will become activated. This is in contrast to the very small numbers of T cells that react to traditional antigens. Each SAg interacts with a characteristic set of Vβ chains, although unrelated SAgs may react with some of the same Vβ chains.

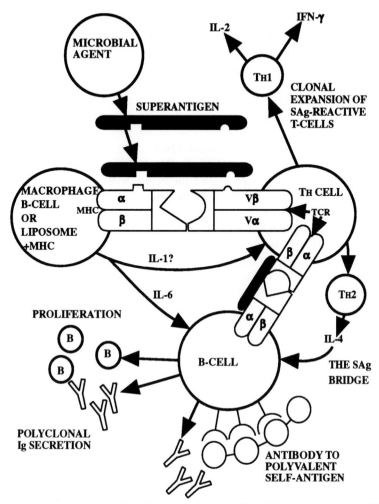

Figure 2. Diagrammatic representation of superantigen-mediated clonal expansion of T cells and polyclonal B-cell activation mediated by the 'superantigen bridge'. From Cole and Atkin (1991) with permission.

A further property of SAgs is their ability to modify the T-cell repertoire *in vivo*. Endogenous mouse retroviral SAgs, when present in mouse strains that possess the appropriate presenting MHC molecule, will result in the deletion of T cells that express the SAg-reactive Vβ chains (Pullen *et al.*, 1988). A similar phenomenon occurs when exogenous bacterial SAg are injected into neonatal or adult mice especially when repeated doses are given (White *et al.*, 1989; McCormack *et al.*, 1993). It has been suggested that this somatic deletion of T cells or 'hole' in the T-cell repertoire could be beneficial to the host by eliminating those T-cell subsets that might ultimately participate in autoimmune disease (Marrack *et al.*, 1993).

A new property of SAgs termed the 'superantigen bridge' has been described for toxic shock syndrome toxin (Mourad *et al.*, 1989) and for MAM (Tumang *et al.*, 1990). In this circumstance, the SAg crosslinks T_H cells via their Vβ TCRs with resting B cells via their MHC molecules, a process which signals B-cell differentiation leading to polyclonal proliferation and immunoglobulin secretion. T-cell help in the form of IL-4 (Cole *et al.*, 1993a) and macrophage production of IL-6 (Homfeld *et al.*, 1990) further contribute to the B-cell activation.

SPECIFIC CHARACTERISTICS OF THE *M. ARTHRITIDIS* SUPERANTIGEN, MAM

The superantigen MAM can be recovered from culture supernatants of *M. arthritidis* (Cole *et al.*, 1981). The molecule which reaches highest titres in senescent cultures is a heat labile, acid-sensitive protein with a molecular weight of 15–30 kDa (Atkin *et al.*, 1986; Kirchner *et al.*, 1986). The high pI value of >9.5 renders the molecule very sticky and it readily adsorbs to glass and plastic as well as to high molecular weight components of mycoplasma culture media and to nucleic acid (Atkin *et al.*, 1986). All strains of *M. arthritidis* examined including both virulent and avirulent strains produce MAM and recent work establishes the molecular weight as 25 000 Da. Computer searches of the gene banks indicate that MAM is phylogenetically unrelated to any other proteins including the staphylococcal, streptococcal and retroviral superantigens (Atkin *et al.*, manuscript in preparation). However, short sequences or motifs were shared between MAM and other SAgs possibly suggesting the location of sites of interaction with lymphocyte molecules (unpublished).

The *M. arthritidis* SAg, MAM, perferentially binds to the conserved murine E_{α} chain of H-2E or to the α chain of the human HLA-DR molecule (Cole and Atkin, 1991). There is also recent evidence that MAM can be weakly presented to T cells by some H-2A molecules (Cole *et al.*, 1993b). Recognition of the MHC/MAM complex is accomplished by a variety of murine Vβ TCRs depending upon the mouse strain used. For example, in Vβ[b] haplotype mice which includes the majority of inbred strains, MAM is recognized by Vβ5.1, 6, 8.1, 8.2 and 8.3 (Cole *et al.*, 1990a; Baccala *et al.*, 1992). In Vβ[a] and Vβ[c], mice that lack various combinations of these Vβ due to genomic and somatic deletions, recognition of T cells bearing Vβ1, 3.1, 7 and 16 can also be demonstrated (Cole *et al.*, 1993b). It is remarkable that the human Vβ TCRs that share the most homology with the above mentioned murine Vβs (Table 1) are all, in fact, activated by MAM (Posnett *et al.*, 1993).

THEORIES OF SUPERANTIGEN TRIGGERING OF AUTOIMMUNE DISEASE

In RA, there is strong evidence to suggest that T cells drive the inflammatory response. Marrack and others (Marrack and Kappler, 1990) have proposed that SAg may cause a clonal expansion of pre-existing self-reactive T cells above the threshold necessary for induction of clinical disease. In a number of experimental models of autoimmune disease, autoreactive T cells clearly play a major role. In experimental allergic encephalomyelitis (EAE), T cells reactive with myelin basic protein appear to control the disease process. Of great interest was the finding that only T cells expressing a limited number of TCRs appeared to be involved (Zamvil *et al.*, 1988). This led to the concept of 'V region disease' as proposed by Heber-Katz and Acha-Orbea (Heber-Katz and Acha-Orbea, 1989) in which T cells bearing specific Vβ TCRs played the dominant role largely irrespective of MHC specificity. Another V region disease is collagen-induced arthritis (CIA) (Courtenay *et al.*, 1980) which is described in detail elsewhere in this volume (Trentham and Dynesius-Trentham, Chapter 23, this volume). In the latter model system, immunization of mice with type II collagen induces a chronic arthritis that is dependent upon a cellular and humoral response to type II collagen. Genetic studies initially suggested that T cells bearing Vβ8 and Vβ6 chain segments were associated with the disease (Banerjee *et al.*, 1988a,b). More recently, Haqqi and coworkers (Haqqi *et al.*, 1992) found additional evidence that T cells bearing Vβ6, 7, 8 and 9 appear to mediate disease, since enrichment of these populations occurs in joints and draining lymph nodes and antibody to Vβ8 decreases the arthritic response (Moder *et al.*, 1993). There is also evidence for involvement of Vβ5.1 in DBA/1 mice since antibody to this TCR can also inhibit arthritis (Chiocchia *et al.*, 1991). Although both collagen-reactive T cells (Holmdahl *et al.*, 1990) and antibody to collagen (Stuart *et al.*, 1984) can independently evoke an arthritic response, both the humoral and cellular arms of the immune response are required for full expression of disease (Seki *et al.*, 1988). The importance of Vβ family expression in the pathogenesis of murine arthritides is discussed in Chapters 19, 21 and 23, this volume.

A second proposed mechanism by which SAgs might induce autoimmunity relates to their ability to initiate B-cell differentiation through a 'superantigen bridge' (Friedman *et al.*, 1991b). The discovery of direct binding of SAgs to MHC molecules on accessory cell surfaces and recognition of this complex by Vβ chain segments of the TCR led to the realization that SAgs might promote an unusual T/B cell collaboration (Tumang *et al.*, 1990) similar to that seen in graft versus host disease (GVHD). In GVHD, donor T_H cells reactive with MHC class II molecules, interact with recipient host B cells inducing polyclonal B-cell activation and an autoimmune response with clinical disease similar to that seen in systemic lupus erythematosus and systemic sclerosis (Gleichmann *et al.*, 1982).

The first indication that SAgs might be capable of stimulating B cells came from the observations of Emery (Emery *et al.*, 1985) who demonstrated that crude preparations of MAM induced peripheral blood lymphocytes from RA patients and from patients with non-inflammatory musculoskeletal disease to secrete higher levels of IgG as compared with lymphocytes cultured alone. Interestingly, they also showed that MAM stimulated the release of IgM RF in lymphocytes from control patients. It was hypothesized that the failure of MAM to increase IgM RF secretion in cells from RA patients might be due to the possibility that MAM-reactive cells were already fully stimulated in these individuals.

In studies to determine whether B-cell activation might proceed via the superantigen bridge, x-irradiated CD4$^+$, MAM-reactive human T cells were tested for helper activity on resting human B cells. It was shown that B cells pulsed with MAM not only activated the MAM-reactive T_H cells, but themselves also underwent differentiation resulting in polyclonal Ig production (Tumang *et al.*, 1990). Similar findings were made by Mourad *et al.* (1989) using the TSST-1 SAg. In subsequent work, it was shown that MAM-reactive BALB/c murine T_H cell lines could also provide help to B cells in the presence of MAM, resulting in both Ig secretion and B-cell proliferation (Tumang *et al.*, 1991; see also Fig. 2). Furthermore, B-cell activation was T_H cell specific since MAM failed to stimulate B cells in the presence of TSST-1 reactive T cells and TSST-1 failed to stimulate B cells in the presence of MAM-reactive T cells

(Tumang *et al.*, 1991). Specific antibody to foreign antigen (sheep red blood cells, SRBC) could also be greatly enhanced when MAM or TSST-1 reactive murine T cells were cultured with SRBC in the presence of MAM or TSST-1. Thus SAgs also have the ability to promote an immune response to T-cell dependent antigens.

IMMUNOREGULATION BY THE MAM SAg *IN VIVO*

A single systemic injection of partially purified MAM (Cole and Wells, 1990) or of bacterial SAg (White *et al.*, 1989) into mice induces a transient toxic effect that is thought to be due to a massive release of cytokines resulting from T-cell activation (Marrack *et al.*, 1990). Animals receiving MAM become lethargic, exhibit ruffled fur, closed eyes and huddle together in the corner of their cage. The mice recover within 2–3 days. The effects of larger or repeated doses of homogeneous MAM remain to be determined.

A marked splenomegaly and lymphadenopathy is seen as early as 24 h, postinjection with MAM. Node lymphocytes expressing Vβ8.1 and Vβ8.2 TCRs are increased in C3H and B10.RIII mice injected with MAM as compared with levels seen in PBS-injected mice (Cole *et al.*, 1993b). Node cells from C57BR mice which lack the Vβ8 family of TCRs exhibit a marked increase in T cells bearing Vβ6. Clonal expansion of specific Vβ TCR bearing T cells has also been noted for other SAgs. However, this expansion is followed by a decrease in the numbers of these T cells possibly due to apoptosis and the surviving cells become anergic to further stimulation (Rellehan *et al.*, 1990; Kawabe and Ochi, 1990; MacDonald *et al.*, 1991). Mice chronically treated with SEB exhibit a total deletion of SEB-reactive Vβ-bearing T cells. In the case of MAM, a single injection also results in a decreased ability of lymphocytes from injected mice to respond to MAM. This decreased response appears to be Vβ specific since responses to SEB are also partially suppressed whereas responses to SEA which utilizes a different set of Vβ TCRs remain largely unaltered (unpublished observations).

Unlike the anergy or deletion seen with the lymphocytes from SEA- or SEB-injected mice, MAM appears to induce a population of T cells with suppressor-like function. Thus, lymphocytes collected from MAM-injected mice can suppress the ability of normal lymphocytes to respond to MAM. Of interest was the finding that the active subset of cells is CD4$^+$ (Cole and Wells, 1990) and that the induced 'suppressor' cells are Vβ specific in their action. Further evidence of altered T-cell function in MAM-injected animals is the finding that treated animals exhibit an inhibition of contact sensitivity to dinitrofluorobenzene and that repeated MAM injections prolong allotypic skin graft survival (Cole *et al.*, 1993a).

B-cell function is also altered in MAM-injected animals. First, there is an increase in responsiveness of lymphocytes to the B-cell mitogen LPS. Second, MAM and SEB result in an increase in antibody-producing cells to SRBC when either SAg is given 2 days postantigenic challenge. Injection of MAM prior to immunization has either no effect or is inhibitory to the immune response to SRBC. Similar observations have been made for other bacterial SAg. Furthermore, splenocytes collected from MAM-injected mice spontaneously secrete higher levels of IgG and IgM than do cells from PBS-injected controls (unpublished observations). All of these findings support the hypothesis that MAM can form a SAg bridge *in vivo* leading to polyclonal B-cell activation and hypergammaglobulinaemia.

How do these changes in T- and B-cell functions relate to cytokine profiles from MAM-injected mice? Consistent with the observed suppression of some T-cell functions, MAM can also suppress the ability of lymphocytes to produce IL-2, a cytokine characteristically produced by T_H1-like cells. A single injection of MAM is sufficient to suppress the IL-2 response by at least 60% through 15 days (Fig. 3). In contrast,

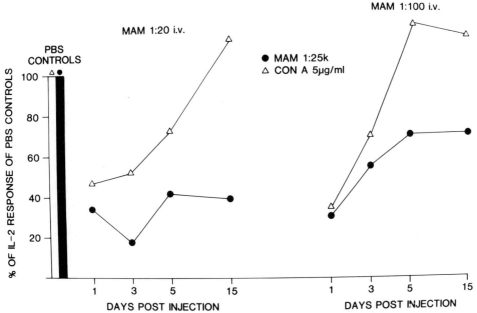

Figure 3. MAM given *in vivo* suppresses lymphocyte production of IL-2. Mice were injected i.v. with 1:20 or 1:100 MAM. After 1–15 days, splenocytes were collected and titred *in vitro* for their ability to produce IL-2 in response to MAM or Con A. IL-2 responses were markedly decreased through 15 days. From Cole *et al.* (1993a), with permission.

MAM can result in a five-fold enhanced ability to produce IL-4, a cytokine produced by T_H2-like cells and which promotes B-cell differentiation (Cole *et al.*, 1993) (Fig. 4). The ability of splenocytes from MAM-injected animals to secrete IL-6, another B-cell differentiation factor produced predominantly by macrophages, was also enhanced by two- to three-fold. It is clear from all of these observations that the i.v. administration of MAM not only expands T cells in a Vβ-restricted manner, but also fundamentally changes immune function from a T_H1-like to a T_H2-like pattern. Mourad and coworkers (1992) have demonstrated similar increases in IL-6 from RA fibroblasts stimulated first with γ-interferon to increase HLA-DR expression and then with the SAg SEA. These cytokine profiles favour development of humoral immunity and could contribute to autoantibody formation (Fig. 2).

EFFECT OF THE SAg MAM ON COLLAGEN-INDUCED ARTHRITIS (CIA)

CIA, a valuable model for RA, is initiated by the immunization of rodents with heterologous type II collagen (Courtenay *et al.*, 1980). Previously, it had been noted

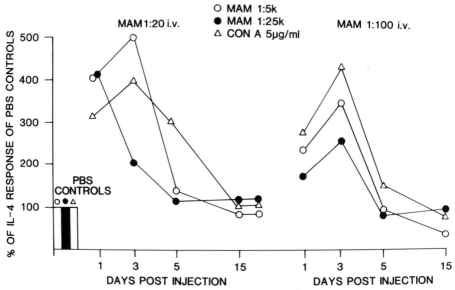

Figure 4. MAM *in vitro* enhances the ability of lymphocytes to produce IL-4. Mice were injected as in Fig. 3. Splenocytes from injected animals exhibited a four- to five-fold increase in their ability to respond to mitogens *in vitro*. From Cole (1993a), with permission.

that there was a marked similarity in the inheritance of susceptibility of rats and mice to CIA and ability of the lymphocytes to respond to the SAg MAM (Cole *et al.*, 1986b). It is now apparent that the major reason for this is in the similarity between Vβ TCR usage by MAM and collagen-reactive T cells. In view of the ability of MAM to expand clonally these same Vβ TCRs *in vivo* and to induce a polyclonal B-cell activation *in vivo*, the next logical step was to determine whether MAM could influence the development of CIA. In the first experiment, male and female ((B10.RIII × RIIIS)F1) × B10.RIII test cross mice, which had received porcine type II collagen 200 days previously and which had largely resolved their arthritis, were challenged in the base of the tail with an emulsion of MAM in Freund's incomplete adjuvant. Male mice developed a small but significant increase in arthritis in comparison with female mice, which are less susceptible to CIA in this cross. No arthritis was seen in mice given adjuvant alone (Cole and Griffiths, 1993).

In similar experiments using mouse strains that also expressed Vβ8, MAM was shown to cause a rapid exacerbation of arthritis when injected i.v. or i.p. into mice whose CIA was in decline (Fig. 5). Mice which lacked Vβ8 but which still expressed Vβ6 and Vβ7 ((C57BR × RIIIS)F1) and which developed a milder form of CIA, also showed a flare in disease when given MAM. Examination of individual mice showed that some animals, which had failed to develop CIA in response to collagen, nevertheless developed arthritis when given MAM 130–180 days later. Systemically administered MAM fails to induce arthritis but when MAM is given intra-articularly to DA rats, a transient arthritis is seen (Cannon *et al.*, 1988). The lesions are characterized by marked hypertrophy of the subsynovium and widespread shedding of the synovial

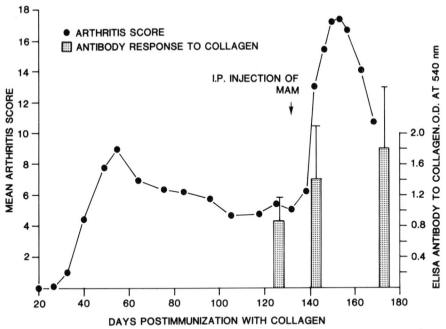

Figure 5. MAM-induced flares of CIA. Mice were immunized with porcine type II collagen at day zero. At 130 days, when the arthritis was past its peak, the animals were injected i.p. with MAM. A rapid increase in disease severity was associated with an enhanced antibody response to collagen. From Cole and Griffiths (1993), with permission.

surface. The lesions heal 14 days postinjection without permanent damage to bone or cartilage. The implication of these observations is that individuals may be sensitized to self antigens without development of overt disease only to develop severe arthritis many months later when exposed to a triggering agent such as a SAg. In another approach, MAM was shown to increase the incidence and severity of CIA, as well as to accelerate the progression of disease when given i.v. to mice suboptimally immunized with collagen (Fig. 6). It thus appears that SAg can trigger, enhance or cause a flare in autoimmune arthritis.

The respective roles of T-cell activation and B-cell differentiation in MAM-induced enhancement of CIA remains to be documented. However, as discussed above, MAM is known to induce a clonal expansion *in vivo* of those Vβ TCR-bearing T cells that contribute to CIA as well as stimulating the B-cell arm of the immune response. Although, in one experiment, MAM-injected mice showed an increase in antibodies to collagen, it remains to be determined whether this response is directly mediated by MAM or indirectly by an increased inflammatory response in the joint. The possibility cannot be excluded that enhanced disease may be due in part to the non-specific effects of lymphokine release from activated T cells and B cells. However, preliminary data indicate that the bacterial SAg, SEA, which uses Vβ TCRs other than those involved in CIA, fails to trigger or enhance CIA in B10.RIII mice as compared with mice injected with PBS. In contrast, SEB which, as for MAM, engages the Vβ8 family of TCRs enhanced disease activity to a similar degree as that seen using MAM.

Another example of SAg-mediated enhancement of experimental arthritis is the

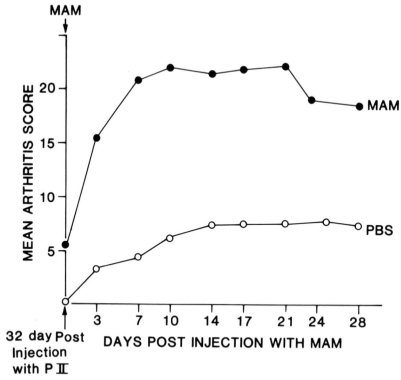

Figure 6. Enhancement of CIA by MAM. Mice in the onset phase of CIA, 32 days postimmunization, were injected i.v. with MAM or PBS. Mice receiving MAM exhibited an accelerated onset of arthritis and of greater severity, as compared with those receiving PBS. From Cole and Griffiths (1993), with permission.

recent work of Schwab *et al.* (1993; see Chapter 22, this volume). These authors demonstrated that the i.v. administration of TSST-1 to rats convalescing from arthritis caused by the injection of streptococcal peptidoglycan polysaccharide, caused an exacerbation of disease activity. T cells are believed to play a major role in this model since antibodies to structural determinants on the α/β TCR inhibit disease (Yoshino *et al.*, 1991) as does treatment with Cyclosporin A (Yocum *et al.*, 1986). Schwab and colleagues demonstrated that a single low dose injection of TSST-1 induced a transient flare in arthritis that resolved within 1 week whereas multiple low dose injections or a single high dose injection resulted in a more chronic sustained disease. The role of specific Vβ chains of the TCR in this model of arthritis has not been established; however, the authors postulated that a superantigenic mechanism of disease enhancement might be responsible since another SAg, *Streptococcal pyogenes* exotoxin-A (SPE-A), was much less effective in this regard.

ROLE OF SAg IN HUMAN RHEUMATIC DISEASES

There is now evidence that SAgs might play a role in several human arthritides including Lyme disease, reactive arthritis and RA. Although *B. burgdorferi*, the agent of Lyme arthritis, is not yet known to possess a SAg, skewing of Vβ TCR expression in humans suffering from this infection has been observed (Lahesmaa *et al.*, 1993). A detailed analysis of T-cell lines reactive with spirochaetal antigens that were isolated from the peripheral circulation of a patient with Lyme arthritis indicated a preferential usage of the Vβ 5.1 TCR, thus suggesting involvement of a Vβ spirochaetal-selective factor. *Yersinia enterocolitica*, one of the intestinal bacteria that play a role in reactive arthritis of humans, may also possess a SAg. Stuart and colleagues (Stuart and Woodward, 1992) showed that culture supernatants and cell extracts of this organism contained a T-cell mitogen, the activity of which was dependent upon AC-bearing class II MHC molecules. Furthermore, T-cell activation was restricted to cells bearing Vβ3, 7, 8.1, 9 and 11 TCRs.

Do MAM-like molecules or other SAgs actively play a role in human arthritis? A number of recent studies suggest that RA might be a 'V region' disease in that there appears to be a skewing of the Vβ TCR repertoire in these patients. Using monoclonal antibody (MAb) or PCR techniques, enrichment of specific Vβ TCR bearing T cells in the synovial fluid, synovium or in the peripheral circulation has been detected. Paliard (1991) detected an increase in the Vβ14 TCR in synovial fluid, but a decrease in the peripheral circulation. Sottini (1991) demonstrated that although there was unrestricted expression of Vβ elements on joint fluid T cells, Vβ expression was limited and two of three patients tested exhibited dominant expression of Vβ7. The absence of Vβ restriction in RA was reported by Brennan and coworkers after using MAbs to Vβ8 and Vβ5 synovial fluid T cells from 10 patients. Eight of the 10 patients examined demonstrated a different pattern of TCR expression in peripheral blood than in their synovial fluid (Brennan *et al.*, 1988). Another single patient, with long-standing RA, was shown, by inverse PCR, to have polyclonal T cells present within the synovium, but also was shown to have a greater than expected representation of Vβ2.1 and Vβ3.1 positive cells (Uematsu *et al.*, 1991). A different approach was taken by Howell (1991) who limited their studies to activated T cells bearing IL-2 receptors isolated from rheumatoid synovial tissue. They found that the majority of patients showed an increase in cells bearing Vβ3, 17 and 14. Friedman (personal communication) also showed a significant increase in Vβ17 both in synovial tissue and in the peripheral circulation of RA patients.

It is noteworthy that most of the Vβ TCR elements that have been found to be enriched on RA synovial lymphocytes are, in fact, those that are used by MAM and those which show the greatest homology with the MAM-reactive murine Vβ TCRs (Table 1). As a result of this, it has been suggested that MAM or MAM-like molecules might play a role in the pathogenesis of human RA (Friedman *et al.*, 1991b; Howell *et al.*, 1991; Cole and Atkin, 1991; Posnett, 1993). Although there have been sporadic reports on the isolation of *Mycoplasma arthritidis* (Jansson *et al.*, 1991) and *M. fermentans* (Williams *et al.*, 1966) from the tissues of human RA patients, these have been unconfirmed by the majority of other investigators (Cole *et al.*, 1985c; Barile *et al.*, 1991). It remains to be determined whether SAgs are produced by any of the species of mycoplasma that normally inhabit humans.

In the human rheumatic diseases there is an association between the occurrence of certain MHC alleles and susceptibility to disease. This association may be exercised at the level of neoantigens, at the time of tolerance breakdown with a resulting recognition of selfreactive antigens or at the time of SAg-mediated triggering of, or enhancement of, disease. Since both antigen and SAg require MHC molecules for

Table 1. Comparison of murine vs. human Vβ usage by MAM. From Cole *et al.* (1993b) with permission

Mouse Vβ TCRs used by MAM	Human equivalents (% homology)[a]	Human Vβ TCRs used by MAM
1[c]	7 (69%)	7[d]
3.1[c]	20[a]/19[b] (70%); 10 (66%)	18[a]/20[bd], 10[d]
5.1[e,c]	1 (67%); 5 (66%)	5[d]
6[f,e,c]	19/17 (73%)	19/17[g,d,e]
7[c]	3 (67%); 15 (68%); 12 (64%)	3[e], 11[e], 12[e]
	14 (65%); 13 (61%); 11 (60%)	13[e], 14[h]
8[f,e,c]	12 (75%); 13 (70%); 3 (66%)	3[e], 11[e], 12[e]
	14 (66%); 15 (64%); 11 (62%)	13[e], 14[h], 15[e]
16[c]	16 (62%); 8 (60%)	8[d]

[a] Nomenclature and homology according to Wilson *et al.* (1988).
[b] Nomenclature according to Toyonaga and Mak (1987).
[c] Cole *et al.* (1993b).
[d] Posnett *et al.* (1993).
[e] Baccala *et al.* (1992).
[f] Cole *et al.* (1990[b])
[g] Friedman *et al.* (1991a)
[h] Marrack (pers. commun.)

recognition, both of these events may be controlled by allelic differences in MHC expression. Each SAg has a hierarchical preference for a specific class II isotype and in some cases for select allotypes (Herman *et al.*, 1990; Scholl *et al.*, 1990). For example, the SEA SAg can activate T cells using any HLA-DR molecule with the exception of HLA-DRw53. This has been explained on the basis of sequence differences within the β chain of HLA-DR and DRw53 as each share a common α chain. Amino acid position 81 seems critical to this recognition as DRB mutants with AA 81 changed to tyrosine lose the ability to present SEA, while DRw53 mutants with AA 81 changed to histidine gain presentation function (Herman *et al.*, 1991).

MAM has been shown to be selective in its response to class II isotypes and engages class II molecules primarily on the basis of their α chains as has been shown for SEB, TSST-1 and Mls-1[a] rather than the α and β chain as was observed for SEA (Dellabona *et al.*, 1990; Herman *et al.*, 1991; Ehrich *et al.*, 1993). H-2Eα and its human homologue HLA-DRα containing class II molecules present much better than H-2Aα when each is paired with identical H-2Eβ proteins (Cole *et al.*, 1990a; Baccala *et al.*, 1992). Recent studies using transgenic mice indicate that the human DQβ molecule (DQB1*0601) when expressed with H-2 Aα is also quite effective in presenting MAM to murine T cells (unpublished observations). Interestingly, this molecule appears to behave like H-2E, since in Eα⁻, B10.M mice that are transgenic for DQB1*0601, T cells bearing Vβ6, 7 and 8.1 are eliminated during thymic ontogeny due to the interaction with the Mls1[a] retroviral SAg (Zhou *et al.*, 1991). However, transgenic cells displaying H-2Eα[f]/DQB1*0601 hybrid molecules differ from H-2Eα[f]/DQB1*0302 molecules in their ability to respond to MAM (unpublished observation) implying that both α and β class II chains contribute to optimal recognition as has previously been demonstrated for TSST-1 (Russell *et al.*, 1991; Braunstein *et al.*, 1992). It remains to be determined whether allelic differences at DRB1 influence presentation by MAM. Such allotypic differences in SAg responsiveness suggest a potential mechanism to account for class II associations with autoimmune disease. For example, an individual with an HLA class II allele containing the 'QKRAAV' (AA 67–75) epitope that is associated with RA (Gregersen *et al.*, 1987), might selectively respond to a specific SAg and thereby develop RA. Amino acids in this region of the β chain have been demonstrated to affect SAg binding (Herman *et al.*, 1991). Thus, SAgs may trigger disease in genetically predisposed individuals, based on class II differences.

If SAgs are involved in the pathogenesis of human RA, an important mechanism of presentation of these SAgs to T cells might be via dendritic cells. Synovial tissues contain relatively large numbers of dendritic cells which are highly effective as APC for SAgs. In fact, dendritic cells which express high levels of MHC molecules are 10–50 times more effective in presenting MAM and other SAgs to T-cell lines (Zvaifler *et al.*, 1985; Bhardwaj *et al.*, 1992). In view of the high avidity of SAgs for dendritic cells, it has been proposed that these cells might be used to isolate SAg-reactive T cells or SAgs bound to dendritic cells isolated from RA tissues (Bhardwaj *et al.*, 1993).

Although SAgs can clearly trigger or exacerbate autoimmune disease where pre-existing anti-self clones are present, there is no evidence as of yet that they can trigger such a response in the normal individual. Viruses, bacteria and mycoplasmas can all cause joint infections with the potential for development of an anti-self response due to acute or chronic infection. Thus, the development of autoimmune disease may be a two step process including separate events; that is, breaking tolerance to self and later, triggering of clinical disease by infection with a SAg-producing organism. In this scenario, since SAgs are very potent, the triggering infection may be subclinical and may be located at a site distant from the target organ.

An alternative hypothesis is that both events may be mediated by the same agent. The mycoplasma model described here is particularly intriguing since *M. arthritidis* can itself cause an acute to chronic arthritic disease of rodents. The role of MAM in this disease is not well defined at present. There is evidence, however, that MAM contributes to the toxicity (Cole *et al.*, 1983) and dermal necrosis (Cole *et al.*, 1985b) seen by administration of live organisms since these symptoms occur only in those mouse strains whose lymphocytes are strongly reactive with MAM. The early immunosuppressive properties of MAM (Cole and Wells, 1990) may well contribute to invasion of the host by *M. arthritidis* and the lack of development of neutralizing or opsonizing antibodies to the organism (Cole *et al.*, 1985c). However, paradoxically, MAM can also act as a B-cell stimulator, which may explain the very early development of non-protective complement-fixing or ELISA antibodies to mycoplasma antigens.

Does MAM exhibit any unique features that would support its potential role in human RA? First, as already described, MAM does activate human T cells bearing Vβ3, 5, 7, 14 and Vβ17. Second, MAM is produced by an organism that itself causes a chronic proliferative arthritis in rodents. Thirdly, there is evidence that MAM may interact in a unique manner with human cells that is distinct from that seen with the staphylococcal SAgs. A number of studies suggest that MAM is far less active in inducing proliferation of human T cells than are the staphylococcal SAg, whereas the staphylococcal toxins are less active than MAM for murine T cells (Cole *et al.*, 1982; Fleischer *et al.*, 1991). This was thought to represent evolutionary adaptations by the SAg secreting organisms to their hosts. A related explanation for the weaker response of human cells is that MAM activates a much smaller percentage of the total population of T cells (Matthes *et al.*, 1988) as compared with that for the staphylococcal SAg

(Fleischer *et al.*, 1991). However, when unseparated human peripheral T cells are reacted with MAM and other SAgs (SEB, SEE and TSST-1) and tested for Ig release, only the MAM-stimulated cultures exhibit marked increases in IgG and IgM. In fact, Ig levels induced by MAM were comparable to those produced by pokeweed mitogen, a B-cell activator (Crow *et al.*, 1992). In view of these results, it was hypothesized that weaker mitogens may favour a shift toward polyclonal B-cell activation and induction of autoimmunity (Crow *et al.*, 1992). Alternative hypotheses are that the MAM-like mitogens may show a greater avidity for MHC molecules than other SAgs or that they might be more effective in transducing activation signals to the B cell.

SUMMARY

SAgs have been hypothesized to play a role in the human autoimmune diseases including RA by clonally expanding anti-self T cells and by triggering polyclonal B cell responses. In this review, we have shown that MAM, a superantigen produced by an organism that causes a chronic proliferative arthritis in rodents, causes *in vivo* expansion of collagen-reactive murine Vβ6 and Vβ8 TCRs and polyclonal activation of B cells. Furthermore, cytokine responses in injected animals shift toward a pattern that would favour the development of a humoral autoimmune response.

Consistent with these properties is the ability of MAM to trigger and accelerate the onset of CIA in mice suboptimally immunized with collagen and to cause rapid flares in arthritis in animals convalescing from a previous episode of CIA. The now proven ability of a SAg to trigger an experimental autoimmune disease and the evidence suggesting that there is a skewing of Vβ chain segments of the TCR in the joints of patients with RA, indicates that the potential role of SAg involvement in the human rheumatic diseases should be actively pursued.

ACKNOWLEDGEMENTS

The authors' work described in this communication was supported by grants from the National Institutes of Health (AI-12103 and AR 02255) and by a grant from the Nora Eccles Treadwell Foundation.

REFERENCES

Acha-Orbea H & Palmer E (1991) M1s-a retrovirus exploits the immune system. *Immunol Today* **12**: 356–361.

Atkin CL, Cole BC, Sullivan GJ, Washburn LR & Wiley BB (1986) Stimulation of mouse lymphocytes by a mitogen derived from *Mycoplasma arthritidis* V. A small basic protein from culture supernatants is a potent T-cell mitogen. *J Immunol* **137**: 1581–1589.

Baccala R, Smith LR, Vestberg M, Peterson PA, Cole BC & Theofilopoulos AN (1992) *Mycoplasma arthritidis* mitogen. V beta engaged in mice, rats, and humans, and requirement of HLA-DR alpha for presentation. *Arthritis Rheum* **35**: 434–442.

Banerjee S, Behlke MA, Dungeon G, Loh DY, Stuart JM, Luthra HS & David CS (1988a) Vβ6 gene of T cell receptor may be involved in type II collagen induced arthritis in mice (abstract). *FASEB J* **2**: A661.

Banerjee S, Haqqi TM, Luthra HS, Stuart JM & David CS (1988b) Possible role of Vβ T cell receptor genes in susceptibility to collagen-induced arthritis in mice. *J Exp Med* **167**: 832–839.

Barile MF, Yoshida H & Roth H (1991) Rheumatoid arthritis: new findings on the failure to isolate or detect mycoplasmas by multiple cultivation or serologic procedures and a review of the literature. *Rev Infect Dis* **13**: 571–582.

Bhardwaj N, Friedman SM, Cole BC & Nisanian AJ (1992) Dendritic cells are potent antigen-presenting cells for microbial superantigens. *J Exp Med* **175**, 267–273.

Bhardwaj N, Hodtsev AS, Nisanian A, Kabak S, Friedman SM, Cole BC et al. (1993) Superantigen reactive T cells are efficiently selected from human blood by dendritic cells. *submitted*

Bisno AL (1993) Rheumatic fever. In Kelley WN, Harris ED, Ruddy S & Sledge CB (eds) *Textbook of Rheumatology*, pp 1209–1220. Philadelphia: WB Saunders.

Braunstein NS, Weber DA, Wang X.-C, Long EO & Karp D (1992) Sequences in Both Class II Major Histocompatibility Complex α and β Chains Contribute to the Binding of the Superantigen Toxic Shock Syndrome Toxin 1. *J Exp Med* **175**: 1301–1305.

Brennan FM, Allard S, Londei M, Savill C, Bolyston A, Carrel S, Maini RN et al. (1988) Heterogeneity of T cell receptor idiotypes in rheumatoid arthritis. *Clin Exp Immunol* **73**: 417–423.

Busche K, Schlesier M, Runge M, Binder A & Kirchhoff H (1990) T cell lines responding to *Mycoplasma arthritidis* and chondrocytes in the *Mycoplasma arthritidis* infection of rats. *Immunobiology* **181**, 398–405.

Cahill JF, Cole BC, Wiley DB & Ward JR (1971) Role of biological mimicry in the pathogenesis induced by *Mycolasma arthritidis*. *Infect Immun* **3**: 24–25.

Cannon GW, Cole BC, Ward JC, Smith JL & Eichwald EJ (1988) Arthritogenic effects of *Mycoplasma arthritidis* T-cell mitogen in rats. *J Rheumatol* **14**: 735–741.

Chiocchia G, Boissier MC & Fournier C (1991) Therapy against murine collagen-induced arthritis with T cell receptor Vβ-specific antibodies. *Eur J Immunol* **21**: 2899–2905.

Choi Y, Kotzin B, Herron L, Callahan J & Marrack P (1989) Interaction of *Staphylococcus aureus* toxin 'superantigens' with human T cells. *Proc Nat Acad Sci USA* **86**: 8941–8945.

Cole BC & Atkin CL (1991) The *Mycoplasma arthritidis* T-cell mitogen, MAM: a model superantigen. *Immunol Today* **12**: 271–276.

Cole BC & Griffiths MM (1993) The mycoplasma superantigen, MAM, triggers and exacerbates auto-immune arthritis. *Arthritis Rheum*, in press.

Cole BC & Wells DJ (1990) Immunosuppressive properties of the *Mycoplasma arthritidis* T-cell mitogen *in vivo*: inhibition of proliferative responses to T-cell mitogens. *Infect Immun* **58**: 228–236.

Cole BC, Ward JR, Jones RS & Cahill JF (1971) Chronic proliferative arthritis of mice induced by *Mycoplasma arthritidis* I. Induction of disease and histopathological characteristics. *Infect Immun* **4**: 344–355.

Cole BC, Daynes RA & Ward JR (1981) Stimulation of mouse lymphocytes by a mitogen derived from *Mycoplasma arthritidis*. I. Transformation is associated with an H-2-linked gene that maps to the I-E/I-C subregion. *J Immunol* **127**: 1931–1936.

Cole BC, Washburn LR, Sullivan GJ & Ward JR (1982) Specificity of a mycoplasma mitogen for lympho-cytes from human and various animal hosts. *Infect Immun* **36**: 662–666.

Cole BC, Thorpe RN, Hassell LA & Ward JR (1983) Toxicity but not arthritogenicity of *Mycoplasma arthritidis* for mice associates with the haplotype expressed at the major histocompatibility complex. *Infect Immun* **41**: 1010–1015.

Cole BC, Naot Y, Stanbridge ES & Wise KS (ed) (1985a). *Interactions of Mycoplasmas and their Products with Lymphoid Cells in vitro. The Mycoplasmas.* London: Academic Press.

Cole BC, Piepkorn MW & Wright EC (1985b) Influence of genes of the major histocompatibility complex of ulcerative dermal necrosis induced in mice by *Mycoplasma arthritidis*. *J Invest Dermatol* **85**: 357–361.

Cole BC, Washburn LR & Taylor-Robinson D (eds) (1985c) *Mycoplasma Induced Arthritis. The Myco-plasmas.* New York: Academic Press.

Cole BC, Araneo BA & Sullivan GJ (1986a) Stimulation of mouse lymphocytes by a mitogen derived from *Mycoplasma arthritidis*. IV. Murine T hybridoma cells exhibit differential accessory cell requirements for activation by *M. arthritidis* T cell mitogen, Concanavalin A, or Hen Egg-white Lysozyme. *J Immunol* **136**: 3572–3578.

Cole BC, Griffiths MM, Sullivan GJ & Ward JR (1986b) Role of RT1 genes in the response of rat lymphocytes to *Mycoplasma arthritidis* T cell mitogen, concanavalin A, and phytohemagglutin. *J Immunol* **136**: 2364–2369.

Cole BC, Kartchner DR & Wells DJ (1989) Stimulation of mouse lymphocytes by a product derived from *Mycoplasma arthritidis*. VII. Responsiveness is associated with expression of a product(s) of the Vβ8 family present on the T cell receptor α/β for antigen. *J Immunol* **142**: 4131–4137.

Cole BC, David CS, Lynch DH & Kartchner DR (1990a) The use of transfected fibroblasts and transgenic mice establishes that stimulation of T cells by the *Mycoplasma arthritidis* mitogen is mediated by E alpha. *J Immunol* **144**: 420–424.

Cole BC, Kartchner DR & Wells DJ (1990b) Stimulation of mouse lymphocytes by a mitogen derived from *Mycoplasma arthritidis* (MAM). VIII. Selective activation of T cells expressing distinct Vβ T cell recep-tors (TCR) from various strains of mice by the 'superantigen' MAM. *J Immunol* **144**: 425–431.

Cole BC, Ahmed EA, Araneo BA, Shelby J, Kamerath C, Wei S, McCall S et al. (1993a) Immunomodu-lation *in vivo* by the *Mycoplasma arthritidis* superantigen, MAM. *Clin Inf Dis* **17**, 5163–5169.

Cole BC, Balderas RA, Ahmed EA, Kono D & Theofilopoulos AN (1993b) Genomic composition and allelic polymorphisms influence Vβ usage by the *Mycoplasma arthritidis* superantigen. *J Immunol* **150**: 3291–3299.

Courtenay JS, Dallman MJ, Dayan AD, Martin A & Mosedale B (1980) Immunization against heterologous type II collagen induces arthritis in mice. *Nature* **283**: 666–668.

Crow MK, Zagon G, Chu Z, Ravina B, Tumang JR, Cole B et al. (1992) Human B cell differentiation induced by microbial superantigens: unselected peripheral blood lymphocytes secrete polyclonal immunoglobulin in response to *Mycoplasma arthritidis* mitogen. *Autoimmunity* **14**: 23–32.

Deacon EM, Mathews JB, Potts AJC, Hamburger J, Bevan IS & Young LS (1991) Detection of Epstein-Barr virus antigens and DNA in major and minor salivary glands using immunocytochemistry and polymerase chain reaction: possible relationship with Sjogren's syndrome. *J Pathol* **163**: 351–360.

Dellabona P, Peccoud J, Kappler J, Parrack P, Benoist C & Mathis D (1990) Superantigens interact with MHC class II molecules outside of the antigen groove. *Cell* **62**: 1115–1121.

Ehrich EW, Devaux B, Rock EP, Jorgensen JL, Davis MM & Chien Y-h (1993) T cell receptor interaction with peptide/major histocompatibility complex (MHC) and superantigen/MHC ligands is dominated by antigen. *J Exp Med* **178**: 713–722.

Emery P, Panyi GS, Welsh KI & Cole BC (1985) Rheumatoid factor and HLA-DR4 in RA. *J Rheumatol* **12**: 217–222.

Firestein GS & Zvaifler NJ (eds) (1992) *Autoimmune Arthropathy: Rheumatoid Synovitis. The Autoimmune Diseases II.* San Diego: Academic Press.

Firestein GS, Xu WD, Townsend K, Broide D, Alvaro-Gracia J, Glasebrook A et al. (1988) Cytokines in chronic inflammatory arthritis. I. Failure to detect T cell lymphokines (interleukin 2 and interleukin 3) and the presence of macrophage colony-stimulating factor (CSF-1) and a novel mast cell growth factor in rheumatoid synovitis. *J Exp Med* **168**: 1573–1586.

Fleischer B, Gerardy-Schahn R, Metzroth B, Carrel CS, Gerlach D & Kohler W (1991) An evolutionary conserved mechanism of T cell activation by microbial toxins: evidence for different affinities of T cell receptor toxin interaction. *J Immunol* **146**: 11–17.

Friedman SM, Crow MK, Tumang JR, Tumang M, Xu YQ, Hodtsev AS et al. (1991a) Characterization of human T cells reactive with the *Mycoplasma arthritidis*-derived superantigen (MAM): generation of a monoclonal antibody against V beta 17, the T cell receptor gene product expressed by a large fraction of MAM-reactive human T cells. *J Exp Med* **174**: 891–900.

Friedman SM, Posnett DN, Tumang JR, Cole BC & Crow MK (1991b) A potential role for microbial superantigens in the pathogenesis of systemic autoimmune disease. *Arthritis Rheum* **34**, 468–480.

Gleichmann E, van Elven EH & Van der Veen JPW (1982) A systemic erythematosus (SLE)-like disease in mice induced by abnormal T-B cooperation. Preferential formation of autoantibodies characteristic of SLE. *Eur J Immunol* **12**: 152–159.

Gregersen PK, Silver J & Winchester RJ (1987) The Shared Epitope Hypothesis: An approach to understanding the molecular genetics of susceptibility to rheumatoid arthritis. *Arthritis Rheum* **30**, 1205–1213.

Haqqi TM, Anderson GD, Banerjee S & David CS (1992) Restricted heterogeneity in T-cell antigen receptor Vβ gene useage in the lymph nodes and arthritic joints of mice. *Proc Nat Acad Sci USA* **89**: 1253–1255.

Harris ED (1993) Etiology and pathogenesis of rheumatoid arthritis. In Kelley WN, Harris ED, Ruddy S & Sledge CB (eds) *Textbook of Rheumatology*, pp 833–874. Philadelphia: WB Saunders.

Heber-Katz E & Acha-Orbea H (1989) The V region disease hypothesis: evidence from autoimmune encephalomyelitis. *Immunol Today* **10**: 164–169.

Herman A, Croteau G, Sekaly RP, Kappler J & Marrack P (1990) HLA-DR alleles differ in their ability to present staphylococcal enterotoxins to T cells. *J Exp Med* **172**: 709–717.

Herman A, Labrecque N, Thibodeau J, Marrack P, Kappler JW & Sekaly RP (1991) Identification of the staphylococcal enterotoxin A superantigen binding site in the beta 1 domain of the human histocompatibility antigen HLA-DR. *Proc Nat Acad Sci USA* **88**: 9954–9958.

Holmdahl R, Andersson M, Goldschmidt TJ, Gustafson K, Jannson L & Mo JA (1990) Type II collagen autoimmunity in animals and provocations leading to arthritis. *Immunol Rev* **118**, 193–232.

Homfeld J, Homfeld A, Nicklas W & Rink L (1990) Induction of interleukin 6 in murine bone-marrow derived macrophages stimulated by *Mycoplasma arthritidis* mitogen MAS. *Autoimmunity* **7**, 317–327.

Howell MD, Diveley JP, Lundeen KA, Esty A, Winters ST, Carlo DJ & Brostoff SW (1991) Limited T-cell receptor β-chain heterogeneity among interleukin 2 receptor-positive synovial T cells suggests a role for superantigen in rheumatoid arthritis. *Proc Nat Acad Sci USA* **88**: 10921–10925.

Hugin AW, Vacchio MS & Morse HC (1991) A virus-encoded 'superantigen' in a retrovirus induced immunodeficiency syndrome of mice. *Science* **252**, 424–427.

Imanishi K, Igarashi H & Uchiyama T (1990) Activation of murine T cells by streptococcal pyrogenic exotoxin A. Requirement for MHC class II molecules on accessory cells and identification of Vβ elements in T cell receptor of toxin reactive T cells. *J Immunol* **14**: 3170–3175.

Jansson E, Makisara P, Vainio K & Vainio K (1971) An 8-year study on mycoplasma in rheumatoid arthritis. *Ann Rheum Dis* **30**, 506–508.

Kawabe Y & Ochi A (1990) Selective anergy of Vβ8+, CD4+ T cells in staphylococcus enterotoxin B-primed mice. *J Exp Med* 1065–1070.

Kirchner H, Brehm G, Nicklas F, Beck R & Herbst F (1986) *Scand J Immunol* **137**: 1581–1589.

Krapf FE, Herrmann M, Leitmann W & Kalden JR (1989) Are retroviruses involved in the pathogenesis of SLE? Evidence demonstrated by molecular analysis of nucleic acids from SLE patients' plasma. *Rheumatol Int* **9**: 115–121.

Lafon M, Lafage M, Martinez-Arends A, Ramirez R. Vuillier F, Charron D et al. (1992) Evidence for a viral superantigen in humans. *Nature* **358**, 507–510.

Lahesmaa R, Shanafelt MC, Allsup A, Soderberg C, Anzola J, Freitas V et al. (1993) Preferential usage of T-cell antigen receptor V region gene segment Vβ5.1 by *Borrelia burgdorferi* antigen-reactive T-cell clones isolated from a patient with Lyme disease. *J Immunol* **150**, 4125–4135.

Laurence J, Hodtsev AS & Posnett DN (1992) Superantigen implicated in dependence of HIV-1 replication in T cells on TCR Vβ expression. *Nature* **358**, 255–259.

Legaard PK, LeGrand RD & Misfeldt ML (1992) Lymphoproliferative activity of *Pseudomonas* exotoxin A is dependent on intracellular processing and is associated with the carboxyl-terminal portion. *Infect Immun* **60**, 1273–1278.

MacDonald HR, Baschieri S & Lees RK (1991) Clonal expansion precedes anergy and death of Vβ8+ peripheral T-cells responding to staphylococcal enterotoxin B *in vivo*. *Eur J Immunol* **21**: 1963–1966.

Marrack P & Kappler J (1990) The staphylococcal enterotoxins and their relatives. *Science* **248**, 705–711.

Marrack PC, Blackman M, Kushnir E & Kappler J (1990) The toxicity of staphylococcal enterotoxin B in mice is mediated by T cells. *J Exp Med* **171**: 455–464.

Marrack P, Winslow GM, Choi Y, Scherer M, Pullen A, White J et al. (1993) The bacterial and mouse mammary tumor virus superantigens; two different families of proteins with the same functions. *Immunol Rev* **131**, 79.

Matthes N, Schrezenmeir H, Homfeld J, Fleischer S, Malissen B & Fleischer B (1988) Clonal analysis of human cells activation by the *Mycoplasma arthritidis* mitogen (MAS). *Eur J Immunol* **18**: 1733–1737.

McCormack JE, Callahan JE, Kappler J & Marrack PC (1993) Profound deletion of mature T-cells *in vivo* by chronic exposure to exogenous superantigen. *J Immunol* **150**: 3785–3792.

Miossec P, Naviliat M, Dupuy A, D'Angeac A, Sany J & Banchereau J (1990) Low levels of interleukin-4 and high levels of transforming growth factor beta in rheumatoid arthritis. *Arthritis Rheum* **33**, 1180–1187.

Moder KG, Luthra HS, Griffiths MM & David CS (1993) Prevention of collagen-induced arthritis in mice by deletion of T cell receptor Vβ8 bearing T cells with monoclonal antibodies. *Br J Rheumatol* **32**: 26–30.

Mourad W, Scholl P, Diaz A, Geha R & Chatila T (1989) The staphylococcal toxic shock syndrome toxin 1 triggers B cell proliferation and differentiation via major histocompatibility complex – unrestricted cognate T/B cell interaction. *J Exp Med* **170**: 2011–2022.

Mourad W, Mehindate K, Schall TJ & McColl SR (1992) Engagement of major histocompatibility complex class II molecules by superantigen induces inflammatory cytokine gene expression in human rheumatoid fibroblast-like synoviocytes. *J Exp Med* **175**, 613–616.

Paliard X, West S, Lafferty JA, Clements JR, Kappler JW, Marrack P et al. (1991) Evidence for the effects of a superantigen in rheumatoid arthritis. *Science* **253**, 325–329.

Posnett DN (1993) Do superantigens play a role in autoimmunity? *Semin Immunol* **5**: 65–72.

Posnett DN, Hodtsev AS, Kabak S, Friedman SM, Cole BC & Bhardwaj N (1993) Interaction of the *Mycoplasma arthritidis* superantigen (MAM) with human T-cells. *Clin Infect Dis* **17** (**supplement**): S170–175.

Pullen AMP, Marrack P & Kappler W (1988) The T-cell repertoire is heavily influenced by tolerance to polymorphic self antigens. *Nature* **335**: 796–801.

Ranki A, Kurki P, Riepponen S & Stephansson E (1992) Antibodies to retroviral proteins in autoimmune connective tissue disease: relation to clinical manifestations and ribonucleoprotein autoantibodies. *Arthritis Rheum* **35**: 1483–1491.

Rellehan BL, Jones LA, Kruisbeek AM, Fry AM & Matis LA (1990) *In vivo* induction of anergy in peripheral Vβ8+ T-cells by staphylococcal enterotoxin B. *J Exp Med* **172**: 1091.

Rose NR & Mackay IR (1992) The immune response in autoimmunity and autoimmune disease. In Rose NR & Mackay IR (eds) *The Autoimmune Diseases II*, pp 1–23. San Diego: Academic Press.

Roudier J, Rhodes G, Peterson J, Vaughan JH & Carson DA (1988) The Epstein-Barr virus glycoprotein gp110, a molecular link between HLA DR4, HLA DR1, and rheumatoid arthritis. *Scan J Immunol* **27**: 367–371.

Russell JK, Pontzer CH & Johnson HM (1991) Both α-helices along the major histocompatibility complex binding cleft are required for staphylococcal enterotoxin A function. *Proc Natl Acad Sci USA* **88**: 7228–7232.

Scholl PR, Diez A, Karr R, Sekaly RP, Trowsdale J & Geha RS (1990) Effect of isotypes and allelic polymorphism on the binding of staphylococcal exotoxins to MHC class II molecules. *J Immunol* **144**: 226–230.

Schwab JH, Brown RR, Anderle SK & Schlievert PM (1993) Superantigen can reactivate bacterial cell wall-induced arthritis. *J Immunol* **150**: 4151–4159.

Seki N, Sudo Y, Yoshioka T, Sugihara S, Fujitsu T, Sakuma, S et al. (1988) Type II collagen-induced murine arthritis. I. Induction and perpetuation of arthritis require synergy between humoral and cell-mediated immunity. *J Immunol* **140**, 1477–1484.

Smith MA & Ryan ME (1988) Parvovirus infections. *Postgraduate Med* **84**, 127–134.

Sottini A, Imberti L, Gorla R, Cattaneo R & Primi D (1991) 'Restricted expression of T cell receptor Vβ but Vα genes in rheumatoid arthritis. *Eur J Immunol* **21**, 461–466.

Stere AC (1989) Lyme disease. *NEJM* **321**, 586–596.

Stuart JM, Townes AS & Kang AH (1984) Collagen autoimmune arthritis. *Ann Rev Immunol* **2**: 199–218.

Stuart PM & Woodward JG (1992) *Yersinia enterocolitica* produces superantigenic activity. *J Immunol* **148**, 225–233.

Taurog JD, Sandberg GP & Mahowald ML (1983) The cellular basis of adjuvant arthritis. II. Characterization of cells mediating passive transfer. *Cellular Immunol* **80**: 148–204.

Tomai MA, Alion JA, Dockter ME, Majumdar G, Spinella DG & Kotbe M (1991) T-cell receptor V gene usage by human T cells stimulated with the superantigen streptococcal M protein. *J Exp Med* **174**, 285–288.

Trentham D & Dynesius-Trentham R (1995) Collagen-induced Arthritis. In *Mechanisms and Models in Rheumatoid Arthritis*. London: Academic Press.

Tumang JR, Cherniack EP, Gietl DM, Cole BC, Russo C, Crow MK & Friedman SM (1991) T helper cell-dependent, microbial superantigen-induced murine B cell activation: polyclonal and antigen-specific antibody responses. *J Immunol* **147**, 432–438.

Tumang JR, Posnett DN, Cole BC, Crow MK & Friedman SM (1990) Helper T cell-dependent human B cell differentiation mediated by a mycoplasmal superantigen bridge. *J Exp Med* **171**, 2153–2158.

Uematsu Y, Wege H, Straus A, Ott M, Bannwarth W, Lanchbury J et al. (1991) The T-cell receptor repertoire in the synovial fluid of a patient with rheumatoid arthritis is polyclonal. *Proc Natl Acad Sci USA* **88**, 8534–8538.

Washburn LR, Cole BC & Ward JR (1980) Chronic arthritis in rabbits induced by mycoplasmas. II. Antibody response and the deposition of immune complexes. *Arthritis Rheum* **23**, 837–845.

Washburn LR, Hirsch S & Voelker LL (1993) Mechanisms of attachment of *Mycoplasma arthritidis* to host cells *in vitro*. *Infect Immun* **61**, 2670–2680.

White J, Herman A, Pullen AM, Kabo R, Kappler JW & Marrack P (1989) The Vβ-specific superantigen staphylococcal enterotoxin B: stimulation of immature T cells and clonal deletion in neonatal mice. *Cell* **56**, 27–35.

Williams MH, Brostoff J & Roitt JM (1966) Possible role of *M. fermentans* in the pathogenesis of rheumatoid arthritis. *Lancet* **2**, 277–280.

Wilson RK, Lai E, Concannon P, Barth RK & Hood LE (1988) Structure, organization and polymorphism of murine and human T-cell receptor α and β chain gene families. *Immunol Rev* **101**, 149.

Yocum DE, Allen JB, Wahl SM, Calandra GB & Wilder RC (1986) Inhibition by Cyclosporin A of streptococcal cell induced arthritis and hepatic granulomas in rats.' *Arthritis Rheum* **29**, 262.

Yoshino S, Cleland L, Mayrhofer G and Brown RR (1991) Prevention of chronic erosive streptococcal cell wall-induced arthritis in rats by treatment with monoclonal antibody against the T cell antigen receptor αβ. *J Immunol* **146**, 4187.

Zamvil SS, Michell DJ, Lee NE, Moore AC, Walker MK, Sakai K et al. (1988) Predominant expression of a T-cell receptor Vβ gene family in autoimmune encephalomyelitis.' *J Exp Med* **167**: 1586–1596.

Zhou P, Anderson GD, Savarirayan S, Inoko H & David CS (1991) Human HLA-DQ beta chain presents minor lymphocyte stimulating locus gene products and clonally deletes TCR V beta 6+, V beta 8.1+ T cells in single transgenic mice. *Hum Immunol* **31**, 47–56.

Zvaifler NJ, Steinman RM, Kaplan G, Lau LL & Rivelis M (1985) Identification of immunostimulatory dendritic cells in the synovial effusions of patients with rheumatic arthritis. *J Clin Invest* **76**, 789–800.

4 Therapy for Rheumatoid Arthritis

G.S. Panayi

INTRODUCTION

Rheumatoid arthritis (RA) is one of the commonest chronic inflammatory diseases of the developed world. As such, it is an important paradigm for the design and evaluation of anti-inflammatory therapies. The ease of access of the synovial membrane (SM) is an additional bonus, as the consequences of therapy can be monitored by sequential biopsies; these can be examined by cell biological (Haworth *et al.*, 1991), immunohistological (Corkill *et al.*, 1991) and molecular methods (Firestein *et al.*, 1990) for changes in cellular composition or expression of cytokines and other molecules thought to be of importance in the inflammatory process.

RA is not only a chronic and disabling disease accompanied by considerable morbidity but it is also associated with a significantly elevated mortality rate comparable to that of triple vessel coronary disease (Pincus and Callahan, 1986). The presently available so-called 'disease-modifying anti-rheumatic drugs' (DMARDs) are rather unsatisfactory, being poorly effective and having considerable and, sometimes, severe and life-threatening side effects (Pincus *et al.*, 1992). Thus, the search for more effective and safer therapies is an urgent task to which considerable effort is being devoted. The search has been aided by the considerable increase in our knowledge of the pathogenesis of RA and our understanding of basic immunology made possible by the developments in cell biology and molecular biology.

PATHOGENESIS OF RHEUMATOID ARTHRITIS

THE T-CELL HYPOTHESIS

RA is believed to be due to a persistent cell-mediated immune response to an as yet undefined antigen(s) which may be endogenous or exogenous (Panayi *et al.*, 1992). Immunohistological examination of the SM shows it to have all the hallmarks of a T-cell driven lesion: an accumulation of predominantly CD4 T cells belonging to the memory phenotype (CD45RO positive) (Pitzalis *et al.*, 1987), activated macrophages (Firestein and Zvaifler, 1987) and synoviocytes or specialized synovial fibroblasts (Haynes *et al.*, 1988). The stimulatory interactions between these cell types lead to the release of a number of inflammatory cytokines and pharmacological mediators.

The association of RA with HLA-DR4 or HLA-DR1 (Lanchbury *et al.*, 1992) reinforces the concept that the disease is due to the activation of T cells. The only known function of HLA-DR molecules is to present processed antigenic peptides to the T-cell receptor (TCR) leading to T-cell activation. The processing and presentation is done by antigen-presenting cells such as specialized dendritic cells, activated

Mechanisms and Models in Rheumatoid Arthritis   Copyright © 1995 Academic Press Ltd
ISBN 0–12–340440–1

B cells and macrophages. All these types of antigen-presenting cells are found within the rheumatoid synovial membrane. Additional evidence for the central role of T cells in RA is provided by the improvement in disease following manipulations which interfere with T-cell function including thoracic duct drainage (Paulus *et al.*, 1977), total lymphoid irradiation (Panayi and Amlot, 1982), lymphacytophoresis (Emery *et al.*, 1986) and cyclosporin A (Panayi and Tugwell, 1993). The T-cell hypothesis in RA has been recently reviewed by us (Panayi *et al.*, 1992). Thus, each component of the trimolecular complex of HLA-DR, antigenic peptide and TCR now forms the target of many immunotherapeutic research programmes.

CELLULAR ACTIVATION IN THE RHEUMATOID SYNOVIUM

The main cells involved in the pathogenesis of RA are T cells, macrophages, synovio-cytes and endothelial cells. All these cells are activated as shown by a number of functional and phenotypic characteristics.

T-cell Activation

T cells are activated as shown by the fact that they are HLA-DR positive, are at G1 of the cell cycle, possess more integrin receptors, such as VLA-4 and 5, on their surface and secrete interleukin-6 (IL-6) (Panayi, 1992). These properties suggest that they are recently activated memory (CD45RO positive) T cells with enhanced adhesive abilities for endothelial cells and increased migratory capacity into tissues; this contention is supported by *in vitro* and *in vivo* experiments (Pitzalis *et al.*, 1988; Pitzalis *et al.*, 1991). Once in the tissues, these cells are retained there because their activated state allows them to adhere firmly to fibrillar components of the connective tissue such as collagen, fibronectin (Rodriguez *et al.*, 1992) and laminin, as well as other cells present within the SM, such as macrophages and synoviocytes, through the process known as heterotypic adhesion. Homotypic adhesion of T cells to T cells is an additional means by which they are retained within the SM (Pitzalis *et al.*, 1988). Lymphocyte adhesion is covered more extensively in Chapter 11, this volume.

Thus, the T cells found within the SM are pre-activated and enter the joint because of their increased adhesive and migratory capabilities. The frequency of T cells specific for RA is probably very low; from what is known of lesions driven by known antigens this will be of the order of 1:500 to 1:3000 (Panayi *et al.*, 1992) but without knowing the 'rheumatoid antigen' it is impossible to determine their frequency. However, their rarity probably explains the failure to detect a consistent oligoclonal population of T cells within the RA SM even with extremely sensitive molecular biological techniques (Marguerie *et al.*, 1992). Furthermore, their scarcity explains the difficulty which has been encountered in detecting the classical T-cell lymphokines, interleukin 2 (IL-2) and interferon γ within the rheumatoid joint (Firestein *et al.*, 1988).

The Mesenchymal Reaction

The mesenchymal reaction is a term applied to the increased numbers of mesenchy-mal cells found within the rheumatoid SM, namely macrophages (Koch *et al.*, 1988; Highton *et al.*, 1989; MacNaul *et al.*, 1990; Koch *et al.*, 1991, 1992), synoviocytes (the specialized fibroblasts) (Haynes *et al.*, 1988; Shiozawa *et al.*, 1989; Case *et al.*, 1989; Lafyatis *et al.*, 1989; Tan *et al.*, 1990; Okada *et al.*, 1990; Sano *et al.*, 1990; MacNaul *et al.*, 1990; Remmers *et al.*, 1991; Unemori *et al.*, 1992; Morales-Ducret *et al.*, 1992; Villiger *et al.*, 1992) and endothelial cells. Indeed, the increased thickness of the synovial lining layer, due to the increased numbers of macrophages and synoviocytes, and the increased numbers of blood vessels are the only established immunohistological criteria which differentiate between RA and osteoarthritis (Farahat *et al.*, 1992). The cells involved in the mesenchymal reaction are activated as demonstrated by several criteria. The one which is of particular relevance from the point of view of the present discussion is the ability of synoviocytes to maintain their activated phenotype after prolonged culture *in vitro*. This raises the important question as to whether rheumatoid synovitis can be initiated by immunological means in an HLA-DR4/1 restricted manner but be subsequently maintained by non-immunological means through the mesenchymal reaction.

One way of answering this question has been by the creation of transgenic mice. Three models are of interest. The first is the TNFα mouse (Keffer *et al.*, 1991) in which there is constitutive hyperproduction of this cytokine in the tissues of the animal including the joint with the development of an erosive arthritis. The second is the mouse transgenic for the *tax* gene of the HTLV-1 virus (Iwakura *et al.*, 1991) which activates the transcription and translation of several cytokine genes and also leads to the development of erosive arthritis. There is a chronic inflammatory cell exudate, including T cells, in the synovium of both these models. Hence, the chronicity of the arthritis in these two transgenic models could still be due to the secondary development of T-cell autoimmunity to some cartilage autoantigen following an acute arthritis due to the hyperproduction of inflammatory cytokines. This biphasic pattern to the development of arthritis has been described in the Lewis rat following the injection of streptococcal cell walls (Sternberg *et al.*, 1989). The relevant experiments are awaited. The third model is the c-fos transgenic mouse (Shiozawa *et al.*, 1992); c-fos is a cellular oncogene which is transcribed early in cell activation particularly in cells of mesenchymal origin. Mice transgenic with c-fos do not have any overt arthritis. Following systemic immunization and intra-articular injection of the antigen there is a florid and destructive synovitis which is characterized by the paucity of T cells in the inflammatory infiltrate of macrophages and synoviocytes. This model is of particular interest and importance since T-cell immunization is clearly necessary for its induction but the number of T cells needed to induce disease is extremely limited. Transgenic models are fully reviewed by Harris in Chapter 27, this volume.

Thus, we may conclude that following activation of T cells by an as yet unknown antigen there is recruitment and activation of the mesenchymal reaction with the release of cytokines such as interleukin 1, tumour necrosis factor α, GM-CSF, interleukin 8, RANTES and platelet-derived growth factor, amongst others, which bring about the inflammatory synovitis with the release of collagenase and other enzymes which cause bone and articular cartilage destruction in the joint. At the apex of this inflammatory cascade is the trimolecular complex of the HLA-DR4/1 molecule presenting the unknown antigenic peptide(s) to the TCR of the disease-specific and disease-causing T cell. The cells involved are the antigen-presenting cell and the T cell. Following this initial activation, the cells involved in the mesenchymal reaction are recruited and activated.

DISEASE-MODIFYING ANTI-RHEUMATIC DRUGS AND THE TREATMENT OF RHEUMATOID ARTHRITIS

The established DMARDs have entered the therapeutic armamentarium largely by accident, argument by analogy or both. To this day their mode of action is unknown – or, rather, too many actions have been proposed for them, mainly on the basis of *in vitro* work. This is a direct consequence of the fact that they were not developed as the result of a strategy directed against a defined target. An example of such a strategy was the development of the non-steroidal anti-inflammatory drugs which have been designed to inhibit specifically the cyclo-oxygenase enzyme. It is salutary to be reminded that, with few exceptions, DMARDs can not be detected in the experimental models of arthritis from which our pathogenetic concepts have been developed. The commonest model, adjuvant arthritis, can be inhibited by non-steroidals which merely demonstrates how complex these models are in their own right. Perhaps the problem lies in the complexity of the actions of DMARDs and the slowness of the onset of their action – many of the experimental models of arthritis being of limited duration. Finally, no DMARD-like drug has successfully entered and stayed in the clinic as a result of screening compounds for anti-inflammatory activity in the experimental models of arthritis. One reason for their withdrawal has been unacceptable toxicity.

However, against this is the fact that these same models are very good at demonstrating the efficacy of immune therapies directed against defined targets. Just three examples will be cited from what is a long list: (a) T-cell vaccination in adjuvant arthritis (Cohen and Weiner, 1988); (b) anti-CD4 monoclonal antibody in collagen arthritis (Chapter 23, this volume); and (c) anti-TNFα monoclonal antibody in collagen arthritis (Brennan *et al.*, 1992 and Chapter 2, this volume). Since the current concept of the pathogenesis of RA postulates that this is an immune-driven disease, therapies developed in other such diseases and in other auto-immune models (such as experimental allergic encephalomyelitis) can be considered for the treatment of RA. One of the major handicaps in the immunotherapy of RA is our ignorance of the antigen or antigens causing or perpetuating the disease. Thus, some very specific therapies directed solely against factors specific for RA, therapies directed against disease-causing T cells for example, are not available to the rheumatologist.

DMARDs should not be considered as something to be consigned to the dustbin of useless treatments. Just as their use arose by accident so the dose and dosing regimens which we employ has come about by the same route. Although combination therapy is often discussed, the examples of its application are unfortunate as the drugs are used at the same dose and with the same dosing regimens as when they are used singly. The result has been increased toxicity without significant improvement in efficacy. Why should this be so?

Since DMARDs are not directed at a single target, since they have a slow onset of activity (they are also known as slow acting drugs (SARDs)), and since they have a persistent effect for weeks after they are discontinued, simple additive approaches to combination therapy are clearly not based on what we know of them. If gold or *d*-penicillamine can have a persistent effect for up to 3 months after discontinuation, then why is gold given weekly or monthly and *d*-penicillamine daily? Perhaps the appropriate approach is not just intermittent and combination therapy but therapy that aims to induce periods of remission in which drugs will not be taken. This strategy would probably reduce toxicity. Whether it would have a better effect on preventing or slowing the development of joint erosions cannot be predicted since we have little evidence that any of our present treatments, used singly, do this long term.

If the 'brave new treatments' based on immunotherapeutic concepts are so exciting and potentially could be so successful, why persist in trying to get more out of the existing therapies? There are two reasons. The first is one of cost; if the new therapies are based on biologics (antibodies, proteins or peptides) then they will be expensive as has been the case with recombinant erythropoietin, interferons and growth factors. The second reason is one of long-term toxicity; we do not know what the long-term consequences are of inhibiting one or more important steps in the host immune defence system.

THE IMMUNOTHERAPY OF RHEUMATOID ARTHRITIS

Despite these strictures, the best long-term hope for patients with RA is the development of new therapies based on targets defined by concepts developed from our understanding of its pathogenesis. Certain definitions are in order.

'Immunotherapy' may be defined as the use of immunologically specific reagents, such as monoclonal antibodies and antigenic peptides, directed against defined targets. Within this broad definition we may distinguish between two types of immunotherapy. The first, 'tolerance-inducing' immunotherapy, aims to bring about an end to the autoimmune process by inducing tolerance. The second, 'anti-inflammatory' immunotherapy, is directed against specific mediators in the inflammatory cascade and does not induce tolerance. Examples of the former would include anti-CD4 antibody therapy and of the latter, antibody therapy directed against TNFα or adhesion molecules. A crucial difference between 'tolerance-inducing' and 'anti-inflammatory' immunotherapy is that the former should be effective after a single or a limited course of treatment while the latter will require repeated courses of treatment probably for the life-time of the patient. With the increaseing sophistication of computer modelling and increasing knowledge of molecular structure/function relationships it may be possible to develop orally active drugs which could replace the biologics which are presently the only known means of delivering immunotherapy.

'Immunomodulation' may be defined as the use of simple drugs which either enhance desirable or suppress undesirable features of the immune response. Corticosteroids, the cytotoxics and cyclosporin A are presently available drugs of this type. With the increasing sophistication of our knowledge of the molecular basis of the immune response, future developments will involve the development of orally active drugs directed against these molecules. Protein kinase C is an important molecule in signal transduction during the stimulation of T cells. Protein kinase C inhibitors have recently been shown to inhibit effectively both T-cell proliferation *in vitro* as well as *in vivo* inflammation due to T-cell activation such as occurs in adjuvant arthritis (Hallam, 1993). Tenidap, an orally active drug produced by Pfizer, inhibits the induced release of interleukin 1, interleukin 6 and, to a lesser extent, TNFα (Otterness *et al.*, 1991; Sipe *et al.*, 1992). The mechanism of action is not known but it appears to act subsequent to receptor triggering. These agents could potentially cause problems as they have a rather wide spectrum of activities and would probably need to be given on a long-term basis.

INDUCTION OF ORAL TOLERANCE

In rodents, the feeding of antigen will induce systemic tolerance to subsequent immunization and has been used as a prophylactic and therapeutic procedure in animal models of human autoimmune disease including arthritis (Staines, 1991). The mode of action of oral tolerance is not clear. One possibility is that the antigen induces the development of antigen-specific CD8 positive T cells in the gut which home to the target issue where they release transforming growth factor β which suppresses immune and inflammatory reactions (Higgins and Weiner, 1988). Another is that peptides, released during digestion of the orally administered antigen, are absorbed into the systemic circulation and directly act on disease-causing T cells to tolerize them (Bitar and Whitacre, 1988). Preliminary results of feeding an extract of myelin to patients with multiple sclerosis have recenly been reported. They show a decrease of T-cell reactivity to myelin basic protein in the patients given active treatment although the degree of clinical improvement obtained was difficult to evaluate (Weiner *et al.*, 1993). The results of a controlled study in which bovine type II collagen is being fed to patients with RA are eagerly awaited (D. Trentham, pers. commun.).

IMMUNOTHERAPY DIRECTED AGAINST THE TRIMOLECULAR COMPLEX

Anti-HLA-DR Immunotherapy

Immunotherapy directed against the HLA-DR component of the trimolecular complex, for example with monoclonal antibodies, has not been reported in human autoimmune disease although retroplacental immunoglobulin, which has been shown to have some ameliorative effect on disease activity in RA, is thought to do so because it contains anti-HLA-DR antibodies (Sany, *et al.*, 1987).

The antigenic peptide, which is held in the groove of the HLA-DR molecule, has been modified so as to block the binding of the disease-causing peptide (Lamont *et al.*, 1990). However, clinical use of this approach may be difficult as there are problems with parenteral delivery of sufficient amounts of blocking peptide and fears for the possible activation of autoimmune clones of T cells by the modified peptide.

Anti-TCR Immunotherapy

Experimental approaches to peptide engineering have shown that alteration of the residues involved in contacting the TCR will bring about inhibition of the disease-causing T cell by the induction of tolerance (Sloan-Lancaster *et al.*, 1993). Lack of knowledge of the nature of the rheumatoid antigen and, consequently, of the TCR interacting with it means that this exciting approach is not open as yet for the immunotherapy of RA. A variant of this approach is the engineering of antigenic peptides which bind to and block the TCR of the disease-causing T cell (Metzler *et al.*, 1993).

As the T cell is merely 'antagonized' and not tolerized, prolonged and, possibly, life-long therapy may have to be given.

T-Cell Vaccination

Closely linked to the use of antagonistic, blocking or tolerizing peptides is therapy directed against the TCR. Monoclonal antibodies directed against monomorphic structures on the TCR have proved successful for the prevention or the treatment of collagen-induced arthritis in the rat (Yoshino et al., 1991). Such immunotherapy has not been used to date for the treatment of RA.

'Vaccination' with disease-causing T cells (Cohen et al., 1983) or with peptides unique to the TCR of the disease-causing T cell (Vandenbark et al., 1991) has been successfully used in experimental arthritis; the vaccination induces T cells which down-regulate the activity of the disease-causing lymphocyte by an anti-idiotypic mechanism. Since the disease-causing T cell in RA has not been cloned, this therapeutic avenue is closed. However, vaccination with activated T cells has been shown to induce regulatory T cells which are antigen non-specific but which inhibit the activity of pathogenic cells; such T cells have been called anti-ergotypic (Lohse et al., 1989). Since the antigen specificity of these cells is irrelevant to their regulatory role, activated T cells have been expanded from the joints of patients, fixed by chemical means and injected back into the patient as a 'vaccine' in order to induce the formation of anti-ergotypic cells (van Laar et al., 1991). Although this treatment is well tolerated, significant clinical and immunological consequences have not been described to date. More T cell 'vaccinations' need to be carried out under controlled conditions before the efficacy of this treatment can be properly assessed.

IMMUNOTHERAPY DIRECTED AGAINST THE T CELL

In addition to the T-cell receptor which confers antigenic specificity, the T cell has a number of other structures on its surface which are involved in T-cell function and activation. Some of these antigens have been used as immunotherapeutic targets.

In probably the first use of monoclonal antibodies for the treatment of RA, we showed that the infusion of mouse or chimaeric antibodies to CD7 produced immunological effects but no clinical benefit (Kirkham et al., 1991, 1992). This is of interest as such antibodies are immunosuppressive and have proved useful in prolonging the lifespan of human renal allografts (Tax et al., 1984; Costantinides et al., 1991). Paradoxically, the negative result has demonstrated that the exquisite specificity of immunotherapeutic reagents can be used to delineate structures which are or are not important in the pathogenesis of RA. Recently, it has been shown that CD7 positive T cells are a unique subset of T cells in their own right (Reinhold et al., 1993) and that they are less likely to be found in the joint as compared to a rejecting allograft (Lazarovits et al., 1992).

Although monoclonal antibodies coupled to the ricin A chain (CD5 Plus) have been shown to be of benefit in RA, further development is apparently not to take place (Strand and Fishwild, 1990). Monoclonal antibody to the interleukin 2 receptor (IL2R) has shown some promise in three patients and further studies are awaited (Kyle et al., 1989). The IL2R is an attractive target as resting T cells do not display it and cannot therefore be affected by therapies directed against it. Using this principle, an immunotoxin of IL-2 conjugated to modified diphtheria toxin has been used with clinical benefit, some patients showing prolonged improvement for weeks after a single course of treatment, with few side effects (Woodworth, 1993). This is targeted cytotoxic therapy and one wonders what its final role in the treatment of RA will be as long-term use will be necessary. The Campath-1H antibody is a humanized rat antibody directed against CDw52 which is an antigen found on T cells but whose exact role in T-cell physiology is unclear. It produces profound and prolonged lymphopenia lasting up to or beyond 1 year. Although there has been clinical improvement reported this has lasted for considerably less time than the lymphopenia (Watts *et al.*, 1993). The discrepancy between the duration of the lymphopenia and the duration of the clinical benefits suggests that the two are not linked. Perhaps the number of T cells needed to maintain the rheumatoid synovitis are few and can still be recruited from the circulation despite the lymphopenia. Perhaps insufficient Campath-IH enters the joint where it may be needed for the effective induction of local lymphopenia; it should be remembered that thoracic duct drainage is effective because of the local rather than for the systemic lymphopenia which it induces. Infective complications, with death of 2 patients, have been reported. The future of this therapy is not clear – it may perhaps be useful as an adjunct to anti-CD4 therapy.

Anti-CD4 therapy, whether used as the mouse or the human/mouse chimaerized antibody, has been extensively investigated in open studies (Herzog *et al.*, 1987, 1989; Wendling *et al.*, 1991). The responses have been highly variable; some patients showing marked and prolonged improvements in disease activity while others have not improved at all. The response is not dependent on the degree of CD4 lymphopenia (Choy *et al.*, 1992), as noted for Campath-1H above, but may be related to the dose of antibody used; most patients appear to be under-dosed on present protocols. Thus, we have evidence that clinical improvement is related to the proportion of synovial T cells which are coated with the antibody (cM-T412) (Choy and Kingsley, 1993). Furthermore, we have shown that antibody may kill disease-causing T cells by inducing apoptosis (Choy *et al.*, 1993).

The use of antibodies directed against T-cell structures requires controlled clinical trials for dose finding, optimum dosing regimens, assessment of efficacy and delineation of side effects. They should be conducted in centres with sufficient immunological expertise not only for adequate monitoring of the effects of the treatment but for investigation of its possible modes of action.

ANTI-INFLAMMATORY IMMUNOTHERAPY

Such immunotherapy is directed against the inflammatory cytokines released during rheumatoid synovitis, the cells and molecules involved in angiogenesis, inflammatory cell adhesion to endothelial cells and cell migration. As an example of anti-inflammatory therapy may be cited the open study in which a chimaeric anti-TNFα antibody has been shown to have marked anti-inflammatory effects on rheumatoid synovitis although retreatment has to be performed every 4 weeks or so (Feldmann, 1993). One of the possible modes of action of this therapy may be to reduce inflammatory cell entry into the joint as TNFα is a very potent activator of endothelial cell adhesion (Haskard *et al.*, 1990). The therapeutic effect of inhibiting cell adhesion and migration has been investigated in an open study in which a monoclonal antibody directed against ICAM-1, a molecule involved in lymphocyte adhesion and migration (Oppenheimer-Marks *et al.*, 1991), has shown clinical benefit in RA (P. Lipsky, pers. commun.; see Chapter 11). It has been recently demonstrated that interleukin 8 is a potent angiogenesis-promoting factor released by activated macrophages within the rheumatoid synovial membrane (Koch *et al.*, 1992). Angiogenesis is undoubtedly an important event in the life history of rheumatoid synovitis as new blood vessels are required for the nutrition of the hyperplastic and hypertrophic synovium. It is therefore encouraging that fumagillin, an orally active compound derived from a product of *A. fumigatus* and its derivatives are potent inhibitors of angiogenesis in the collagen-induced arthritis model (Peacock *et al.*, 1992); the results of clinical trials with such drugs are eagerly awaited. It should not be forgotten that healthy cartilage releases a potent angiogenesis inhibiting factor and that diseased cartilage, such as that from rheumatoid joints, is unable to do so (Moses *et al.*, 1990, 1992); perhaps therapy directed to restoring this function of articular cartilage may prove beneficial in preventing long-term cartilage destruction in RA.

SUMMARY AND FUTURE PROSPECTS

There is little doubt that many molecules, cells and processes involved in inflammation will be used increasingly in the future as immunotherapeutic targets of relevance to RA. The eventual place of therapies based on such targets for the clinical management of RA will depend on the results of properly conducted clinical trials as well as the cost of the treatments themselves.

The therapeutic agents which are making the running at the present are biologics, namely monoclonal antibodies or recombinant proteins, which pose problems in designing adequate dose-finding and dosing regimens. Since these agents have been rationally designed, it is imperative that they are studied in centres with the appropriate immunological expertise so as to ascertain 'proof of concept' should they prove to be effective. Trials of new therapeutic agents in RA, whether biologics or conventional drugs, raise an important ethical and an important practical issue. The ethical issue arises over the question of carrying out placebo controlled studies over months and even 1–2 years and thereby denying patients the best available treatment. The practical issue concerns the sheer number of therapeutic agents undergoing or about to undergo clinical trial, some nine as a rough estimate. The complexity and duration of drug trials, as presently executed in RA, makes this a daunting task.

I believe that a new approach is needed in the design and execution of such therapeutic clinical trials. First, such trials should be comparison trials against the best established treatment for the ethical reasons advanced above. Second, such trials should be relatively short-term studies not extending beyond 6 months with long-term toxicity and efficacy studies being carried out after marketing; this should not be a problem since it is likely that these agents will be used in specialist centres or hospitals in the first instance. Third, simplified clinical assessment criteria are needed to reduce the time, cost and complexity of clinical trials; it is encouraging that European and North American rheumatologists are actively collaborating in assessing the effectiveness and sensitivity of using only a limited number of clinical and laboratory measures of disease activity in therapeutic trials. These last two considerations should speed-up as well as improve the quality of therapeutic trials in RA.

REFERENCES

Bitar DM & Whitacre CC (1988) Suppression of experimental autoimmune encephalomyelitis by the oral administration of myelin basic protein. *Cell Immunol* **112**: 364–370.

Brennan FM, Maini RN & Feldmann M (1992) TNF alpha – a pivotal role in rheumatoid arthritis? *Br J Rheumatol* **31**: 293–298.

Case JP, Lafyatis R, Remmers EF, Kumkumian GK & Wilder RL (1989) Transin/stromelysin expression in rheumatoid synovium. A transformation-associated metalloproteinase secreted by phenotypically invasive synoviocytes. *Am J Pathol* **135**: 1055–1064.

Choy EHS & Kingsley G (1993) Anti-CD4 therapy in rheumatoid arthritis. *Clin Exp Rheum* **11 (supplement 8)**: S147–S149.

Choy EHS, Chikanza IC, Kingsley GH, Corrigall VM & Panayi GS (1992) Treatment of rheumatoid arthritis with single dose or weekly pulses of chimaeric anti-CD4 monoclonal antibody. *Scand J Immunol* **36**: 291–298.

Choy EHS, Pitzalis C, Adjage J, Forrest L, Kingsley G & Panayi G (1993) Apoptosis of antigen specific CD4 lymphocytes may be a mechanism of action of anti-CD4 monoclonal antibodies (mAb). *Clin Exp Rheum* **11 (supplement 8)**: S188 (Abstract).

Cohen IR & Weiner HL (1988) T cell vaccination. *Immunol Today* **9**: 332–335.

Cohen PL, Naparstek Y, Ben-Nun A & Cohen IR (1983) Lines of T lymphocytes induce or vaccinate against autoimmune arthritis. *Science* **219**: 56–58.

Corkill MM, Kirkham BW, Haskard DO, Barbatis C, Gibson T and Panayi GS (1991) Gold treatment of rheumatoid arthritis decreases synovial expression of the endothelial leukocyte adhesion receptor ELAM-1. *J Rheumatol* **18**, 1453–1460.

Costantinides Y, Kingsley GH, Pitzalis C & Panayi GS (1991) Inhibition of lymphocyte proliferation by a monoclonal antibody (RFT2) against CD7. *Clin Exp Immunol* **85**: 164–167.

Emery P, Smith GN & Panayi GS (1986) Lymphocytaphoresis – a feasible treatment for rheumatoid arthritis. *Br J Rheumatol* **25**: 40–43.

Farahat MNMR, Yanni G, Poston R & Panayi GS (1992) Immunohistological and functional differences in rheumatoid and osteoarthritic synovial membranes. *Br J Rheumatol* **31**: S1–S10.

Feldmann M (1993) TNF-α in rheumatoid arthritis and prospects of anti-TNF therapy. *Clin Exp Rheum* **11/ S-8**: S173.

Firestein GS & Zvaifler NJ (1987) Peripheral blood and synovial fluid monocyte activation in inflammatory arthritis. II. Low levels of synovial fluid and synovial tissue interferon suggest that gamma-interferon is not the primary macrophage activating factor. *Arthritis Rheum* **30**: 864–871.

Firestein GS, Xu WD, Townsend K, Broide D, Alvar-Garcia JM, Glasebrook A et al. (1988) Cytokines in chronic inflammatory arthritis. I. Failure to detect T cell lymphokines (interleukin 2 and interleukin 3) and presence of macrophage colony-stimulating factor (CSF-1) and a novel mast cell growth factor in rheumatoid synovitis. *J Exp Med* **168**: 1573–1586.

Firestein GS, Alvaro-Garcia JM & Maki R (1990) Quantitative analysis of cytokine gene expression in rheumatoid arthritis. *J Immunol* **144**: 3347–3353.

Hallam TJ (1993) Functional significance of protein kinase C in human T-cell activation: a new therapeutic class? *Clin Exp Rheum* **11 (supplement 8)**: S131–S134.

Haskard DO, Thornhill MH, Kyan-Aung U, Kingsley GH, Pitzalis C & Panayi GS (1990) Cytokine induced changes in the endothelial cell surface membrane: significance for lymphocyte traffic during inflammation. In Melchers F (ed) *Progress in Immunology VII*, p 780. Berlin: Springer Verlag.

Haworth C, Brennan FM, Chantry D, Turner M, Maini RN & Feldmann M (1991) Expression of granulocyte–macrophage colony-stimulating factor in rheumatoid arthritis: regulation by tumor necrosis factor alpha. *Eur J Immunol* **21**: 2575–2579.

Haynes BF, Grover BJ, Whichard LP, Hale LP, Nunley JA, McCollum DE et al. (1988) Synovial microenvironment–T cell interactions. Human T cells bind to fibroblast-like synovial cells *in vitro*. *Arthritis Rheum* **31**: 947–955.

Herzog C, Walker C, Pichler W, Aeschlimann A, Wassmer P, Stockinger H et al. (1987) Monoclonal anti-CD4 in arthritis. *Lancet* **ii**: 1461–1462.

Herzog C, Walker C, Miller W, Riever P, Reiter C, Riethmuller G et al. (1989) Anti-CD4 antibody treatment of patients with rheumatoid arthritis: I. Effect on clinical course and circulating T cells. *J Autoimmun* **2**: 627–642.

Higgins PJ & Weiner HL (1988) Suppression of experimental autoimmune encephalomyelitis by oral administration of myelin basic protein and its fragments. *J Immunol* **140**: 440–445.

Highton J, Smith M & Bradley J (1989) Cells of the monocyte/macrophage series in peripheral blood and synovial fluid in inflammatory arthritis. A preliminary study of cellular phenotype. *Scand J Rheumatol* **18**: 393–399.

Iwakura I, Tosu M, Yoshida E, Takiguchi M, Sato K, Kitajima et al. (1991) Induction of inflammatory arthropathy resembling rheumatoid arthritis in mice transgenic for HTLV-1. *Science* **253**: 1026–1027.

Keffer J, Probert L, Cazlaris H, Goergopoulos S, Kaslaris E, Kioussis D et al. (1991) Transgenic mice expressing human tumor necrosis factor: a predictive genetic model of arthritis. *EMBO J* **10**: 4025–4031.

Kirkham BW, Pitzalis C, Kingsley GH, Chikanza IC, Sabharwal S, Barbatis C et al. (1991) Monoclonal antibody treatment in rheumatoid arthritis: clinicial and immunological effects of a CD7 monoclonal antibody. *Br J Rheumatol* **30**: 459–463.

Kirkham BW, Thien F, Pelton BK, Pitzalis C, Amlot P, Denman AM et al. (1992) Chimeric CD7 monoclonal antibody therapy in rheumatoid arthritis. *J Rheumatol* **19**: 1348–1352.

Koch AE, Polverini PJ & Leibovich SJ (1988) Functional heterogeneity of human rheumatoid synovial tissue macrophages. *J Rheumatol* **15**: 1058–1063.

Koch AE, Kunkel SL, Burrows JC, Evanoff HL, Haines GK, Pope RM et al. (1991) Synovial tissue macrophage as a source of the chemotactic cytokine IL-8. *J Immunol* **147**: 2187–2195.

Koch AE, Polverini PJ, Kunkel SL, Harlow LA, DiPietro LA, Elner VM et al. (1992) Interleukin-8 as a macrophage derived mediator of angiogenesis. *Science* **258**: 1798–1801.

Kyle V, Coughlan RJ, Tighe H, Waldmann H and Hazleman BL (1989) Beneficial effect of monoclonal antibody to interleukin 2 receptor on activated T cells in rheumatoid arthritis. *Ann Rheum Dis* **48**: 428–429.

Lafyatis R, Thompson NL, Remmers EF, Flanders KC, Roche NS, Kim SJ et al. (1989) Transforming growth factor-beta production by synovial tissues from rheumatoid patients and streptococcal cell wall arthritic rats. Studies on secretion synovial fibroblast-like cells and immunohistologic localization. *J Immunol* **143**: 1142–1148.

Lamont AG, Sette A, Fujinami R, Colon SM, Miles C & Grey HM (1990) Inhibition of experimental autoimmune encephalomyelitis induction in SJL/J mice by using a peptide with high affinity for IA5 molecules. *J Immunol* **145**: 1687–1693.

Lanchbury JS, Sakkas LI & Panayi GS (1992) Genetic factors in rheumatoid arthritis. In Smolen JR, Kalden JR & Maini RN (eds) *Rheumatoid Arthritis: Recent Research Advances*, p 17. Berlin: Springer Verlag.

Lazarovits AI, White MJ & Karsh J (1992) CD7-T cells in rheumatoid arthritis. *Arthritis Rheum* **35**: 615–624.

Lohse AW, Mor F, Karin N & Cohen IR (1989) Control of experimental autoimmune encephalomyelitis by T cells responding to activated T cells. *Science* **244**: 820–822.

MacNaul KL, Hutchinson NI, Parsons JN, Bayne EK & Tocci MJ (1990) Analysis of IL-1 and TNF-alpha gene expression in human rheumatoid synoviocytes and normal monocytes by *in situ* hybridization. *J Immunol* **145**: 4154–4166.

Marguerie C, Lunardi C & So A (1992) PCR-based analysis of TCR repertoire in human autoimmune diseases. *Immunol Today* **13**: 336–338.

Metzler B, Pairchild PJ & Wraith DC (1993) MHC binding peptides as therapeutic agents. *Clin Exp Rheum* **11 (supplement 8)**: S45–S46.

Morales-Ducret J, Wayner E, Elices MJ, Alvaro-Garcia JM, Zvaifler NJ & Firestein GS (1992) α4/β1 integrin (VLA-4) ligands in arthritis: vascular cell adhesion molecule expression in synovium and on fibroblast-like synoviocytes. *J Immunol* **149**: 1424–1438.

Moses MA, Sudhalter J & Langer R (1990) Identification of an inhibitor of neovascularisation from cartilage. *Science* **248**: 1408–1410.

Moses MA, Sudhalter J & Langer R (1992) Isolation and characterization of an inhibitor of neovascularisation from scapular chondrocytes. *J Cell Biol* **119**: 475–482.

Okada Y, Morodomi T, Enghild JJ, Suzuki K, Yasui A, Nakanishi I, Salvesen G & Nagase H (1990) Matrix metalloproteinase 2 from human rheumatoid synovial fibroblasts. Purification and activation of the precursor and enzymic properties. *Eur J Biochem* **194**: 721–730.

Oppenheimer-Marks N, Davis LS, Bogue DT, Ramberg J & Lipsky PE (1991) Differential utilization of ICAM-1 and VCAM-1 during the adhesion and transendothelial migration of human T lymphocytes. *J Immunol* **147**: 2913–2921.

Otterness IG, Bliven ML, Downs JT, Natoli EJ & Hanson DC (1991) Inhibition of interleukin 1 synthesis by tenidap: a new drug for arthritis. *Eur Cytokine Netw* **3**: 277–283.

Panayi GS (1992) The immunopathogenesis of rheumatoid arthritis. *Rheumatol Review* **1**: 63–74.

Panayi GS & Amlot PL (1982) Total lymphoid irradiation in rheumatoid arthritis. *Lancet* **1**: 25–27.

Panayi GS & Tugwell P (1993) The use of cyclosporin A in rheumatoid arthritis: proceedings of an international consensus meeting. *Br J Rheumatol* **32 (supplement 1)**.

Panayi GS, Lanchbury JS & Kingsley GH (1992) The importance of the T cell in initiating and maintaining the chronic synovitis of rheumatoid arthritis. *Arthritis Rheum* **35**: 729–735.

Paulus HE, Machleder HI, Levine S, Yu DTY & MacDonald NS (1977) Lymphocyte involvement in rheumatoid arthritis. Studies during thoracic duct drainage. *Arthritis Rheum* **20**: 1249–1262.

Peacock DJ, Banquerigo ML & Brahn E (1992) Angiogenesis inhibition suppresses collagen arthritis. *J Exp Med* **175**: 1135–1138.

Pincus T & Callahan LF (1986) Taking mortality in rheumatoid arthritis seriously – predictive markers, socioeconomic status and comorbidity. *J Rheumatol* **13**: 841–845.

Pincus T, Marcum SB & Callahan LF (1992) Longterm drug therapy for rheumatoid arthritis in seven rheumatology private practices: II. Second line drugs and prednisone. *J Rheumatol* **19**: 1885–1894.

Pitzalis C, Kingsley GH, Murphy J & Panayi GS (1987) Abnormal distribution of the helper-inducer and suppressor-inducer T lymphocyte subsets in the rheumatoid joint. *Clin Immunol Immunopathol* **45**: 252–258.

Pitzalis C, Kingsley GH, Haskard DO & Panayi GS (1988) The preferential accumulation of helper-inducer T lymphocytes in inflammatory lesions: evidence for regulation by selective endothelial and homotypic adhesion. *Eur J Immunol* **18**: 1397–1404.

Pitzalis C, Kingsley GH, Covelli M, Meliconi R, Markey A and Panayi GS (1991) Selective migration of the human helper-inducer memory T cell subset: confirmation by *in vivo* cellular kinetic studies. *Eur J Immunol* **21**: 369–376.

Reinhold U, Abken H, Kukel S, Moll M, Muller R, Oltermann I et al. (1993) CD7-T cells represent a subset of normal human blood lymphocytes. *J Immunol* **150**: 2081–2089.

Remmers EF, Sano H, Lafyatis R, Case JP, Kumkumian GK, Hla T et al. (1991) Production of platelet derived growth factor B chain (PDGF-B/c-sis) mRNA and immunoreactive PDGF B-like polypeptide by rheumatoid synovium: coexpression with heparin binding acidic fibroblast growth factor-1. *J Rheumatol* **18**: 7–13.

Rodriguez RM, Pitzalis C, Kingsley GH, Henderson EM, Humphries MJ and Panayi GS (1992) T-lymphocyte adhesion to fibronectin: a possible mechanism for T cell accumulation in the rheumatoid joint. *Clin Exp Immunol* **89**: 439–445.

Sano H, Forough R, Maier JA, Case JP, Jackson A, Engleka K et al. (1990) Detection of high levels of heparin binding growth factor-1 (acidic fibroblast growth factor) in inflammatory arthritic joints. *J Cell Biol* **110**: 1417–1426.

Sany J, Clot J, Combe B, Franchimont P, Malaise M, Hauwaert C et al. (1987) Treatment of rheumatoid arthritis. Comparative study of the effect of immunoglobulins G eluted from the placenta and of veno-globulins. [French]. *Presse Medicale – Paris* **16**: 723–724.

Shiozawa S, Shiozawa K, Tanaka Y, Morimoto I, Uchihashi M, Fujita T et al. (1989) Human epidermal growth factor for the stratification of synovial lining layer and neovascularisation in rheumatoid arthritis. *Ann Rheum Dis* **48**: 820–828.

Shiozawa S, Tanaka Y, Fujita T & Tokuhisa T (1992) Destructive arthritis without lymphocyte infiltration in H2-c-fos transgenic mice. *J Immunol* **148**: 3100–3104.

Sipe JD, Bartle LM & Loose LD (1992) Modification of proinflammatory cytokine production by the antirheumatic agents tenidap and naproxen. A possible correlate with clinical acute phase response. *J Immunol* **148**: 480–484.

Sloan-Lancaster J, Evavold BD & Allen PM (1993) Induction of T-cell anergy by altered T-cell-receptor ligand on live antigen-presenting cells. *Nature* **363**: 156–159.

Staines NA (1991) Oral tolerance and collagen arthritis. *Br J Rheumatol* **30**: 40–43.

Sternberg EM, Young WS, Bernardini R, Calogeno AE, Chrousos GP, Gold PW et al. (1989) A central nervous system defect in biosynthesis of corticotropin-releasing hormone is associated with susceptibility to streptococcal cell wall-induced arthritis in Lewis rats. *Proc Natl Acad Sci USA* **86**: 4771–4775.

Strand V & Fishwild D (1990) Treatment of rheumatoid arthritis with an anti-CD5 immunoconjugate: clinical and immunologic findings and preliminary results of treatment. *Arthritis Rheum.* **33**: S25 (abstract).

Tan PL, Farmiloe S, Yeoman S & Watson JD (1990) Expression of the interleukin 6 gene in rheumatoid synovial fibroblasts. *J Rheumatol* **17**: 1608–1612.

Tax WJM, Tidman NH, Janossy G, Trejdosiewicz L, Willems R, Leeuwenberg J et al. (1984) Monoclonal antibody (WT 1) directed against a T cell surface glycoprotein: characteristics and immunosuppressive activity. *Clin Exp Immunol* **55**: 427–436.

Unemori EN, Hibbs MS & Amento EP (1992) Constitutive expression of a 92-kD gelatinase (type V collagenase) by rheumatoid synovial fibroblasts and its induction in normal human fibroblasts by inflammatory cytokines. *J Clin Invest* **88**: 1656–1662.

van Laar JM, Miltenburg AMM, Verdonk MJ, Daha MR, de Vries RRP & Breedveld FL (1991) T cell vaccination in rheumatoid arthritis. *Br J Rheumatol* **30**: 28–29.

Vandenbark AA, Chou YK, Hashim G & Offner H (1991) *Br J Rheumatol* **30**: 20–23.

Villiger PM, Terkeltaub R & Lotz M (1992) Production of Monocyte Chemoattractant Protein-1 by inflamed synovial tissue and cultured synoviocytes. *J Immunol* **149**: 722–727.

Watts RA, Isaacs JD, Hale G, Hazleman BL & Waldmann H (1993) CAMPATH-1H in inflammatory arthritis. *Clin Exp Rheum* **11/S-8**: S165.

Weiner HL, Mackin GA, Matsui M, Orav EJ, Khoury SJ, Dawson DM et al. (1993) Double-blind pilot trial of oral tolerization with myelin antigens in multiple sclerosis. *Science* **259**: 1321–1324.

Wendling D, Wijdenes J & Racadot T (1991) Utilisation therapetique d'un anti corps monoclonal anti-CD4 dans la polyarthrite reumatoide refractaire. Resultats preliminaires. *Rev. Rhum* **58**: 13–17.

Woodworth TG (1993) Early clinical studies of IL-2 fusion toxin in patients with severe rheumatoid arthritis and recent onset insulin-dependent diabetes mellitus. *Clin Exp Rheum* **11/S-8**: S177.

Yoshino S, Cleland LG & Mayrhofer G (1991) Treatment of collagen-induced arthritis in rats with a monoclonal antibody against the alpha/beta T cell antigen receptor. *Arthritis Rheum* **34**: 1039–1047.

Pathology of
Rheumatoid Arthritis

5 Histopathology of the Rheumatoid Joint

A.J. Freemont

INTRODUCTION

Rheumatoid arthritis is perhaps better described as rheumatoid disease, a multisystem disorder in which synovial joints are the most commonly involved organ system. In very general terms there are three major pathological entities in rheumatoid disease; local tissue inflammation, the rheumatoid nodule and a vasculitis.

Local tissue inflammation consists of a mixed inflammatory cell infiltrate in which lymphocytes, plasma cells and macrophages predominate. It is associated with local tissue damage and reparative fibrosis. The number of polymorphs within the infiltrate is variable, being greatest in early lesions and in 'acute flares'.

Histologically the rheumatoid nodule is a serpiginous area of tissue necrosis surrounded by radially orientated (pallisaded) lines of macrophages (Collins, 1937). When the nodule occurs in fibrous connective tissues, as it most commonly does, the collagen necrosis appears to be complete, but when viewed between crossed polarizers residual collagen fibres can be seen crossing the areas of necrosis.

The vasculitis in rheumatoid disease may affect the arterial or venous sides of the circulation (Scott *et al.*, 1981). In arteries there are two major types of vasculitis: (a) a necrotizing arteritis, in which mural polymorphs are the characteristic feature, leading to vascular occlusion and tissue infarction; and (b) a subacute or lymphocyte/macrophage mediated arteritis which may cause either ischaemia or infarction. On the venous side of the circulation the most common lesion is a leukocytoclastic vasculitis (venulitis). In this lesion polymorphs are present in the wall of the venule, but, in addition, there is polymorph breakdown witnessed by finely particulate nuclear dust in and about the vessel wall. Both arterial, necrotizing and venular vasculitis are manifestations of immune complex deposition/formation, with complement activation, polymorph chemotaxis and polymorph mediated tissue injury.

JOINT DISEASE

Within joints of patients with rheumatoid disease, chronic (lymphocyte mediated) or active chronic (lymphocyte and polymorph mediated) tissue inflammation are the predominant mechanisms leading to the tissue changes, rheumatoid nodule formation and vasculitis being rare (Cruikshank, 1954; Gardner, 1972). Because the inflammatory process targets synovium specifically, of all the joints in the body, by far the most commonly affected are the synovial, or diarthrodial joints.

Rheumatoid disease is typicaly a polyarthropathy affecting the metacarpophalyngeal and metatarsophalyngeal joints and then with decreasing frequency, the wrists, ankles, knees, shoulders, elbows and hips. The synovial joints of the spine including

Mechanisms and Models in Rheumatoid Arthritis
ISBN 0–12–340440–1

the neurocentral joints of the cervical spine and the median atlanto-axial joint (which often incorporates a synovial sac between the posterior surface of the dens of the axis and the transverse ligament of the axis) are also commonly involved in the disease process (Bywaters, 1982).

In any individual the disease may be in different stages of evolution in different joints. The evolution can be thought of as having three progressive stages – acute (characterized by hyperaemia, oedema and a polymorph-rich infiltrate), chronic (characterized by a chronic inflammatory cell infiltrate, tissue damage and fibrosis) and end stage (a postinflammatory stage of fibrosis, scarring and secondary events such as the development of osteoarthritis). There may also be transitionary states.

For the sake of simplicity the following description will concentrate upon the 'classical' appearance of the rheumatoid joint in the chronic phase, the acute and end stage phases will be described later and separately.

THE HISTOPATHOLOGY OF SYNOVIAL JOINTS IN THE 'CHRONIC' OR 'CLASSICAL' PHASE OF RHEUMATOID DISEASE

Synovial joints are complex structures which allow bone ends to angulate, slide and twist relative to one another. The structure of the joint has evolved to permit this variety of movements. The joint consists of the bone ends covered by articular cartilage and surrounded by a fibrous capsule. The capsule (together with the muscles acting across the joint) gives stability to the joint and in places the dense capsular fibrous tissue is thickened to form ligaments which are strategically positioned to provide additional support in sites of recurrent loading. The capsule is lined by synovium which is no more than vascular fibrous or adipose tissue covered, in the normal joint, by an incomplete layer of specialized synovial cells of two types, the type A and type B synoviocytes, which have special phagocytic and biosynthetic properties respectively. The synovium is reflected on to the periosteal surface of any intra-articular bone but does not cover cartilage. The synovium is involved in producing the synovial fluid which has lubricating and nutrient functions.

In rheumatoid disease all these structures may become abnormal and the pathological changes in each will be described separately.

SYNOVIAL CHANGES IN RHEUMATOID DISEASE

The synovium is believed to be the seat of the changes that occur in the joint. Macroscopically the normally flat synovium becomes thrown into villi (Fig. 1), or finger-like processes, and may appear brown as a consequence of accumulation of haemosiderin pigment (Collins, 1949; Fassbender, 1975).

When sectioned and examined microscopically the villi are seen to consist of a core of fibro-adipose tissue covered by multilayered synoviocytes. The core of each villus contains, and is often expanded, by aggregates of inflammatory cells (Fig. 2). The subvillous synovial subintima also contains numerous inflammatory cells. Throughout the synovium there is a change in the number and type of blood vessels. The three components of the synovium that are important in understanding the histopathology of rheumatoid disease are the synoviocytes, the inflammatory infiltrate and the vasculature.

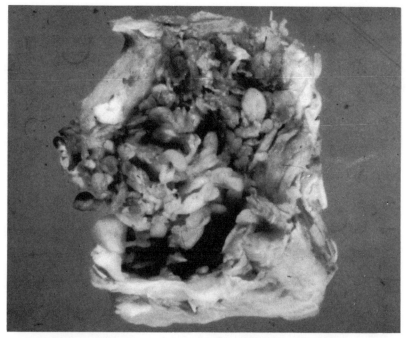

Figure 1. Macroscopic view of villous rheumatoid synovium.

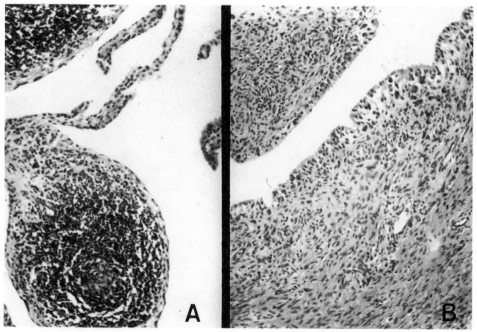

Figure 2. Rheumatoid synovium showing villi with lymphocyte aggregates (A) and synoviocyte hyperplasia (B).

Synoviocyte Layer

Synoviocytes

In rheumatoid disease the synoviocytes are both hypertrophic (large) and hyperplastic (increased in number) (Fig. 3). The increase in synoviocyte number and size results in

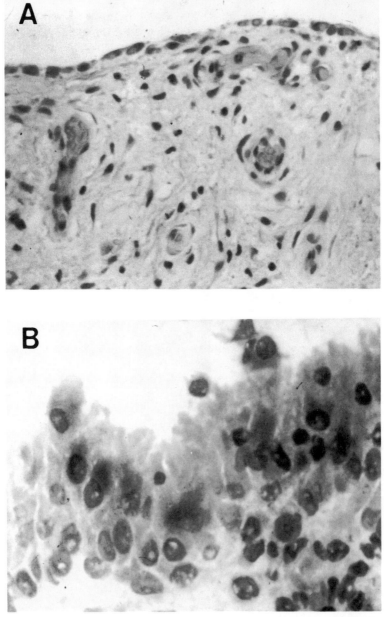

Figure 3. (A) Normal synovium with an incomplete layer of synoviocytes. H and E ×150. (B) Synoviocyte hypertrophy and hyperplasia in rheumatoid synovium. H and E ×200.

the formation of a multicellular layer covering the surface of the synovium. The most superficial cells have long microvilli projecting from their surfaces. Whilst both type A and type B synoviocytes are increased in number careful ultrastructural, immuno-histochemical and histochemical investigations have shown that the major increase is amongst the type A cells (Eulderink, 1982).

Inflammation within the synoviocyte layer

In rheumatoid disease the synoviocyte layer often contains inflammatory cells which, unlike the inflammatory infiltrate in the subintima, frequently consists of polymorphs, presumably in the transit from blood to synovial fluid. In active disease particularly, it is possible to see focal, 'explosive' lesions on the surface of the synovium where large numbers of polymorphs appear to be pouring into the fluid. The presence of poly-morphs in the synoviocyte layer is more common in certain of the seronegative spondylarthropathies than rheumatoid disease.

Fibrin and rice bodies

Frequently the synovial surface is covered by a layer of fibrin. This material, as fibrinogen, exudes from the synovial microvasculature, most commonly in active chronic inflammation. It polymerizes to fibrin within the joint where it adheres to all the surfaces. That on the synovium is often of sufficient quantity and present for sufficient time to be absorbed into the synovial villi where it undergoes organization. If not absorbed it may, mixed with synovial fluid lipids and glycoproteins, form rounded aggregages between 2 and 7 mm in diameter called 'rice bodies' (Albrecht et al., 1965; Popert et al., 1982) which can be aspirated from the joint using a wide bore needle.

'Ulceration', superficial necrosis, heminodules and propagating synovial fissures

In places the surface of the synovium may be denuded of synoviocytes, a pattern sometimes and wrongly called ulceration. In these areas fibrin and necrotic debris are in contact with the synovial surface which consists of granulation tissue (Fig. 4), which more frequently than not, contains inflammatory cells. These presumably represent areas of superficial damage to the synovium and evolving secondary tissue repair processes.

Sometimes these areas of tissue necrosis form a half-moon shaped structure with its straight surface along the synovial surface and with macrophage rich granulation tissue at its periphery (Fig. 5). This very closely resembles a halved rheumatoid nodule but it is not clear if the pathogenesis of these two lesions is the same.

Occasionally, towards the bases of villi, these areas of necrosis appear more ribbon-like and penetrate more deeply into the subintima. In some of these the necrotic debris disappears and the cleft so formed comes to be lined by synoviocytes. Some believe this to be the origin of villi and whether strictly true or not it certainly leads to an increase in the folding of the synovial surface. Three dimensional reconstructions of synovia showing these changes lends support to the concept that this may be the mechanism by which villi form (Edwards et al., 1983).

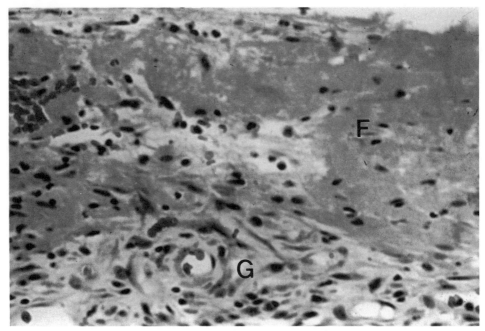

Figure 4. Fibrin (F) overlying granulation tissue (G). H and E ×100.

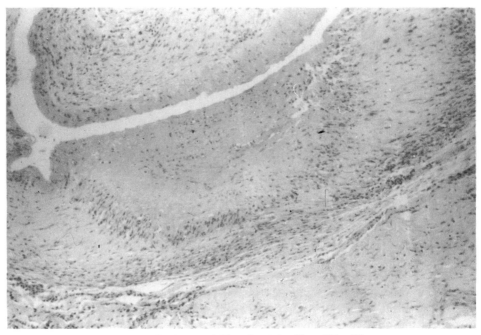

Figure 5. A synovial heminodule. H and E ×25.

Bone and cartilage fragments within the synovium

Because rheumatoid disease is a destructive arthropathy the synovial surface and the adjacent superficial subintima may contain fragments of cartilage and bone eroded from the articular surfaces and then absorbed from the synovial fluid into the synovium (Fig. 6). Sometimes the fragments of bone are so small that they amount to no more than spherulites of crystalline hydroxyapatite. The cartilage and bone may stimulate a multinucleated giant cell reaction, and the smaller apatite spherulites a macrophage response.

The Core of the Villi

Morphology of villi

The shape and size of villi varies enormously even within a single joint. Commonly the villi contain chronic inflammatory cells. Lymphocytes may have a follicular distribution and the follicles may contain germinal centres. Plasma cells usually surround the follicles. As the inflammatory process within the villi – and indeed throughout the synovium – is that of chronic inflammation, it is commonly associated with the tissue fibrosis. Therefore, it is not unexpected, particularly in long-standing inflammation, to find that in rheumatoid synovium, some of the villi have a dense fibrous core. These villi may become detached and lose their synoviocyte covering, forming fibrous loose bodies within the joint (Freemont and Denton, 1991).

Synovial Inflammation

Inflammatory cells

Depending upon the phase of the disease the rheumatoid synovium contains a mixed inflammatory cell infiltrate in which the major cell types are polymorphs, lymphocytes, plasma cells and macrophages.

Polymorphs

In early disease and in inflammatory flares polymorphs accumulate in the synovial membrane. They will also be seen if infection or crystal deposition disease is superimposed upon the rheumatoid disease (Fig. 7) (see later).

Many of the polymorphs contain phagocytosed immune complexes and are called 'ragocytes' (Hollander *et al.*, 1965). These cells are much more clearly seen in synovial fluid. Whether they play a part in rheumatoid tissue damage is still disputed but the processes of apoptosis and subsequent cytophagocytosis by which polymorphs are usually cleared from tissues is impaired in rheumatoid disease. How this may influence disease progression is discussed under synovial fluid.

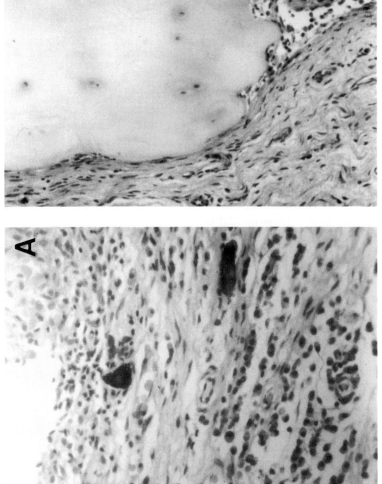

Figure 6. Synovium containing bone fragments (A) and cartilage (B). H and E ×100.

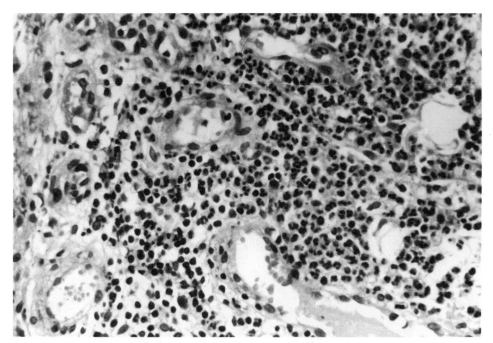

Figure 7. Acutely inflamed synovium in early rheumatoid disease. H and E ×200.

Lymphocytes

As in all the chronic synovitides lymphocytes easily outnumber all other inflammatory cells within the synovium in rheumatoid disease. When their number is relatively low they have a perivascular distribution throughout the synovium, with the exception of the superficial subintima where they tend to be more diffusely distributed. Increased numbers are arranged in sheets or in follicles which may contain germinal centres (Ziff, 1974) (Fig. 8).

The lymphocytes can be shown by immunohistochemistry to be predominately of the T-cell lineage (see Chapters 7 and 11, this volume). The helper/suppressor ratio is considerably higher than in normal peripheral blood (typically 5–10:1 vs. 2:1; Zvaifler and Silver, 1985). When follicles are present, B and T lymphocytes are mixed.

Plasma cells

As in most inflammatory arthropathies the majority of plasma cells react for cytoplasmic IgG, and a significant proportion (approximately 20–40%) are positive for IgA (Youinou *et al.*, 1984). Uniquely amongst the inflammatory arthropathies in rheumatoid disease, even in its chronic phase, >10% of the plasma cells are positive for cytoplasmic IgM (Freemont and Rutley, 1986).

Macrophages

These are the major non-lymphoid cells within the inflamed synovium. The majority of these cells are HLADr positive in tissue sections (Igushi *et al.*, 1986; see also

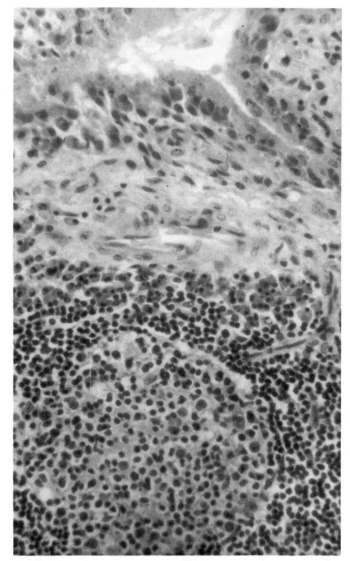

Figure 8. Classical chronic rheumatoid inflammation. There is synoviocyte hypertrophy and a lymphoid follicle containing a germinal centre and surrounded by plasma cells. H and E ×200.

Chapter 7, this volume). Their functions are diverse and are discussed elsewhere within this volume.

Dendritic macrophages

Within the rheumatoid synovium is a group of morphologically distinct cells with a stellate or dendritic morphology. Their phenotype has been carefully studied in tissue sections and this has shown certain similarities to circulating dendritic cells and the interdigitating cells of lymph nodes (Poulter *et al.*, 1983).

Mast cells

Other inflammatory cells are present within the synovium, but their significance is uncertain. Latterly the mast cell has been regarded with some interest because of the multiplicity of potential activities, inflammatory and non-inflammatory that it could mediate (Bromley *et al.*, 1984; see also Chapter 6, this volume). Mast cell accumulation in synovium is not restricted to rheumatoid disease or even to the inflammatory arthropathies making assessment of the importance of these cells in synovial inflammation and associated tissue changes difficult to interpret (Dean *et al.*, 1994).

Amyloid

Like all chronic inflammatory disorders, rheumatoid disease predisposes to the development of amyloid. Amyloid is a generic term describing a protein that accumulates because its normal alpha helical structure is replaced by a less degradable beta pleated sheet configuration. In rheumatoid disease the protein is the acute phase reactant serum protein A which forms amyloid A (AA: Peyps, 1988) that is deposited in the synovium, particularly in walls of blood vessels. It is amorphous and eosinophilic when viewed with the light microscope and reacts with the stain Congo Red (Puchtler *et al.*, 1962). Deposition of amyloid within blood vessel walls leads to poor vascular function and relative tissue ischaemia.

Synovial Vasculature

Haemic vasculature

Although the distribution and nature of the blood vessels varies from joint to joint, in general terms it consists of a complex anastomosing network of microvessels (arterioles, capillaries and venules) that permeates the synovium with capillaries forming an increasingly high proportion of the vessels the nearer one approaches to the surface. Even so there is always a layer of synoviocytes or matrix between the capillary wall and/or the synovial fluid.

When compared with normal the number of vessels per unit volume of synovium is increased in rheumatoid disease. This is most noticeable in the subintima. The villi are also very vascular. In areas of heavy lymphocytic inflammation the vessels change their morphology, chemistry and function to form vessels identical to lymph node high endothelial venules (Freemont *et al.*, 1984; Freemont, 1987). These vessels, which are specialized for promoting lymphocyte traffic from the blood into the synovium, can be recognized by their plump endothelial cells, thickened vascular basement membrane and their constant association with lymphocytes, which includes lymphocytes within their lumina, wall and basement membrane, and about their periphery (Freemont, 1988). The trafficking of leukocytes within the rheumatoid joint is discussed by Oppenheimer-Marks and Lipsky in Chapter 11, this volume.

Vasculitis within synovium is surprisingly uncommon but occasionally it occurs giving rise to synovial infarction.

Lymphatic vasculature

The lymph vessels of the synovium and the changes that occur to them in disease are poorly characterized (Davies, 1946).

Although all the changes described above may be encountered in rheumatoid synovium it is essential to recognize that there is gross variation in the histolological appearances of the synovium in different joints and even within the same joint. The factors influencing the dramatically different patterns of cellular and matrix responses within adjacent parts of the same area of synovium are not understood.

THE CARTILAGE IN RHEUMATOID ARTHRITIS

Normal Cartilage

Normal cartilage consists of a meshwork of type II collagen fibres that encapsulates aggregates of partially hydrated, hydrophilic glycosaminoglycans. The expansion of the glycosaminoglycans by ingress of water from synovial fluid is resisted by the collagen fibres, making the cartilage very hard. In histological sections the cartilage consists of eosinophilic fibrils in which are chondrocytes surrounded by very broad, and often merging, zones of haematoxophilic glycosaminoglycan rich matrix. The synovium does not normally overlie articular cartilage.

Rheumatoid Disease

In rheumatoid disease the inflamed synovium is no longer under those normal control mechanisms that inhibit synovial overgrowth of cartilage. The synovium starts to encroach upon the edge of the cartilage at the periphery of the joint. As the synovium overgrows it there is destruction and loss of cartilage (Fig. 9).

There are two basic disease processes underlying cartilage erosion: (a) destruction of cartilage by synovium (Fig. 10); and (b) chondrocyte destruction of their domainal cartilage, a process sometimes called chondrocytic chondrolysis (Mitchell and Shepherd, 1970), in which the earliest manifestation is enlargement of the chondrocyte lacunae (Fig. 11).

There have been several mechanisms proposed to explain synovial destruction of cartilage. Histological examination of the encroaching synovium (pannus) as it overgrows the cartilage shows that at the synovium/cartilage interface endothelial cells of small vessels, macrophages, polymorphs or mast cells may be the dominant feature (Fig. 12). Various mechanisms implicating these cells in the erosive process have been suggested and investigated (Mohr and Wessinghage, 1978; Bromley *et al.*, 1984). All could be implicated either directly or indirectly by releasing or causing the release of degradative enzymes. Chondrocytic chondrolysis is explained on the basis of release of cytokines that stimulate chondrocyte synthesis of collagenase.

Adjacent to the erosion front there is loss of perichondrocytic haematoxophilia, suggesting that in this area there is an alteration in chondrocyte function. This may represent a change to, for instance, collagenase synthesis, but the finding of dead chondrocytes abutting on to the erosion front suggests that it may represent cell dysfunction as a prelude to cell death.

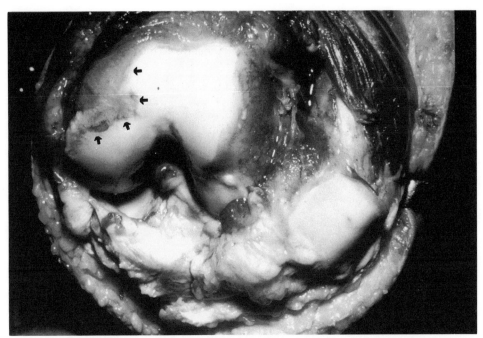

Figure 9. An opened knee from a patient with rheumatoid disease. There is erosion of the articular cartilage of the lower end of the femur (arrowed).

As the pannus and its associated cartilage destruction advance so the erosive process may lead to loss of the full thickness of the cartilage and even breakdown of underlying calcified cartilage and bone (Bromley *et al.*, 1985).

The cartilage and subchondral bone plate may also be eroded from the side adjacent to the marrow. The juxta-articular marrow loses haemopoietic cells and develops an infiltrate not dissimilar to that within the synovium, except that here macrophages represent a larger proportion of the infiltrate. Part of this unusual process is the formation and activation of multinucleated cells which will erode bone (osteoclasts), and similar cells that will erode calcified and non-calcified cartilage. These are known as chondroclasts (Bromley and Wooley, 1984; Fig. 13).

Thus attacked from both sides the cartilage is rapidly lost and, even if not completely lost, irreparably damaged.

BONE IN RHEUMATOID DISEASE

Juxta-articular Osteopenia

The osteoclastic resorption of bone is not restricted to the subchondral bone plate but there is a field change within the marrow in periarticular bone associated with a generalized increase in osteoclasis (and, to a lesser extent, osteoblastic activity) along all of the trabeculae within that region. This leads to trabecular osteopenia (Gardner,

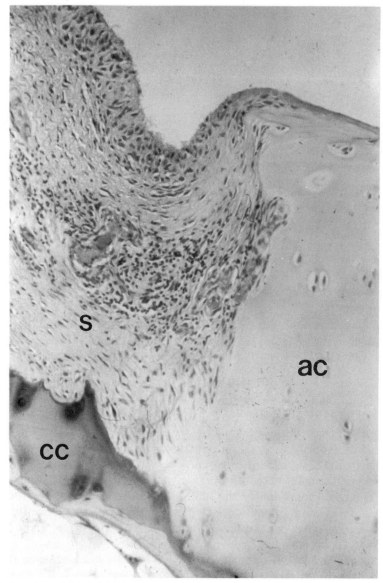

Figure 10. Erosion of the full thickness of articular cartilage (ac) by synovium (s). On the left only calcified cartilage (cc) remains. H and E ×80.

1986). It is believed that in rheumatoid disease osteoclasis is stimulated by IL-1 produced by the inflammatory cells.

Pseudocysts

Occasionally juxta-articular bone loss appears cystic on X-ray. These 'cysts' are not true cysts but erosion cavities filled with oedematous or myxoid fibrovascular tissue

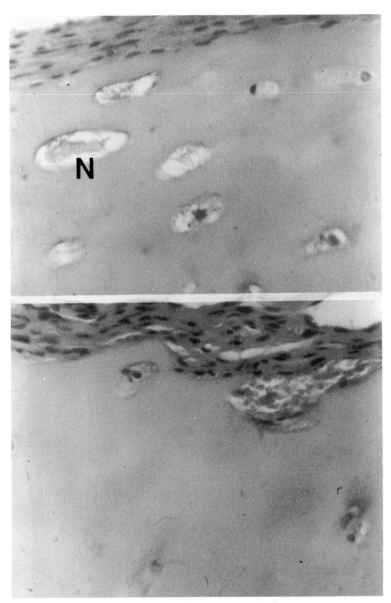

Figure 11. Pannus overlying cartilage is causing erosion. In the upper picture there is also chondrocytic chondrolysis (compare the osteocyte lacunae with those in the lower picture). Some of the chondrocytes are necrotic (N). H and E ×150.

that often communicate with eroded superficial cartilage. They are associated with lymphoplasmacytic inflammatory cell aggregates in the bone marrow.

Marginal erosions

Where the synovium is reflected over periosteal bone close to the insertion of the capsule, high levels of IL-1 released from local aggregates of inflammatory cells lead

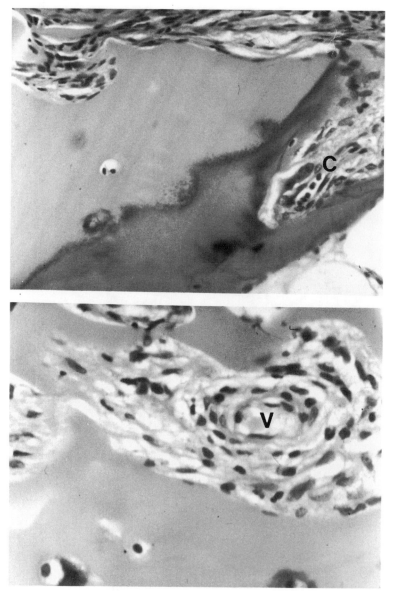

Figure 12. Two patterns of cartilage erosion. In the upper picture there is erosion of cartilage by pannus and calcified cartilage by a chondroclast (c). H and E ×100. In the lower picture the erosive front is very vascular (v). H and E ×150.

to active periosteal osteoclasis (Fig. 14) and the formation of the typical peripheral rheumatoid erosion (Bromley and Woolley, 1984).

Infarction

Of all the components of the joint avascular necrosis occurs most commonly in bone. This may be due to a vasculitis within end arteries supplying a region of juxta-articular bone or may be secondary to therapy (Williams *et al.*, 1988).

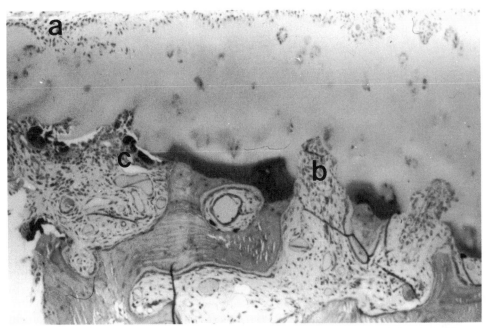

Figure 13. Cartilage erosion from 'above' (a) and 'below' (b). There is an inflammatory infiltrate in the subchondral marrow and chondroclastic erosion (c). H and E ×80.

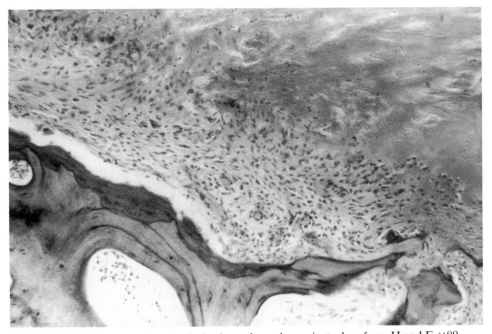

Figure 14. Erosion of periarticular bone from the periosteal surface. H and E ×80.

The cellular response of bone in rheumatoid arthritis is reviewed by Skerry and Gowen in Chapter 10, this volume.

BONE MARROW

Many of the changes seen in the bone marrow adjacent to articular surfaces have already been described. But there is one that is not specific to rheumatoid disease but nevertheless is characteristic even in the absence of excessive osteoclasis. The marrow at a little distance from the articular surface frequently shows loss of haemopoietic cells, oedema and occasional aggregates of lymphocytes. This may be particularly useful diagnostically when trying to decide if osteoarthritis is secondary to rheumatoid disease or not.

CAPSULE AND LIGAMENTS

The stability of the joint depends upon the structural integrity of the capsule and its ligamentous thickening. In turn the capsule only functions normally when the intra-articular structures are themselves normal allowing it to remain under tension. In rheumatoid disease loss of articular cartilage, as a consequence of erosion by pannus, leads to a closer approximation of the bone ends when the joint is in compression. In this position the capsule is no longer held under tension and lateral movement of the articular surfaces over one another can occur. When this happens the capsule is at risk of traumatic injury.

The joint capsule may also be involved in the inflammatory process, by extension from the adjacent synovium and this in its turn may lead to tissue damage and reparative scarring. The weakened capsule adds to the increased instability of the joint allowing the articular surfaces to move abnormally and excessively relative to one another, a process known as subluxation (Fig. 15). Subluxation may be no more than a cause of morbidity in most sites but should the dens of the axis sublux due to rheumatoid erosion of the transverse ligament of the atlas (Fig. 16) forced cervical flexion and extension can result in direct compression or embarrassment of the vasculative to the high spinal cord and death (Whaley and Dick, 1968). The cervical spine is also at risk because erosive destruction of the neurocentral joints can lead to subluxation of the vertebral bodies on one another with angulation and narrowing of the cervical spinal canal (Fig. 17).

SYNOVIAL FLUID

Synovial fluid is best regarded as a hypocellular, avascular liquid connective tissue in free chemical connection with synovium and cartilage (Freemont and Denton, 1991). Normal synovial fluid is present in small amounts, is viscid and contains less than 100 cells per cubic millimetre, most of which are synoviocytes or altered chondrocytes derived from synovium and cartilage, or rare lymphocytes and macrophages that have migrated into the fluid from the synovium.

In disease the volume of synovial fluid often increases and its composition and cellularity change. Some of the cellular changes are typical of rheumatoid disease and others reflect the degree of disease activity. It is during exacerbations of disease

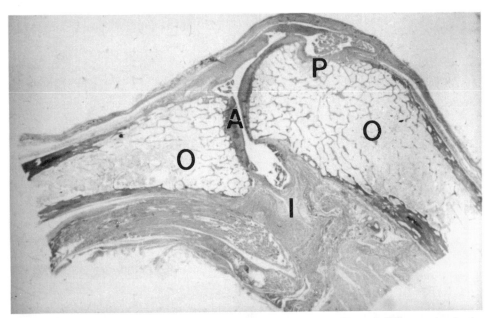

Figure 15. Subluxation of a metacarpal over a proximal phalanx. There is inflammation in the capsule (I), loss of articular cartilage (A), periarticular erosion (P) and medullary osteopenia (O). H and E ×10.

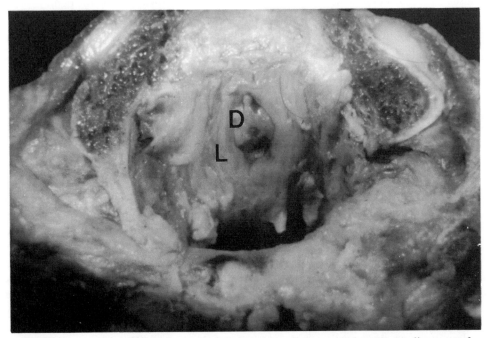

Figure 16. Protrusion of the dens of the axis (D) through the eroded transverse ligament of the atlas (L).

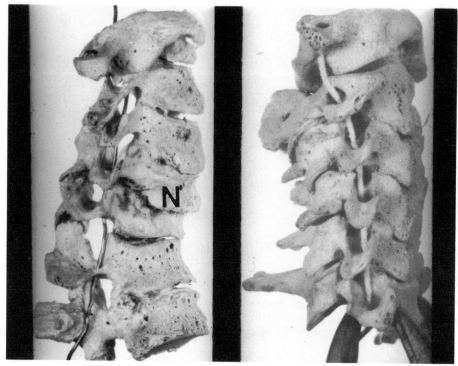

Figure 17. Gross destruction of the vertebral bodies adjacent to the neurocentral joints (N) causing distortion of the spinal anatomy. Compare with the normal spine on the right.

activity that the joints most commonly become distended with synovial fluid and it is at this time that aspiration is usually undertaken.

Typical Synovial Fluid Findings

Rheumatoid disease is essentially an erosive, destructive, primary inflammatory arthropathy and the synovial fluid findings reflect this.

The nucleated cell count is between 1500 and 50 000+ cells per millimetre (Cruikshank, 1954), the cells being predominantly polymorphs (Davies and Freemont, 1990; Fig. 18), a sharp contrast to the synovial inflammatory cell infiltrate.

If an unstained, undiluted sample of fresh synovial fluid (the 'wet prep') is examined by pseudophase, phase or Normarski phase light microscopy fragments of cartilage and bone, and crystals of hydroxyapatite eroded from the articular surfaces can be seen.

Immune complexes within the synovial fluid are phagocytosed by polymorphs and macrophages. The phagocytosed complexes can be visualized as apple green/black intracellular inclusions in the wet prep. The phagocytes containing these inclusions are called ragocytes (Hollander *et al.*, 1965). Ragocytes are found in many of the primary inflammatory arthropathies; but a ragocyte count in excess of 70% of all nucleated cells within the fluid is diagnostic of rheumatoid disease (Freemont and Denton, 1991). It should be noted that this level of ragocyte count can also be found in some

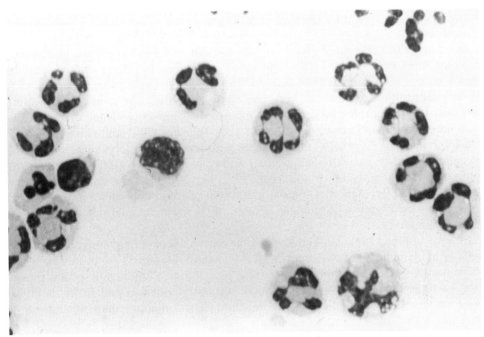

Figure 18. The synovial fluid in rheumatoid disease is populated mainly by polymorphs. Modified Giemsa ×500.

'secondary inflammatory arthropathies' – notably septic arthritis, and acute crystal arthritis, but organisms or crystals are also present in the fluid.

Cytocentrifugation of the synovial fluid specimen allows the various cell types within the fluid to be identified and, where possible, quantified. As already mentioned the predominant cell in most samples of synovial fluid aspirated from the joints of patients with rheumatoid disease is the polymorph (55–90% of all nucleated cells) the remainder being a mixture of lymphocytes (some of which are activated and enlarged) macrophages, mast cells and synoviocytes. The normal fate of infiltrating polymorphs is that they beome apoptotic (Kerr *et al.*, 1984), in which state they can remain for 24 h isolated from their environment, unresponsive to external events. At the end of this time apoptotic polymorphs suddenly disintegrate releasing their powerful digestive enzymes into the synovial fluid. Usually this is prevented as the apoptotic cells are digested and neutralized by specialized macrophages to form cytophagocytic macrophages (CPM). In rheumatoid disease, for reasons that are not clear, CPM formation is inhibited (Jones *et al.*, 1993). CPM cannot form and the apoptotic polymorphs remain within the fluid until they disintegrate when there is a release of their potent digestive products. This may contribute to cartilage degradation. The counterargument that polymorphs do not contribute to cartilage degradation is discussed in a number of chapters in this volume, particularly Chapters 9 and 18.

In approximately 9% of patients, lymphocytes are the most common cell within the synovial fluid aspirate (Davies *et al.*, 1988). This finding is not restricted to a single joint or to a specific phase of the disease, but runs true for the individual no matter which joint is aspirated or when. The disease progression in the joints of these patients is less aggressive with a longer time from presentation to the development of end-stage disease.

In addition to these major types of cells the synovial fluid in rheumatoid disease contains small numbers of cells found in no other disorder. They include multinucleate cells – both plasma cells and synoviocytes, and conventional, mononuclear plasma cells (although these are very rare considering the number in the synovium), *tart* cells (a polymorph containing a phagocytosed lymphocyte with a recognizable chromatin pattern), immunoblasts, *mott* cells (plasma cells containing numerous Russell bodies), *Reider* cells (macrophages with a distinctive lobulated nucleus surrounding a central pale attenuated area) and cells containing *Dohle* bodies (aggregates of microfilaments) (Freemont *et al.*, 1991; Fig. 19). The important factor linking many of these cells is that they form as a consequence of abnormalities in the cytoskeleton or cell membranes, presumably because of the nature of environment within the rheumatoid joints.

Several authors have described low concentrations of committed antigen-presenting cells within synovial fluid of patients with rheumatoid disease. These cannot be recognized morphologically within cytocentrifuge preparations, but have a specific phenotype that can be detected immunohistochemically. Henderson and Edwards (1987) have reviewed their significance and function. Their number does not appear to correlate with clinical features or therapy.

THE HISTOPATHOLOGY OF SYNOVIAL JOINTS IN THE EARLY PHASE

The features described above refer predominantly to the classical, chronic inflammatory process typical of rheumatoid disease. As already stated the disease process varies in activity with time and this is reflected in the histopathology of the joint. The histological appearances are particularly different from the chronic phase in early and end stage disease.

The histopathology of the joints in patients with early rheumatoid disease is not as well described as in classical or end stage disease, simply because recognition is difficult and biopsy, particularly of the articular surfaces, rare (Kulka *et al.*, 1955).

In the very earliest stages of the disease erosion of the cartilage and bone is not a feature, although marginal cartilage erosion occurs at a much earlier stage than is generally appreciated (Lipson, 1984). The earliest changes occur in the synovium. It is inflamed although, as might be expected, the inflammatory infiltrate is not as heavy as later. The notable difference, however, is the large number of polymorphs which can be identified within the synovial subintima. There is synoviocyte hypertrophy and hyperplasia in even the earliest biopsied lesions (Revell, 1987).

The synovial fluid shows no significant differences in early and established disease.

THE HISTOPATHOLOGY OF THE END STAGE JOINT IN RHEUMATOID DISEASE

The hallmarks of late disease are a decrease in inflammation and profound, irreparable damage to articular surfaces consequent upon the rheumatoid process. This

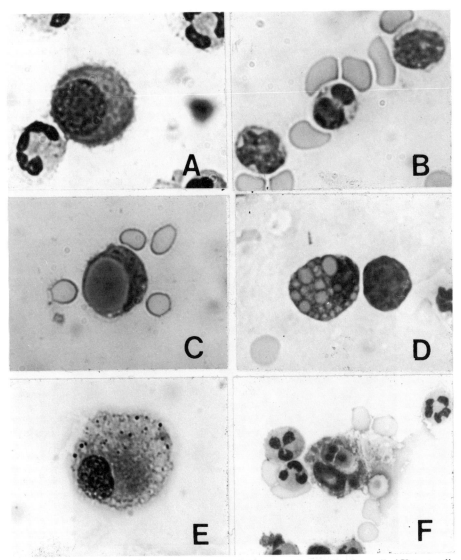

Figure 19. A selection of synovial fluid cells. (A) Plasma cell; (B) Reider cell; (C) tart cell; (D) mott cell; (E) synoviocyte; (F) CPM. Giemsa ×300 to ×600.

damage together with the abnormal loading of the joint secondary to subluxation causes rapid and profound development of osteoarthritis. The pattern of the osteoarthritis may be the same as that seen in conventional weight-bearing joints. This will include eburnation, subarticular bone sclerosis and cyst formation and the development of peripheral osteophytes (Fig. 20).

Equally common is a rather different and characteristic pattern of osteoarthritis. In this the shape of the articular surface is preserved but the cartilage is lost from the entire articular surface (Fig. 21). Frequently the subarticular bone plate is also lost. The articulating surface now consists of trabecular ends separated by highly vascular

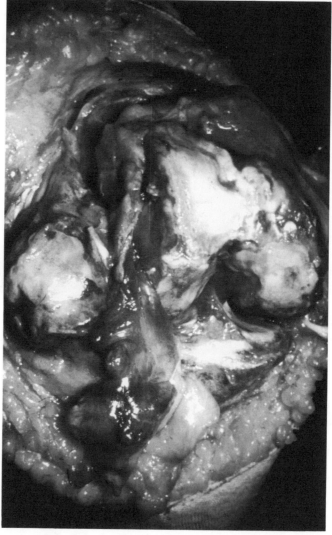

Figure 20. Gross erosion and secondary osteoarthritis of end stage rheumatoid disease of the knee.

fibrocartilaginous and fibrous tissue containing aggregates of inflammatory cells (Fig. 22). In this pattern of osteoarthritis there are few, if any, osteophytes. Even in clinically quiescent ('burnt out') disease lymphoid aggregates may still be found within the marrow up to several centimetres from the joint margin.

Patients who have advanced to end stage disease have often experienced infarction of their articular surface, either as a consequence of the vasculitic component of their primary disease or following therapy. These patients have a third pattern of disruption of the articular surface. Here the articular surface is destroyed focally, and the shape is considerably distorted and irregular. Trabecular ends and sheets of fibrous tissue represent the articular surface (Fig. 23).

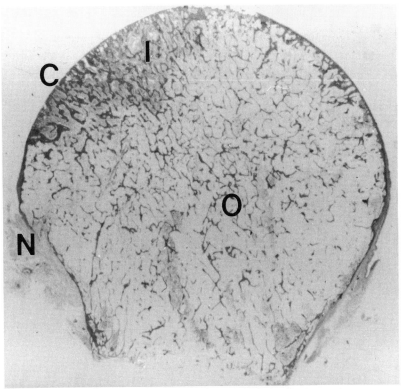

Figure 21. Rheumatoid disease of the humeral head. The shape of the head is preserved but there is total loss of cartilage (C) and no osteophytes (N). There is trabecular osteopenia (O) and an infarct (I). H and E ×4.

Synovial Fluid

The synovial fluid findings in end stage disease mirror the changes elsewhere within the joint. The cell count is usually low (<1000 cells/mm: Cruickshank, 1954) and the cells are predominately lymphocytes and macrophages. The fluid contains much debris from the damaged articular surface and synovium including cartilage, bone and fibrotic synovial villi.

Joint Replacement

End stage disease often necessitates treatment with prosthetic implantation. The surgery, the presence of the implant, and the subsequent and inevitable breakdown of the implant lead to a new set of appearances characterized by giant cell response to introduced and locally derived foreign debris.

As might be expected of any chronic disease, other arthropathies might be superimposed upon the rheumatoid process. The two most important are infection and crystal deposition disease.

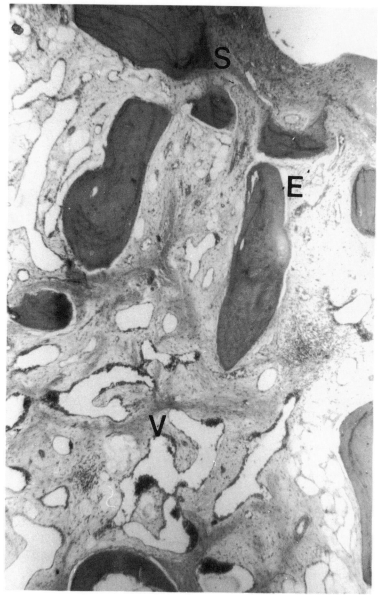

Figure 22. End stage rheumatoid disease. There is loss of cartilage and the subchondral bone plate (S), the articular surface consisting of trabecular ends (E) covered by fibrous tissue. The marrow is very vascular (V). H and E ×20.

SUPERIMPOSED ARTHROPATHIES

Infective Arthritis and Rheumatoid Disease

The immunosuppressive properties of the disease itself and some of its treatment modalities leave the patient with rheumatoid disease susceptible to infection. Even

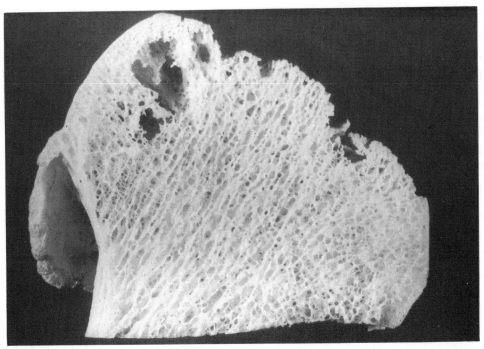

Figure 23. A macerated femoral head. There is gross destruction of the femoral head and the changes of secondary osteoarthritis.

untreated patients are at a high risk of developing sepsis within a diseased joint and in patients on immunosuppresant treatment non-bacterial articular infections with organisms such as fungi is also a risk.

The most common infection is a septic arthritis. The synovial inflammatory infiltrate changes and polymorphs dominate the pattern. There is acute synovial necrosis with nuclear debris of a type not seen normally in rheumatoid disease. The synovial fluid cell count increases and polymorphs increase to constitute more than 95% of the nucleated cells. More than 95% of the nucleated cells are ragocytes. The release of polymorph enzymes leads to further cartilage degradation and chondrocyte death. Polymorphs infiltrate the cartilage and within as little as 24 h of the onset of symptoms total destruction of the cartilage may have occurred (Curtiss, 1969).

A careful search for infective organisms is therefore indicated in tissue and synovial fluid from the joints of all rheumatoid patients in whom there is a clinical suspicion of infection.

Other forms of infective arthritis, such as tuberculous and fungal arthritis, occur with increased prevalence in patients with rheumatoid disease. The typical granulomata caused by these organisms are quite different to the inflammatory lesions of rheumatoid disease none of which are true granulomata.

Patients with inflamed rheumatoid joints are more likely to develop a reactive type of arthropathy, usually in a previously diseased joint, than is the general population. The major distinguishing feature of a superimposed reactive arthritis is the presence of CPM in the synovial fluid, even though in the underlying disease their formation is inhibited.

Crystals and Rheumatoid Disease

Hydroxyapatite from the damaged articular surface is a common finding in the synovium and synovial fluid of patients with rheumatoid disease, as is the presence of crystals of calcium pyrophosphate dihydrate in elderly patients with relatively quiescent disease. It is said that gout and rheumatoid disease do not co-exist. Although not entirely true it is an exceptionally rare occurrence. The difficulty lies in distinguishing coincidental crystal deposition from a crystal arthritis superimposed on the rheumatoid disease. When an acute crystal arthropathy is present, crystal aggregates will be found in the synovium and cartilage and intracellular crystals in the synovium and synovial fluid.

DISORDERS OF PERIARTICULAR STRUCTURES

Periarticular Cysts and Bursae

There is a tendency in rheumatoid disease for the development of periarticular cysts and bursae. These may become lined by a structure identical to rheumatoid synovium and distended with rheumatoid 'synovial fluid' (Wagner and Abgarowicz, 1970). With disease chronicity these cysts become distended with thick, turbid fluid heavily laden with crystals of cholesterol and cholesterol ester. The lining incorporates large numbers of lipid-laden macrophages and the cells within the bursal fluid consist predominantly of macrophages many of which have phagocytosed tiny lipid droplets (Freemont and Denton, 1991). Rheumatoid nodule-like lesions are more common in the walls of bursae than in synovia (Fig. 24). There is both intra- and extracellular iron. This and the cholesterol bear witness to recurrent haemorrhage into the bursa.

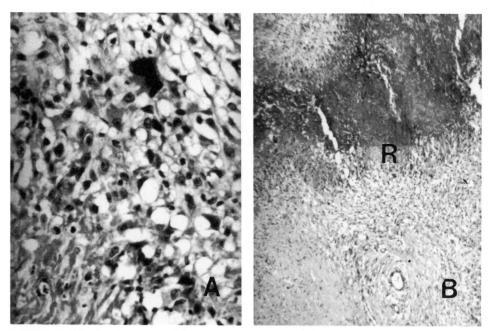

Figure 24. (A) Lipophages and (B) a rheumatoid nodule (R) in the wall of a para-articular bursa. H and E (A) ×100, (B) ×20.

Tendons and Tenosynovium

The inflammatory process seen in articular synovium may also occur in the synovium of tendon sheaths (tenosynovium). The tenosynovium becomes thickened distorting the overlying skin (Fig. 25). Inflammatory cells, inflammatory mediators and tissue

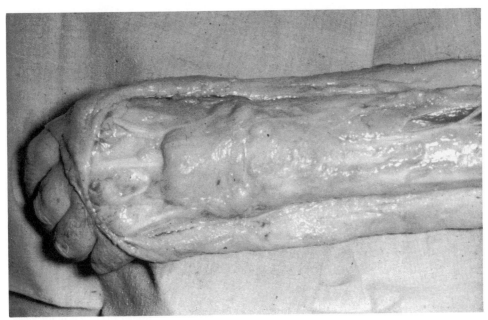

Figure 25. Thickened tenosynovium of the extensor tendons of the forearm from a patient with rheumatoid disease.

degrading enzymes are released from the tenosynovium into the tenosynovial fluid and together with inflammatory lesions within the tendon can lead to weakness and rupture of the tendon often with associated necrosis (Gardner, 1972; Razzano *et al.*, 1973).

CONCLUSIONS

This short review of the histopathology of the rheumatoid joint should be used as a reference point for the following chapters on the cellular and molecular mechanisms of the pathology of RA and the various chapters describing animal models of this most complex of diseases.

REFERENCES

Albrecht M, Marinetti GV, Jacox RF & Vaughan JH (1965) A biochemical and electron microscopy study of rice bodies from rheumatoid patients. *Arthritis Rheum* **8**: 1053–1063.

Bromley M & Woolley DE (1984) Chondroclasts and osteoclast at subchondral sites of erosion in the rheumatoid joint. *Arthritis Rheum* **27**: 968–975.

Bromley M, Fisher WD & Wooley DE (1984) Mast cells at sites of cartilage erosion in the rheumatoid joint. *Ann Rheum Dis* **43**: 76–79.

Bromley M, Bertfield H, Evanson JM & Woolley DE (1985) Bidirectional erosion of cartilage in the cartilage in the rheumatoid knee joint. *Ann Rheum Dis* **44**: 676–681.

Bywaters EGL (1982) Rheumatoid and other diseases of the cervical interspinous bursae, and changes in the spinous processes. *Ann Rheum Dis* **41**: 360–370.

Collins DH (1937) The subcutaneous nodule of rheumatoid arthritis. *J Rheumatol* **14**: 97–115.

Collins DH (1949) *The Pathology of Articular and Spinal Diseases*. London: Edward Arnold.

Cruickshank B (1954) The arteritis of rheumatoid arthritis. *Ann Rheum Dis* **13**: 136–146.

Curtiss PH (1969) Cartilage damage in septic arthritis. *Clin Orthop Rel Res* **64**: 87–90.

Davies DV (1946) The lymphatics of the synovial membrane. *J Anat* **80**: 21–23.

Davies MJ & Freemont AJ (1990) Synovial fluid cytology in rheumatoid arthritis. *International Medicine for the Specialist* **11**: 121–128.

Davies MJ, Denton J, Freemont AJ & Holt PJL (1988) Comparison of serial synovial fluid cytology in rheumatoid arthritis: delineation of subgroups with prognostic implications. *Ann Rheum Dis* **47**: 559–562.

Dean G, Hoyland JA, Denton J, Donn RP & Freemont AJ (1994) Mast cells in the synovium and synovial fluid in osteoarthritis. *Br J Rheumatol* (in press).

Edwards JCW, Mackay A, Moore AR & Willoughby DA (1983) The mode of formation of synovial villi. *Ann Rheum Dis* **42**: 585–590.

Eulderink F (1982) The synovial biopsy. In Berry CL (ed) *Bone and Joint Disease*, pp 26–72. New York: Springer-Verlag.

Fassbender HG (1975) *The Pathology of Rheumatoid Diseases*. Berlin: Springer-Verlag.

Freemont AJ (1987) Molecules controlling lymphocyte-endothelial interactions in lymph nodes are produced in vessels of inflamed synovium. *Ann Rheum Dis* **46**: 924–928.

Freemont AJ (1988) HEV-like vessels in lymphoid and non-lymphoid tissues. *Int Tissue React* **X(2)**: 85–88.

Freemont AJ & Denton J (1991) In Austin Gresham G (ed) *Atlas of Synovial Fluid Cytopathology. Current Histopathology Vol 18.* Dordrecht: Kluwer Academic.

Freemont AJ & Rutley C (1986) Distribution of immunoglobulin heavy chains in diseased synovia. *J Clin Pathol* **39**: 731–735.

Freemont AJ, Jones CJP, Bromley M & Andrews P (1984) Changes in vascular endothelium related to lymphocyte collections in diseased synovia. *Arth Rheum* **26**: 1427–1433.

Freemont AJ, Denton J, Chuck A, Holt PJL & Davies M (1991) Diagnostic value of synovial fluid microscopy: a reassessment and rationalisation. *Ann Rheum Dis* **50**: 101–107.

Gardner DL (1972) *Pathology of Rheumatoid Arthritis*. London: Edward Arnold.

Gardner DL (1986) Pathology of rheumatoid arthritis. In Scott JT (ed) *Copeman's Textbook of Rheumatic Diseases*, 6th edn, pp 604–652. Edinburgh: Churchill Livingstone.

Henderson B & Edwards JCW (1987) *The Synovial Lining in Health and Disease*. London: Chapman & Hall.

Hollander JL, McCarty DL, Astorga G & Castro-Murillo E (1965) Studies of the pathogenesis of rheumatoid joint inflammation. 1. The 'RA cell' and a working hypotheses. *Ann Intern Med* **62**: 271–280.

Hutton CW, Hinton C & Dieppe PA (1987) Inter-articular variation of synovial changes in knee arthritis: biopsy study comparing changes in patellofemoral synovium and the medial tibiofemoral synovium. *Br J Rheumatol* **26**: 5–8.

Igushi T, Kuroska M & Ziff M (1986) Electronmicroscopic study of HLA-DR and monocyte/macrophage staining cells in the rheumatoid synovial membrane. *Arthritis Rheum* **29**: 600–613.

Jones S, Denton J, Holt PLJ & Freemont AJ (1993) Possible clearance of polymorph leukocytes from synovial fluid by cytophagocytic mononuclear cells; implications for the pathogenesis of inflammatory arthritides. *Ann Rheum Dis* **52**: 121–126.

Kerr JRF, Bishop CJ & Searle J (1984) Apoptosis. In Anthony PP & McSween RNM (eds) *Recent Advances in Histopathology 12*, pp 1–15. Edinburgh: Churchill Livingstone.

Kulka JP, Bocking D, Ropes MW & Bauer W (1955) Early joint lesions of rheumatoid arthritis: report of eight cases, with knee biopsies of less than one year's duration. *Arch Pathol* **59**: 129–150.

Lipson SJ (1984) Rheumatoid arthritis of the cervical spine. *Clin Orthop Rel Res* **182**: 143–149.

Mitchell N & Shepard N (1970) The ultrastructure of articular cartilage in rheumatoid arthritis. *J Bone Joint Surg* **52-A**: 1405–1423.

Mohr W & Wessinghage D (1978) The relationship between polymorphonuclear granulocytes and cartilage destruction in rheumatoid arthritis. *Zeitschrift fur Rheumaforschung* **37**: 81–86.

Peyps MB (1988) Amyloids. In Santer M (ed) *Immunological Disease* (4th edn), pp 111–156. Boston: Little, Brown and Co.

Popert AJ et al. (1982) Frequency of occurrence, mode of development and significance of rice bodies in rheumatoid joints. *Ann Rheum Dis* **41**: 109–117.

Poulter LW et al. (1983) The involvement of interdigitating (antigen-presenting) cells in the pathogenesis of rheumatoid arthritis. *Clin Exp Immunol* **51**: 247–254.

Puchtler H, Sweat F & Levine M (1962) On the binding of Congo Red by amyloid. *J Histochem Cytochem* **10**: 355–364.

Razzano CD, Wilde AH & Phalen GS (1973) Bilateral rupture of the infrapatellar tendon in rheumatoid arthritis. *Clin Orthop Rel Res* **91**: 158–161.

Revell PA (1987) The synovial biopsy. In Anthony PP & McSween RNM (eds) *Recent Advances in Histopathology (No. 13)*, pp 79–93. Edinburgh: Churchill Livingstone.

Scott DGI, Bacon PA & Tribe CR (1981) Systemic rheumatoid vasculitis: a clinical and laboratory study of 50 cases. *Medicine* **60**: 288–297.

Wagner T & Abgarowicz T (1970) Microscopic appearance of Baker's cyst in cases of rheumatoid arthritis. *Rheumatologia* **8**: 21–60.

Whaley K & Dick WC (1968) Fatal subaxial dislocation of cervical spine in rheumatoid arthritis. *BMJ* **2**: 31.

Williams IA et al. (1988) Survey of the long-term incidence of osteonecrosis of the hip and adverse medical events in rheumatoid arthritis after high dose intravenous methylprednisolone. *Ann Rheum Dis* **47**: 930–933.

Youinou RY, Morrow JW, Lettin AWF, Lydyard PM & Roitt IM (1984) Specificity of plasma cells in the rheumatoid synovium. *Scand J Immunol* **20**: 307–315.

Ziff M (1974) Relation of cellular infiltration of rheumatoid synovial membrane to its immune response. *Arthritis Rheum* **17**: 313–319.

Zvaifler NJ & Silver RM (1985) Cellular immune events in the joints of patients with rheumatoid disease. In Gupta CJ & Talal N (eds) *Immunology of Rheumatic Diseases*, pp 517–542. New York: Plenum Medical.

6 Cellular Mechanisms of Cartilage Destruction

David E. Woolley

INTRODUCTION

Extensive proteolytic degradation of articular cartilage is a characteristic feature of joint destruction in rheumatoid arthritis (RA). This prolonged and often inexorable process is generally irreversible and is commonly associated with invasive, hypertrophied synovial pannus tissue comprised of synoviocytes and various inflammatory cells. Over the last 30 years numerous studies by pathologists and researchers have identified a spectrum of histopathological features and a variety of specific cell types at sites of cartilage erosion (Kulka *et al.*, 1955; Ball, 1969; Fassbender, 1975; Gardner, 1978; Mohr, 1984; Harris, 1989). Quite often the temptation has been to describe a 'pattern' or sequence of events leading to pannus development and/or cartilage loss. These hypotheses, despite being based on legitimate histological observations, have often resulted in disagreement and debate rather than gaining general acceptance. Some examples of the theories presented include the concept of synoviocyte transformation into erosive 'immature mesenchymal cells' (Fassbender, 1975, 1983), the importance of neutrophils in early erosions of small joints (Mohr and Wessinghage, 1978; Mohr, 1986), the contributions of dedifferentiated chondrocytes to the early development of pannus tissue (Mitrovic, 1985) and the sequential progression from the erosive early pannus of fibroblastic/macrophagic cells to an end-stage fibrotic scar tissue (Fassbender and Simmling-Annefeld, 1983; Takasugi and Inoue, 1988).

The histopathology of the rheumatoid lesion presented in most rheumatology textbooks invariably illustrates tissue sections derived from small joints. It is generally assumed that small joint histopathology is likely to be similar to that for large joints, but this is seldom the case. This chapter presents some histological observations of cartilage erosion sites using a variety of immunological and histochemical techniques. The basic questions which are essential for a better understanding of joint destruction in RA may be summarized as follows:

1. Which enzymes and specific cell types are responsible for cartilage erosion?
2. Is there a recognized pattern or sequence of cellular events for progressive joint destruction?
3. Which microenvironmental factors modulate proteinase expression at sites of cartilage erosion?

DEVELOPMENT OF PANNUS TISSUE

There is much debate and speculation concerning how pannus tissue develops. The junction between synovial tissue, cartilage and bone is considered of fundamental

Mechanisms and Models in Rheumatoid Arthritis
ISBN 0–12–340440–1

importance for the development of pannus and early cartilage erosions in rheumatoid joints (Fassbender, 1975). A recent histological analysis of this marginal tissue from normal joints has indicated that it closely resembles, and is in continuity with, adjacent synovial tissue, being comprised of both macrophages and type B synoviocytes (Allard *et al.*, 1990). The conventional view is that pannus develops from the adjacent synovial membrane with the sequential incorporation of inflammatory cells and neo-vascularization (Fassbender, 1975, 1983; Shiozawa *et al.*, 1983). However, other authors argue that dedifferentiated chondrocytes form the initial pannus (Mills, 1970; Barrie, 1981; Mitrovic, 1985) or that chondrocytes may partly contribute to its formation (Ziff, 1983; Cooke *et al.*, 1985; Allard *et al.*, 1987; Takasugi and Inoue, 1988). Although many authors have contributed to this debate, the four main schools of thought are briefly summarized below.

Fassbender (1975, 1983) is of the opinion that fibrin exudates are important for the initiation of local proliferation by synovial connective tissue cells which subsequently invade cartilage matrix and subchondral bone. These cells have been described as 'immature mesenchymal cells' having tumour-like morphology and erosive properties, but lacking neovascularization. Subsequently these cells become more fibroblastic-like with the addition of vascularization and the appearance of a few macrophages and lymphocytes. A permanent fibrous pannus develops with collagen deposition and increased numbers of macrophages, but with few lymphocytes, mast cells and neutrophils. Eventually the final mature pannus is characterized by dense collagenous scar tissue with few fibroblasts. While enlargement of chondrocytic lacunae is frequently observed in arthritides of long duration, Fassbender (1985) does not favour the concept of a chondrocyte contribution to the developing erosive pannus tissue.

Shiozawa (1985) is in general agreement with Fassbender's views, stating that chondrocytes do not play a major role in pannus formation, but they may contribute to the composition of non-invasive, fibrous pannus where the junction with cartilage is not clearly demarcated and may be continuous with the cartilage matrix. This latter observation has been confirmed and supported by Allard *et al.* (1987) who demonstrated that a 'transitional fibroblastic zone' at the cartilage–pannus junction represented chondrocyte-derived cells and matrix as demonstrated by the production of the glycosaminoglycans, keratan and chondroitin sulphate. Similarly, localization studies of lysozyme and S-100 protein indicated that, in a minority of knee joint specimens, chondrocytes were occasionally identified in fibrous pannus tissue (Takasugi and Inoue, 1988). Such observations may well represent 'healing' or 'repair' mechanisms since they are often associated with fibrous, rather quiescent, pannus tissue, typical of the chondroid metaplasia described by Mohr (1984, 1986) as late stage, reparative tissue.

Mitrovic (1985) on the other hand has attributed the formation of pannus tissue to the fibrous 'metaplasia' of hyaline cartilage where chondrocytes activated by inflammatory cytokines dedifferentiate, enlarge their lacunae, coalesce and finally break onto the cartilage surface to form a fibrous pannus. This subsequently becomes invaded by inflammatory cells from synovial fluid to form the inflamed synovial tissue. Thus pannus invasion consists primarily of local dedifferentiation of structurally organized tissues such as cartilage, bone and tendon in response to rheumatoid inflammation; the specialized cells lose their phenotype and acquire fibroblastic characteristics to destroy the cartilage.

Lastly, many studies have emphasized the role of polymorphonuclear neutrophils (PMNs) in cartilage erosion. PMNs have been described at the cartilage–pannus junction of small joint specimens showing early cartilage erosions (Mohr and Wessinghage, 1978; Mohr and Menninger, 1980; Mohr, 1986). Our own studies on rheumatoid knee joint specimens have only occasionally shown PMNs at the cartilage–pannus junction, but when seen it was apparent they had actively invaded the cartilage matrix (Bromley and Woolley, 1984a). By contrast, many pathologists are of the opinion that because PMNs are rarely seen in pannus tissue their contribution to cartilage degradation may be minimal (Fassbender, 1975; Vernon-Roberts, 1983; Harris, 1989).

THE RHEUMATOID LESION

There is no question that a wide spectrum of histological observations of the rheumatoid lesion is regularly encountered, not only between specimens but also within the same specimen. Figure 1 illustrates three examples of cartilage erosion by what is described as 'cellular' pannus tissue. These specimens were obtained from knee arthroplasties which of necessity represented late stage disease. However, by contrast to the 'cellular' pannus–cartilage junctions shown in Fig. 1, other tissue blocks from different sites of the same specimen showed thickened fibrous pannus tissue with relatively few fibroblasts (Bromley and Woolley, 1984a). Thus within the same specimen wide variations in joint histopathology are evident. Since this chapter is to focus on the cellular invasion and erosion of cartilage, little more will be said of the fibrous pannus tissue, except to state that this apparently quiescent form of pannus was observed in approximately 50% of all knee specimens examined.

The photomicrographs of the cartilage–pannus junctions in Fig. 1 illustrate that cells at the cartilage interface quite often present a different appearance to those of the supporting pannus. The cellular density and morphology observed at cartilage erosion sites in Fig. 1(b) and (c) clearly indicate microenvironments in which cellular activity is likely to be different to that of the fibrous overlay containing polarized fibroblastic-like cells. This concept of 'microenvironmental erosion sites' becomes more apparent when enzyme localization studies are taken into account.

CARTILAGE-DEGRADING ENZYMES

Collagen and proteoglycan are the two major components of cartilage and each requires specific enzymes for degradation. Several enzymes are known to attack proteoglycan, especially the serine proteinases derived from granulocytes, and the metalloproteinase stromelysin produced by synoviocytes and chondrocytes. Extracellular degradation of cartilage collagen fibrils is a complex process since the macromolecular organization involves combinations of collagen types II, XI and IX, each of which is vulnerable to different enzymes (Gadher et al., 1988, 1990). The breakdown of fibrillar collagen, which provides the skeletal framework for articular cartilage, invariably results in an irreversible loss of cartilage which cannot be repaired with its original properties. Collagenase is recognized as the prime rate-limiting enzyme for collagen fibril degradation (Woolley, 1984; Krane et al., 1990), although other enzymes may facilitate its action and can accelerate the rate of collagenolysis

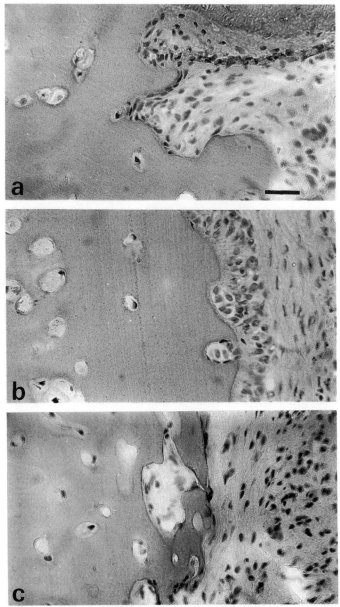

Figure 1. Photomicrographs of rheumatoid knee lesions to illustrate the variations observed for the distribution and morphology of cells at cartilage erosion sites. (a) Photomicrograph showing bone/cartilage: pannus junction with chondrocytes showing minimal chondrolytic activity. (b) Photomicrograph of cartilage–pannus junction showing differences in both the cellular morphology and distribution at the cartilage interface compared to the supporting fibroblastic pannus tissue. Note chondrocytes with enlarged lacunae apparently contributing to chondrolysis. (c) Photomicrograph of cartilage–pannus junction to illustrate a localized microenvironment containing cells with little fibrous tissue compared to the adjacent fibroblastic pannus tissue. Chondrocytes close to the junction appear atypical with evidence of chondrolytic activity. All tissue sections stained with methylene blue-azure II; bar = 50 μm.

(Woolley, 1984). The enzymology of cartilage and bone destruction is reviewed by both Poole *et al.* (Chapter 9, this volume) and Cawston (Chapter 17, this volume).

A role for lysosomal cathepsins in cartilage degradation has been strongly supported, but these enzymes are now thought to provide a predominantly intracellular contribution to matrix degradation via phagolysosomes with their acidic pH environment. The cysteine proteinases cathepsin B and cathepsin L have been shown to degrade cartilage collagens II, IX and XI (Maciewicz *et al.*, 1990) and proteoglycan aggregates (Nguyen *et al.*, 1990); and cathepsin B has been localized in synovial cells closely associated with the cartilage and bone of rheumatoid joints (Trabandt *et al.*, 1990). Both macrophages and activated fibroblasts contain lysosomes, and phagocytosis of cartilage and collagenous components has been demonstrated at sites of matrix resorption by synoviocytes (Harris *et al.*, 1977) and chondroclasts (Bromley and Woolley, 1984b). Thus, under specific conditions and in certain specimens the lysosomal cysteine proteinases could make a significant contribution to matrix degradation.

PROTEINASES AT CARTILAGE–PANNUS JUNCTIONS

Using FITC-immunolocalization techniques on cartilage–pannus junctions collagenase was demonstrated in approximately 40% of all cellular junctions examined (Woolley *et al.*, 1977). Whereas synovial tissue remote from the cartilage interface showed relatively few cells expressing collagenase, the enzyme was more frequently observed at cartilage erosion sites in a patchy distribution (Woolley *et al.*, 1980). Figure 2(a) shows immunoreactive collagenase concentrated at the cartilage–pannus interface; only occasionally were chondrocytes close to the junction found to be positive for this enzyme, and deeper chondrocytes were consistently negative for collagenase synthesis. Compared to collagenase, stromelysin was more frequently demonstrated in pannus tissue and junctional specimens (Fig. 2(b) and (c)), but again it was more commonly observed at sites of cartilage erosion. The local concentration of stromelysin at the edges of articular cartilage, and the demonstration of enzyme production by rounded cells at the cartilage interface is shown in Fig. 2. However, most specimens showed relatively few cells producing enzyme at the time of sampling, indicating that synthesis of these metalloproteinases is a transient, intermittent process rather than a persistent, autonomous activity (Woolley, 1984).

Histochemical studies of other proteinases have also added weight to the concept of localized, rather than widespread, production of degradative enzymes. Mast cell tryptase, a major component of mast cell granules, has often been demonstrated extracellularly at cartilage erosion sites (Figs 3(a) and 4(a)). The aggregation of mast cells at the rheumatoid lesion is an interesting phenomena (Bromley *et al.*, 1984; Woolley *et al.*, 1989), and tryptase release may have importance for the activation of metalloproteinase precursors such as prostromelysin (Gruber *et al.*, 1989). Intracellular acid phosphatase is demonstrated in Fig. 3(b) where cells apparently attacking the cartilage contain significant quantities of this lysosomal enzyme. It seems probable that the erosive cells at the interface are macrophages, but the important realization was that other macrophages away from the cartilage erosion site contained relatively little acid phosphatase. Similarly, non-specific esterase activity at the cartilage–pannus junction (Fig. 3(c)), an enzyme produced both by macrophages (Bromley and

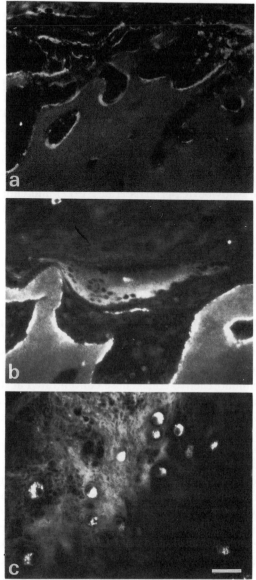

Figure 2. Photomicrographs to demonstrate the cartilage-degrading enzymes collagenase and stromelysin at cartilage erosion sites derived from rheumatoid knee specimens using FITC-immunolocalization. (a) Photomicrograph of immunoreactive collagenase at the cartilage–pannus junction. Collagenase was rarely observed in chondrocytes, and relatively little enzyme was demonstrable in the overlying pannus tissue (Woolley *et al.*, 1977). (b) Photomicrograph of immunoreactive stromelysin at cartilage erosion sites. Note the enzyme is largely restricted to the erosive edge of the cartilage matrix with relatively few cells positive for stromelysin. (c) Photomicrograph of immunoreactive stromelysin at the cartilage–pannus junction with cells and tissue of the pannus appearing positive for enzyme. By contrast the cartilage (on right) is negative although a few chondrocytes also appear to express stromelysin. The demonstration of both collagenase and stromelysin at cartilage erosion sites is invariably patchy, with many junctional specimens being devoid of enzyme. Indirect FITC-immunolocalization technique using a Zeiss Photomicroscope III. Bar = 25 μm for all micrographs.

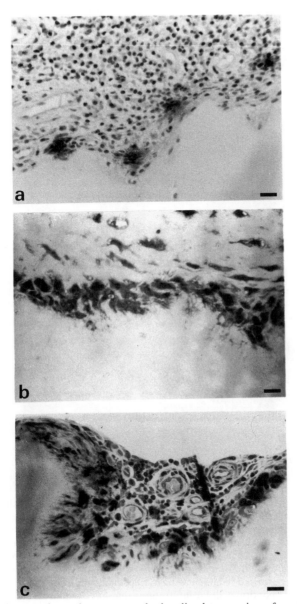

Figure 3. Photomicrographs to demonstrate the localized expression of proteinases at the cartilage–pannus junction of rheumatoid knee joints. (a) Extracellular mast cell tryptase associated with the cartilage–pannus junction. Demonstrated by the APAAP technique using monoclonal antibody to human tryptase. Bar = 30 μm. (b) Localized production of acid phosphatase at sites of cartilage erosion, probably produced by macrophages and some activated fibroblasts. Acid-phosphatase staining as described by Bromley and Woolley (1984b). Bar = 15 μm. (c) Non-specific esterase (α-naphthyl acetate esterase) activity confined to cells apparently invading and eroding articular cartilage. Enzyme demonstrated as described by Bromley and Woolley (1984a). Bar = 30 μm.

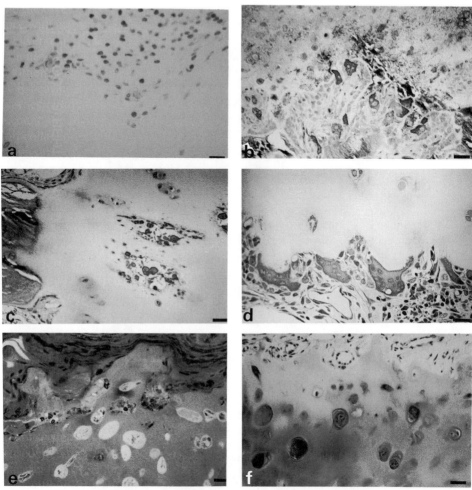

Figure 4. Photomicrographs to illustrate the various cellular mechanisms that may participate and contribute to the degradation of articular cartilage of rheumatoid knee joints. (a) Mast cells visualized by immunoreactive tryptase. The extracellular distribution of this enzyme is indicative of mast cell activation and granule release. APAAP technique and haematoxylin counterstain. Bar = 25 μm. (b) Osteoclastic resorption of subchondral bone and calcified cartilage. The multinucleated osteoclasts are stained for acid phosphatase and subchondral osteolytic activity has exposed hyaline cartilage to cellular infiltrations of bone-derived cells. Bar = 70 μm. (c) Subchondral cellular infiltrations that have penetrated the hyaline cartilage. Note that chondrolysis is associated with capillaries and acid-phosphatase positive cells (probably macrophages and activated chondrocytes). Tidemark zone on left. Bar = 50 μm. (d) Subchondral lesion showing multinucleated chondroclasts stained for acid phosphatase, attached to hyaline cartilage (Bromley and Woolley, 1984b). Bar = 25 μm. (e) Low power photomicrograph to illustrate chondrocyte-mediated chondrolysis. Note grossly enlarged chondrocytic lacunae subjacent to mast cell aggregates. Acid toluidine blue staining. Bar = 100 μm. (f) Low-power photomicrograph to illustrate localized proteoglycan or glycosaminoglycan synthesis by articular chondrocytes close to the cartilage–pannus junction. Same specimen as (e). Acid toluidine blue staining. Bar = 100 μm.

Woolley, 1984a) and activated fibroblasts (Gadher and Woolley, 1987), was also a common observation at cartilage erosion sites. Thus it seems reasonable to postulate that the macrophagic and fibroblastic phenotype is subject to change, especially in response to local microenvironmental factors which bring about the activation of catabolic processes. Such changes in proteinase expression by the macrophage population may be partly explained by developmental stages of mononuclear phagocytes (Shapiro *et al.*, 1991).

Although much emphasis has been placed on macrophages, fibroblasts and neutrophils as cells that have an effective role in cartilage destruction, the contribution of other cell types such as mast cells and multinucleated cells has often been underestimated (see Bromley *et al.*, 1984, 1985). Mast cells have a potent repertoire of preformed proteinases such as tryptase, chymase, carboxypeptidase and plasminogen activator, as well as many important mediators including histamine, heparin and cytokines (Woolley *et al.*, 1989; Galli, 1990). Thus the demonstration of mast cell tryptase in extracellular sites at the cartilage–pannus junction (Fig. 4(a)) also implies that other granule-derived enzymes and mediators are released in these locations (Norrby and Woolley, 1993).

SUBCHONDRAL CARTILAGE EROSION

Subchondral cartilage erosions have often been underestimated in large joint pathology even though generalized osteoporosis and juxta-articular bone loss are common features of late stage rheumatoid disease (Mills, 1970; Gardner, 1978; Ishikawa *et al.*, 1984; Leisen *et al.*, 1988; Bogoch *et al.*, 1988). During our studies on rheumatoid knee joints we became aware that approximately 40% of specimens showed extensive subchondral erosions of both bone and cartilage (Bromley and Woolley, 1984b; Bromley *et al.*, 1985). Increased numbers of multinucleated osteoclasts were often observed in osteolytic lesions (Fig. 4(b)) where the eventual breakdown of calcified cartilage resulted in penetration of hyaline cartilage by cellular infiltrations of bone-derived cells. Interestingly, this subchondral attack of the cartilage reflects a different cellular composition to that of the synovial pannus tissue (Bromley *et al.*, 1985). Figure 4(c) shows the cellular invasion of hyaline cartilage by acid-phosphatase positive cells and small blood vessels. However, a major feature of subchondral lesions are the multinucleated chondroclasts which show erosive attachments to the cartilage matrix (Fig. 4(d)). Chondroclasts are defined as multinucleate, acid-phosphatase positive cells with ruffled borders specifically associated with either calcified or hyaline cartilage, in contradistinction to osteoclasts which are exclusively associated with mineralized bone (Bromley and Woolley, 1984b). Chondroclasts were observed in approximately 30% of large joint specimens where they appeared to make a major contribution to the subchondral cartilage erosions of large joints, but we have rarely found these cells associated with small joint pathology (Woolley, 1992). By contrast, Leisen *et al.* (1988) have reported osteoclastic activity as a major component in the degradation of calcified cartilage and subchondral bone of metacarpal joints.

CHONDROCYTES AND CARTILAGE DEGRADATION

Several investigators have drawn attention to the importance of the chondrocyte in bringing about cartilage matrix degradation (Cooke *et al.*, 1985; Mitrovic, 1985). Our histological studies of large joints have shown that about 25% of specimens show significant chondrolysis by chondrocytes. One example is shown in Fig. 4(e) where the enlarged chondrocytic lacunae are associated with a pannus junction containing local concentrations of mast cells (Woolley *et al.*, 1985). Serial sectioning of such specimens indicated that these superficial lacunae were not in continuity with invasive pannus tissue and suggested that chondrocytes had been activated to bring about local lytic activity. By contrast, adjacent junctional areas of the same specimen revealed chondrocytes close to the pannus interface showing no signs of chondrolytic activity, and others where the synthesis of new glycosaminoglycans was evident (Fig. 4(f)), presumably in an attempt to repair earlier proteoglycan depletion (see Mitchell and Shepard, 1978). Thus within a single large joint specimen, chondrocytes were observed to participate in both catabolic and metabolic activities, probably indicating chondrocyte responsiveness to different local signals, and again emphasizing the microenvironmental nature of cartilage loss and repair.

It is well known that normal cartilage is generally resistant to invasion by a variety of tumour cells and blood vessels, a property explained by the presence of 'anti-invasion factors' (Kuettner *et al.*, 1978). Indeed, it has also been described as 'immunologically privileged' due to its avascular nature (Champion *et al.*, 1983), and is known to be a rich source of proteinase inhibitors (see Bromley *et al.*, 1985). The clear invasion of cartilage shown here by both synovial and bone-derived cells might suggest that 'rheumatoid' cartilage has become deficient in some of these properties. Thus the bidirectional erosion of cartilage might reflect changes in either the cartilage matrix components or their immunogenicity, as judged by the production of autoantibodies to specific cartilage components (Morgan, 1990). At present the nature of any compositional or structural changes in the cartilage of rheumatoid joints remains unclear.

T CELLS AND THE RHEUMATOID LESION

Our histological studies have rarely demonstrated T lymphocytes at sites of cartilage erosion, but many specimens contained some lymphocytic infiltration in pannus tissue remote from the cartilage junction (Bromley *et al.*, 1985). It is generally recognized that T lymphocytes are essential for initiating the inflammatory process (Cush and Lipsky, 1991); but their extended role in the maintenance and development of pannus tissue has been questioned (Firestein and Zvaifler, 1990; Firestein, 1991). Some have argued that T cells are not important for chronic synovitis and cartilage erosion, this being driven by an excessive and autonomous monokine production by the macrophage-like synoviocyte population (Firestein, 1991). Such a concept was supported by a study of radiological progression in RA joints where the number of macrophages, but not lymphocyte populations, infiltrating the synovial membrane was found to correlate with joint deterioration (Yanni *et al.*, 1991; Bresnihan, 1992). However, since the effects of T-cell lymphokines are known to stimulate or recruit such cells as macrophages, B cells, fibroblasts, mast cells and neutrophils, especially in relation to the production of autoantibodies, cytokines and prostaglandins, it seems probable that T cells continue to influence the pathophysiology of the pannus tissue, albeit at a distance from sites of cartilage erosion (see Gaston, 1993). The immunohistology of the rheumatoid synovium is described in Chapter 7, this volume).

BIDIRECTIONAL ATTACK OF ARTICULAR CARTILAGE

The bidirectional attack frequently observed in large joint pathology often demonstrated different cell types above and below the cartilage. Whereas macrophages and fibroblasts are the predominant cells of cartilage–synovial pannus junctions, multinucleated cells, macrophages and small blood vessels are the major components of the subchondral erosion front (Fig. 5). Multinucleated cells with acid phosphatase activity have never been observed at synovial pannus–cartilage junctions, and are considered unique to subchondral erosions. The diagrammatic illustration shown in Fig. 6 attempts to summarize our histochemical analyses of over 100 cellular junctions obtained from knee joint specimens. Although local concentrations of macrophages and fibroblasts were observed at cartilage erosion sites for most specimens, no regular pattern of cartilage erosion has emerged. Some specimens showed local accumulations of mast cells or neutrophils in discrete microfoci along cartilage–pannus junctions, often interspersed with macrophages or fibroblasts as the predominant cell type for some junctional specimens (Bromley and Woolley, 1984a; Woolley et al., 1985). Such observations indicate that the cellular composition at sites of cartilage erosion is very variable. These observations are best explained by microenvironments characterized by local cellular interchange which resemble inflammatory cycles along the cartilage erosion front. As yet we do not know the sequence of events, nor the relative time that each cell type occupies a particular location, but this cellular turnover and production of degradative enzymes is probably regulated by locally produced mediators.

Figure 7 illustrates the different patterns of cartilage erosion observed for large and small rheumatoid joint pathology. The low-power micrographs both show bidirectional attack on the articular cartilage, but whereas the large joint is usually characterized by a discontinuous pannus – each erosive front containing a different composition of erosive cells – the small joint pathology illustrates a continuous pannus tissue brought about by the 'capping' or 'underpinning' process (Uehlinger, 1971; Barrie, 1981; Wyllie, 1983). Whilst these two patterns of cartilage erosion are commonly observed for a significant proportion of large and small rheumatoid joints, respectively, other patterns and cellular permutations are often encountered.

MICROENVIRONMENTAL NATURE OF CARTILAGE DEGRADATION

So how can the observations reported here, and the quite disparate theories of pannus development and cartilage loss described in 'Development of pannus tissue', be reconciled? Firstly they are all largely based on morphological observations using a limited number of histochemical staining techniques. However, the major reason for the nonconformity of the hypotheses probably relates to the availability of tissue specimens from patients at different stages of the disease process, and to basic differences between small and large joint pathology. Most studies are limited to late-stage disease where arthroplasty is the last resort, thus bypassing the cellular events which may be more characteristic of early lesions. But is it correct to expect a unitary explanation for the development of pannus tissue and/or the cellular mechanisms of cartilage erosion? The great variations seen in tissue morphology at cartilage erosion sites from any large joint specimen strongly suggest that both erosive and reparative mechanisms are

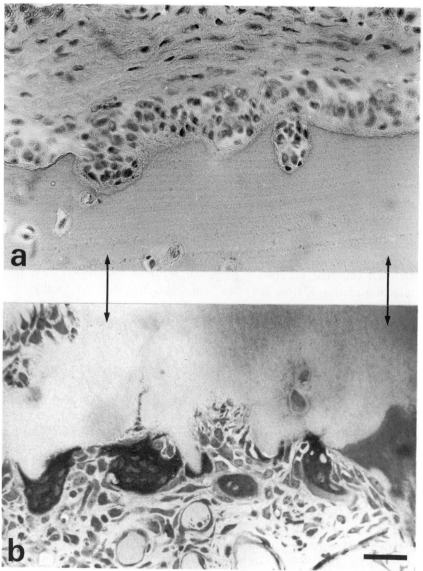

Figure 5. Bidirectional cartilage erosion, as illustrated by different cell types, is a common observation for large rheumatoid joint pathology. (a) Synovial pannus–cartilage junction showing localized foci of cartilage-degrading cells. Note the microenvironmental nature of localized matrix degradation, as judged by the different morphology and distribution of cells at erosion sites compared to the supporting pannus tissue. (b) Subchondral erosion of hyaline cartilage in the same specimen as (a), showing multinucleated chondroclasts, macrophages and small blood vessels as the common components of the resorptive interface. Note remnants of tidemark zone on far right. Acid phosphatase staining with methylene blue : azure II as counterstain. Bar = 50 µm.

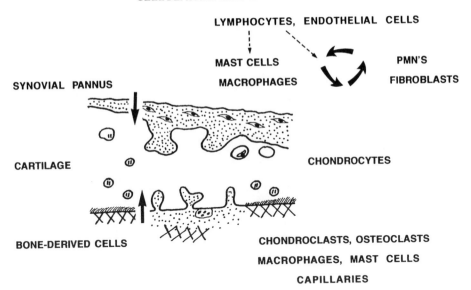

Figure 6. Diagram to illustrate the bidirectional erosion of cartilage which is a common feature of large joint pathology. The predominant cell types observed at the synovial pannus–cartilage junctions are variable but usually represent macrophages, fibroblasts, mast cells and neutrophils. Such observations are best explained by *microfocal inflammatory cycles.* By contrast, the predominant cells of the subchondral lesion are recognized as multinucleated chondroclasts/osteoclasts, macrophages and small blood vessels. Lymphocytes are seldom seen in close association with cartilage and were rarely seen in subchondral lesions (Bromley and Woolley, 1984a,b). Chondrolytic activity by chondrocytes was observed for only a minority of large joint specimens (*c.* 25%).

functional at different sites of the same specimen. This is best explained as microenvironmental activity which, in all probability, is regulated by locally derived mediators such as cytokines and prostanoids. Thus the 'patchy' demonstration of metalloproteinase expression, the local overexpression of glycosaminoglycan synthesis observed for some chondrocytes, the local increase in fibrous collagen deposits and chondroid metaplasia may all reflect local cellular responses to microenvironmental signals.

The view expressed here is that individual cartilage erosion sites are spatially and temporally separated, with the predominant cell type, identified at the time of sampling, subject to change brought about by locally co-ordinated signals. The cytokines, growth factors, neuropeptides, prostanoids, complement, immune complexes and local degradation products may all contribute to the local recruitment and regulation of specific cell functions. Many of these factors are derived from inflammatory cells that may occupy the rheumatoid lesion, and the enhanced production of cytokines in rheumatoid patients has been demonstrated by several studies (Lipsky *et al.*, 1989; Feldmann *et al.*, 1990; Arend and Dayer, 1990; Brennan *et al.*, 1991). The proinflammatory cytokines tumour necrosis factor α (TNFα) and interleukin-1 (IL-1) have been shown to play important roles in cartilage and bone degradation (see Feldmann *et al.*, 1990; Oyajobe and Russell, 1992); and TNFα has also been assigned a pivotal role in the pathogenesis of rheumatoid arthritis (Brennan *et al.*, 1992). Indeed, TNFα expression by cells of the monocyte/macrophage lineage has recently been demonstrated both in synovial tissue and at the cartilage–pannus junction (Chu

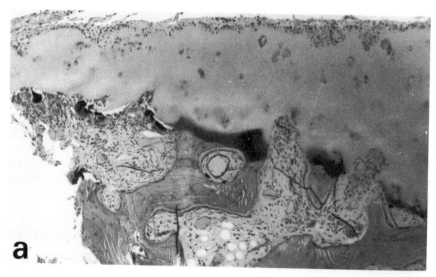

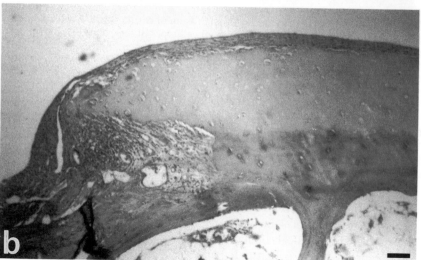

Figure 7. Large and small rheumatoid joints often show different patterns of cartilage degradation. (a) Bidirectional cartilage degradation observed in a rheumatoid knee specimen. Note cartilage erosion by overlying synovial pannus tissue as well as subchondral cellular infiltrations of hyaline cartilage and breaching of calcified tidemark zone. (b) 'Capping' of cartilage by a continuous synovial pannus tissue observed in a metacarpophalangial joint. Initial synovial erosions undercut the cartilage by resorption of subchondral bone with subsequent envelopment of the cartilage surface. Multinucleated osteoclasts/chondroclasts are less frequently seen in small joint pathology. Bar = 150 μm.

et al., 1991; see Chapter 2, this volume). Similarly, IL-1 and its receptor have been demonstrated in pannus cells at the cartilage–pannus junction, and also in some chondrocytes (Deleuran *et al.*, 1992). While these studies add weight to the concept of cytokine-driven degradation processes, the frequency of extracellular secretion of both TNFα and IL-1 remains uncertain, as too is the local availability of receptor antagonists and 'repair' cytokines such as transforming growth factor-β_1 (TGF-β_1) which may counter the TNFα and IL-1 stimulatory effects for proteinase expression. The recent demonstration of TNFα, IL-1α, IL-6, granulocyte-macrophage colony-stimulating factor (GM-CSF) and TGF-β in pannus cells at cartilage erosion sites showed that most cytokine-containing cells appeared to be macrophages (Chu *et al.*, 1992). By contrast, only TGF-β_1 was demonstrated in junctional regions with a fibrous, fibroblastic pannus tissue, and none of the cytokines was detected in synovial tissue from normal joints. Moreover, chondrocytes from all specimens were reported to be positive for IL-1α, TNFα, IL-6, GM-CSF and TGF-β_1, where it was suggested they may contribute to normal cartilage homeostasis (Chu *et al.*, 1992). In this context an association between IL-1α and TNFα production and stromelysin expression by human articular chondrocytes was reported by Shinmei *et al.* (1991). The role of growth factors in rheumatoid joint pathology is discussed in Chapter 12, this volume.

This concept of microenvironmental proteinase production is therefore dependent upon a complex sequence(s) of cellular events brought about by specific local signals derived from both cells, extracellular matrix and possibly immune complexes. Such signals are capable of initiating and promoting the activation, recruitment and proliferation of specific cells at sites of cartilage erosion. This applies not only to the cartilage–pannus junction but also to subchondral erosion sites where the factors mediating osteoblastic and osteoclastic activity have similarly been reviewed (Oyajobe and Russell, 1992; MacDonald and Gowen, 1992; see also Skerry and Gowen, Chapter 10, this volume). Thus the permutations of both cellular- and site-derived signals that may be operational at any one time are likely to regulate different cellular activities at discrete sites throughout the affected joint. Since such local regulation is likely to occur at both early and late stages of pannus formation and cartilage destruction, it is difficult to see how any of the proposed hypotheses described in 'Development of pannus tissue' can fully explain the rheumatoid lesion of most specimens.

CONCLUDING REMARKS

The questions originally posed in the Introduction can only be part-answered at present since the histological evidence for cartilage destruction suggests that many degradative mechanisms are possible.

The enzymes involved in cartilage degradation, of necessity, relate to the cells that occupy erosion sites. Whereas metalloproteinases are the predominant enzymes of mesenchymal cells such as synovial fibroblasts and chondrocytes, the serine proteinases are more commonly expressed by granulocytes such as PMNs and mast cells. Macrophages and mast cells not only have a broad repertoire of degradative enzymes, but also have the potential to produce the pro-inflammatory cytokines and mediators that stimulate proteinase expression by neighbouring cells.

While macroscopic patterns of cartilage erosion may be recognized, these are often quite different for the histopathology of large and small rheumatoid joints, and are often confounded by the specific stage of the disease process. At the microscopic level there appears to be great variation in the predominant cell types that occupy cartilage erosion sites, particularly well demonstrated in the bidirectional erosion of large joints where the subchondral erosion site contains cells considered unique to this erosive front.

Owing to the wide spectrum of histological observations reported for the rheumatoid lesion it is unlikely there is a unitary explanation for pannus development and cartilage erosion. The opinions expressed here favour the formation of discrete microenvironments in which cellular interactions driven by locally produced mediators and matrix components regulate both catabolic and reparative activities. Cartilage loss probably reflects an imbalance in these two processes, especially since cartilage matrix does not appear to be replenished with its original properties.

ACKNOWLEDGEMENTS

Many thanks are due to my colleagues Michael Bromley and Lynne Tetlow for all their contributions, to Harvey Bertfield and Michael Morris for the regular supply of surgical material, and to Tracy Bent and Margaret Williamson for preparation of the typescript. Special thanks also to David and Joan Cowie, Langrigg for providing such excellent facilities. This work has been supported by the Arthritis & Rheumatism Council.

REFERENCES

Allard SA, Muirden KD, Camplejohn KL & Maini RN (1987) Chondrocyte-derived cells and matrix at the rheumatoid cartilage–pannus junction identified with monoclonal antibodies. *Rheumatol Int* 7: 153–159.

Allard SA, Bayliss MT & Maini RN (1990) The synovium-cartilage junction of the normal human knee. *Arthritis Rheum* 33: 1170–1179.

Arend WP & Dayer JM (1990) Cytokines and cytokine inhibitors or antagonists in rheumatoid arthritis. *Arthritis Rheum* 33: 305–315.

Ball J (1969) Pathological aspects of rheumatoid arthritis. In Hijmans W, Paul WD & Herchel H (eds) *Early Synovectomy in Rheumatoid Arthritis*, pp 23–27. Amsterdam: Excepta Medica Foundation.

Barrie HJ (1981) Histological changes in rheumatoid disease of the metacarpal and metatarsal heads as seen in surgical material. *J Rheumatol* 8: 246–257.

Bogoch E, Gschwend N, Bogoch B, Rahn B & Perren S (1988) Juxtaarticular bone on experimental arthritis. *J Orthop Res* 6: 648–656.

Brennan FM, Field M, Chu CQ, Feldmann M & Maini RN (1991) Cytokine expression in rheumatoid arthritis. *Br J Rheumatol* 30: 76–80.

Brennan FM, Maini RN & Feldmann M (1992) TNFα – a pivotal role in rheumatoid arthritis? *Br J Rheumatol* 31: 293–298.

Bresnihan B (1992) The synovial lining cells in chronic arthritis. *Br J Rheumatol* 31: 433–436.

Bromley M & Woolley DE (1984a) Histopathology of the rheumatoid lesion: identification of cell types at sites of cartilage erosion. *Arthritis Rheum* 27: 857–863.

Bromley M & Woolley DE (1984b) Chondroclasts and osteoclasts at subchondral sites in the rheumatoid joint. *Arthritis Rheum* 27: 968–975.

Bromley M, Fisher WD & Woolley DE (1984) Mast cells at sites of cartilage erosion in the rheumatoid joint. *Ann Rheum Dis* 43: 76–79.

Bromley M, Bertfield H, Evanson JM & Woolley DE (1985) Bidirectional erosion of cartilage in the rheumatoid knee joint. *Ann Rheum Dis* 44: 676–681.

Champion BR, Sell S & Poole AR (1983) Immunity to homologous collagens and cartilage proteoglycans in rabbits. *Immunology* 48: 605–616.

Chu CQ, Field M, Feldmann M & Main RN (1991) Localisation of tumour necrosis factor α in synovial tissue and at the cartilage–pannus junction in patients with rheumatoid arthritis. *Arthritis Rheum* 34: 1125–1132.

Chu CQ, Field M, Allard S, Abney E, Feldmann M & Maini RN (1992) Detection of cytokines at the cartilage/pannus junction in patients with rheumatoid arthritis: implications for the role of cytokines in cartilage destruction and repair. *Br J Rheumatol* 32: 653–661.

Cooke TDV, Suni M & Maeda M (1985) Deleterious interactions of immune complexes in cartilage of experimental immune arthritis: the erosion of pannus-free hyaline cartilage. *Clin Orthop* **183**: 235–245.

Cush JJ & Lipsky PE (1991) Cellular basis for rheumatoid inflammation. *Clin Orthop Rel Res* **265**: 9–22.

Deleuran BW, Chu CQ, Field M, Brennan FM, Katsikis P, Feldmann M et al. (1992) Localisation of interleukin-1α, type 1 interleukin-1 receptor and interleukin-1 receptor antagonist in the synovial membrane and cartilage/pannus junction in rheumatoid arthritis. *Br J Rheumatol* **31**: 801–809.

Fassbender HG (1975) *Pathology of Rheumatic Diseases*, pp 75–137. Heidelberg: Springer-Verlag.

Fassbender HG (1983) Histomorphological basis of articular cartilage destruction in rheumatoid arthritis. *Coll Rel Res* **3**: 141–155.

Fassbender HG (1985) Is pannus a residue of inflammation? (Letter). *Arthritis Rheum* **27**: 956–957.

Fassbender HG & Simmling-Annefeld M (1983) The potential aggressiveness of synovial tissue in rheumatoid arthritis. *J Pathol* **139**: 399–406.

Feldmann M, Brennan FM, Chantry D, Haworth C, Turner M, Abney E et al. (1990) Cytokine production in the rheumatoid joint: implications for treatment. *Ann Rheum Dis* **49**: 480–486.

Firestein GS (1991) The immunopathogenesis of rheumatoid arthritis. *Curr Opinion Rheumatol* **3**: 398–406.

Firestein GS & Zvaifler NJ (1990) How important are T cells in chronic rheumatoid synovitis? *Arthritis Rheum* **33**: 768–773.

Gadher SJ & Woolley DE (1987) Comparative studies of adherent rheumatoid synovial cells in primary culture: characterisation of the dendritic (stellate) cell. *Rheumatol Int* **23**: 13–22.

Gadher SJ, Eyre DR, Duance VC, Wotton SF, Heck LW, Schmid TM et al. (1988) Susceptibility of cartilage collagens type II, IX, X and XI to human synovial collagenase and neutrophil elastase. *Eur J Biochem* **175**: 1–7.

Gadher SJ, Eyre DR, Wotton SF, Schimd TM & Woolley DE (1990) Degradation of cartilage collagens type II, IX, X and XI by enzymes derived from human articular chondrocytes. *Matrix* **10**: 154–163.

Galli SJ (1990) Biology of Disease. Microenvironmental regulation of mast cell development and phenotypic heterogeneity. *Lab Invest* **62**: 5–33.

Gardner DL (1978) Pathology of rheumatoid arthritis. In Scott JT (ed) *Copemans' Textbook of Rheumatic Diseases*, 6th edn, pp 199–250. Edinburgh: Churchill Livingstone.

Gaston H (1993) Synovial lymphocytes and the aetiology of synovitis. *Ann Rheum Dis* **52**: 517–521.

Gruber BL, Marchese MJ, Suzuki K, Schwartz LB, Okada Y, Nagase H et al. (1989) Synovial procollagenase activation by human mast cell tryptase. Dependence upon matrix metalloproteinase 3 activation. *J Clin Invest* **84**: 1657–1662.

Harris ED (1989) Pathogenesis of rheumatoid arthritis. In Kelley WN, Harris ED & Sledge CB (eds), pp 905–942. Philadelphia: WB Saunders.

Harris ED, Glauert AM & Murtey AHG (1977) Intracellular collagen fibres at the pannus–cartilage junctions in rheumatoid arthritis. *Arthritis Rheum* **20**: 657–665.

Ishikawa H, Ohno O & Hirohata K (1984) An electron microscopic study of the synovial-bone junction in rheumatoid arthritis. *Rheumatol Int* **4**: 1–8.

Krane SM, Conca W, Stephenson ML, Amento EP & Goldring MB (1990) Mechanisms of matrix degradation. *Ann NY Acad Sci* **580**: 340–354.

Kuettner KE, Pauli BU & Soble L (1978) Morphological studies on the resistance of cartilage to invasion by osteosarcoma cells *in vitro* and *in vivo*. *Cancer Res* **38**: 277–287.

Kulka JP, Bocking D, Ropes MW & Bauer WE (1955) Early joint lesions of rheumatoid arthritis. *Arch Pathol Lab Med* **59**: 129–150.

Leisen JCC, Duncan H, Riddle JM & Pitchford W (1988) The erosive front: a topographic study of the junction between the pannus and the subchondral plate in the macerated rheumatoid metacarpal head. *J Rheumatol* **15**: 17–22.

Lipsky PE, Davis LS, Cush JJ & Oppenheimer-Marks (1989) The role of cytokines in the pathogenesis of rheumatoid arthritis. *Springer Semin Immunopathol* **11**: 123–162.

MacDonald BR & Gowen M (1992) Cytokines and bone. *Br J Rheumatol* **31**: 149–155.

Maciewicz RA, Wotton SF, Etherington DJ & Duance VC (1990) Susceptibility of the cartilage collagens type II, IX and XI to degradation by the cysteine proteinases, cathepsin B and L. *FEBS Lett* **269**: 189–193.

Mills K (1970) Pathology of the knee joint in rheumatoid arthritis: a contribution to the understanding of synovectomy. *J Bone Joint Surg* **52B**: 746–756.

Mitchell NS & Shepard N (1978) Changes in proteoglycan and collagen in cartilage in rheumatoid arthritis. *J Bone Joint Surg* **60A**: 349–354.

Mitrovic D (1985) The mechanism of cartilage destruction in rheumatoid arthritis (letter). *Arthritis Rheum* **28**: 1192–1193.

Mohr W (1984) *Gelnkkrankheiten. Diagnostik und Pathogenese. Makroskopischer und histologischer strukturveranderungen.* Stuttgart: Georg Thieme Verlag.

Mohr W (1986) Pathobiochemistry of cartilage destruction. *J Clin Chem Clin Biochem* **24**: 949–951.

Mohr W & Menninger H (1980) Polymorphonuclear granulocytes at the pannus–cartilage joint in rheumatoid arthritis (letter). *Arthritis Rheum* **23**: 1413–1414.

Mohr W & Wessinghage D (1978) The relationship between polymorphonuclear granulocytes and cartilage destruction in rheumatoid arthritis. *Z Rheumatol* **37**: 81–86.

Morgan K (1990) What do anti-cartilage antibodies mean? *Ann Rheum Dis* **49**: 62–65.

Nguyen Q, Mort JS & Roughley PJ (1990) Cartilage proteoglycan aggregate is degraded more extensively by cathepsin L than by cathepsin B. *Biochem J* **266**: 569–573.

Norrby K & Woolley DE (1993) Role of mast cells in mitogenesis and angiogenesis in normal tissue and tumour tissue. *Adv. in the Biosciences* **89**: 71–116.

Oyajobe BO & Russell RGG (1992) Bone remodelling, cytokines and joint disease. In Kuettner K (ed) *Articular Cartilage and Osteoarthritis*, pp 333–348. New York: Raven Press.

Shapiro S, Campbell EJ, Senior RM & Welgus HG (1991) Proteinases secreted by human mononuclear phagocytes. *J Rheumatol* **18**: 95–98.

Shinmei M, Masuda K, Kikuchi T, Shimomura Y & Okada Y (1991) Production of cytokines by chondrocytes and its role in proteoglycan degradation. *J Rheumatol* **18** (**supplement** 27): 89–91.

Shiozawa S (1985) Reply to letter by Dr Mitrovic. *Arthritis Rheum* **28**: 1193–1195.

Shiozawa S, Shiozawa K and Fujita T (1983) Morphologic observations in the early phase of the cartilage–pannus junction: light and electron microscopic studies of active cellular pannus. *Arthritis Rheum* **26**: 472–478.

Takasugi S & Inoue (1988) Pannus tissue at the cartilage–synovium junction in rheumatoid arthritis. *Acta Med Okayama* **42**: 83–95.

Trabandt A, Aicher WK, Gay RE, Sukhatme VP, Nilson-Hamilton M, Hamilton RT et al. (1990) Expression of the collagenolytic and Ras-induced cysteine proteinase cathepsin L and proliferation-associated oncogenes in synovial cells and MRL/1 mice and patients with rheumatoid arthritis. *Matrix* **10**: 349–361.

Uehlinger E (1971) Bone changes in rheumatoid arthritis and their pathogenesis. In Muller W, Harwerth HG & Fehr K (eds) *Rheumatoid Arthritis: Pathogenic Mechanisms and Consequences in Therapeutics*, pp 25–36. London: Academic Press.

Vernon-Roberts R (1983) Rheumatoid joint pathology re-visited. In Carson-Dick W & Moll JMH (eds) *Recent Advances in Rheumatology 3*, pp 73–95. New York: Churchill Livingstone.

Woolley DE (1984) Mammaliam collagenases. In Piez KA & Reddi AH (eds) *Extracellular Matrix Biochemistry*, pp 119–157. New York: Elsevier.

Woolley DE (1992) Mast cells and histopathology of the rheumatoid lesion. In Balint G (ed) *Rheumatology, State of the Art*, pp 112–114. New York: Elsevier.

Woolley DE, Crossley MJ & Evanson JM (1977) Collagenase at sites of cartilage erosion in the rheumatoid joint. *Arthritis Rheum* **20**: 1231–1239.

Woolley DE, Tetlow LC & Evanson JM (1980) Collagenase immunolocalisation studies of rheumatoid and malignant tissues. In Woolley DE & Evanson JM (eds) *Collagenase in Normal and Pathological Connective Tissues*, pp 105–125. Chichester: John Wiley.

Woolley DE, Bromley M & Evanson JM (1985) Reply to Dr Cooke (letter). *Arthritis Rheum* **28**: 1197–1198.

Woolley DE, Bartholomew JS, Taylor DJ & Evanson JM (1989) Mast cells and rheumatoid arthritis. In Galli SJ & Austin KF (eds) *Mast Cell and Basophil Differentiation and Function in Health and Disease*, pp 183–193. New York: Raven Press.

Wyllie JC (1983) Histopathology of the subchondral bone lesion in rheumatoid arthritis. *J Rheumatol* **10**: 26–28.

Yanni G, Whelan A, Feighery C & Bresnihan B (1991) Greater monocyte/macrophage numbers in rheumatoid synovial membrane predict a worse radiological outcome. *Arthritis Rheum* **34**: S117.

Ziff M (1983) Factors involved in cartilage injury. *J Rheumatol* **11** (**supplement**): 13–25.

7 Immunohistochemistry of Rheumatoid Synovium

J.C.W. Edwards and L.S. Wilkinson

INTRODUCTION

The immunofluorescent technique was first described in 1950 (Coons and Kaplan, 1950) but its use for identification of cell type and function in synovium really began with the localization of collagenase by Woolley *et al.* in 1977. The general use of immunohistochemistry on synovial tissue did not occur until a few years later, at the time of the development of cell specific monoclonal antibodies (Edwards, 1980; Duke *et al.*, 1982).

Immunohistochemistry reached synovium late because no clear diagnostic value was seen in synovial histology, and indeed, disease assessment remains largely clinical. None the less, in terms of understanding the cellular interactions involved in the disease, immunohistochemistry has made a major contribution. A 'snapshot' of cells in a tissue section does not prove that any particular interaction is going on, but it does give an indication of what interactions may be occurring, and perhaps more importantly, those that are probably not. Thus, T cells are rarely seen in contact with intimal synoviocytes or chondrocytes and intimal macrophages do not show the range of gene expression that might be expected in response to γ-interferon (Bröker *et al.*, 1990).

For a time, monoclonal antibodies were seen as the definitive tools. More recently, the relative advantages of different techniques has become apparent and monoclonals are seen as part of a battery of tools including enzyme cytochemistry, conventional polyclonal antisera, *in situ* hybridization for mRNA and non-immunoglobulin based ligand-binding techniques. The range of conjugation and visualization techniques has greatly increased with the use of avidin–biotin systems, multiple fluorochromes, enzyme conjugates, haptens such as digoxigenin, gold particles and other metal enhancement systems. Different systems are useful in different circumstances and their relative merits for the analysis of synovial tissue are discussed at the end of this chapter.

When monoclonal antibodies first appeared there was a hope that they would provide markers of cell type of complete specificity and sensitivity. The aim was to identify 'helper T cells' or 'dendritic cells'. It has become clear that most gene products are expressed by a range of cells to a different degree under different conditions of maturation or stimulation. Thus CD4 is expressed both on lymphocytes and macrophages. When present on a cell carrying CD3, it indicates that the cell is in a position to interact with MHC Class II via a T-cell receptor; an interaction that may or may not involve a 'helper' function.

Similarly, the concept of 'activation markers' is becoming obsolete, since 'activation' implies that a cell can only respond to stimuli in one way. It is now clear that cells such as macrophages and fibroblasts can be stimulated by different mediators to express a number of different patterns of gene products. Thus, to understand the state

Mechanisms and Models in Rheumatoid Arthritis
ISBN 0–12–340440–1

of responsiveness of a given cell may require comparison of expression of several gene products and the use of multiple labelling techniques.

CELLULAR PATTERNS IN SYNOVIAL TISSUE

As described in Chapter 5 of this volume, synovium consists of a surface layer of cells, comprising both macrophages and fibroblast-like synoviocytes, beneath which is a connective tissue stroma or subintima (Edwards, 1987). In the normal tissue the subintima contains numerous venules and capillaries, scattered macrophages, fibroblasts and mast cells and, in adipose synovium, large numbers of adipocytes. Small numbers of T lymphocytes may also be present (Lindblad and Hedfors, 1987). In disease the tissue becomes infiltrated with lymphocytes, plasma cells, macrophages and to a lesser extent neutrophils. The general pattern of cellular infiltration is indicated in the ideogram (Plate II).

MACROPHAGES

Macrophages are present in normal synovium both in the intimal layer and within the subintima. In disease macrophage numbers increase markedly and their range of marker expression varies at different sites in the tissue (Hogg *et al.*, 1985; Salisbury *et al.*, 1987; Bröker *et al.*, 1990).

Intimal macrophages in normal synovium stand out as the major non-specific esterase (NSE) positive cells in the tissue. Macrophages present in the subintima show weaker NSE activity and also tend to have less cytoplasm. Macrophages at all sites in the tissue are CD68 positive, and other cells are negative. Unfortunately, this clear distinction is not present in disease (see below). In normal tissue, macrophages are in the minority in the intima and may be absent for stretches of 100 μm or more in sections.

The range of gene expression of normal intimal macrophages has not been studied in as much detail as that of macrophages in diseased tissue, largely because of shortage of truly normal tissue. However, the prominent NSE activity seen in these cells, their relatively large size and also the absence of α4 integrin expression (Edwards *et al.*, 1993a), suggests that they are not simply resting cells but have responded to some sort of stimulus. Their close proximity to fibroblastic synoviocytes, which constitutively express VCAM-1 may be relevant, since Gharavi *et al.* (1993) have shown that macrophages cocultured with VCAM-1 expressing fibroblasts are sensitized to the production of tumour necrosis factor in response to inflammatory mediators.

In rheumatoid arthritis (RA) intimal macrophages increase in numbers and are usually in the majority (although there can be great variation in the proportions of the two cell types within a single specimen) (Plate III). This contrasts with osteoarthritis, in which more than 50% of intimal cells are synoviocytes (Edwards and Wilkinson, in preparation).

The apparent thickness of the intima in RA is partly an artefact of oblique sectioning of a complex villous surface (the intima may appear five or more cells thick, when three is probably the usual maximum). Moreover, the distinction between intimal and deep cells becomes unclear. Rheumatoid intima is often stratified with a layer of macrophages lying superficial to the synoviocytes. Beneath the synoviocytes macrophages are again present in a third zone which may appear to be continuous with the intima but is best regarded is distinct. Synoviocyte markers such as VCAM-1 (Wilkinson *et al.*, 1993a) are useful in identifying the true extent of the intima (Plate IV) (see also Chapter 8, this volume).

Rheumatoid intimal macrophages are consistently NSE positive, CD14 dull, and CD64 dull, whereas subintimal macrophages are more often strongly CD14, CD64 positive and only weakly NSE positive (Bröker *et al.*, 1990), although scattered cells showing strong NSE activity are present in all layers of the tissue. All macrophages in rheumatoid tissue appear to be CD68 positive, but within the intima fibroblastic synoviocytes may carry modest amounts of CD68 as well (Wilkinson *et al.*, 1992). This is not surprising, since CD68 is associated with lysosomes and synoviocytes carry large numbers of lysosomes in diseased tissue. Cultured fibroblasts can show quite strong CD68 expression. The prominent expression of CD68 on macrophages is thus useful for identification under some conditions but must be interpreted with caution.

Rheumatoid intimal macrophages show prominent expression of a wide range of membrane antigens found on stimulated leukocytes, including MHC class II (Duke *et al.*, 1982), as might be expected from such cells in an inflammatory environment. One of the difficulties encountered in interpreting the distribution of membrane antigens in the intima is that the two cell types carry interdigitating processes which form a mesh between the cells. This means that a membrane antigen present on only one cell type may appear to be present around all intimal cells. This may have given rise to confusion in the past over the nature of animal cell populations and the extent of MHC class II expression in particular. This point is considered again below in the technical section.

Rheumatoid intimal macrophages show prominent acid phosphatase activity and fibroblastic synoviocytes relatively lower levels. Tartrate-resistant acid phosphatase activity is restricted to strongly CD68 positive giant cells found within or just beneath the intima, and clusters of closely associated mononuclear cells (Wilkinson *et al.*, 1993b). These cells also express the vitronectin receptor and thus have histochemical features associated with osteoclasts (Plate V). Whether they can truly be classified as osteoclasts depends somewhat on definition, but may become clearer when information is available about their calcitonin receptor status. The rather different-shaped giant cells found in the deep stroma of pigmented villonodular synovitis tissue are known to be calcitonin receptor positive. Interestingly, the intimal macrophage giant cells in rheumatoid arthritis may coexist with synoviocyte giant cells which rarely show more than four nuclei (Wilkinson *et al.*, 1993b).

Cells carrying macrophage markers occur within lymphocyte clusters and within the stroma of rheumatoid synovium (Duke *et al.*, 1982; Bröker *et al.*, 1990). The nature of macrophages and related cells within lymphocyte clusters remains unclear as will be discussed in more detail in the following section on antigen-presenting cells. Macrophages in the deep stroma away from lymphocyte clusters tend to be organized in loose groups around venules and frequently contain haemosiderin. They have an elongated outline very similar to neighbouring fibroblasts and a small proportion can be seen to be in contact with VCAM-1 positive stromal fibroblasts via cytoplasmic processes (Wilkinson *et al.*, 1993a).

Palmer and colleagues (Palmer *et al.*, 1987) have described a subset of macrophages in rheumatoid synovium and nodular tissue, associated with areas of necrosis, which stain strongly with an antibody (5.5) to the MRP8/14 heterodimeric complex of S100 calcium-binding proteins. Some of this staining may relate to neutrophil debris, since MRP8/14 is prominent in neutrophil cytoplasm, but a significant part of the staining appears to be intrinsic to the macrophages. Whether MRP8/14 plays a role in necrosis or whether it is simply a marker of a macrophage response to local cell death remains to be established.

The relationship between synovial macrophage subpopulations in terms of life history is a matter of debate. The simplest view is that all synovial macrophages derive from blood-borne monocytes and that their functional status within the tissue is determined by the microenvironment around the vessel through which they migrate. It seems likely that intimal macrophages move up to the surface having migrated through superficial venules, and may change their behaviour on arrival at the surface. However, the above view may be too simple. There is some evidence that, at least in mice, there are two populations of macrophages, those that are seeded in the tissue early in life and which form a resident population and those that are recruited during inflammation. This may be particularly relevant to tissues with specialized 'resident' forms, such as the Kuppfer cells of the liver. The resident population is seen as having a limited potential to divide and maintain itself in response to locally produced growth factors.

It is possible that there is a resident macrophage population in synovium and that during inflammation a distinct subset of macrophages appears. Naito has shown that osteopetrotic mice which lack CSF-1 have no synovial macrophages (Naito et al., 1991). Normal intimal macrophages have been suggested to be resident on the basis that they do not reappear in OP mouse synovium following infusion of CSF-1 (Cecchini, pers. commun.). It is, therefore, conceivable that some of the increase in intimal cell numbers seen in disease is due to local division. However, the lack of evidence of macrophage division in synovium, based on the use of the Ki67 antibody (Revell et al., 1987), suggests that macrophage numbers increase by immigration. There is no way of distinguishing a resident and an immigrant population in human tissues except on the basis of what are considered by most to be simply markers of maturation, and to date no evidence has been found for two macrophage phenotypes in the intima of inflamed synovium.

OTHER ANTIGEN-PRESENTING CELLS

Although typical phagocytic macrophages are effective antigen-presenting cells they are viewed as less efficient than so-called dendritic antigen-presenting cells. Terminology is difficult in this area. There are two quite distinct types of dendritic antigen-presenting cell. The first type show prominent expression of MHC class II and appear to be bone-marrow derived. They include the interdigitating dendritic cells (IDC) of T cell areas in lymphoid tissue and the Langerhans cells of skin. The second type are follicular dendritic reticulum cells (FDRC), which do not express class II but express complement receptors, VCAM-1 and a molecule recognized by the antibody R4/23. FDRC are probably derived from resident stromal cells and form a dense meshwork of processes in lymphoid follicle centres.

Within synovium the situation is further confused by the fact that normal fibroblast-like synoviocytes are 'dendritic' and the collagenase secreting fibroblasts found in rheumatoid synovium are even more so, thus the term dendritic has several unrelated connotations. Synoviocytes express VCAM-1 but not the R4/23 epitope (Wilkinson *et al.*, 1993a). FDRC do not have high uridine diphosphoglucose dehydrogenase (UDPGD) activity. Thus, although expression of VCAM-1 may be linked in some way to a dendritic cell shape, synoviocytes and FDRCs are otherwise not particularly closely related in terms of function. Interestingly, the unknown molecule recognized by the antibody 67 is also present on both synoviocytes and cells within germinal centres (Palmer *et al.*, 1985).

A number of workers have provided evidence for the presence of IDCs in rheumatoid synovium (Salisbury *et al.*, 1987; Wilkinson *et al.*, 1990). The antibody RFD1 appears to mark such cells preferentially in lymphoid tissue. Even in normal synovium a few RFD1 positive cells can be found, which do not appear to be typical macrophages, in that they are CD68 negative. However, these are extremely sparsely scattered in the intima. In rheumatoid synovium intimal macrophages are frequently RFD1 positive and a few RFD1 positive CD68 negative cells can be found. Large RFD1 positive cells are seen within lymphocyte aggregates which lack CD68 and other mature macrophage marker, RFD7. However, as is the case in lymphoid tissue, large CD68 positive macrophages are also present and contribute to the overlapping mesh of cell processes. Cells with features of FDRC are also present in at least some samples of rheumatoid synovium. At the centres of lymphocyte aggregates, in association with B lymphocytes, are large spidery cells which express VCAM-1 as do FDRC and in well-formed aggregates these cells express the R4/23 epitope. When true germinal centres are present, the distribution of VCAM-1 and R4/23 is identical, as found in lymphoid tissue (Wilkinson *et al.*, 1993a).

It has to be said that with current optical and sectioning techniques it is not always possible to be sure of the identity of cells responsible for the mesh of staining seen in lymphoid aggregates. While cells with features of FDRC appear to be distinct, it is uncertain whether there is a black and white distinction between macrophages and IDC, just as there may be an overlap between macrophages and osteoclasts. IDC and macrophages may well have a common origin and diverge in terms of function in the peripheral tissues in response to their microenvironment. Segregation of the two phenotypes may be blurred within inflamed tissue.

LYMPHOCYTES

Rheumatoid synovium consistently contains increased numbers of lymphocytes and in some samples up to 80% of the tissue may be taken up by a dense accumulation of lymphocytes and plasma cells. However, in some samples lymphoid cells are relatively sparse. As discussed below, this may actually be associated with more aggressive destructive disease, as suggested originally by Fassbender (1975).

Lymphocytes may be scattered loosely in the tissue, gathered in small clusters or larger aggregates with a distinct follicular structure. In about 10% of samples from patients with established disease there are fully formed secondary follicular structures with germinal centres.

Early attempts to classify the lymphocytes in rheumatoid synovium made use of the ability of T cells to form 'E' rosettes with sheep red cells (van Boxel and Paget, 1975; Meijer *et al.*, 1976). Studies of disaggregated cells had shown T cells to outnumber B cells and application of sheep red cells to sections also suggested that T cells were predominant. However, the rosette technique did not allow for identification of individual cells in tissue sections.

Early monoclonal antibody studies confirmed that T cells were in the majority (Duke *et al.*, 1982) and also showed that in large lymphocyte aggregates T and B cells were arranged within follicular structures in a way similar to that seen in lymphoid tissue. Small aggregates are composed almost exclusively of T cells, with occasional B cells at the centre, often around a central venule with plump endothelial cells. Larger aggregates tend to have a central group of B cells, in the largest structures forming the germinal centre. Wherever B cells are present at the centre of T cell aggregates associated cells are found expressing VCAM-1 (a similar pattern occurs in labial tissue from patients with Sjögren's syndrome) (Edwards *et al.*, 1993a). Small lymphocytes diffusely scattered in the tissue stroma are mostly T cells although in some samples they may be outnumbered by B-cell derived plasma cells.

T CELLS

The majority of the T cells present are CD4 positive (Duke *et al.*, 1982). It is worth noting that although macrophages show less bright CD4 staining they may outnumber T cells in the tissue, and identification of CD4 positive T cells requires double labelling with CD3 and CD4. This has possible implications for the use of monoclonal anti-CD4 antibodies as therapeutic agents. CD8 positive cells are less numerous and tend to occur loosely scattered in the subintimal stroma rather than in aggregates.

T cells carry a surface molecule, CD45, which occurs in two forms, CD45RO and CD45RA. Cells carrying CD45RO are considered to carry immunological memory and to have been primed by interaction with antigen. CD45RA cells are, in contrast, seen as immunologically naive. The great majority of cells in the synovium in RA are CD45RO positive (Pitzalis *et al.*, 1987) and double labelling studies have confirmed the predominant T cell phenotype is, as expected, CD4$^+$CD45RO$^+$. The CD45RO status of rheumatoid synovial T cells could be taken as indicative of a specific antigen-driven response within the tissue. However, considering the chronicity of the lesion it may be that CD45RO positivity is to be expected from the longstanding presence of cells in the tissue.

The T-cell receptor is polymorphic and a number of studies have examined the pattern of Vβ region subclasses expressed in rheumatoid tissue (Paliard *et al.*, 1991). Paliard found lower rates of Vβ 14 expression in peripheral blood T cells as compared to T cells derived from joints but Howell (Howell *et al.*, 1991) found a wide range of Vβ mRNA and no evidence of preferential Vβ 14 usage in the joint (see Chapters 2 and 3, this volume).

A small proportion of T cells express a receptor composed of γ and δ rather than α and β chains. Brennan (Brennan *et al.*, 1988) found a higher proportion of γ/δ than α/β bearing cells in rheumatoid synovium when compared to peripheral blood. However, this has not been a universal finding. Smith and coworkers (Smith *et al.*, 1990) found few γ/δ T cells in rheumatoid synovial tissues but noted a relative increase in the A13 as opposed to the BB3 subset. Recent studies have described the expression of a variety of other T-cell products associated with antigen recognition and proliferation (see Chapter 2, this volume).

B CELLS AND PLASMA CELLS

B lymphocytes, as indicated by markers such as CD19 and CD22, are found chiefly at the centres of larger T-cell aggregates in close association with cells expressing VCAM-1 and, in fully formed germinal centres, R4/23 (Edwards *et al.*, 1993a). Plasma cells are, in contrast, found diffusely distributed outside the tight lymphocyte clusters within the subintimal stroma. Their numbers vary, but in some cases they appear to make up the majority of all nucleated cells. Cells producing all three major immunoglobulin classes can be demonstrated immunochemically in rheumatoid synovia (Revell and Mayston, 1982) although IgA-secreting cells are very much in the minority. No generally applicable method for identifying antibody specificity in cells in sections is available, although it is theoretically feasible and T-cell specificities have been demonstrated in other contexts using labelled antigen-binding techniques. Rheumatoid factor activity in rheumatoid synovial plasma cells has been studied using the binding of heat aggregated IgG (HAIG) to pepsin-treated sections (McCormick, 1963). Binding of HAIG can be demonstrated in this way, but Revell (pers. commun.) has shed doubt on the specificity of the binding and it may be that the presence of antibody within a solid phase (the section) alters the binding kinetics.

The possibility of restricted clonality and preferential use of certain Vh genes has been addressed using antibodies to κ and λ light chains. Although preferential Vh gene usage has been reported by some authors, the general view is the B-cell response in rheumatoid tissue is consistent with a broad polyclonal antigen-driven response.

POLYMORPHS

Polymorphs are readily identifiable immunochemically by the presence of elastase or X hapten. They can also be identified by their peroxidase activity using the same reagents used for developing peroxidase conjugates in immunoperoxidase techniques with a modified incubation protocol. Polymorphs are very rare in normal synovium but are consistently present in rheumatoid synovium in small numbers, chiefly between the superficial venular net and the tissue surface. Fewer neutrophils are demonstrable by peroxidase activity than by elastase content and whereas elastase may be seen as a halo around polymorph rests in the tissue, peroxidase activity tends to be limited to intact cells, suggesting that peroxidase is rapidly inactivated once released from the cell. However, at the centre of rheumatoid nodules and within fibrin on the surface of rheumatoid synovium active extracellular peroxidase can be seen (Edwards *et al.*, in preparation). The significance of this is uncertain but a failure to control extracellular activity of the enzyme could have implications for the generation of altered self antigens.

RESIDENT CELLS

Resident synovial cells and in particular the intimal synoviocytes are considered in more detail in Chapter 8, this volume. In recent years the ability to separate synoviocytes from macrophages immunochemically has allowed the delineation of synoviocyte gene expression in some detail. Synoviocytes have a high activity of uridine diphosphoglucose dehydrogenase, high content of prolyl hydroxylase, prominent expression of the adhesion molecules VCAM-1, CD44 and β1 integrin and the unknown antigen recognized by antibody 67, and are associated with a number of specialized matrix components, as described below (Edwards, 1994).

VESSELS

Small vessels are often difficult to identify with standard stains such as haematoxylin and eosin. Immunohistochemistry has proved useful for the demonstration of blood vessel distribution in synovium and the presence of endothelial cell gene products; in particular the adhesion molecules. The monoclonal antibody EN4 probably binds to all vessels but binds to isolated non-vascular cells as well. This is not usually a problem if used in the context of a nuclear counterstain and appreciation of morphology. The lectin *Ulex europaeus* agglutinin 1 (UEA1) is also a useful pan-endothelial marker which binds to few if any other cells (Wilkinson and Edwards, 1991a). A variety of avidin–biotin and immunochemical linking systems are available for UEA1 which make it useful for multiple labelling. UEA1 staining tends to spread throughout the vessel wall, whereas EN4 only stains the endothelial layer, and this may affect choice of reagent.

Lymphatics bind UEA1 but fail to bind the antibody PAL-E, which binds to venules, or anti-desmin, which binds to arterioles. Double labelling with UEA1 and a PLA-E/anti-desmin cocktail can thus demonstrate lymphatics specifically (Wilkinson and Edwards, 1991a). In normal synovium lymphatics are present closely associated with arterioles and venules. In rheumatoid tissue lymphatics are more difficult to find (Plate VI) and it seems likely that many are destroyed during the chronic inflammatory process although radiographic studies have suggested that clearance from synovial fluid to large lymphatics may be enhanced in rheumatoid synovium by the presence of abnormal communications.

There have been divergent accounts of changes in vascularity in the synovium in RA. The general impression is of very vascular tissue, yet morphometric studies have shown a loss of superficial vessels (Stevens *et al.*, 1991). It seems likely that the increase in apparent vascularity reflects an increase in the thickness of the tissue immediately deep to the intima, which is heavily supplied with venules. In normal tissue vessel numbers drop off rapidly more than $200\,\mu m$ beneath the surface. In rheumatoid tissue the vascularized zone may be much thicker.

A large number of studies have been made of the expression of adhesion molecule such as ICAM-1, E-selectin, VCAM-1 and CD44 on rheumatoid synovial vessels. These are reviewed in Chapter 12 of this volume. ICAM-1 is present on normal vessels and increases with inflammation. Increased expression is seen in rheumatoid tissue both on vessels and other cells. Immunoreactive E-selectin is also present in small amounts on some normal synovial venules, but no more than in dermis (Fairburn *et al.*, 1993). Its expression is increased in inflammatory states, including rheumatoid synovium. Very little vascular VCAM-1 is present in normal synovium, and what there is tends to be on cells peripheral to the endothelial layer. This low level of staining contrasts with the bright staining seen on synoviocytes, even in inflamed tissue.

NERVES

Immunohistochemical and non-immunoglobulin based histochemical techniques have recently been used to great effect to define the neural components of synovium and are described in detail in Chapter 18, this volume.

CONNECTIVE TISSUE MATRIX AND OTHER EXTRACELLULAR COMPONENTS

Immunochemistry and non-immunoglobulin based techniques can be used effectively to study extracellular matrix as long as it is appreciated that the accessibility of matrix components to reagents is variable. Hyaluronan may occur in a free soluble form, which cannot satisfactorily be immobilized in tissue sections (fixatives make it clump above the section). It may also occur bound to proteoglycan in such a way that it is unavailable for histochemical probe binding. Hyaline cartilage matrix components can be difficult to stain, perhaps because of the charge density of sulphated glycosamino-glycans. For some reason immunochemical demonstration of collagen type I is also difficult, possibly because of its low immunogenicity in its native state or poor avail-ability of epitopes in the fibril form. Traditional collagen stains such as picrosirius red are often more useful. Minor collagens can be demonstrated more satisfactorily.

Matrix products include various types of collagen, elastin, non-fibrous glycopro-teins, hyaluronan, sulphated glycosaminoglycan species and small proteoglycan core proteins such as decorin and biglycan. In normal synovium collagen type III is present in the intima, but in rheumatoid tissue is absent from the most superficial layer of cells (Scott *et al.*, 1984), perhaps because of the stratification of the intima with macro-phages at the surface. mRNA for collagen III is almost entirely confined to the intima in normal tissue but is more generally present throughout the tissue in rheumatoid samples (Noble *et al.*, 1993). Changes in other minor collagens known to be present in the intima (Ashhurst *et al.*, 1991) have not been studied in detail in rheumatoid tissue. Of the non-fibrous proteins tenascin is perhaps of particular interest, being present close to the intima in normal tissue, but more generally in rheumatoid samples (McCachren and Lightner, 1992).

Sulphated glycosaminoglycan species are difficult to identify in their native state and are best analysed following chondroitinase digestion, which leaves disaccharide stubs attached to the core protein moiety which are recognized by a series of anti-bodies. In normal synovium chondroitin 4 sulphate is generally distributed in the tissue but chondroitin 6 sulphate is limited to vascular basement membranes and, perhaps surprisingly, the luminal surface of the intima. This intimal band is usually lost in rheumatoid tissue (Worrall *et al.*, 1994).

Antibodies to hyaluronan (HA) have been found to be unsatisfactory for histo-chemical staining. HA is much more satisfactorily demonstrated using an aggrecan core protein HA binding region based probe. Stainable hyaluronan is confined to the intima in normal synovium but is more generally distributed in rheumatoid tissue (Pitsillides *et al.*, 1994).

Immunochemistry has been used to demonstrate the presence of foreign or altered material in synovium. Bacterial elements have been sought over a long period of time, but without consistently positive results. Hughes *et al.*, 1991 have described chlamydial elements in the synovium of patients with chronic inflammatory polyarthritis. Bacterial components such as lipid A have also been described in rheumatoid synovium. The difficulty with such studies has always been the problem of excluding a crossreactivity with altered host material. Unfortunately it is never possible to exclude such crossreactivities totally with immunochemical techniques. For this reason efforts to detect bacterial material have tended to move towards demonstration of bacterial DNA using polymerase chain reaction techniques. Although highly sensitive these techniques are also not without the possibility of false positive results and no consensus has been established about the presence of significant quantities of bacterial DNA in rheumatoid tissue.

Immunochemistry can be used to analyse changes in tissue matrix occurring as part of rheumatoid disease. Fibrin deposition can be observed with standard stains but immunochemical methods improve specificity and sensitivity. Fibronectin can be demonstrated in large quantities in rheumatoid tissue, in association with the intima and in particular with areas of fibrin incorporation or deposition (Scott *et al.*, 1981). An antibody to terminal *N*-acetylglucosamine residues on glycoproteins has been used to demonstrate the appearance of this abnormal sugar residue in rheumatoid tissue (Sharif *et al.*, 1990) (Plate VII). The presence of the residue is, however, common to tissues from other inflammatory states associated with tissue necrosis or remodelling and may reflect the effects of extracellular enzymes or reactive oxygen species derived from scavenging cells.

SOLUBLE SECRETORY PRODUCTS: CYTOKINES AND PROTEINASES

Immunolocalization of soluble secretory products has not proved easy and interpretation must be cautious. The amounts of such products present in cell cytoplasm may not reflect secretory rates, particularly if, as has been suggested, products such as cytokines and proteases are secreted in short bursts. Estimates of total content of tissue eluates may well be more informative.

There are further problems in interpretation of cytokine immunoreactivity in tissue. Cytokines tend to be present in very small amounts, at the limit of immunochemical detection. They may also be of low immunogenicity. Under these conditions the overriding problem is that of crossreactivity. Many anti-cytokine antibodies crossreact with other antigens in tissue sections, giving varying staining patterns. Polyclonal antisera may be more sensitive but excluding crossreactivity for polyclonal reagents is essentially impossible. Monoclonal antibodies may be more reliable, but it is almost certainly necessary to find several antibodies known to bind to different epitopes on the cytokine, which nevertheless give the same staining pattern, before immunostaining can be considered reliable (Wilkinson and Edwards, 1991b).

There is a consensus that increased amounts of TNFα, IL-1, IL-6 and a number of growth factors are present in rheumatoid synovium, both in cells in the intima and in the deep stroma. Some of these findings are described in more detail in Chapters 2 and 14, this volume.

Metalloproteinase localization is limited by the weakness of the immunochemical signal. Reynolds and Hembry (1992) have devised a method for increasing sensitivity of staining by pre-incubation of tissues with monensin. However, this raises certain practical and theoretical problems, in particular the change in rates of production of such enzymes that may occur once tissue is explanted. Nevertheless, the technique appears to be useful. Woolley and colleagues have also studied metalloproteinase distribution in some detail, with the use of double labelling for cell identification (see Chapter 6, this volume, for this and a general analysis of the enzymes involved in pannus progression). The consensus is that collagenase-producing cells are present in rheumatoid synovium both within the intima, the subintima and at the front of advancing pannus. Gelatinase positive cells tend to be present scattered in the sub-intima. Stromelysin is found bound diffusely to collagenous matrix in proximity to positively stained cells, often within or close to the intima.

RHEUMATOID NODULES

A minority of patients with RA develop nodular necrobiotic lesions. There has been an interesting debate about the relationship between the genesis of these lesions and that of synovitis. As indicated in Chapter 5, this volume, there are certain shared features and within joints synovial intimal cells can sometimes be seen to blend imperceptibly into the palisading cells which are characteristic of the margin of the necrotic zone of nodules.

If the necrotic centre of the nodule is seen as analogous to a rheumatoid synovial space, which itself often contains necrotic fibrin laden 'rice bodies', a similar sequence of zones can be identified moving outwards into the tissue of both types of lesion. A layer of large cells (intima or palisade) is followed by a zone rich in rounded macro-phages and small blood vessels, with clusters of lymphocytes and scattered plasma cells further out. A few neutrophils occur within the surface layers of the living tissue but are chiefly found within the synovial space or necrotic centre, in varying states of disintegration. The most obvious difference between the nodule and rheumatoid synovitis, apart from the geometry, is the relative paucity of lymphocytes and, in particular, plasma cells, although in some cases significant clusters of T cells can be seen.

The relationship between palisading cells and synovial intimal cells has recently been clarified. Palisading cells were previously classified as fibroblasts or histiocytes, at a time when these terms reflected morphology rather than any clear evidence of lineage or function. In the 1980s a number of workers (Hedfors *et al.*, 1983; Palmer *et al.*, 1987) observed that a significant proportion of the cells expressed macrophage markers. Recently we have shown that, like intimal cells, palisading cells are a dual population, consisting of both macrophages and fibroblasts (Plate VIII). However, the fibroblasts show no indication of synoviocyte differentiation (Edwards *et al.*, 1993b). Interestingly, in the rare situation where a nodule has cavitated and its internal surface relined with cells these may show synoviocyte differentiation.

The necrotic centre of rheumatoid nodules seems to be a sump for the accumulation of a wide variety of bits of cells and matrix. It is possible to demonstrate collagen, cell organelles, immunoglobulin and fibrin, for instance. Of particular interest perhaps is the remarkably strong staining for neutrophil components such as elastase and myelo-peroxidase, the latter in a demonstrably active form (Edwards *et al.*, in preparation). The importance of neutrophil suicide within nodules may perhaps be underestimated. MRP8/14 is also present within the necrotic centre in large quantities (Palmer *et al.*, 1987). One set of molecules that are notably absent from the centre are glycosaminoglycans (GAGs) such as hyaluronan and chondroitin sulphates, possibly because of the action of neutrophil enzymes. This lack of basophilic GAGs may partly explain the strongly eosinophilic nature of the necrotic material.

DIAGNOSTIC AND PROGNOSTIC VALUE OF SYNOVIAL IMMUNOCHEMISTRY

Histological analysis of synovium from patients with inflammatory joint disease has never become a routine clinical procedure because of a lack of evidence that it provides useful diagnostic or prognostic information. Synovial histology is chiefly of value in the demonstration of uncommon conditions such as tuberculosis, sarcoidosis (and only in the few cases in which granulomata are found), tumours and tumour-like conditions, amyloid arthropathy and involvement with systemic infiltrative disease. Immunohistochemistry may contribute to this in terms of analysis of cytokeratin expression in so-called synovial sarcomata, which have now been clearly demonstrated to be unrelated to synoviocytes (Salisbury and Isaacson, 1985; Smith et al., in preparation), and specific amyloid components, such as beta 2 microglobulin in subjects with renal disease.

Histochemical and immunohistochemical analysis of synovium in inflammatory joint disease probably can be of prognostic value, but good prospective studies have not been reported. One particular problem is that of variability of tissue from within a single joint. Our own observations on tissue taken at total joint replacement suggest that a wide variety of appearances can be found in a single joint, varying from near normality to necrosis with heavy fibrin deposition to more organized tissue containing large numbers of lymphocytes. It is clear that any meaningful sampling must involve the use of standard sites. Bresnihan and coworkers have indicated that using standard site specific biopsy procedures, biopsy appearances are sufficiently consistent to be useful (Rooney et al., 1988). Using synovial biopsies Veale et al. (1993) have recently demonstrated a difference in total macrophage numbers between rheumatoid and psoriatic arthritic tissues. Mulherin et al. (1993) have also suggested that macrophage numbers in synovium are the best prognostic indicator of subsequent erosion – a finding that would agree with the general experience of many.

Currently, diagnostic synovial histology is largely restricted to haematoxylin and eosin staining. It could be argued that if synovial tissue is to be examined histologically at all a technique for detecting macrophages is called for as a minimum. Morphology is valueless as a guide to macrophage identity. Our current practice is to use an assessment of NSE activity double labelled with an antibody to prolyl hydroxylase of VCAM-1 (APAAP/fast blue) on 4-μm sections, which gives good visualization of the two intimal cell types in particular (the relative merits of synoviocyte markers is discussed further in Chapter 8, this volume). This method shows a clear difference between intimal populations in established rheumatoid and osteoarthritic tissues and could perhaps be usefully applied to early tissue samples.

COMPARISON WITH FINDINGS IN OTHER INFLAMMATORY LESIONS AND WITH LYMPHOID TISSUE

It is difficult to judge the specificity of immunohistochemical findings in rheumatoid synovium against chronic inflammatory lesions in other organs such as gut or skin. In these tissues not only the resident cells but the normal leukocyte-derived populations within the tissue are quite different in type and density. Comparison with other chronic inflammatory conditions of synovium has revealed rather little difference. However, Revell and Mayston (1982) found fewer IgM-secreting plasma cells in ankylosing spondylitic synovium than in rheumatoid tissue. Polymorphs are more commonly described in large numbers in Reiter's tissue and intimal macrophage numbers may be lower in psoriatic synovitis (Veale *et al.*, 1993).

In comparison with forms of arthritis in which the irritant is other than an antigenic stimulus, such as osteoarthritis (OA) and gout the number of lymphocytes tends to be greater but the proportion of T and B cells may not be different, suggesting that the importance of T cell numbers as a clue to rheumatoid pathogenesis may be over-stressed. Increased intimal macrophage numbers and vascular proliferation may be more important. Rheumatoid synovial tissue has been regarded by some as an ectopic lymphoid organ. This is supported by the presence of large numbers of lymphoid cells, which are often organized into follicle-like clusters. However, it is worth noting that there are a number of important dissimilarities between the two types of tissue. Lymphoid organs have specialized routes of entry for recirculating lymphoid cells. Lymph nodes have an afferent lymphatic. Cell traffic is determined by the expression of specific adhesion molecules on the endothelium of these afferent vessels. Rheumatoid synovium has no afferent lymphatic supply and no area corresponding to the nodal paracortex. Specialized vessels expressing cytokine inducible adhesion molecules tend to occur at the centre of T-cell aggregates and it is likely that cellular influx occurs at these sites, both for T and B cells. This is in contrast to the situation in lymph node in which both types of cell are thought to reach follicles from the periphery (Lortan *et al.*, 1987). Another important difference between rheumatoid synovium and lymph node is the presence in synovium of large numbers of plasma cells.

TECHNIQUES OF IMMUNOHISTOCHEMISTRY APPLIED TO SYNOVIUM

In a tissue in which cells of different types are closely apposed, immunohistochemistry is limited in value unless individual cells expressing the gene product of interest can be identified. This effectively means that double labelling is necessary for most studies. Moreover, section thickness is critical. This particularly applies to the intimal layer, which contains two types of cell, macrophages and synoviocytes which cannot be reliably identified on the basis of morphology. To ensure that tissue is suitable for as many labelling techniques as possible certain guidelines for tissue preparation should be followed, which it may be useful to outline here. Frozen tissue is the most versatile, but some other methods of preparation will be considered later.

Rheumatoid synovial tissue probably does not deteriorate significantly for most purposes if kept cool for an hour or two, but freezing within 20 min is recommended, and for messenger RNA studies freezing in the operating suite within minutes of removal is advised. Samples up to 5 mm in size should be immersed rapidly in isopentane or hexane previously cooled to $-70°C$ with solid carbon dioxide or to freezing point with liquid nitrogen. Direct immersion in liquid nitrogen is unsatisfactory. Once frozen, tissue can be stored in small hermetically sealed containers at $-70°C$ for many months, and most antigens are satisfactorily demonstrated after 2 years or more of storage. In large or poorly sealed containers the tissue dessicates and may become unusable after a much shorter time.

Interpretation of synovial histology is critically dependent on being able to distinguish the biological (intimal) surface from cut surfaces. This is not easy, since the biological surface may be devoid of cells in some tissues. A continuous undulating surface, devoid of 'whiskers' is usually biological, but where there is fibrin deposition and tissue remodelling an experienced eye is required. It is worth noting that samples proffered by surgeons as 'synovium' may turn out to have no identifiable biological surface back in the laboratory (it may have been destroyed by diathermy!). In animal work marking the biological surface with India ink can be useful, and for normal human tissue mounting on cork to ensure sectioning at right angles to the surface is feasible. However, for rheumatoid tissue this is usually impractical and it has to be remembered that the surface is usually going to be cut obliquely, with a consequent apparent increase in intimal thickness.

The value of synovial immunohistochemistry is highly dependent on section thickness. The maximum useful thickness for distinguishing the cytoplasmic domains of intimal cells is $7\,\mu m$ and increasingly we are finding that reliable interpretation requires a thickness of not more than $4\,\mu m$. Thicker sections ($10\,\mu m$) have certain advantages for quantitative cytochemistry, but are unsuitable for identification of cell type. Rheumatoid synovium is heterogeneous and not infrequently contains mineral fragments, so cutting sections of this thickness requires a good quality cryostat such as Bright or Reichart Jung with a cutting temperature of $-30°C$.

Sections are usually dried under a fan for 20–30 min before any fixation. Tissues containing large numbers of lymphocytes sometimes develop a blurred appearance when stained with enzyme conjugates, and lose their nuclear morphology with haematoxylin. This appears to be due to the rehydration of hydrophilic macromolecules during incubations to form a gel overlying the section. It can usually be avoided by careful drying and, if necessary, 30 s at the end of drying on a hot plate at 60°C.

Fixation depends on the antigen(s) to be identified but acetone is the most widely used fixative. Metalloproteinases are particularly fixative sensitive. Sections $4\,\mu m$ thick do not require permeabilization for most intracellular antigens but Triton is sometimes recommended for antigens within subcellular organelles.

The details of individual immunochemical techniques are outside the scope of this chapter. However, since study of the synovial intima is very much dependent on the use of double labelling techniques it may be of value to discuss some of the factors that determine choice of combination. Different techniques are useful for different combinations of markers. Three types of double labelling technique are available for light microscopy; double immunofluorescence, double labelling using enzymatic techniques and a combination of an enzymatic technique with fluorescence. Double immunofluorescence is unrivalled for precision of localization and the option for analysing the two colour images both separately and superimposed. Its disadvantages include impermanence and lack of visual clues to tissue structure. Quantification is limited by the tendency of fluorochromes to fade whilst being measured.

Enzymatic techniques may either assess enzyme activity present within the cell of interest, or the activity of an enzyme conjugated to an immunochemical reagent. Chromogens used with enzymatic techniques can be assessed by microdensitometry, giving a reproducible quantitative (for endogenous enzyme activity), or semiquanti-

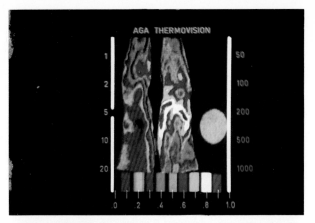

Plate I An infrared thermograph of the knees of a patient with rheumatoid arthritis. One knee is inflamed as is demonstrated by the white and yellow coloration over the knee joint indicating increased warmth secondary to inflammation.

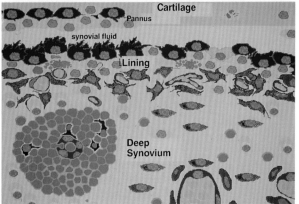

Plate II Ideogram of cell infiltration in rheumatoid synovium. NSE$^+$ macrophages (plum) are prominent in the lining layer and CD14$^+$ macrophages (pink, blue outline) are present in the deeper layers. Lymphocytes are present in clusters (lower left) and also scattered in the deep tissue, together with plasma cells (showing pale perinuclear golgi zone). Vessels are shown in tan (red cells in yellow), including one with high endothelium amongst the lymphocytes.

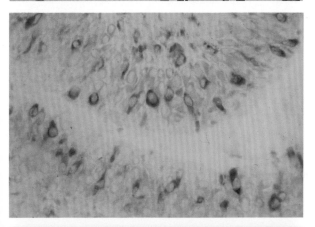

Plate III Rheumatoid synovial intima showing NSE$^+$ macrophages (brick red) and prolyl hydroxlase containing fibroblastic synoviocytes, visualized with alkaline phosphatase and fast blue. Final magnification ×250.

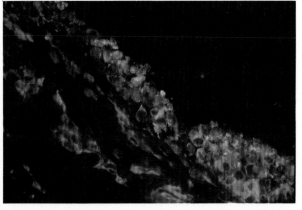

Plate IV Rheumatoid synovial intima showing CD68$^+$ macrophages (rhodamine, red) and VCAM-1$^+$ fibroblastic synoviocytes (fluorescein, green). Final magnification ×250.

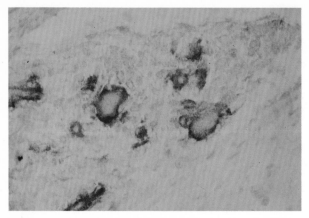

Plate V Rheumatoid synovium showing vitronectin receptor positive giant cells and mononuclear precursors (alkaline phosphatase/fast red). Macrophages at other sites in the tissue were vitronectin receptor negative. Final magnification ×250.

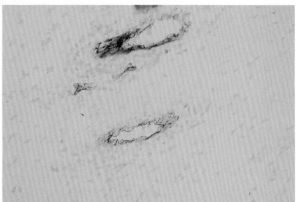

Plate VI Rheumatoid synovial subintima showing an arteriole (lower centre) stained with UEA1 (peroxidase/DAB, tan colour) and a venule (top centre) double labelled with UEA1 and PAL-E (β-galactosidase, turquoise colour). In normal tissue a UEA1$^+$/PAL-E$^-$ thin-walled lymphatic would be seen in association, but here is absent. Final magnification ×250.

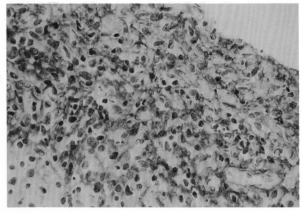

Plate VII Rheumatoid synovial surface showing extensive abnormal accumulation of material carrying terminal N-acetylglucosamine residues, stained here with monoclonal antibody GN7 (peroxidase/DAB, tan colour). Final magnification ×250.

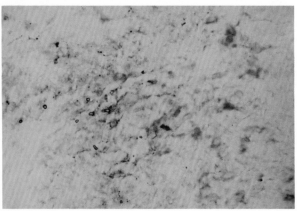

Plate VIII Rheumatoid nodule palisading cells. These comprise both NSE$^+$ macrophages (brick red) and prolyl hydroxylase containing fibroblasts. The latter were shown to be VCAM-1 and UDPGD negative on serial sections. Final magnification ×250.

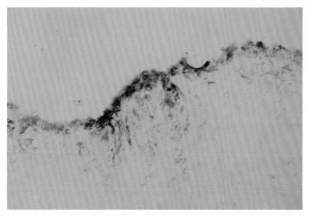

Plate IX Normal synovium showing the two intimal cell populations. NSE$^+$ macrophages appear as brick red. VCAM-1$^+$ synoviocytes appear as blue. Final magnification ×125.

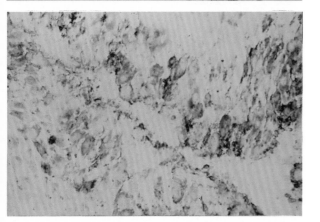

Plate X Oblique section of rheumatoid synovial intima reacted for UDPGD activity, showing synoviocytes (blue) with cytoplasmic processes intermingled with negative cells. Subintimal cells show minimal UDPGD activity. Final magnification ×250.

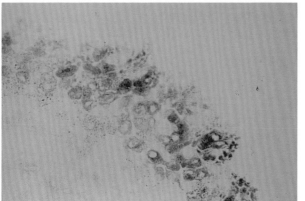

Plate XI Rheumatoid synovial intima folded around a cleft (running bottom right to top left) showing NSE$^+$ macrophages (brick red) and VCAM-1$^+$ synoviocytes (blue). Final magnification ×250.

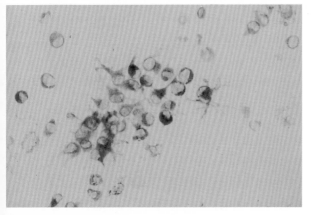

Plate XII Fresh cytospin preparation of cells disaggregated from osteoarthritic synovium. A clump of intimal cells are seen, retaining their close apposition. The synoviocytes show strong UDPGD activity (blue). The macrophages show prominent CD68 expression (red). Final magnification ×250.

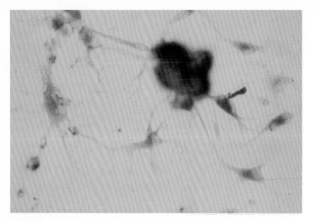

Plate XIII Fibroblastic cells derived from synovium in tissue culture, following the addition of glass particles (seen as grey). The fibroblastic cells in contact with particles have retained the high UDPGD activity (blue) and branching morphology of intimal synoviocytes. Final magnification ×250.

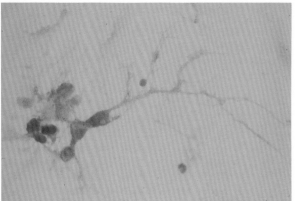

Plate XIV Similar culture to Plate XIII, showing two branching fibroblastic cells in contact with particles expressing VCAM-1 (red). Other cells, for example lower left, showed minimal VCAM-1 expression and an elliptical shape under phase contrast. Final magnification ×250.

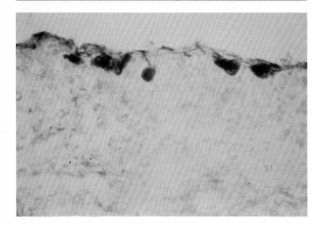

Plate XV Tissue lining a loose total hip replacement prosthesis showing a clearly defined layer of cells of high UDPGD activity (blue) on the surface. Final magnification ×250.

tative (for immunostaining) result. Enzymatic techniques work best when the two reagents produce colour in different cells since overlap is difficult to interpret. Thus enzymatic techniques for cell identification tend to be most helpful as negative labels to compare with markers in a different cell type.

Although cell-membrane bound molecules are popular for identification of leukocyte populations they cause problems with double labelling when cells of different types are closely apposed. To see a negative cell amongst many positive cells requires that it is contact with another negative cell on at least one side. Cytoplasmic markers are much more satisfactory, especially those that are close to the nucleus. By producing a central 'signet ring' appearance within the cell such markers assist in cell counting as well avoiding confusion with other cells. Cytoplasmic enzymes such as NSE, UDPGD, prolyl hydroxylase, elastase, phosphatases and ATPase are useful in this respect.

Although it is easier to interpret double labelling when the two stains show reciprocal rather than concordant distribution, to be satisfied that a molecule is preferentially expressed on one of two cell types we prefer to use both approaches. For colocalization, a combination of a fluorochrome with an enzyme product allows the two stains to be viewed without interference. Care has to be taken to avoid chromogens which quench fluorescence or which themselves fluoresce.

Endogenous enzyme activities in the tissue such as UDPGD tend to be developed first, because they suffer during long incubations, although NSE is remarkably robust. Direct conjugation, biotinylation and the use of subclass specific second antisera give a wide range of options for double immunochemistry. Triple labelling is only feasible when looking for recriprocal staining patterns and when at least one marker is robust, such as the ligand on vessels for *Ulex europaeus* lectin. Information on three markers can, alternatively, be gained by using cocktails, if for instance a cell positive for one marker but negative for two others is sought.

An ever-present problem with immunochemistry is crossreactivity or non-specific binding. Common examples of non-specific binding sites are mucus, keratin, mast cells, eosinophils (especially in gut) and vascular wall cells. There are no problem sites unique to synovium but vessels and mast cells can be troublesome. Loss of staining following absorption of the antibody with antigen is no guarantee of specificity and the only good evidence that staining is bona fide is that it can be reproduced with several reagents, preferably of different immunoglobulin classes from different animal sources.

Although thin sections assist in the identification of individual cells carrying membrane antigens within a closely packed mass there are times when the distance between cells is less than the resolution of the light microscope. This is particularly relevant to lymphocyte aggregates and it may be very difficult to establish which cells are expressing a particular molecule, even when double fluorescence is used. It is often necessary to use information from eluted cells to confirm which cell types are likely to be carrying specific antigens. There are potential pitfalls with this since molecules such as VCAM-1 are readily lost from cells during tissue digestion. Confocal microscopy might be expected to help with separating cells of different types in a close mesh, but currently the results on tissue sections are disappointing. A 4-μm section shows very little variation in staining pattern when subjected to further optical sectioning. The confocal image is short of ideal, partly because of the digitizing process and partly because of loss of visual clues which we unconsciously use to 'clean up' directly viewed fluorescence images. In theory, confocal microscopy should be useful for whole tissue preparations, and it will give a three dimensional image of synovial intima stained with a simple fluorochrome such as eosin. Unfortunately the repeated incubations required for more sophisticated labelling generate problems. The confocal system is also limited to fluorescence (or at least epi-illumination).

The combination of immunohistochemistry and electronmicroscopy has important advantages, but also major drawbacks. Electronmicroscopy allows clear separation of cell outlines. Thus, immunoelectronmicroscopy has been used to analyse the presence of class II on intimal cell populations and confirm that it is largely restricted to the macrophages (Mapp and Revell, 1988). The main problems are loss of sensitivity and difficulties with sampling bias. Much of the interpretation of immunochemistry in synovium depends on being able to see the various areas of the tissue in a single section and compare relative abundance of different markers. This is not possible with electronmicroscopy because of the very small size of section that can be viewed. Electron microscopy is also labour intensive and retains only a limited place.

SUMMARY

Immunohistochemistry has proved useful in identifying the cellular players in the rheumatoid game, and their physical relationship to each other. It has shown where molecules are present capable of mediating cellular interactions and where they are not. It allows certain hypotheses regarding pathogenesis to be discarded, but it can only assist in identifying the true mechanism of the disease in conjunction with *in vivo* or *in vitro* interventional experiments. Recent developments in therapy using inhibitors to a wide variety of putative mediators provide scope for such studies *in vivo*. With the increase in sophistication in immunochemistry over the last few years it is to be hoped that such a dual approach will bear fruit in the not too distant future.

REFERENCES

Ashhurst DE, Bland YS & Levick JR (1991) An immunohistochemical study of the collagens of rabbit synovial interstitium. *J Rheumatol* **18**: 1669–1672.

Brennan FM, Londei M, Jackson A, Hercend T, Brenner MB, Maini RN et al. (1988) T cells expressing γδ chain receptors in rheumatoid arthritis. *J Autoimmunity* **1**: 319–326.

Bröker B, Edwards JCW, Fanger M & Lydyard P (1990) The prevalence and distribution of macrophages bearing FcRI, FcRII and FcRIII in synovium. *Scand J Rheumatol* **19**: 123–135.

Coons AH & Kaplan MH (1950) Localization of antigen in tissue cells. *J Exp Med* **91**: 1–13.

Duke O, Panayi GS, Poulter L & Janossy G (1982) An immunohistological analysis of lymphocyte populations and their microenvironment in the synovial membranes of patients with rheumatoid arthritis using monoclonal antibodies. *Clin Exp Immunol* **49**: 22–29.

Edwards JCW (1980) Synovial lining cells; derivation from bone marrow and surface Ia. *Proceedings of the Combined Annual Provincial Meeting of the RSM Section of Rheum. and Rehab.*, p. 6. BARR and Heberden Society.

Edwards JCW (1987) Structure of synovial lining. In Henderson B & Edwards JCW (authors) *The Synovial Lining in Health and Disease*, pp 31–40. London: Chapman & Hall.

Edwards JCW (1994) The nature and origins of synovium. *J Anat*, in press.

Edwards JCW, Wilkinson LS, Speight P & Isenberg DA (1993a) Vascular cell adhesion molecule 1 and a4 and b1 integrins in lymphocyte aggregates in Sjögren's syndrome and rheumatoid arthritis. *Ann Rheum Dis* **52**: 806–811.

Edwards JCW, Wilkinson LS & Pitsillides AA (1993b) The palisading cells of rheumatoid nodule: comparison with synovial intimal cells. *Ann Rheum Dis* **52**: 801–805.

Fairburn K, Kunaver M, Wilkinson LS, Cambridge G, Haskard DO & Edwards JCW (1993) Intercellular adhesion molecules in normal synovium. *Br J Rheumatol* **32**: 302–306.

Fassbender HG (1975) *Pathology of Rheumatic Diseases.* Berlin: Springer-Verlag.

Gharavi E, Pudiak D & Looney RJ (1993) VCAM-1 on fibroblasts induces TNFa production by monocytes. *American College of Rheumatology Scientific Abstracts* **S94**.

Hedfors E, Klareskog L, Lindblad S, Forsum U & Lindahl G (1983) Phenotypic characterisation of cells within subcutaneous rheumatoid nodules. *Arthritis Rheum* **26**: 1333–1339.

Henderson B (1982) The contribution made by cytochemistry to the study of the metabolism of the normal and rheumatoid synovial lining cell (synoviocyte). *Histochem J* **14**: 527–544.

Hogg N, Palmer DG & Revell PA (1985) Mononuclear phagocytes of normal and rheumatoid synovial membrane identified by monoclonal antibodies. *Immunology* **56**: 673–681.

Howell MD, Diveley JP, Lunden KA, Esty A, Winters ST, Carlo DJ et al. (1991) Limited T cell receptor beta chain heterogeneity among interleukin-2 receptor positive synovial T cells suggests a role for superantigen in rheumatoid arthritis. *Proc Natl Acad Sci* **88**: 10921–10925.

Hughes RA, Hyder E, Treharne JD & Keat AC (1991) Intra-articular chlamydial antigen and inflammatory arthritis. *Quart J Med* **80**: 575–588.

Lindblad S & Hedfors E (1987) The synovial membrane in healthy individuals – immunohistochemical overlap with synovitis. *Clin Exp Immunol* **69**: 41–47.

Lortan JE, Rowbottom CA, Oldfield S & MacLennan IC (1987) Newly produced virgin B cells migrate to secondary lymphoid organs but their capacity to enter follicles is restricted. *Eur J Immunol* **17**: 1311–1316.

Mapp PI & Revell PA (1988) Ultrastructural characterisation of macrophages in the synovial lining. *Rheumatol Int* **8**: 171–176.

McCachren SS & Lightner VA (1992) Expression of human tenascin in synovitis and its regulation by interleukin-1. *Arthritis Rheum* **35**: 1185–1196.

McCormick JN (1963) An immunofluorescence study of rheumatoid factor. *Ann Rheum Dis* **22**: 1–10.

Meijer CJLM, van de Putte LBA, Eulderink F, Kleinjan R, Lafeber G & Bots GTAM (1976) Character-istics of mononuclear cell populations in chronically inflamed synovial membranes. *J Pathol* **121**: 1–11.

Mulherin D, Fitzgerald O & Bresnihan B (1993) Radiologic progression of rheumatoid arthritis over six years correlates with macrophage numbers in the synovium. *American College of Rheumatology Scientific Abstracts* **S86**.

Naito M, Hayashi S, Yoshida H, Mishikawa S, Shulz LD & Takahashi K (1991) Abnormal differentiation of tissue macrophages in osteopetrosis (op) mice defective in the production of macrophage colony stimulating factor. *Am J Pathol* **139**: 657.

Noble DP, Pitsillides AA, Dudhia J & Edwards JCW (1993) *In situ* hybridisation for decorin, collagens type I and III mRNA in normal, rheumatoid and osteoarthritic synovial lining. *Br J Rheumatol* **32** (**supplement 1**): 38.

Paliard X, West SG, Lafferty JA, Clements JR, Kappler JW, Marrack P et al. (1991) Evidence for the effects of a superantigen in rheumatoid arthritis. *Science* **253**: 325–329.

Palmer DG, Selvendran Y, Allen C, Revell PA & Hogg N (1985) Features of synovial membrane identified with monoclonal antibodies. *Clin Exp Immunol* **59**: 529–538.

Palmer DG, Hogg N, Allen CA, Highton J & Hessian P (1987) A mononuclear phagocyte subset associated with cell necrosis in rheumatoid nodules: identification with monoclonal antibody 5.5. *Clin Immunol Immunopathol* **45**: 17–28.

Pitsillides AA, Worrall JG, Wilkinson LS, Bayliss MT & Edwards JCW (1994) Hyaluronan concentration in non-inflamed and rheumatoid synovium. *Br J Rheumatol*, in press.

Pitzalis C, Kingsley GH, Murphy J & Panayi GS (1987) Abnormal distribution of the helper-inducer and suppressor-inducer memory T cell subsets in the rheumatoid joint. *Clin Immunol Immunopathol* **45**: 252–258.

Revell PA & Mayston V (1982) Histopathology of the synovial membrane of peripheral joints in ankylosing spondylitis. *Ann Rheum Dis* **41**: 579–586.

Revell PA, Mapp PI, Lalor PA & Hall PA (1987) Proliferative activity of cells in synovium as demonstrated by a monoclonal antibody, Ki67. *Rheumatol Int* **7**: 183–186.

Reynolds JJ & Hembry RM (1992) Immunolocalisation of metalloproteinases and TIMP in normal and pathological tissues. *Matrix* **Supplement 1**: 375–382.

Rooney M, Condell D, Quinlan W, Daly L, Whelan A, Feighery C et al. (1988) Analysis of histologic variation of synovitis in rheumatoid arthritis. *Arthritis Rheum* **31**: 956–963.

Salisbury AK, Duke O & Poulter LW (1987) Macrophage-like cells of the pannus area in rheumatoid arthritic joints. *Scan J Rheumatol* **16**: 263–272.

Salisbury JR & Isaacson PG (1985) Synovial sarcoma. *J Pathol* **147**: 49–57.

Scott DL, Delamere JP & Walton KW (1981) The distribution of fibronectin in the pannus in rheumatoid arthritis. *Br J Exp Pathol* **62**: 362–367.

Scott DL, Salmon M & Walton KW (1984) Reticulin and its related structural connective tissue proteins in the rheumatoid synovium. *Histopathology* **8**: 469–479.

Sharif M, Rook G, Worrall JG, Wilkinson LS & Edwards JCW (1990) Terminal N-acetylglucosamine in chronic synovitis. *Br J Rheumatol* **29**: 25–31.

Smith M, Bröker BM, Moretta L, Ciccone E, Grossi CE, Edwards JCW et al. (in press). γδT cells and their subsets in blood and synovial tissue from rheumatoid arthritis patients. *Scand J Immunol* **32**: 585–593.

Stevens CR, Blake DR, Merry P, Revell PA & Levick JR (1991) A comparative study by morphometry of the microvasculature in normal and rheumatoid synovium. *Arthritis Rheum* **34**: 1508–1513.

van Boxel JA & Paget SA (1975) Predominantly T cell infiltrate in rheumatoid synovial membranes. *NEJ Med* **293**: 517–520.

Veale D, Yanni G, Rogers S, Barnes L, Bresnihan B & Fitzgerald O (1993) Reduced synovial membrane macrophage numbers, ELAM-1 expression, and lining layer hyperplasia in psoriatic arthritis as compared with rheumatoid arthritis. *Arthritis Rheum* **36**: 893–900.

Wilkinson LS & Edwards JCW (1989) Microvascular distribution in normal human synovium. *J Anatomy* **167**: 129–136.

Wilkinson LS & Edwards JCW (1991a) Demonstration of lymphatics in synovium. *Rheumatol Int* **11**: 151–155.

Wilkinson LS and Edwards JCW (1991b) Binding of antibodies raised against tumour necrosis factor alpha to blood vessels in inflamed synovial tissue. *Rheumatol Int* **11**: 19–25.

Wilkinson LS, Worrall JG, Sinclair HS & Edwards JCW (1990) Immunohistochemical reassessment of accessory cell populations in normal and diseased human synovium. *Br J Rheumatol* **29**: 4, 259–263.

Wilkinson LS, Pitsillides AA, Worrall JG & Edwards JCW (1992) Light microscopic characterisation of the fibroblastic synovial lining cell (synoviocyte). *Arthritis Rheum* **35**: 1179–1184.

Wilkinson LS, Edwards JCW, Poston R & Haskard DO (1993a) Cell populations expressing VCAM-1 in normal and diseased synovium. *Lab Invest* **68**: 82–88.

Wilkinson LS, Pitsillides AA & Edwards JCW (1993b) Giant cells in arthritic synovium. *Ann Rheum Dis* **52**: 182–184.

Woolley DE, Crossley MJ & Evanson JM (1977) Collagenase at sites of cartilage erosion in the rheumatoid joint. *Arthritis Rheum* **20**: 1231–1239.

Worrall JG, Bayliss MT & Edwards JCW (1994) Zonal distribution of sulphated proteoglycans in normal and rheumatoid synovium. *Ann Rheum Dis*, in press.

Cellular Mechanisms in
Rheumatoid Arthritis

8 Fibroblastic Synovial Lining Cells (Synoviocytes)

J.C.W. Edwards

CELL POPULATIONS IN SYNOVIUM

Normal synovial tissue contains all the resident cells of soft connective tissue, including fibroblasts, macrophages, adipocytes, mast cells, nerve fibres, occasional polymorphs and lymphocytes, and vascular cells, including pericytes. In addition, synovium is characterized by a surface layer of cells, or intima, immediately beneath which is a zone of relatively high vascularity (Key, 1932; Edwards, 1987).

The normal synovial intima consists of flattened or cuboidal overlapping cells, rarely more than three deep (Plate IX). It is not present on all areas of the tissue, some areas being devoid of any surface cells. The intima contains two distinct cell types. Cells of one type are macrophages by all available criteria (see Chapter 7, this volume). The other cells resemble fibroblasts in size, nuclear/cytoplasmic ratio, chromatin pattern and cytoplasmic ultrastructure (Barland *et al.*, 1962). These latter cells can be referred to as fibroblast-like synoviocytes, or simply synoviocytes, since they are the only type of cell which so far has been identified as specific to synovium.

In the past, nomenclature has been confused because of the difficulties of distinguishing cell types when they are so closely packed together. The presence of two intimal cell types was initially demonstrated by electronmicroscopic studies (Barland *et al.*, 1962). These studies predated the modern concept of a monocyte-derived macrophage lineage. For reasons that are not clear the macrophages were described merely as 'macrophage-like' or type A cells, although they conformed to all ultrastructural criteria for macrophages. The synoviocytes were termed type B cells. Apparently intermediate forms were reported in diseased tissue (Ghadially and Roy, 1967; Kinsella *et al.*, 1970) but not from normal tissue. Graabaeck (1982) failed to find evidence of intermediate forms in a detailed electronmicroscopic study of normal tissue using serial sectioning.

Organelle content in both macrophages and fibroblasts can change significantly in disease, and tends to converge, with an increase in rough endoplasmic reticulum in macrophages and an increase in lysosomal content in fibroblasts, particular in those from synovium (Fraser *et al.*, 1979). Thus, the presence of cells of intermediate ultrastructure is not surprising. It serves to indicate that ultrastructure is not a reliable gold standard for differentiating these cell types in diseased tissue. With the advent of a wider range of immunochemical and cytochemical techniques which will differentiate the two cell types by the presence of individual gene products relating to specific functions (see Plates V, and VII) (Wilkinson *et al.*, 1992), the ultrastructural typing of intimal cells is effectively obsolete.

A number of publications refer to three cell types in rheumatoid synovial tissue, (I–III) the third type being an MHC class II expressing dendritic antigen-presenting cell (Burmester *et al.*, 1983). However, this classification is based on cells eluted from the

Mechanisms and Models in Rheumatoid Arthritis
ISBN 0–12–340440–1

tissue, which will include a wide range of subintimal cells and cannot be equated with the intimal layer. There is evidence of a very small number of CD68 negative cells expressing the class II related marker RFD1 in normal synovial intima, but these cells probably make up less than 1% of the total (Wilkinson *et al.*, 1990). In diseased tissue a clear distinction between macrophages and dendritic antigen-presenting cells has not been achieved. The issue of specialized antigen-presenting cells is dealt with in more detail in Chapter 7, this volume.

FIBROBLASTIC CELLS

In terms of the biology of synovial resident cells, the interest focuses on the intimal fibroblast-like synoviocyte and its relationship to other types of fibroblast. Discussion of this issue has to start with the admission that the term fibroblast may cover a range of cells of differing function which may be difficult to distinguish with current techniques. The term implies a cell in loose rather than hard connective tissue with the ability to make fibrous matrix components and collagen in particular. Unfortunately, the term is often used by histologists to mean a long thin cell in connective tissue. Fibroblasts are often long and thin, but so are many stromal macrophages, and immunohistochemistry shows that cell shape is a poor guide to identity.

To date there is no totally satisfactory cytochemical marker for fibroblasts. Antibodies to the β subunit of prolyl hydroxylase, which is involved in collagen synthesis, are readily available (Hoyhtya *et al.*, 1984), but significantly amounts of the β subunit of the enzyme are also present in non-collagen synthesizing cells with prominent protein synthesizing capacity (e.g. plasma cells). In practice such antibodies do pick out fibroblasts in both normal and inflamed tissue (see Plate V), but at least in theoretical terms this marker is less than ideal. Antibodies to procollagens or C peptide fragments may prove more useful. Currently, identification is best achieved by a combination of absence of leukocyte-related markers, site, morphology and prolyl hydroxylase content. This tends to mean that study of any further functional marker in cells identified as fibroblasts requires cross referencing of several double labelling techniques in serial sections.

SYNOVIOCYTE SPECIALIZATION

Synoviocytes are distinguished from other fibroblasts in being present on an internal connective tissue surface. They are not mesothelial cells, since they lack the basement membrane and abutting, rather than overlapping, arrangement of peritoneal or pleural cells. They have multiple processes, giving then a stellate shape in normal tissue (McDonald and Levick, 1988) and often a polarized octopus or sea-anemone like shape in diseased tissue, with the arms extending to the tissue surface.

Until recently it has been difficult to be sure that synoviocytes and other fibroblasts are distinct in terms of function, although synthesis of synovial fluid hyaluronan has always been ascribed to synoviocytes (Hadler, 1981). Recent cytochemical and immunochemical studies using double labelling techniques to differentiate macrophages and fibrolastic cells have shown that synoviocytes are indeed distinct both in terms of ability to synthesize hyaluronan, as judged by activity of the enzyme uridine diphosphoglucose dehydrogenase, and expression of VCAM-1 (Wilkinson *et al.*, 1992,

1993a). They also appear to show a degree of specialization in terms of synthesis of several other matrix components and adhesion molecules.

The ability of synovium to synthesize hyaluronan has long been recognized (Yielding *et al.*, 1957). However, it had not been clear whether only the intimal layer of cells were responsible or whether all of the fibroblasts deeper in the tissue shared this property. Certain observations belie too simple an analysis. Canoso and colleagues found that superficial synovial bursae contained very little hyaluronan (Canoso *et al.*, 1983) and large amounts of hyaluronan (in our hands up to 20 mg/ml) are found in the fluid within ganglia, which lack an intima (Ghadially, 1983).

Hyaluronan synthesis is dependent on a series of enzymatic steps, which generate a long-chain polymer of alternating glucuronate and *N*-acetylglucosamine residues. Before polymerization can occur, the monosaccharides must be available in UDP-conjugated form. UDP-*N*-acetylglucosamine is also utilized in the synthesis of glycoproteins and its availability is not thought to be a limiting factor. UDP-glucuronate is used only for the synthesis of hyaluronan and chondroitin sulphates in connective tissue cells and its availability is likely to be critical to the rate of hyaluronan synthesis (McGarry and Gahan, 1985). The availability of UDP-glucurinate is dependent on its synthesis from UD-glucose by UDP glucose dehydrogenase (UDPGD). The final copolymerization of the two monosaccharide species is achieved by hyaluronan synthase (Prehm, 1983).

In normal synovium, synoviocytes (i.e. non-macrophage intimal cells) differ from all other cells in the tissue in having a high activity of UDPGD (Wilkinson *et al.*, 1992), demonstrable *in situ* by cytochemistry. Quantitative microdensitometry indicates that the activity is four to nine times that of other cells. In rheumatoid tissue the differential between intimal synoviocyte and deep fibroblast UDPGD activity may be less clear cut (activity ratio 2.5:1), but is still clearly evident (Plate X). Synoviocytes also show a high content of hyaluronan synthase, as demonstrated immunochemically (see Plate VII) (Worrall *et al.*, 1992). Thus, the specialized synthetic capacity of these cells is confirmed.

The extracellular matrix immediately surrounding intimal cells differs from that in the deeper tissue. It shows few collagen bundles and much of it appears either amorphous or finely fibrillar by electronmicroscopy (Ghadially, 1983). Immunochemistry suggests that intimal matrix is rich in minor collagens including types III, V and VI (Ashhurst *et al.*, 1991). Normal intimal matrix also contains proteoglycan bearing chondroitin-6-sulphate, which is otherwise usually restricted to basement membranes in connective tissue (Worrall *et al.*, 1994). Similarly, tenascin is present in synovial intima (McCachren and Lightner, 1992). It is likely that synoviocytes are responsible for most of the synthesis of intimal matrix, although evidence for this is often circumstantial. For instance, intimal cells taken as a whole show a higher content of messenger RNA for collagen type III and decorin than cells in the subintima (Noble *et al.*, 1993). Since macrophages do not produce these molecules in significant amounts it is likely that the RNA is within synoviocytes. An unidentified molecule, recognized by the monoclonal antibody 67 raised by Hogg and coworkers, stains material surrounding synoviocytes (Stevens *et al.*, 1990), but its composition and function are not known.

In addition to specialized matrix synthesis synoviocytes show prominent expression of the adhesion molecules VCAM-1 (Plates II, IV and XI) CD44 and β1 integrin

(Wilkinson *et al.*, 1993a; Henderson *et al.*, 1993; Edwards *et al.*, 1993a). Many cell types normally express CD44, and a range of β1 integrins, and the expression on synoviocytes is only relatively prominent. However, the constitutive expression of VCAM-1 by synoviocytes is much more unusual. Follicular dendritic reticulum cells in lymphoid tissue also constitutively express VCAM-1 (Rice *et al.*, 1991), as do a small proportion of vascular wall cells, but the great majority of fibroblastic cells in normal tissue do not.

VCAM-1 binds to the α4β1 integrin heterodimer (VLA-4) which is present on many macrophages. This raises the possibility that synoviocytes are involved in im-mobilizing macrophages in the intimal layer. Somewhat surprisingly, staining for the α4 integrin chain in synovial intima is minimal. Staining for the β1 chain is prominent (El Gabalawy and Wilkins, 1992), but the preferential β1 chain expression appears to be on synoviocytes (Edwards *et al.*, 1993a) possibly in conjunction with the α5 chain as the fibronectin receptor VLA-5. The functions of these adhesion molecule systems in the intima remain to be clarified, but the constitutive expression of VCAM-1 on synoviocytes raises an interesting possibility in terms of the susceptibility of synovium to chronic inflammation in autoimmune disease (see Chapter 7, this volume).

SYNOVIAL FIBROBLASTIC CELLS *IN VITRO*

The literature on synovial fibroblastic cells in culture has for a long time been difficult to interpret because passageable adherent cells derived from synovial tissue by diges-tion or explants contain an unknown mixture of synoviocytes and subintimal fibro-blasts. Certain features suggest that such cells are largely derived from the synoviocyte layer. They tend to be more kite-shaped or stellate than the ribbon-like fibroblasts of dermis. They can produce large amounts of hyaluronan (Castor *et al.*, 1962). Fibro-blasts from a variety of other sources will also produce hyaluronan in culture but synovial fibroblasts appear to produce a higher proportion of hyaluronan in relation to other glycosaminoglycans. Fibroblasts derived from synovium also tend to produce more collagenase and prostaglandin in response to IL-1, but it is not clear whether this reflects normal synoviocyte function *in vivo*.

In terms of the two features that distinguish synoviocytes from subintimal fibro-blasts most clearly in tissue sections, the findings *in vitro* are complex. UDPGD activity is high in a proportion of fibroblastic cells in fresh cytospin preparations (Plate XII) (Wilkinson *et al.*, 1992) but is rapidly lost in culture. Moreover, until recently, UDPGD activity in prolonged cultures often seemed capricious, with cells at the edges of the culture showing more activity than those at the centre – an observation first made by De Luca (pers. commun.). Reports of VCAM-1 expression by synovial fibroblastic cells in culture have varied from expression only on cytokine stimulation (Marlor *et al.*, 1992) to constitutive expression by approximately 30% of cells (Morales-Ducret *et al.*, 1992). Recent observations in the Synovial Biology Unit at University College London suggest that up to 75% of fibroblastic cells derived from both rheumatoid and osteoarthritic tissue will express VCAM-1, but fibroblasts from dermis showed no significant VCAM-1 expression under the same conditions. How-ever, the level of VCAM-1 expression by synovial cells in culture does not compare with that seen on intimal synoviocytes in tissue sections, at least as judged immuno-chemically, and falls further with time.

By chance, it was observed that in some synovial fibroblastic cell cultures groups of cells with high UDPGD activity persisted. These cells were in contact with alizarin red positive particles believed to be hydroxyapatite fragments of bone origin carried over during disaggregation of arthritic tissues. Further cultures were seeded with synthetic hydroxyapatite or glass particles and in both cases cells in contact with such mineral particles showed high activity of UDPGD (Plate XIII). Furthermore these cells retained a stellate morphology, with several long branching processes, and showed prominent expression of VCAM-1 (Plate XIV). Thus, they show the characteristic features of intimal synoviocytes (Croft *et al.*, in preparation).

These observations suggest that although synovial fibroblastic cells may have a propensity to express VCAM-1 in the absence of stimulation, the normal expression of VCAM-1 by synoviocytes reflects some site specific mechanical or geometric signal perceived by the cell through contact with its matrix. It is unlikely that *in vivo* the signal comes from a mineral particle. The particles probably simply mimic the physiological signal, possibly because it has something to do with physical discontinuity of the cell's environment. The suggestion, therefore, is that although synovial fibroblastic cells in culture may reflect intimal synoviocyte function to a degree, this is variable and may be dependent both on the proportion of synoviocytes in the original digest and the length of time in culture. It may be possible to restore synoviocyte function using a physical stimulus, but the precise requirements for this stimulus are not known, nor is it known whether fibroblasts from other sources will respond to such stimuli and develop synoviocyte features.

SYNOVIOCYTE ORIGINS

Joint synovium develops in the embryo from cells present in the early skeletal anlage at sites known as interzones (O'Rahilly and Gardner, 1978). In common with perichondrium and in contrast with other nearby cells, these sites show prominent expression of CD44 (Edwards *et al.*, 1993b). This raises the possibility that both intimal synoviocytes and subintimal cells differ from other fibroblasts in their range of gene expression because of their anatomical origins. However, since normal subintimal cells at no stage of development show the special features of synoviocytes, this suggestion has no experimental support to date. Moreover, VCAM-1 expression has not so far been seen in foetal joint tissues other than on blood vessels, apparently developing postnatally.

Historical evidence suggests that synovium can also form at sites of tissue shearing stresses away from embryologically predetermined sites such as joints and tendon sheaths. Experimental pseudoarthroses form a 'synovial' membrane (Kupper *et al.*, 1978) as do adventitious bursae (Collins, 1949). Fibroblastic cells with synoviocyte features have been found to develop on adventitious connective tissue surface, but only under certain circumstances, possibly associated with surface movement. Connective tissue surfaces generated by subcutaneous injection of air in rodents show no rise in UDPGD activity in surface cells (Wilkinson *et al.*, 1993b). In contrast, cells on the surface of tissues lining loose artificial joint prostheses, which may form a layer resembling synovial intima (Goldring *et al.*, 1983), show high UDPGD activity and VCAM-1 expression (Plate XV) (Edwards, 1994). Cells on the surface of tissue lining a plastic implant in human subcutaneous tissue subjected to repeated movement showed high UDPGD activity but no increase in VCAM-1 expression. Similar, but immobile, implants in sheep showed no such rise in UDPGD activity. Interestingly, both high UDPGD activity and VCAM-1 expression have been seen on cells lining adventitious spaces in rheumatoid nodules (Edwards *et al.*, 1993a) but not in the palisading layer.

One important conclusion from these findings is that UDPGD activity and VCAM-1 expression, although often associated are to an extent independently regulated. This is consistent with findings in rheumatoid arthritic synoviocytes which show up-regulation of VCAM-1 expression but a reduction in UDPGD activity (Wilkinson *et al.*, 1992, 1993a). Even within normal human synovial intima UDPGD activity and VCAM-1 expression show a significant degree of independent variation in individual cells.

It appears that cells of high UDPGD activity will appear on the surface of a soft connective tissue lining in contact with a hard surface over which the tissue moves. Although the regenerate lining present around hip prostheses is at a site previously occupied by synovium the general view is that cells repopulating such a surface are unlikely to derive from pre-existent intimal cells, but rather from cells within the surrounding connective tissue stroma (Mitchell and Blackwell, 1968). This must always remain open to doubt, but the appearance of cells of high UDPGD activity around the plastic implant in human tissue away from a site of pre-existing synovium gives clearer evidence that these cells can develop from non-synovial populations.

PROLIFERATION

The ability of synoviocytes to proliferate, and their physiological rate of division, remain difficult to establish. In disease the number of intimal cells increases significantly. It is now clear that in inflammatory disease many of the extra cells are immigrant macrophages (Henderson *et al.*, 1988), but considering the great increase in synovial surface area there is probably an increase in the total number of synoviocytes as well. In mechanical joint disease most of the increased number of intimal cells are synoviocytes (see Chapter 7, this volume). Measurements of the rate of proliferation of intimal cells in rheumatoid synovium have indicated rates to be low. In studies using Feulgen cytophotometry (Henderson, 1987), the proportion of cells carrying more than one diploid complement of chromatin was 4% or less. Using monoclonal antibodies to proliferation markers, such as Ki67 (Revell *et al.*, 1987), labelling rates were very low (1:2000–1:30000). These findings have led to the suggestion that synoviocytes derive from precursor fibroblastic cells in the subintima rather than from other intimal cells. This is consistent with the idea that synoviocyte differentiation is an option for any fibroblastic cell under the right local conditions, rather than being predetermined in a restricted population during embryogenesis. Very occasionally cell division is seen in the intima, and in animal models Fuelgen studies indicate that division does occur at an early stage (Henderson, 1987) suggesting that under certain conditions proliferation within the lining does occur.

Fassbender has suggested that as part of the rheumatoid arthritic lesion connective tissue cells undergo what may be described as mesenchymoid transformation (Fassbender, 1975); that is to say they appear to proliferate and at the same time take on an undifferentiated morphology. These cells are by and large not at the tissue surface and should not be equated with intimal cells. Nevertheless, in rheumatoid tissue the distinction between intimal and subintimal cells often becomes blurred and it may be that common changes occur in cells throughout the depth of the tissue. With the advent of immunohistochemical techniques it has become clear that these sheets of 'undifferentiated cells' are a mixture of macrophages and fibroblasts and their resemblance to embryonic mesenchyme is probably fortuitous.

MOLECULAR CONTROL OF GENE EXPRESSION IN SYNOVIOCYTES

The transcription factors controlling synoviocyte function are not currently known. Fibroblastic cells from rheumatoid synovium express c-fos and egr-1 *in vitro* and this has been related to collagenase production (Trabandt *et al.*, 1992). C-fos and jun-B mRNA has been localized to synoviocytes in rheumatoid arthritic tissues by *in situ* hybridization (Kinne *et al.*, 1993) on the basis of codistribution with mRNA for collagens in intimal cells. In other fibroblasts NFκB has been implicated in the up-regulation of VCAM-1 expression but no clear evidence is available in respect to intimal synoviocytes. The signals involved in VCAM-1 expression, high UDPGD activity and other specialized functions in normal synoviocytes are not known. It seems unlikely that NFκB is involved in VCAM-1 expression in normal tissue since cytokines such as tumour necrosis factor are not detectable in normal tissue and in rheumatoid tissue, where tumour necrosis factor can be found, VCAM-1 expression and UDPGD activity are dissociated.

RELATIONSHIP OF SYNOVIOCYTES TO PANNUS FIBROBLASTS

In RA a film of variably vascular fibrous tissue migrates across and replaces the articular cartilage surface. The cells of this pannus are probably of mixed origin. Some may be derived from chondrocytes which have dissolved their own matrix. (When cartilage is transplanted to subcutaneous tissue chondrocytes resorb their matrix, proliferate and migrate into the surrounding tissue (Sedgwick *et al.*, 1986). Fibro-blastic cells from synovium also appear to invade but so far there is no indication whether they are intimal synoviocytes or not. Pannus rarely shows a clearly defined surface or intimal layer, often consisting of a disorganized mass of large cells of both macrophage and fibroblast type. It has been suggested that binding of pannus to cartilage may be mediated by β1 integrins (Shiozawa *et al.*, 1992), which are promi-nently expressed on synoviocytes, but other fibroblasts carry these ligands and it may be that the precise origin of the pannus fibroblasts is not critical to their destructive potential.

REFERENCES

Ashurst DE, Bland YS & Levick JR (1991) An immunohistochemical study of the collagens of rabbit synovial interstitium. *J Rheumatol* **18**: 1669–1672.

Barland P, Novikoff AB & Hamerman D (1962) Electron microscopy of the human synovial membrane. *J Cell Biol* **14**: 207–216.

Burmester GR, Locher P, Koch B, Winchester RJ, Dimitriu-Bona A, Kalden JR et al. (1983) The tissue architecture of synovial membranes inflammatory and non-inflammatory joint diseases. *Rheumatol Int* **3**: 173–181.

Canoso JJ, Stack MT & Brandt K (1983) Hyaluronic acid content of deep and superficial subcutaneous bursae of man. *Ann Rheum Dis* **42**: 171–175.

Castor CW, Prince RK & Dorstewitz EL (1962) Characteristics of human fibroblasts cultivated *in vitro* from different anatomical sites. *Lab Invest* **11**: 703.

Collins DH (1949) *The Pathology of Articular and Spinal Diseases.* London: Edward Arnold.

Edwards JCW (1987) Structure of synovial lining. In Henderson B & Edwards JCW (eds) *The Synovial Lining in Health and Disease*, pp 17–39. London: Chapman & Hall.

Edwards JCW (1994) The nature and origins of synovium. *J Anat*, in press.

Edwards JCW, Wilkinson LS & Pitsillides AA (1993a) The palisading cells of rheumatoid nodule: comparison with synovial intimal cells. *Ann Rheum Dis* **52**: 801–805.

Edwards JCW, Wilkinson LS & Pitsillides AA (1993b) Cell distribution and behaviour associated with the formation of joint cavities. *American College of Rheumatology Scientific Abstracts* **S265**.

El-Gabalawy & Wilkins J (1992) b1(CD29) integrin expression in rheumatoid synovial membranes: an immunohistologic study of distribution patterns. *J Rheumatol* **20**: 231–237.

Fassbender HG (1975) Rheumatoid arthritis. In *Pathology of Rheumatic Diseases*, pp 118–119. Berlin: Springer Verlag.

Fraser JRE, Clarris BJ & Baxter E (1979) Patterns of induced variation in the morphology, hyaluronic acid secretion, and lysosomal enzyme activity of cultured human synovial cells. *Ann Rheum Dis* **38**: 287–294.

Ghadially FN (1983) *Fine Structure of Synovial Joints.* London: Butterworths.

Ghadially FN & Roy S (1967) Ultrastructure of synovial membrane in rheumatoid arthritis. *Ann Rheum Dis* **26**, 426–443.

Goldring SR, Schiller AL, Roelke M, Rourke CM, O'Neill DA, Harris WH et al. (1983) The synovial-like membrane at the bone–cement interface in loose total hip replacements and its proposed role in bone lysis. *J Bone Joint Surg (A)* **65**: 575–584.

Graabaeck PM (1982) Ultrastructural evidence for two distinct types of synoviocyte in rat synovial membrane. *J Ultrastruct Res* **78**: 321–339.

Hadler N (1981) The biology of the extracellular space. In Hasselbacher P (ed) *The Biology of the Joint. Clin Rheum Dis* **7**(1): 71–98.

Henderson B (1987) Cell turnover in the synovial lining. In Henderson B & Edwards JCW (eds) *The Synovial Lining in Health and Disease*, pp 75–100. London: Chapman & Hall.

Henderson B, Revell P & Edwards JCW (1988) Synovial lining cell hyperplasia in rheumatoid arthritis: dogma and fact. *Ann Rheum Dis* **47**: 348–349.

Henderson KJ, Pitsillides AA, Edwards JCW & Worrall JG (1993) Reduced expression of CD44 in rheumatoid synovial cells. *Br J Rheumatol* **32** (**Abst supplement 1**): 25.

Hoyhtya M, Myllya R, Siuva J, Kivirkko KL & Tryggvason K (1984) Monoclonal antibodies to human prolyl-4-hydroxylase. *Eur J Biochem* **141**: 477–482.

Key JA (1932) The synovial membrane of joints and bursae. In *Special Cytology* Vol 2, pp 1055–1076. New York: PB Hoeber.

Kinne RW, Boehm S, Iftner T, Algner T, Bravo R, Kroczek RA et al. (1993) Expression of jun-B and c-fos proto-oncogenes by activated fibroblast-like cells in synovial tissue of rheumatoid arthritis and osteoarthritis patients. *American College of Rheumatology Scientific Abstracts* **s264**.

Kinsella TD, Baum J & Ziff M (1970) Studies of isolated synovial lining cells of rheumatoid and nonrheumatoid synovial membranes. *Arthritis Rheum* **13**: 734–753.

Kupper W, Creutzig A, Gerdtz KG, Creutzig H & Ostern HJ (1978) Creation of a reaction-less pseudarthrosis on ulna of dog. *Res Exp Med* **172**: 167–176.

Marlow CW, Webb DL, Bombara MP, Greve JM & Blue ML (1992) Expression of vascular cell adhesion molecule-1 in fibroblast-like synoviocytes after stimulation with tumour necrosis factor. *Am J Pathol* **140**: 1055–1060.

McCachren SS & Lightner VA (1992) Expression of human tenascin in synovitis and its regulation by interleukin 1. *Arthritis Rheum* **35**: 1185–1196.

McDonald JN & Levick JR (1988) Morphology of surface synoviocytes in situ at normal and raised joint pressure, studied by scanning electron microscopy. *Ann Rheum Dis* **47**: 232–240.

McGarry A & Gahan PB (1985) A quantitative cytochemical study of UDPDglucose: NAD oxidoreductase activity during stelar differentiation in *Pisum sativum* L. c Meteor. *Histochemistry* **83**: 551–554.

Mitchell N & Blackwell P (1968) The electron microscopy of regenerating synovium after subtotal synovectomy in rabbits. *J Bone Joint Surg* **50**: 675–686.

Morales Ducret J, Wayner E, Elices MJ, Alvaro Garcia A, Firestein G & Zvaifler N (1992) a_4/b_1 integrin (VLA-4) ligands in arthritis: vascular cell adhesion molecule expression in synovium and on fibroblast-like synoviocytes. *Arthritis Rheum* **149**: 1424–1431.

Noble DP, Pitsillides AA, Dudhia J & Edwards JCW (1994) *In situ* hybridisation for decorin, collagens type I and III mRNA in normal, rheumatoid and osteoarthritic synovial lining. *Br J Rheumatol* **32** (**Abst supplement 1**): 38.

O'Rahilly R & Gardner E (1978) The embryology of movable joints. In Sokoloff L (ed) *The Joints and Synovial Fluid*, Vol 1, pp 105–176. New York: Academic Press.

Prehm P (1983) Synthesis of hyaluronan in differentiated teratocarcinoma cells. II. Mechanisms of chain growth. *Biochem J* **211**: 191–198.

Revell PA, Mapp PI, Lalor PA & Hall PA (1987) Proliferative activity of cells in synovium as demonstrated by a monoclonal antibody, Ki67. *Rheumatol Int* **7**: 183–186.

Rice GE, Munro JM, Corless C & Bevilacqua MP (1991) Vascular and non-vascular expression of INCAM-110; a target for mononuclear leucocyte adhesion in normal and inflamed human tissues. *Am J Pathol* **138**: 385–393.

Sedgwick AD, Moore AR, Edwards JCW & Willoughby DA (1986) Degradation of cartilage in contact with soft tissue. *Int J Tissue React* **8**(4): 309–319.

Shiozawa S, Yoshihara R, Kuoroki Y, Fujita T, Shiozawa K & Imura S (1992) Pathogenic importance of fibronectin in the superficial region of articular cartilage as a local factor for the induction of pannus extension over rheumatoid articular cartilage. *Ann Rheum Dis* **51**: 869–873.

Stevens CR, Mapp PI & Revell PA (1990) A monoclonal antibody (Mab 67) marks type B synoviocytes. *Rheumatol Int* **10**: 103–106.

Trabandt A, Aicher WK, Gay RE, Sukhatme VP, Fassbender HG & Gay S (1992) Spontaneous expression of immediate-early response genes c-fos and egr-1 in collagenase-producing rheumatoid synovial fibroblasts. *Rheumatol Int* **12**: 53–59.

Wilkinson LS, Worrall JG, Sinclair HS & Edwards JCW (1990) Immunohistochemical reassessment of accessory cell populations in normal and diseased human synovium. *Br J Rheumatol* **29**: 4, 259–263.

Wilkinson LS, Pitsillides AA, Worrall JG & Edwards JCW (1992) Light microscopic characterisation of the fibroblastic synovial lining cell (synoviocyte). *Arthritis Rheum* **35**: 1179–1184.

Wilkinson LS, Edwards JCW, Poston R & Haskard DO (1993a) Cell populations expressing VCAM-1 in normal and diseased synovium. *Lab Invest* **68**: 82–88.

Wilkinson LS, Moore AR, Pitsillides AA, Willoughby DA & Edwards JCW (1993b) Comparison of surface fibroblastic cells in subcutaneous air pouch and synovial lining: differences in uridine diphosphoglucose dehydrogenase activity. *J Exp Pathol* **74**: 113–115.

Worrall JG, Baylis MT & Edwards JCW (1994) Zonal distribution of sulphated proteoglycans in normal and rheumatoid synovium. *Br J Rheumatol* in press.

Yielding KL, Tomkins GM & Bunim JJ (1957) Synthesis of hyaluronic acid by human synovial tissue slices. *Science* **125**: 1300–1300.

9 Cellular Biology of Cartilage Degradation

A. Robin Poole, Mauro Alini and
Anthony P. Hollander

INTRODUCTION

In conjunction with synovial fluid, articular cartilage provides an almost frictionless surface in diarthrodial joints that is very strong, reversibly deformable, and permits normal articulation. Damage to and loss of these cartilages, such as occurs in arthritis, leads to loss of joint function.

Adult human articular cartilage is composed of chondrocytes (less than 5% by volume) and an extensive complex extracellular matrix (Poole, 1993), which is synthesized by these cells and can be degraded by them, probably as or more potently than any other cell type. Careful regulation of matrix synthesis and degradation (together these processes represent turnover) is an integral requirement for the maintenance of a healthy, fully functional cartilage. In arthritis, the normal turnover of this matrix, which is thought to be primarily mediated by the chondrocytes, is impaired as a result of abnormal environmental stimuli. These are both chemical (particularly in rheumatoid arthritis (RA) and include cytokines, generated by inflamed synovium and cells in synovial fluid) and mechanical stimuli. The latter play an important role in the development of osteoarthritis (OA) resulting from joint incongruity or damage to joint tissues leading to altered loading of cartilage. Changes in matrix turnover can lead to net degradation or net accretion of matrix. The attendant remodelling that causes degradation involves both damage to the collagen fibrillar network (loss of tensile properties) and loss of the large proteoglycan aggrecan (loss of compressive stiffness), as well as involving the other numerous constituents from which this matrix is organized (see Poole, 1993). Net degradation may also occur as a result of impaired synthesis, as in RA.

In this chapter we review recent advances in our understanding of cartilage degeneration/degradation *in vitro* and *in vivo*. We discuss how degradation relates to the environment of the cell and matrix turnover, in physiology and pathology.

MECHANISMS OF MATRIX DEGRADATION

TISSUE PROTEINASES

Extensive studies in the last decade have confirmed earlier indications that cartilage degradation primarily results from the extracellular activity of tissue proteinases (Poole, 1990; Woessner, 1991; Matrisian, 1992) (Table 1). Chondrocytes can synthesize and secrete a large number of these proteinases which, together (not singly), degrade the extracellular matrix of cartilage.

Mechanisms and Models in Rheumatoid Arthritis
ISBN 0–12–340440–1

Table 1. Cartilage proteinases, substrates, pH optima, and natural inhibitors. Modified from Poole (1993) with permission

Proteinase classes and names	Natural activator	Cartilage substrates	pH	Inhibitor
Metallo				
Interstitial collagenase MMP-1 (52→42, 24)[a]	Stromelysin Plasmin Kallikrein Cathepsin B	Collagen types II and X (not IX, XI); denatured type II, aggrecan	Neutral	TIMP-1 > TIMP-2
Neutrophil collagenase[b] (MMP-8 (75→58)	As interstitial collagenase (?)	Collagen type II	Neutral	TIMP-1, TIMP-2
Gelatinases 72 kDa MMP-2 (72→66) 92 kDa MMP-9 (92→86)	Plasmin elastase (MMP-2)	Denatured type II collagen type X and XI, elastin	Neutral	TIMP-2 > TIMP-1
Stromelysin-1 MMP-3 (57→48, 28)	Plasmin Cathepsin B	Aggrecan, fibronectin type IX and XI collagens, procollagens, link protein g decorin, elastin	4.8–8.0	TIMP-1 > TIMP-2
Stromelysin-2 MMP-10 (57→44)	As stromelysin-1 (?)	As stromelysin-1 (?)	4.8–8.0	TIMP-1 > TIMP-2
Stomelysin-3 MMP (-11) (51→44)	Unknown	Unknown	Unknown	TIMP-1/TIMP-2
Matrilysin (PUMP) MMP-7 (28→19)	As stromelysin-1	Aggrecan	Neutral	TIMP-1/TIMP-2
Macrophage metalloelastase MMP-12 (53→21)	Unknown	Elastin Fibronectin	Neutral	Unknown
Serine				
Plasmin (from plasminogen)[c]	Plasminogen activators (UPA, TPA) Plasmin, cathepsin B Kallikrein[c]	Prometalloproteinases	Neutral	α$_2$-anti-plasmin
Tissue plasminogen activator (from pro TPA)	Cathepsin B Kallikrein	Plasminogen	Neutral	Protease nexin I, PAI-1
Urokinase-type plasminogen activator (from pro UPA)	Cathepsin B Kallikrein	Plasminogen	Neutral	Protease nexin I, PAI-1

Elastase[b]	None	Type II, IX, X, XI collagens, aggrecan, fibronectin	Neutral	α_1-PI
Cathepsin G[b]	None	TIMP, aggrecan, elastin, type II collagen	Neutral	α_1-PI
Kallikrein[c]	Factor XII$_a$, XII$_f$	Procollagenase, prostromelysin (?) progelatinase (?)	Neutral	α_1-PI
Cysteine				
Cathepsin B	None	Procollagen type II, type II collagen (telopeptides), aggrecan, link protein	5.0–6.5	Cystatins
Cathepsin L	None	Link protein, elastin, type II collagen (telopeptides), aggrecan	4.0–6.5	Cystatins
Cathepsin S	None	Probably as cathepsin B	Neutral	Cystatins
Aspartate				
Cathepsin D	None	Aggrecan, denatured type II collagen	3.0–6.0	α_2-macroglobulin

[a] Proenzyme → active enzyme (molecular sizes, kDa).
[b] From polymorphonuclear leukocytes (neutrophils).
[c] From plasma.
α_1-PI, α1-proteinase inhibitor; PAI-1, plasminogen activator inhibitor-1.

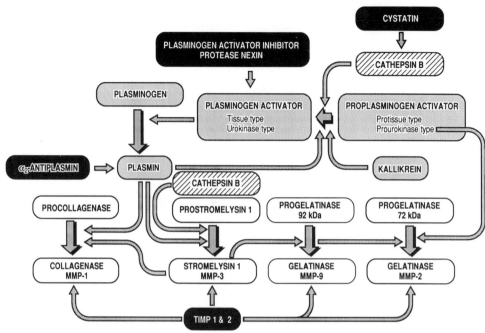

Figure 1. Proteinase–inhibitor interactions regulating metalloproteinase activity. Proteinases of the same class are indicated by boxes of the same kind. Closed boxes represent the inhibitors. Activation of one proteinase by another and their inhibition are indicated by the arrows. Modified from Poole (1993) with permission.

Most attention has been focused recently on metalloproteinases (Table 1; Fig. 1). These function at both neutral and moderately acid and alkaline pH. Whether matrilysin is present in articular cartilage remains unclear.

ACTIVATION OF PROMETALLOPROTEINASES

Metalloproteinases share common structural features (Docherty and Murphy, 1990) (Fig. 2). All require a zinc atom at the active site. They are synthesized and secreted as inactive proenzymes which are activated in the extracellular matrix. This activation may involve a mechanism called the 'cysteine switch' (van Wart and Birkedal-Hansen, 1990; Springman et al., 1990), whereby an initial 'exogenous' proteolytic or free radical cleavage leads to a change in molecular conformation resulting from disengagement of a cysteine residue (near the amino terminus) from the zinc atom in the active site (Fig. 3). This results in secondary autocleavage(s), or cleavage by another proteinase leading to full activation. Thus, by way of example, activation of prostromelysin involves removal of a portion of the prodomain by plasmin destabilizing the association with zinc of the cysteine residue in the conserved PRCGV(or N)PD sequence. This altered conformation permits autoproteolysis by stromelysin, leading to removal of the entire prodomain. This may extend to cleavage and removal of significant portions of the molecule (Marcy et al., 1991). Alternatively, procollagenase can be partially activated by plasmin to produce a molecule which is further cleaved by

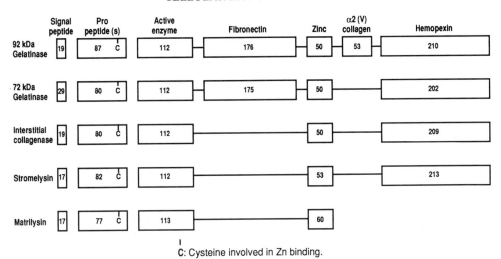

C: Cysteine involved in Zn binding.

Figure 2. Domain structures of human prometalloproteinases. The number of amino acid residues is shown in each domain where domains are absent, the connection of remaining domains is indicated by a single line. 'C' located in the propeptide indicates the approximate position of the cysteine involved in the cysteine switch. The fibronectin-like domain, the zinc-containing active site, the α2(V) collagen-like domain and the hemopexin-like domain are shown. Sequence data are published in Docherty and Murphy (1990). From Woessner (1991) with permission.

stromelysin-1, with removal of the prodomain to produce 'superactivation' of collagenase (Murphy *et al.*, 1987; Brinckerhoff *et al.*, 1990). The 92-kDa gelatinase is also activated by stromelysin (Ogata *et al.*, 1992; Okada *et al.*, 1992). Stromelysin-1 can also activate the 72-kDa gelatinase in conjunction with aminophenyl mercuriacetate (Miyazaki *et al.*, 1992). Hence it may act as a coactivator.

Plasmin has been reported to be a very poor activator of the 72-kDa and 92-kDa gelatinases (Murphy *et al.*, 1989; Okada *et al.*, 1990; Moll *et al.*, 1990; Chen *et al.*, 1991), although others have more recently shown that urokinase type plasminogen activators (PA) can activate the 72-kDa gelatinase (Keski-Oja *et al.*, 1992). The presence of plasminogen in chondrocyte cultures causes increased matrix degradation in the presence of interleukin-1 (IL-1). This implicates plasmin activity, derived from plasminogen activator by plasminogen (Collier and Ghosh, 1988; Cruwys *et al.*, 1990). Because of the large size of plasminogen (90 kDa), it is unlikely that plasminogen can penetrate healthy cartilages, other than the more permeable aggrecan-deficient superficial zone of articular cartilages. Ordinarily, the proteoglycan aggrecan renders the matrix impermeable to most molecules larger than about 60 kDa (Maroudas, 1976). But in arthritis, loss of aggrecan molecules and the resultant increased matrix permeability would favour plasminogen penetration. Whether this molecule can be synthesized by chondrocytes is not known.

Both PAs, namely the urokinase and tissue types (Campbell *et al.*, 1988) and the plasminogen activator-1 (PA-1) inhibitor (Campbell *et al.*, 1991) are produced by chondrocytes, and in increased amounts on stimulation with IL-1. Since cell surfaces bear receptors for urokinase-type PA, plasminogen and plasmin (see Vassalli *et al.*, 1991) these enzymes probably operate in pericellular site. Plasminogen activators

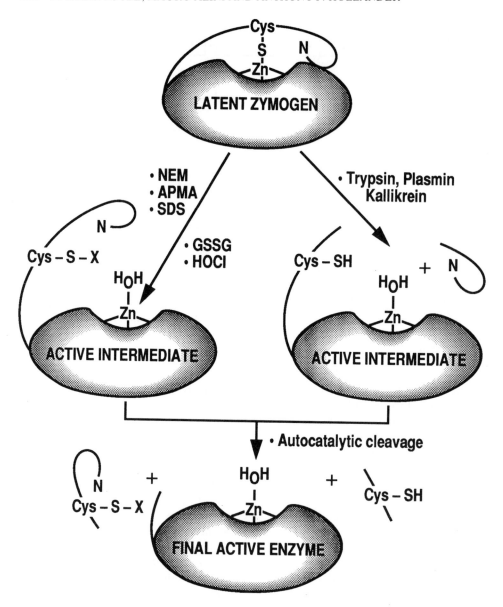

Figure 3. Cysteine switch mechanism of prometalloproteinase activation, as proposed by Springman *et al.* (1990). Cysteine in the prodomain (see Fig. 2) binds to zinc to maintain latency. Reagents that react with sulphydryl groups bind covalently to cysteine and produce an active intermediate. These include organomercurials such as aminophenyl mercuriacetate (APMA), *N*-ethylmaleimide (NEM), oxidized glutathione (GSSG), hydrochlorous acid (HOCl) and sodium dodecyl sulphate (SDS). Alternatively, proteolytic enzymes (serine proteinases) can cleave the propeptide towards the amino terminus. These also include elastase and cathepsin G. In the second step the active enzyme can be autocatalytically cleaved to remove the propeptide and confer permanent activity. From Woessner (1991) with permission.

therefore have the potential to play an important role in matrix degradation but their involvement in cartilage degradation remains unproven.

The cysteine proteinase cathepsin B can activate prostromelysin-1 (Murphy *et al.*, 1992b) at near neutral pH (J.S. Mort and A.R. Poole *et al.*, in preparation). It is also reported to activate prourokinase-type PA (Kobayashi *et al.*, 1991). Recently, inhibition of cysteine proteinases (Buttle and Saklatvala, 1992; Buttle *et al.*, 1992), and specifically cathepsin B (Buttle *et al.*, 1993), and metalloproteinases (Seed *et al.*, 1993; Mort *et al.*, 1993; Buttle *et al.*, 1993) with synthetic inhibitors was shown to arrest matrix degradation, *in vitro*, implicating both classes of proteinases at the levels indicated in Fig. 1. Thus, we envisage, in some situations, a complex interactive cascade of cysteine and metalloproteinases, metalloproteinase activation involving cysteine proteinases, resulting in matrix degradation. But whereas an inhibitor of cathepsin B can inhibit IL-1 stimulated degradation, it has no effect on retinoic acid-stimulated degradation (Buttle *et al.*, 1993). Since in both systems degradation is inhibited by a metalloproteinase inhibitor it would seem that cathepsin B may not always be involved in the activation of metalloproteinases, such as prostromelysin-1, but metalloproteinases are always involved. For further information concerning metalloproteinase activation mechanisms, consult Nagase *et al.* (1991).

PROTEINASE INHIBITORS

The activities of these proteinases are regulated by class-specific proteinase inhibitors (Table 1, Fig. 1). The balance between active (activated) proteinase and active inhibitor determines the amount of net proteolysis. In osteoarthritic cartilage, the contents of the tissue inhibitors of metalloproteinases (TIMP-1 and TIMP-2) (Yamada *et al.*, 1987; Dean *et al.*, 1989), serine proteinase inhibitors (Yamada *et al.*, 1987) and cysteine proteinase inhibitors (Martel-Pelletier *et al.*, 1990) are reduced, in comparison to proteinase content, favouring enhanced proteolysis, a pathobiological characteristic of arthritis. Similarly, in the hypertrophic zone of the growth plate there is increased degradation (Dean *et al.*, 1985, 1990) and net loss of type II collagen (Alini *et al.*, 1992) resulting from increased production of procollagenase, prostromelysin and progelatinase (Dean *et al.*, 1985; Brown *et al.*, 1989), coupled with a reduction in TIMP (Brown *et al.*, 1989), which favours enhanced proteolysis (Dean *et al.*, 1985, 1990). Thus, enhanced degradation in both growth plate and in osteoarthritic cartilages results from an imbalance in proteinase inhibitor activity. However, there are, as yet, no convincing results to indicate that one of these naturally occurring inhibitors can arrest the degradation of cartilage matrix. The role of proteases in RA is dealt with in detail by Cawston in Chapter 17, this volume.

FREE RADICALS

Free radicals have long been implicated in damage to connective tissues in inflammation and arthritis. But data supporting a role for these radicals were, until recently, lacking. Chondrocytes can generate hydrogen peroxide from which free radicals can be readily generated (see below) (Tiku *et al.*, 1990). Nitric oxide synthase is present and can be induced by IL-1 and tumour necrosis factor α (TNFα) (Palmer *et al.*, 1993). Hyaluronic acid is very susceptible to cleavage by free radicals, particularly superoxide (Greenwald and Moy, 1980; Halliwell and Gutteridge, 1986) and hydroxyl (Wong *et al.*, 1981) radicals. Therefore in the absence of demonstratable hyaluronidase activity in cartilage, the reduction in the molecular size of hyaluronic acid with increasing age (Thonar *et al.*, 1978; Holmes *et al.*, 1988) and that observed following synthesis by chondrocytes (Ng *et al.*, 1992), is likely due to chondrocyte-generated free radicals. Hydroxyl radical (°OH), formed from hydrogen peroxide in the presence of transition metals (such as copper and zinc), can cleave link protein at a site between two histidine residues near the amino terminus (Roberts *et al.*, 1987, 1989). This probably results from transition metal binding between these histidines, catalysing a Fenton-type or Haber–Weiss reaction (Halliwell and Gutteridge, 1986). The core protein of aggrecan is also cleaved by the °OH radical (Roberts *et al.*, 1989). Careful studies employing free radical scavengers are needed to determine how important these radicals are in causing damage to matrix molecules in cartilage.

Neutrophils can produce quantities of hypochlorous acid (HOCl) which can activate latent neutrophil procollagenase and progelatinase as well as inactivating inhibitors of these and other proteinases (Weiss *et al.*, 1985, 1989). Hypochlorous acid can also activate the 92-kDa progelatinase (Okada *et al.*, 1992a). It is conceivable that this activation involves oxidation of the cysteine-switch residue. Therefore nitric oxide, hypochlorous acid, as well as other free radicals, may together or singly activate some or all of the latent metalloproteinases. Moreover oxygen-derived free radicals can potently degrade cartilage matrix alone or in the presence of free radical-activated neutrophil procollagenase (Burkhardt *et al.*, 1986). But neutrophils may not play a major role in producing cartilage damage in acute inflammation as suggested by the studies of Pettipher *et al.* (1989, 1990) and Dodge and Poole (1989). Their effects may be less obvious and remain to be identified. The involvement of free radicals in the pathology of RA is reviewed by Halliwell in Chapter 15 of this volume.

COLLAGEN CLEAVAGE

Collagenase is the only proteinase that can cleave the triple helix of type II collagen in cartilage and type I and III collagens in other tissues. A three-quarter·fragment (TC^A) and a one-quarter (TC^B) fragment are produced from the collagen α chains (Fig. 4). The former is clearly recognizable in bovine articular cartilages cultured with IL-1 (Dodge and Poole, 1989), implicating collagenase in the degradation of type II collagen. This leads to unwinding of the triple helix which can be detected in normal and arthritic cartilages immunohistochemically (Dodge and Poole, 1989; Mort *et al.*, 1993) and by immunoassay (Hollander *et al.*, 1994). Normal healthy adult human articular cartilages may contain up to 3% of their total collagen in an unwound (non-helical) molecular form. But in the bovine foetus this percentage is increased to about 10%. This may reflect in part the increased cleavage that occurs during the process of remodelling which is an integral feature of the growth process.

Increased cleavage of the more superficial type II collagen at and close to the articular surface is a feature of ageing and early changes in OA cartilage (Fig. 5) (Dodge and Poole, 1989). In OA this damage is observed in the same sites where increased expression of the stromelysin-1 gene and, to a lesser degree, the insterstitial collagenase gene are detected by *in situ* hybridization (Nguyen *et al.*, 1992). Overall, there is increased expression of mRNA for collagenase, stromelysin-1 and both the

COLLAGEN FIBRIL

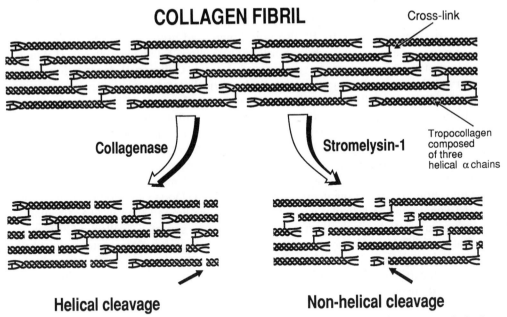

Figure 4. Cleavage of type II collagen by mammalian collagenase (MMP-1) and stromelysin-1 (MMP-3). Modified from Poole (1993) with permission.

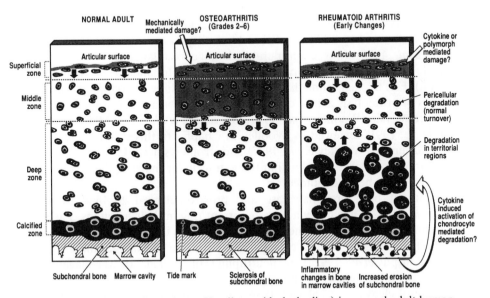

Figure 5. Sites of degradation of type II collagen (dark shading) in normal adult human articular cartilage and in arthritis detected with a polyclonal antiserum to epitopes on the CB8 and CBII peptides of type II collagen. Subchondral changes in bone are shown. The direction of progression of collagen cleavage with further degeneration is indicated by solid arrows. Modified from Poole (1993) with permission.

72-kDa and 92-kDa gelatinases in OA (Mohtai et al., 1993). Using immunohisto-chemistry, Okada et al. (1992b) also noted increased production of stromelysin-1 in these more superficial sites where fibrillation develops following collagen II damage and loss of the proteoglycans aggrecan and decorin. Collagen II degradation is then observed deeper in the matrix, starting in pericellular sites adjacent to the more superficial band of collagen II damage. It spreads out from the cell involving territorial and interterritorial sites. Thus, collagen II degeneration progresses deeper into the cartilage into the mid and deep zones in OA as the cartilage becomes progressively more degenerate (Dodge and Poole, 1989; Hollander et al., 1994) (Fig. 5).

This contrasts to RA, where type II collagen cleavage is usually first seen in peri-cellular and territorial sites adjacent to the calcified matrix and subchondral bone around chondrocytes of the deep zone (Figs 5 and 6) (Dodge and Poole, 1989). In RA early damage to the articular surface is much more limited than in OA: fibrillation, which occurs in OA as a result of damage to the more superficial collagen fibrils, is not a feature of RA, probably because of the less extensive damage to these fibrils. Diffuse damage to collagen fibrils through the cartilage matrix is a feature of more advanced cartilage degeneration in RA (Dodge and Poole, 1989). This clearly involves damage to pre-existing collagen fibrils (Dodge et al., 1991). Collectively, these observations suggest that in RA the cellular events in the adjacent juxta-articular bone, which produces an extensive osteopenia, may result in the production of 'prodegradative' cytokines, such as IL-1 and TNFα (see section on cytokines/growth factors in this chapter), which act not only on osteoblasts/osteoclasts, but also upon these deep zone chondrocytes close to the bone (Figs 5 and 6). The role of cytokines in bone remodelling in RA is discussed by Skerry and Gowen in Chapter 10, this volume.

The chondrocyte clearly has the potential to degrade type II collagen, as evidenced by the damage caused by addition of IL-1 to cartilage in culture (Dodge and Poole, 1989; Mort et al., 1993). In RA considerable damage to collagen II is observed in sites immediately adjacent to pannus invading cartilage (A. Hollander et al., manuscript in preparation) (Fig. 6), suggesting that both direct and indirect (chondrocyte-mediated) mechanisms of proteolysis are involved. The synovium is a potent source of collage-nase and stromelysin (Woolley et al., 1977; Gravallese et al., 1991; McCrachen, 1991; Firestein et al., 1991, reviewed by Woolley in Chapter 6, this volume). Adjacent to pannus, collagenase (Woolley et al., 1977) and stromelysin-1 (Hasty et al., 1990) can be detected in chondrocytes and within the extracellular matrix, where collagen and other molecules are being degraded.

The ability of both procollagenase and prostromelysin-1 to bind to collagen (Murphy et al., 1992a) must play a very important role in their functions. Particularly since it permits accumulation of these latent proteinases in extracellular sites awaiting activation. The ability to bind to collagen resides in the carboxy-terminal regions of interstitial (Murphy et al., 1992a) and neutrophil (Hirose et al., 1993) collagenases and stromelysin-1 (Murphy et al., 1992a).

Triple helical cleavage of collagen II resulting from the activity of the neutrophil collagenase may be of limited importance, as discussed above. Moreover, experimen-tal studies of beige mice, which are deficient in elastase and cathepsin G, have revealed that antigen-induced arthritis leads to as much cartilage proteoglycan (aggre-can) loss as in normal mice (Pettipher et al., 1990). Loss of articular cartilage aggrecan

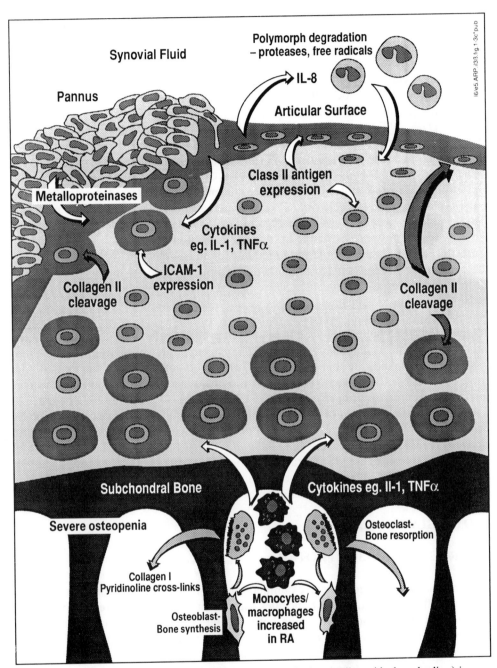

Figure 6. Sites of degradation of type II collagen in articular cartilage (darker shading) in rheumatoid arthritis and its relationship to synovial pannus, joint fluid and changes in subchondral bone.

in acute inflamed joints in rabbits is also independent of polymorphonuclear leukocyte (neutrophil) accumulation (Pettipher *et al.*, 1989). It would therefore seem that the role of the polymorph in cartilage degradation is secondary to that of chondrocyte and synovial-mediated degradation.

Collagen II can also be cleaved in the non-helical telopeptide regions where inter-molecular crosslinks are located (Fig. 4). Thus stromelysin-1 (Wu *et al.*, 1991), cathepsin B (Burleigh *et al.*, 1974) and the polymorph proteinases elastase and cathepsin G (Starkey *et al.*, 1977) can all cleave in these non-helical sites, probably leading to loss of tensile properties, as in the case of elastase (Bader *et al.*, 1981). The relative importance of stromelysin-1 and interstitial collagenase in collagen cleavage remains to be clearly established. But when articular cartilage is cultured with IL-1, the biosynthesis of matrix molecules, such as collagen II, is inhibited (Tyler and Benton, 1988; Goldring *et al.*, 1988, 1990). Thus the increased extractability of collagen II α chains, which is observed under these conditions (Dodge and Poole, 1989), suggests the activity of a proteinase capable of cleaving in the non-helical telopeptide domains. Since this activity is inhibitable by a metalloproteinase inhibitor (Mort *et al.*, 1993), the activity of stromelysin-1, or another metalloproteinase, is implicated. Even if stromelysin-1 does not significantly cleave type II collagen, the ability of stromelysin-1 to superactive procollagenase (Murphy *et al.*, 1987; Brinckerhoff *et al.*, 1990) still makes it a very important enzyme in collagenolysis.

Unwound triple helical collagen is readily cleaved by either the 72-kDa or 92-kDa gelatinases (Table 1) and also by interstitial collagenase and stromelysin-1. But there is no evidence to indicate that any of these other metalloproteinases can degrade the triple helix of type II collagen. Thus, their roles in collagen degradation are viewed as secondary rather than primary.

Relatively little is known of the degradation of other collagens in cartilage. Type IX collagen is, however, not cleaved by interstitial collagenase. But stromelysin-1 can cleave this molecule extensively (Okada *et al.*, 1989). Since abnormal expression of α_1(IX) chains can cause degenerative changes in cartilage (Nakata *et al.*, 1993), damage to type IX collagen by this proteinase would be an important contributing component to loss of cartilage function in arthritis.

PROTEOGLYCAN CLEAVAGE

AGGRECAN AND LINK PROTEIN

A number of recent studies have examined the cleavage of the core protein of aggrecan and of link protein. These molecules form macromolecular aggregates with hyaluronic acid (HA), binding occurring between the G1 globular domain of aggrecan, link protein and HA (Fig. 7). *In vitro* analyses first revealed that aggrecan is initially cleaved proteolytically to release a very high molecular weight product essentially similar in size to intact aggrecan but no longer capable of aggregation with HA (Campbell *et al.*, 1986). In adult human and bovine cartilages, this cleavage, in the interglobular domain between the G1 and G2 globular domains (Fig. 7) (Fosang *et al.*, 1991a; Sandy *et al.*, 1991b; Flannery *et al.*, 1992), occurs between residues Glu 373 and Ala 374, both *in vivo* (Sandy *et al.*, 1992) and *in vitro* (Sandy *et al.*, 1991a,b; Loulakis *et al.*, 1992; Ilic *et al.*, 1992) (Fig. 8). The interglobular domain is also

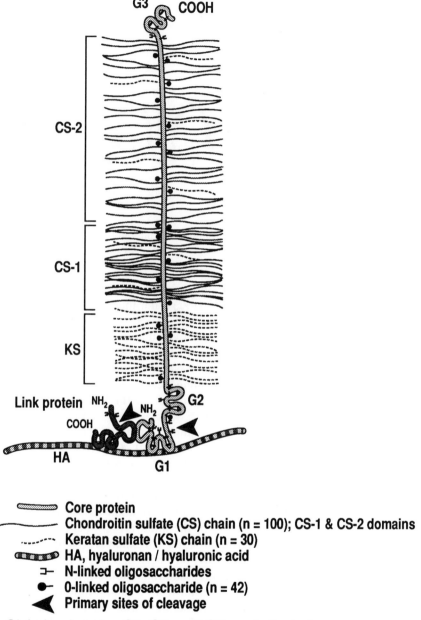

Figure 7. Main sites of cleavage (arrowheads) in aggrecan and link protein. Modified from Poole (1993).

cleaved by matrilysin, the 72-kDa and 92-kDa gelatinases, cathepsin B and interstial collagenase (Hughes *et al.*, 1991; Fosang *et al.*, 1992) (Fig. 8). Naturally occurring cleavage sites here and elsewhere in the molecule, such as in the chondroitin sulphate

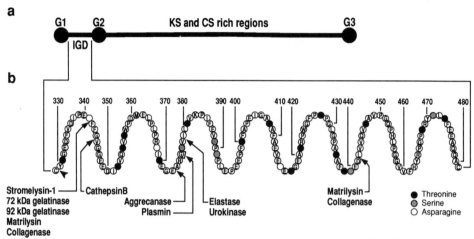

Figure 8. Sites of cleavage of aggrecan core protein in the interglobular domain between G1 and G2 by tissue proteinases. Modified from Fosang *et al.* (1992) with permission.

rich region, have characteristic features suggesting that one common proteinase is responsible (Loulakis *et al.*, 1992; Ilic *et al.*, 1992) other than stromelysin-1 (Fosang *et al.*, 1991a; Flannery *et al.*, 1992).

In proteoglycan aggregates, Nguyen, Roughley and Mort and their colleagues have shown that link proteins are mainly cleaved in the exposed amino terminal region (Figs 7 and 9) where natural cleavages sites have been identified. Within the disulphide-bonded loop closest to the amino terminus, cleavages can occur between residues 65 and 66, and between 72 and 73 (Nguyen *et al.*, 1991). Stromelysin-1, cathepsin B, cathepsin G, stromelysin-2, collagenase, 72-kDa and 92-kDa gelatinases all produce fragments of link protein with *N*-termini identical to those produced *in situ* and *in vivo* (Nguyen *et al.*, 1991, 1993). Cathepsin L (Nguyen *et al.*, 1990) and hydroxyl radicals (Roberts *et al.*, 1987) can also cleave within the amino-terminal disulphide-bonded loop. Using antibodies prepared to the amino-terminal sequence that is produced on cleavage of link protein by stromelysin-1, it is apparent that whereas this proteinase-generated cleavage site is commonly observed in neonatal cartilage it is much less commonly found in the adult (Hughes *et al.*, 1992). These observations confirm earlier amino terminal sequencing analyses (Nguyen *et al.*, 1989, 1991). Collectively, it would seem that either stromelysin-1 is less involved in degradation of proteoglycan aggregates in the adult and that another proteinase(s) is more active, or that altered cleavage sites may result from changes in molecular structure and aggregation due to differences in posttranslational modification of proteins, such as altered glycosylation, that occur in ageing. For example, the interglobular region of aggrecan between G1 and G2 contains keratan sulphate (Barry *et al.*, 1992). In the foetus and newborn, there is much less keratan sulphate on aggrecan core than is present in the adult (Roughley and White, 1980). Thus accessibility of proteinases to the core protein may be regulated by the glycosaminoglycans or oligosaccharides as sites of glycosylation vary with age, thereby influencing cleavage sites.

Although newly synthesized aggrecan molecules contain the G3 globular domain, rotary shadowing analyses have revealed that only a proportion of molecules possess

a

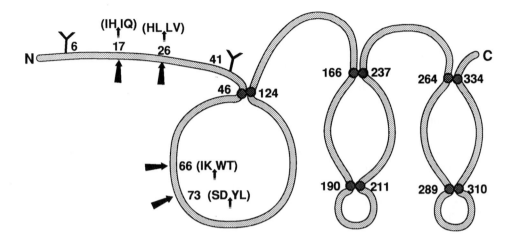

b

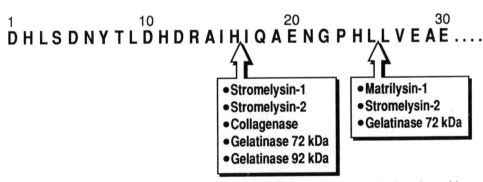

Figure 9. Sites of cleavage in human adult link protein. a, natural sites; b, sites cleaved by metalloproteinases. The residues that become amino termini on cleavage are shown as well as sequence before and after cleavage site. Modified from Nguyen *et al.* (1991, 1993) with permission.

this domain in adult cartilage (Paulsson *et al.*, 1987; Mörgelin *et al.*, 1988). Its removal is no doubt the result of proteolytic 'trimming' in the extracellular matrix. Further evidence for extracellular proteolysis is provided by the progressive accumulation of extracellular keratan sulphate-rich and chondroitin sulphate-rich degradation products with increasing age (Franzen *et al.*, 1981; Webber *et al.*, 1987; Poole *et al.*, 1993a). In OA, degradation products are even smaller in early disease (Rizkalla *et al.*, 1992). These degradation products retained, in part, by their ability to bind to hyaluronan, increase in content especially in the deep zone (Baylis and Ali, 1978; Franzen *et al.*, 1981). When the hyaluronan is lost in OA, so are the aggrecan molecules

(Rizkalla *et al.*, 1992), since they no longer have sufficient binding sites within the extracellular matrix.

In ageing (Roughley *et al.*, 1985), as well as in OA, there is a preponderance of these degradation products containing the G1 globular domain. In arthritis, these degradation products are released into synovial fluid (Witter *et al.*, 1987) in increased amounts (Dahlberg *et al.*, 1992). The content of the G1 globular domain is more common in rheumatoid joints with more advanced cartilage damage (Saxne and Heinegård, 1992), probably due to increased matrix degradation producing a cartilage matrix richer in these degradation products. In earlier disease molecules containing the glycosaminoglycan-rich region predominate.

In vitro, the release of the proteoglycan aggrecan from cartilage matrix occurs prior to that of type II collagen degradation products (Dingle *et al.*, 1975; A. Hollander *et al.*, manuscript in preparation) suggesting that proteoglycans are more susceptible to degradation and loss from the extracellular matrix. However, measurement of collagen fragment release is not an accurate indication of collagen II cleavage *in situ*, since degradation of collagen leading to unwinding of the triple helix in the extracellular matrix precedes a significant increased release of collagen II fragments when cartilage is cultured with IL-1 (A. Hollander *et al.*, manuscript in preparation). Yet denaturation of type II collagen is effectively secondary to detectable loss of the proteoglycan aggrecan. But whereas these proteoglycans can be replaced by active biosynthesis and contents are generally maintained in a disease such as OA, localized loss occurs at and close to the articular surface in the early disease (Fig. 5), but in the mid and deep zones (Rizkalla *et al.*, 1992), there is a compensatory increase in content and these molecules are lost only in advanced disease (A.R. Poole *et al.*, manuscript in preparation). In contrast, there is a net loss of collagen at all stages of OA although this is not observed in RA (Hollander *et al.*, 1994).

The release of aggrecan from articular cartilages stimulated by IL-1 can also be arrested by a hydroxamate inhibitor of metalloproteinases (Seed *et al.*, 1993; Mort *et al.*, 1993; Buttle *et al.*, 1993). Thus, metalloproteinases are also directly implicated in the degradation of aggrecan. Although metalloproteinases may be involved in the cleavage of this molecule, inhibition of a putative activator(s) of prometalloproteinases can also lead to inhibition of their cleavage. Thus, inhibitors of cysteine proteinases can arrest the rapid release of aggrecan induced by IL-1 but not that induced by retinoic acid (Buttle *et al.*, 1993). Whether cysteine proteinases act solely as activators of metalloproteinases or can also cleave aggrecan and collagens in the extracellular matrix remains to be established.

Following traumatic joint injury, such as meniscal tear or cruciate ligament rupture, there is a rapid (within 1 week) increase in aggrecan fragments in synovial fluid (Lohmander *et al.*, 1989; Lohmander, 1991). These then return to levels just above normal within about 10–20 weeks. Joint injuries of this kind often eventually lead to clinical post-traumatic OA, where aggrecan levels are elevated in synovial fluids (Dahlberg *et al.*, 1992). Chondrocytes appear to sense a change in matrix loading, caused probably by joint instability created by traumatic injury, and respond by increased turnover of the proteoglycan aggrecan. These degradative changes may initially involve primarily the pericellular matrix where newly synthesized molecules are present: later, as pathology develops, resident molecules are also degraded (Figs 11 and 12).

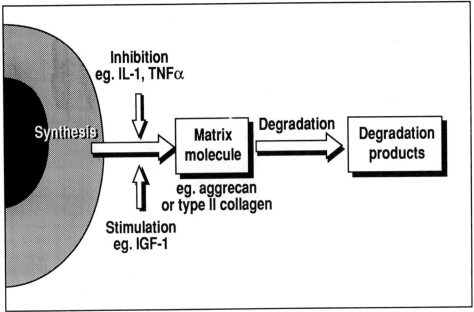

Figure 10. Degradation of newly synthesized matrix molecules can be dependent upon the rate of synthesis. This can be influenced by cytokines as indicated. A cell is shown on the left of the figure. Thus degradation products detected by immunoassay may reflect how synthesis (not just degradation) is influenced by environmental cytokines (see also Fig. 12).

DECORIN

The proteoglycan decorin binds to collagen fibrils as they form and can regulate fibril diameter: fibrils that form in the presence of decorin are of reduced diameter (Vogel and Trotter, 1987). In normal adult articular cartilage, collagen fibrils are much thinner at the articular surface (Ratcliffe *et al.*, 1984) where decorin is most concentrated (Poole *et al.*, 1986). It is in these sites, where collagen fibrils are aligned in parallel to the surface (Weiss *et al.*, 1968), that the tensile properties of adult articular cartilage are maximal (Kempson *et al.*, 1973; Akizuki *et al.*, 1986; Roth and Mow, 1980). Whether decorin plays a role in determining these tensile properties is not known. But in early OA, the damage to these fibrils (Dodge and Poole, 1989), leading to a loss of tensile properties (Kempson *et al.*, 1973; Akizuki *et al.*, 1986), is associated with a net loss of decorin from these more superficial sites (Poole, 1993) (Fig. 11). There is a concomitant increase in content within the middle and deep zones (Poole, 1993), where tensile properties are commonly maintained (Kempson *et al.*, 1973). In RA, there is also net loss of this proteoglycan associated with cleavage, again especially in the superficial zone (Witsch-Prehm *et al.*, 1992). Degradation of decorin probably results, in part at least, from the extracellular activity of stromelysin-1 (Nakano and Scott, 1988).

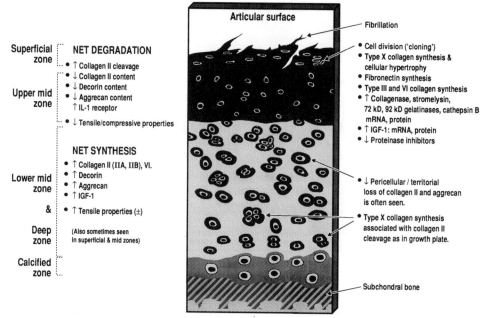

Figure 11. General changes in articular cartilage in osteoarthritis (Mankin grade 2–7). Increases (↑) and decreases (↓) in content, synthesis or mRNA and mechanical properties are indicated.

REGULATION OF MATRIX TURNOVER BY CYTOKINES/GROWTH FACTORS: THE BALANCE BETWEEN SYNTHESIS AND DEGRADATION

Net degradation of cartilage matrix likely results from imbalances in the synthesis, activation and inhibition of proteinases coupled with impaired synthesis and incorporation of molecules within the extracellular matrix, resulting in net loss of structural matrix molecules. Ordinarily, a balance is carefully maintained and regulated. Controlled proteolysis is a feature of normal physiology as evidenced by the release of type II collagen and aggrecan fragments and other cartilage matrix molecules into healthy synovial fluid and peripheral blood which can be detected by immunoassay (see review by Poole, 1994). This physiological turnover of matrix (which is most pronounced during growth) likely involves a rapidly turning-over pool of matrix molecules which are probably mainly in close proximity to the chondrocyte in the pericellular domain (Fig. 12). Thus, whether 'resident' structural molecules (remote from the cell surface) are involved in this measurable turnover and release of cartilage molecules *in vivo* in healthy people is not known at present. But in pathology, such as arthritis, there is unquestionably excessive damage to and removal of resident molecules. This is evidenced morphologically (Mitchell and Shepard, 1978) and immunohistochemically (Dodge and Poole, 1989; Dodge *et al.*, 1991) detectable damage to articular cartilage collagen fibrils in RA and in OA. In both OA and RA, degradation of collagen II is increased over that observed in normal articular cartilage (Hollander *et al.*, 1994). That this also involves enhanced degradation of new synthesized molecules requires examination but is a likely possibility. Thereby excessive proteinase

DEGRADATION OF TYPE II COLLAGEN AND AGGRECAN

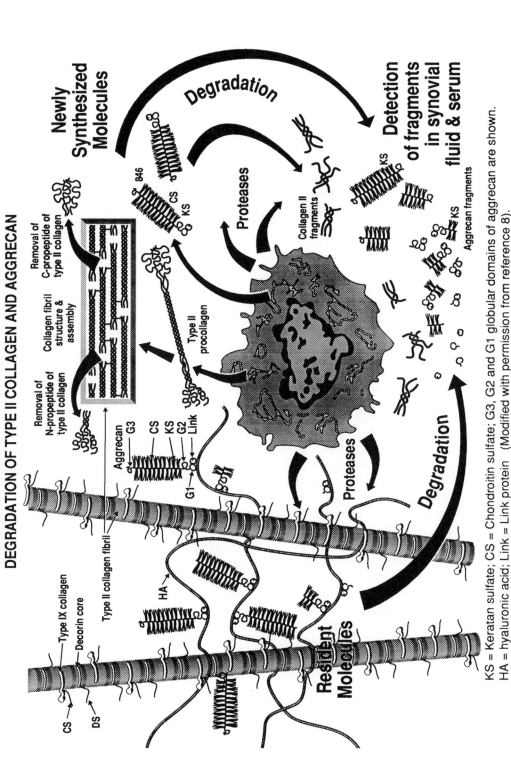

Figure 12. Synthesis and degradation of matrix molecules by chondrocytes. Degradation of newly synthesized molecules may occur in predominantly pericellular sites; in pathology damage to 'resident' molecules is also observed. Reproduced with permission from Poole *et al.* (1993). KS, Keratan sulphate; CS, chondroitin sulphate; G3, G2 and G1, globular domains of aggrecan are shown; HA, hyaluronic acid; Link, link protein.

KS = Keratan sulfate; CS = Chondroitin sulfate; G3, G2 and G1 globular domains of aggrecan are shown. HA = hyaluronic acid; Link = Link protein   (Modified with permission from reference 8).

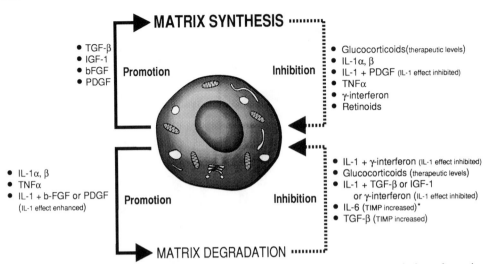

Figure 13. Cytokines and other molecules influencing the synthesis and degradation of matrix by chondrocytes. Degradation of newly synthesized molecules may occur in predominantly pericellular sites; in pathology damage to 'resident' molecules is also observed. Modified from Poole (1993) with permission.

activity can not only cause degradation of preassembled matrix, but would also negate effective repair of damaged matrix. The role of growth factors in RA pathology is discussed by Zagorski and Wahl in Chapter 12, this volume.

Cytokines can significantly influence this balance between synthesis and degradation. Some of these are shown in Fig. 13. Insulin-like growth factor-1 (IGF-1) is probably the most potent anabolic molecule present in serum (McQuillan *et al.*, 1986; Luytens *et al.*, 1988) and synovial fluid (Schalkwijk *et al.*, 1989a), being capable of stimulating the synthesis of major structural matrix molecules in adult articular cartilage. In contrast, the cytokines TNFα (Ikebe *et al.*, 1988; Goldring *et al.*, 1990) and IL-1α,β (Tyler, 1985a; Goldring *et al.*, 1988, 1990; Benton and Tyler, 1988) can, individually or together, potently inhibit matrix synthesis (of type II collagen and aggrecan) at concentrations one-tenth to one-hundredth less than those that stimulate cartilage degradation (Arner and Pratta, 1989). Consequently, loss of the proteoglycan aggrecan from human cartilage can be stimulated by IL-1 without an increase in the rate of degradation of proteoglycan (Nietfield *et al.*, 1990). Thus, inhibition of cartilage matrix synthesis alone can create pathology. Therapeutic levels of glucocorticoids can also potently damage cartilage through inhibition of matrix synthesis of this kind (Chandler and Wright, 1958; Mankin and Conger, 1966).

IL-1α,β, especially 1α (Saklatvala *et al.*, 1984; Tyler, 1985b), and TNFα (Saklatvala, 1986; Lefebvre *et al.*, 1990; Mitchell and Cheung, 1991) can, *in vitro*, potently enhance cartilage degradation. This occurs via increased transcription of metalloproteinases, especially stromelysin-1 in human articular cartilage *in vitro* (Nguyen *et al.*, 1992) and in rabbits *in vivo* (Hutchinson *et al.*, 1992). In the case of TNFα this may involve stimulation of plasminogen activator synthesis (Lefebvre *et al.*, 1990), as well as enhanced transcription of collagenase and stromelysin (Mitchell and Cheung, 1991). Under these conditions, TIMP-1 expression is increased or relatively unchanged. IL-1β also stimulates cathepsin B activity in articular chondrocytes (Baici and Lang, 1990). Cysteine proteinase synthesis and secretion may also be regulated by TNFα.

Interestingly, IGF-1 negates the degradative activities of IL-1 and TNFα, protecting cartilage against the effects of these molecules (Tyler, 1989; Fosang *et al.*, 1991b). In OA, although circulating levels of IGF-1 are reduced (Denko *et al.*, 1990) there is evidence for the increased expression of the IGF-1 gene and enhanced synthesis of this molecule in cartilage (Middleton and Tyler, 1992). This may correlate with the enhanced matrix biosynthesis observed in this disease (Mankin and Lippiello, 1970; Thompson and Oegema, 1979). Likewise, the lack of responsiveness to IGF-1 of cartilage in experimental inflammatory arthritis (Schalkwijk *et al.*, 1989b) could also result from the inhibitory *in vivo* effects on matrix synthesis of 'excessive amounts' of the cytokines IL-1 and TNFα.

Although transforming growth factor $β_1$ (TGFβ$_1$) has been reported to inhibit cartilage proteoglycan synthesis (van der Kraan *et al.*, 1992), exogenous TGFβ can, like IL-6 (Lotz and Guerne, 1991) protect against cartilage degradation induced by IL-1 (Chandrasekhar and Harvey, 1988). In immature cartilages it can potently stimulate matrix synthesis of aggrecan (Morales and Roberts, 1988). This has not been shown for skeletally mature cartilages. This protection probably involves stimulation of proteoglycan synthesis and an increase in the synthesis of TIMP, as is seen in fibroblasts (Edwards *et al.*, 1987; Overall *et al.*, 1989). Also TGFβ produces down-regulation of IL-1 receptor expression on chondrocytes (Harvey *et al.*, 1991; Rédini *et al.*, 1993) and downregulation of metalloproteinases through a TGFβ-sensitive element on the metalloproteinase genes (see section in this chapter on transcription).

The fact that IL-1α,β (Ollivierre *et al.*, 1986; Tiku *et al.*, 1992), TNFα (Henderson *et al.*, 1993), as well as IGF-1 (Middleton and Tyler, 1992) and TGFβ (Ellingsworth *et al.*, 1986) are expressed and synthesized by chondrocytes, means that the product of autocrine and paracrine effects of these molecules may play very significant roles in regulating cartilage metabolism. γ-Interferon can also potently inhibit the induction by IL-1 of metalloproteinases in human articular chondrocytes (Andrews *et al.*, 1990) yet in this case it inhibits collagen synthesis in cartilage (Goldring *et al.*, 1986).

In combination with other cytokines IL-1 can exhibit even more potent activity. Thus, a combination of IL-1 and basic fibroblast growth factor (bFGF) (Phadke, 1987) or platelet-derived growth factor (PDGF) (Smith *et al.*, 1991) can enhance the degradative activity of IL-1 whereas bFGF (Makower *et al.*, 1988) and PDGF (Prins *et al.*, 1982) alone can stimulate matrix synthesis (Poole, 1993). The effect of bFGF (Chin *et al.*, 1991) and PDGF (Smith *et al.*, 1990) is to upregulate IL-1 receptors but, in the case of PDGF, without changing receptor affinity. In OA, receptors for IL-1 on articular chondrocyte may be increased (Martel-Pelletier *et al.*, 1992). But PDGF negates the inhibitory effect of IL-1 on proteoglycan synthesis in chondrocytes (Harvey *et al.*, 1993). It is likely that TGFβ and IGF-1, which both down-regulate IL-1 activity (see above), may also regulate IL-1 receptor expression, by analogy with TGFβ's effect on fibroblasts (Dubois *et al.*, 1990).

TNFα can more potently influence transcriptional and translational events when present in combination with IL-1 (Goldring *et al.*, 1990). Using antibodies to IL-1α, IL-1β and TNFα, studies of the effects of synovial fluids from patients with arthritis on the metabolism of human cartilage have revealed that synovial fluids which stimulate matrix degradation may rely on the presence of IL-1α or IL-1β or a combination of IL-1β and TNFα depending upon the fluid (Hollander *et al.*, 1991). Since combinations of these cytokines alone do not necessarily stimulate degradation, it is likely that other cytokines are also required. The failure of the IL-1 receptor antagonist to prevent products of synovial cells from stimulating expression of chondrocyte collagenase and stromelysin (Bandara *et al.*, 1992), also suggests that cytokines other than IL-1 are present in synovial fluids that can stimulate matrix degradation.

Contrary to common belief, the degradation of type II collagen and aggrecan in adult human articular cartilage is often stimulated by IL-1α,β (Ismaiel *et al.*, 1992; Mort *et al.*, 1993). But human adult cartilage is less sensitive than many animal cartilages, such as nasal septum, for reasons yet unclear. Only some normal human articular cartilages may respond (38%) although the majority of articular cartilages taken from patients with OA and RA show a response, as indicated by the enhanced loss of proteoglycan from arthritic cartilages (Ismaiel *et al.*, 1992).

IL-1 can clearly cause potent degradative changes *in vitro*. The same is observed *in vivo*. Thus injection of IL-1 into rabbit knees produces polymorph infiltration and loss of aggrecan (Pettipher *et al.*, 1986; Page Thomas *et al.*, 1991; McDonnell *et al.*, 1992). This is accompanied by increased expression and synthesis of stromelysin-1 in synovium and cartilage (Hutchison *et al.*, 1992) and accumulation of this molecule in synovial fluids (McDonnell *et al.*, 1992). Intra-articular TNFα causes polymorph infiltration in rabbit knees. It is markedly less potent than IL-1, but at suboptimal doses both cytokines synergize to produce more polymorph infiltration (Henderson and Pettipher, 1989). In mice, increased matrix degradation (van de Loo and van den Berg, 1990) and inhibition of cartilage proteoglycan synthesis (van Beuningen *et al.*, 1991) are both produced by IL-1. The medial femoral–tibial compartment is most sensitive, especially the medial tibial plateau (van Beuningen *et al.*, 1991), which shows more pronounced degenerative changes in OA. Traditionally, these changes have been thought to relate to less complete coverage of the cartilage surfaces by the meniscal fibrocartilage but they may result from differences in chondrocyte sensitivity to environmental cytokines.

These effects of IL-1 are longer-lasting at the level of inhibition of proteoglycan synthesis (van de Loo and van den Berg, 1990). Inhibitory intra-articular effects of IL-1 on synthesis are observed in rabbits (Page Thomas *et al.*, 1991) and in rats, both young and old (Chandrasekhar *et al.*, 1992) but are more pronounced in older mice (van Beuningen *et al.*, 1991). A role for IL-1 in inhibiting proteoglycan synthesis in antigen-induced arthritis in mice is indicated by the removal of this inhibition by antibodies to IL-1 (van de Loo *et al.*, 1992). The reader is referred to Chapter 13, this volume, for a discussion by Firestein on naturally occurring cytokine inhibitors and their role in RA pathology and treatment.

The depletion of proteoglycan in human cartilage caused by inhibition of synthesis is strongest in young cartilages (Nietfeld *et al.*, 1990). The inhibition of systemic cartilage matrix synthesis may be of special importance in the degeneration of articular cartilage in RA where levels of these synovial cytokines are increased over those found in OA. In RA patients, levels of fragments of the proteoglycan aggrecan are reduced in serum (Poole *et al.*, 1990; Spector *et al.*, 1992; Manincourt *et al.*, 1993; Poole *et al.*, 1994) and in synovial fluids (Saxne *et al.*, 1988) when inflammation is increased. Also, in OA joints increased inflammation can influence aggrecan turnover resulting in reduced matrix proteoglycan release (measured as keratan sulphate) (Poole et al., 1994). Thus low levels of cytokines, such as IL-1 and TNFα, that can inhibit matrix synthesis producing less substrate available for degradation may account for this inverse relationship between proteoglycan aggrecan fragments and inflammation (Fig. 10). These molecules may primarily represent a rapid turnover pool in the pericellular domain. In contrast, the direct correlation between aggrecan release and inflammation in synovial fluids in RA (Poole et al., 1994) may reflect degradation of resident 'longer lasting' molecules.

We know little, as yet, of the effects of neuropeptides on cartilage metabolism. But substance P, which is found in increased concentrations in inflamed joints such as in RA (Menkes et al., 1993), can increase collagenase production by chondrocytes (Halliday et al., 1993). Other studies have previously shown that intra-articular infusion of substance P can stimulate cartilage loss (Levine et al., 1984), possibly by stimulating synovial cell collagenase production (Lotz et al., 1988). More studies of these neuropeptides are needed to explore the link between cartilage metabolism and sensory nerves serving the joint. The potential role of neuropeptides in RA pathology is reviewed by Mapp and Blake (Chapter 16, this volume).

MOLECULAR MECHANISMS OF CYTOKINE SIGNALLING IN CHONDROCYTES WITH SPECIAL REFERENCE TO METALLOPROTEINASES

INTERMEDIARY PATHWAYS

This area has attracted much interest in recent years especially in connection with IL-1. Given that a cell surface receptor-mediated event is first required for cell activation by IL-1, subsequent signalling appears to be protein kinase c (PKC) independent: staurosporine, a PKC inhibitor, does not block the stimulation of collagenase synthesis by IL-1 and has no effect on prostaglandin E_2 production (Conca et al., 1989). This contrasts to the observed blockage by H-7, another PKC inhibitor, of IL-1 induction of stromelysin mRNA in rheumatoid synovial fibroblasts (Case et al., 1990). Other indications for PKC-independent pathways in chondrocytes apply to the effects of IL-1 on stimulation of proteoglycan degradation and inhibition of proteoglycan synthesis since PKC-deficient cells are equally responsive to IL-1, although PKC activation can down-regulate the action of IL-1 (Arner and Pratta, 1991).

TRANSCRIPTIONAL REGULATION

Few studies have been made of chondrocytes so our knowledge comes mainly from work on other cells (Matrisian, 1992). The promoter regions of the genes for human and rat stromelysin-1 and -2 and human interstitial collagenase have common regulatory regions activated by IL-1 and TNFα. The genes all contain TATA elements approximately 30 nucleotides upstream from the transcriptional start site. All have AP-1 and PEA-3 sites within the most proximal 210 bp. These sites, alone or in combination possibly with other sites, regulate basal and induced transcription. The activating transcriptional factors include the proto-oncogenes c-fos and c-jun (which can transactivate the AP-1 element) and c-ets (which transactivates the PEA-3 element). Interestingly, the 72-kDa gelatinase (Frisch et al., 1990; Matrisian, 1992) and neutrophil collagenase genes lack the TATA box and AP-1 sites, whereas collagenase, stromelysin-1, the 92-kDa gelatinase and the urokinase plasminogen activator genes all contain these elements.

TNFα produces a prolonged increase of c-jun contrasting with transient increases elicited by a phorbol ester (Brenner *et al.*, 1989). IL-1 activates a promoter transcriptional regulating element (TRE) binding site (Quinones *et al.*, 1989; Lafyatis *et al.*, 1990) and transiently induces both c-jun and c-fos expression (see also Conca *et al.*, 1989). Induction of metalloproteinase gene expression can be down-regulated by glucocorticoids (Clark *et al.*, 1987; Frisch and Ruley, 1987) as well as TGFβ (Edwards *et al.*, 1987; Overall *et al.*, 1989). Both can block at the transcriptional level, TGFβ inhibiting stromelysin-1 through an upstream sequence in the stromelysin-1 promoter referred to as the TGFβ inhibitory element (Kerr *et al.*, 1988). This sequence binds a nuclear protein complex that contains FOS. Induction of c-fos expression is required for the effect. All-*trans* retinoic acid inhibits IL-1 and phorbol ester induction of collagenase by inhibiting induction of FOS, but not c-jun expression (Lafyatis *et al.*, 1990). Okadaic acid, which inhibits protein phosphatases and therefore inhibits the activities of protein kinases, markedly increases steady-state levels of collagenase mRNA via the AP-1 consensus sequence in the collagenase promoter and other sequences upstream of the AP-1 consensus site (Kim *et al.*, 1990). Again c-fos expression is stimulated whereas c-jun is less affected. Whether these same regulatory elements operate in chondrocytes remains to be established, but it is a likely possibility.

DEGRADATION PRODUCTS OF MATRIX MOLECULES CAN STIMULATE MATRIX DEGRADATION BY CHONDROCYTES AND OTHER CELLS

The interaction of the chondrocyte with its extracellular matrix involves receptor-mediated binding of matrix molecules to the cell surface. The receptor for type II collagen (anchorin) (Pfaffle *et al.*, 1988; Fernandez *et al.*, 1988) and the CD44 hyaluronic acid receptor (Aruffo *et al.*, 1990) have both been identified. In addition, chondrocytes, like other cells, possess receptors for fibronectin and fragments thereof containing the RGD amino acid sequence. Werb and her colleagues (1989), working with synovial fibroblasts, first discovered that addition of a hexapeptide containing the RGD sequence, as well as fragments of fibronectin, or monoclonal antibodies to the fibronectin receptor, would induce gene expression of collagenase and stromelysin-1. Subsequently, addition of fibronectin fragments, as well as the RGD peptide, to chondrocytes was found to cause up to a 50-fold enhancement of gelatinolytic and collagenolytic activities as well as a 23-fold increase in aggrecan fragment release (Homandberg *et al.*, 1992). It is likely that fragments of other molecules which bind in a receptor-mediated fashion to chondrocytes may also produce similar effects.

The mechanisms whereby degradation products of structural extracellular matrix molecules can produce these changes is presently unclear. But it may well prove to be related to the use of receptor-mediated mechanisms by chondrocytes to sense mechanical changes in their extracellular matrix. Microfilament bundles, candidates for the intracellular relay of receptor signals, are not detectably altered in their organization (Werb *et al.*, 1989). Cells can distinguish between 'inactive' intact molecules and the 'stimulatory' fragments of fibronectin. Whereas monovalent molecules are inactive in solution, multimetric or immobilized molecules are active. Thus receptor aggregation appears to be required.

Similar effects are also produced by extracellular matrix molecules in other cell types. Biswas and Dayer (1979) originally revealed that interstitial collagenase production by skin fibroblasts and synovial cells is stimulated by both native and denatured forms of types I, II and III collagens. Human monocytes also produce increased amounts of mononuclear cell factor (IL-1) in the presence of native human collagens I, II and III (Dayer *et al.*, 1980, 1982). The CB11 peptide of type II collagen (Goto *et al.*, 1988) as well as degradation products of the proteoglycan aggrecan (Gurr *et al.*, 1990) can stimulate increased IL-1α,β production by monocytes/macrophages.

These observations reveal that both intact and degraded matrix molecules can have profound effects on cytokine and proteinase synthesis and release by both stromal and inflammatory cells. Thus these observations indicate that once fragmentation of matrix molecules occurs in a pericellular site around the chondrocyte, degradation products may further enhance matrix degradation. Since an increased content of fibronectin is observed in OA cartilages (Wurster and Lust, 1984; Miller *et al.*, 1984), degradation products of this molecule produced in pericellular sites may have profound effects on proteinase and cytokine synthesis.

MECHANICAL FORCES REGULATE MATRIX TURNOVER

The chondrocyte is exquisitely sensitive to changes in its extracellular environment that involve changes in compressive loading (review, Poole, 1993). How this regulation occurs is unclear but likely involves receptor-mediated signals transmitted indirectly by pressure 'transducers' in the extracellular matrix, such as the collagen fibrillar network, as well as direct effects on cell metabolism. The anchorin CII receptor for type II collagen may function in this way. Cartilage matrix synthesis (Palmoski and Brandt, 1984; van Kampen *et al.*, 1985) and degradation (Sah *et al.*, 1991) can be inhibited or stimulated by changes in compressive loading according to the nature of the applied load (see also review Poole, 1993). Static compressive loading (and increased osmotic pressure) results in a decreased water content, increased concentrations of sulphate and carboxyl group counterions, namely K^+, H^+, and Ca^{2+} and a decreased concentration of free SO_4^{2-} (Schneiderman *et al.*, 1986; Urban and Bayliss, 1989). This decrease in free SO_4^{2-} concentration can inhibit proteoglycan synthesis. The concentration of hydrogen ions will also increase locally under loading as these molecules are compressed. Therefore the pH of the extracellular matrix is likely altered when changes in charge density are produced. It has been calculated that at 50% compression the extracellular pH is reduced by about 0.5 unit (Gray *et al.*, 1988). Thus in the pericellular environment, where proteoglycan density is at its highest, compression may cause the pH to be as low as pH 6.0–6.5 (Poole, 1993). This would favour the activity of cysteine proteinases and yet still permit metalloproteinase activity. Damage to the pericellular matrix would also serve to change the mechanical environment of the cell and alter the balance between synthesis and degradation.

Alterations in the mechanical stability of a knee joint produced by cruciate ligament rupture, immobilization, excessive activity or meniscal tear(s) can each, in time, in animals and people cause loss and degeneration of articular cartilages in that joint leading to the development of OA (see review Poole, 1993). The rapid changes in aggrecan metabolism that occur in humans within days of traumatic inquiry to menisci or cruciate ligaments (Lohmander, 1991) likely result from alterations in joint cartilage loading.

ENHANCED DEGRADATION OF CARTILAGE MATRIX ACCOMPANIES EXPRESSION OF THE HYPERTROPHIC PHENOTYPE

In skeletal growth (growth plate) and fracture repair, expression of the hypertrophic phenotype by chondrocytes is characterized by synthesis of type X collagen which is secreted into the extracellular matrix where it associates, in part at least, with type II collagen fibrils (Schmid and Linsenmeyer, 1985; Gibson et al., 1986; Leboy et al., 1988; Poole and Pidoux, 1989). This immediately precedes calcification of cartilage matrix around these cells. The hypertrophic cell is capable of rapidly digesting its extracellular matrix leading to an enlargement in cell volume. This results from degradation and loss of type II collagen (Alini et al., 1992) which is accompanied by a net increase in synthesis of collagenase, 72-kDa gelatinase and stromelysin-1 over TIMP synthesis (Dean et al., 1985; Brown et al., 1989). The calcification of cartilage matrix which follows type X collagen synthesis is closely associated with the presence of extracellular matrix vesicles formed from the plasma membrane (Poole, 1991; Howell and Dean, 1992). These vesicles are enriched in metalloproteinase(s) of unknown identity (Katsura and Yamada, 1986; Dean et al., 1992). This increase in matrix degradation and expression of the hypertrophic phenotype is inhibited by TGF-β (Kato et al., 1988) and bFGF (Kato and Iwamoto, 1990). These changes are summarized in Fig. 14.

In OA, expression of type X collagen is often observed, particularly in association with 'clones' or clusters of chondrocytes close to sites of cartilage fissuring and fibrillation (Thomas et al., 1991; von der Mark et al., 1992; Walker et al., 1993). The extent of these changes in OA remains to be more clearly established although partial calcification of cartilage matrix is frequently a feature of this disease (Wilkins et al., 1983; Gordon et al., 1984; Pritzker et al., 1987), suggesting that a process of endochondral ossification can occur in OA as articular cartilages degenerate.

The hormonal/cytokine events which trigger expression of the hypertrophic phenotype are just beginning to be understood. Further work is required to determine whether these molecules involved in growth and fracture repair are also definitely involved in pathological 'degradative' changes in articular cartilages in arthritis.

DEGENERATIVE CHANGES IN ARTICULAR CARTILAGE IN AGEING AND IN OSTEOARTHRITIS

As cartilage ages so the structures and properties of the extracellular matrix change. The tensile properties, due largely to its collagen fibrils, alter. The tensile properties are greatest in the superfical zone of knee articular cartilage. They increase up to the third decade of life, and then decrease markedly with increasing age (Kempson, 1982). This accompanies the appearance of detectable damage to the collagen II fibrils at the articular surface (Stockwell et al., 1983; Dodge and Poole, 1989; Hollander et al., 1994). Loss of tensile strength is even more pronounced in OA (Kempson et al.,

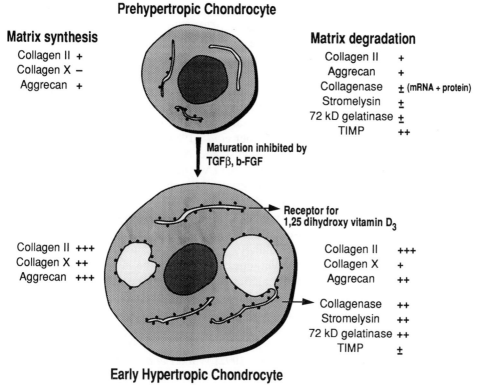

Figure 14. Expression of the hypertrophic phenotype (e.g. in growth plate) is accompanied by increased proteolysis, particularly of type II collagen. Relative rates of synthesis of matrix molecules and/or proteinases as indicated.

1973; Akizuki *et al.*, 1986). In more advanced OA these changes are associated with a net loss of type II collagen (Mankin and Lippiello, 1970; Venn and Maroudas, 1977; Dodge *et al.*, 1991; Hollander *et al.*, 1994) and increased damage to the triple helix of 'resident' type II collagen molecules (Dodge and Poole, 1989; Hollander *et al.*, 1994), resulting in fibrillation and fissuring of cartilage. This is accompanied by a net loss of the proteoglycan decorin at the articular surface (Poole, 1993). The decorin molecules are normally closely associated with the collagen fibrils (Poole *et al.*, 1986; Witsch-Prehm *et al.*, 1992) and they are lost as these fibrils are damaged.

These degenerative changes involving the collagen fibrils resulting in a progressive loss of tensile properties are not observed in articular cartilage of the talus of the ankle (Kempson, 1991). This is of special interest since the incidence of OA in the ankle joint is very much lower than in the knee. Furthermore, the importance of these collagen fibrils is highlighted by the fact that genetically determined abnormalities in type II (Ala-Kokko *et al.*, 1990; Katzenstein *et al.*, 1990; Eyre *et al.*, 1991) and type IX (Nakata *et al.*, 1993) collagen structure in humans and mice, respectively, lead to the premature development of OA, of the familial kind in the case of the Col 2 gene.

In advanced OA (when collagen II damage is extensive) there is a net loss of hyaluronan as well as aggrecan (Sweet *et al.*, 1977; Thonar *et al.*, 1978; Thompson and Oegema, 1979; Rizkalla *et al.*, 1992; A.R. Poole *et al.*, manuscript in preparation).

This is associated with a reduction in the rate of aggrecan synthesis, which is elevated early in the disease (Mankin and Lippiello, 1970; Thompson and Oegema, 1979). These changes result from damage to the collagen preventing interaction and retention of these molecules with collagen fibrils. Loss of aggrecan leads to a loss of the equilibrium modulus (determined by compressive testing): this is ordinarily more pronounced in ageing (Armstrong and Mow, 1982). This change may, through biomechanical effects, result in reduced synthesis. Ageing itself results in the progressive accumulation of fragments of aggrecan, many of which bind to hyaluronan (Bayliss and Ali, 1978; Franzen et al., 1981; Webber et al., 1987). These are most commonly found deep in the articular cartilage (Bayliss and Ali, 1978; Franzen et al., 1981), where degradation products accumulate. In OA, the sizes of these fragments are further reduced in early phase 1 (Mankin grades 2–6) disease, whereas they increase in size over normal fragments in phase II (Mankin grades 7–13) disease (Rizkalla et al., 1992). This suggests that there is net degradation occurring in phase 1 and net synthesis of new molecules in phase 2. Biosynthesis of these proteoglycans increases in early human OA (Mankin and Lippiello, 1970; Thompson and Oegema, 1979) even though there is localized reduced synthetic potential in the superficial zone when pronounced matrix damage occurs (Lafeber et al., 1992). This is accompanied by a general increase in synthesis of type II collagen in both human (Lippiello et al., 1977; F. Nelson, A.R. Poole and co-workers, unpublished) and experimental OA (Eyre et al., 1980; Hui-Chou and Lust, 1982). In human OA, this is accompanied by the abnormal synthesis of type III collagen (Aigner et al., 1993) and type X collagen (Thomas et al., 1991; von der Mark et al., 1992; Walker et al., 1993) and in increased content of type VI collagen (Ronzière et al., 1990), the latter also being seen in experimental OA (McDevitt et al., 1988).

Clearly major alterations in collagen synthesis are a feature of OA. The development of OA is accompanied by increased synthesis of proteinases such as cathepsin B (Bayliss and Ali, 1978; Martel-Pelletier et al., 1990), stromelysin-1 (Nguyen et al., 1992; Okada et al., 1992), collagenase (Ehrlich et al., 1977; Pelletier et al., 1983), the 72-kDa gelatinase (Mohtai et al., 1993) and the 92-kDa gelatinase (Mohtai et al., 1993). This occurs first in the superficial zone (Nguyen et al., 1992; Okada et al., 1992b), and is accompanied by collagen II cleavage and loss of the proteoglycans decorin and aggrecan. There is an overall decrease in OA cartilages in the contents of inhibitors of cysteine proteinases (Martel-Pelletier et al., 1990), serine proteinases (Yamada et al., 1987) and metalloproteinases (Yamada et al., 1987; Dean et al., 1989). Overall with the net loss of TIMP there is an increase in proteolysis (Yamada et al., 1987; Dean et al., 1989). These changes are summarized in Fig. 11. They are often reflected by increased release of fragments of the proteoglycan aggrecan into synovial fluid (Lohmander et al., 1989; Lohmander, 1991; Dahlberg et al., 1992). Serum increases in these molecules have been reported (Thonar et al., 1985; Sweet et al., 1988) although others have not been able to confirm these increases using similar detection methods (Spector et al., 1992; Poole et al., 1994).

The role of the synovium in these cartilages changes in OA is still not well understood. Inflammation is clearly identifiable at arthroscopy but is much less acute and less chronic than that seen in RA. Increased levels of myeloperoxidase in synovial fluid over those in serum are indicative of local intra-articular influx and degranulation of polymorphonuclear leukocytes (P. Dieppe et al., manuscript in preparation). Much increased levels of stromelysin-1, and to a lesser degree, of interstitial collagenase have been observed (Lohmander *et al.*, 1993). These increases in metalloproteinases are greater than those of TIMP both in amount and molar ratio. The content of the urokinase-type plasminogen activator and its inhibitor are also elevated in synovial fluids over those in plasma (Brommer *et al.*, 1992) as is the activity of the synovial enzyme, especially in seropositive rheumatoid patients (Brommer *et al.*, 1992). These differences correspond to the increased radiologically detected joint destruction.

CARTILAGE AND SYNOVIAL CHANGES IN RHEUMATOID ARTHRITIS AND OTHER INFLAMMATORY ARTHRITIDES ASSOCIATED WITH MATRIX DEGRADATION

In RA, the increased production of IL-1 (Miyasaka *et al.*, 1988; Westacott *et al.*, 1990), TNFα (Yoshida *et al.*, 1992). TNFα receptors (Roux-Lombard *et al.*, 1993) as well as the interstitial collagenase and stromelysin (Westacott *et al.*, 1990; Gravallese *et al.*, 1991; McCrachen, 1991; Firestein *et al.*, 1991; Walakovits *et al.*, 1992; Clark *et al.*, 1993) in chronic inflamed synovium and in synovial fluid are thought to play important roles in cartilage destruction (Fig. 6). Unlike OA, erosive synovial/pannus ingrowth and destruction of bone and ligaments as well as articular cartilage, are integral features of the disease. The erosive ingrowth of pannus may be related to cartilage collagen degradation and the stimulation by IL-1 of chondrocyte IL-8 synthesis (Lotz *et al.*, 1992; Recklies and Golds, 1992), a potent angiogenic molecule (Koch *et al.*, 1992). This would favour synovial cell/monocyte-based 'pannus' formation *in vitro* (Ishikawa *et al.*, 1991). Adjacent to the edge of this 'invasive' pannus tissue is the most pronounced destruction of type II collagen observed in RA (Fig. 6). This can be seen both morphologically (Harris *et al.*, 1970, 1977; Kobayashi and Ziff, 1975) and immunohistochemically using antibodies to denatured type II collagen (A. Hollander *et al.*, manuscript in preparation). Within such sites in extracellular matrix can be detected both collagenase (Woolley *et al.*, 1977) and stromelysin (Hasty *et al.*, 1990). This is associated with increased expression by synovium of these proteinase (see above) and abnormal expression of the integrin ICAM-1 on chondrocytes (Davies *et al.*, 1991, 1992). Class II antigens are also expressed elsewhere in the cartilage (Burmester *et al.*, 1983), being inducible with γ-interferon (Goldring *et al.*, 1986). These cell surface changes suggest altered interactions of chondrocytes with the extracellular matrix. ICAM-1 expression can also be induced by culture with IL-1, TNFα or interferon-γ (Davies *et al.*, 1991), suggesting that there is an active release of cytokines in these sites.

Remote from pannus and synovium, degradation of type II collagen can be detected (Kimura *et al.*, 1977; Mitchell and Shepard, 1978; Dodge and Poole, 1989; Hollander *et al.*, 1994). This is observed at the articular surface but is usually more pronounced in the deep zone of cartilage adjacent to subchondral bone (Mitchell and Shepard, 1978; Dodge and Poole, 1989; Dodge *et al.*, 1991) (Figs 5 and 6). The reasons for this may relate to the increased turnover of subchondral bone seen in RA (Uhlinger, 1971). This is associated with increased bone resorption and infiltration of mononuclear cells (Takashima *et al.*, 1989). This resultant highly osteoporotic state may be the consequence of an inflammatory process centred within the bone driven by the release of cytokines such as IL-1 and TNFα (Fig. 6). Cytokines may 'spill over' and activate adjacent chondrocytes leading to the degenerative changes we have described. Active erosion of cartilage from subchondral sites (Tateishi, 1973; Bromley and Woolley, 1984; Bromley *et al.*, 1985) may involve a similar activation of chondrocytes to that seen elsewhere adjacent to pannus. Moreover, synovial and bone proteinases may penetrate articular cartilages and, in the case of latent metalloproteinases, may be activated by chondrocyte proteinases. Whether this happens is not known. This invasion edge contains chondroclasts and blood vessels, suggestive of an active angiogenic process such as that seen in the growth plate. This may relate, in part, to increased IL-8 production. Eventually, damage to type II collagen is seen throughout cartilage matrix in RA.

The fact that the damage to collagen II at the articular surface is usually less pronounced than that in the deep zone suggests that damage by polymorphonuclear leukocytes in synovial fluid, mediated by free radicals, polymorph (neutrophil) collagenase, cathepsin G and elastase, may be less important than expected. In fact, other experimental studies have revealed that in inflammatory arthritis damage to articular cartilage in rabbits and mice (Pettipher *et al.*, 1989, 1990) can occur independently of the presence of a normal complement of polymorphs.

Articular cartilage metabolism changes in RA in such a way that this can be detected *in vivo* by analyses of degradation products released from cartilage into synovial fluid and serum (Ratcliffe *et al.*, 1988; Poole *et al.*, 1993a; Poole *et al.*, 1994; Poole, 1994; Poole and Dieppe, 1994). In early rapid erosive disease serum levels of cartilage oligomeric protein (COMP, a thrombospondin-like molecule) are elevated compared to levels in patients with early but slowly erosive disease (Forslind *et al.*, 1992). In reactive arthritis, levels of COMP in synovial fluids correlate with those in serum (Saxne *et al.*, 1993) indicating that measurements of this molecule in serum may be reflective of changes in articular cartilages. In more advanced RA, articular cartilage is more degraded. This is reflected in smaller aggrecan fragments released into the synovial fluid (Saxne and Heinegård, 1992) with the G1 globular domain becoming more common. A chondroitin sulphate epitope (846) found on the largest aggrecan molecules (Rizkalla *et al.*, 1992) is also frequently elevated in established RA (Poole *et al.*, 1994). But in rapid erosive disease levels are reduced below normal levels and those in slow erosive disease (T. Saxne *et al.*, manuscript in preparation). Since this reduction probably results from impaired synthesis (Fig. 10), this suggests that there is impaired biosynthesis of proteoglycan molecules in cases of acute inflammation. This is further indicated by the reduced levels of aggrecan fragments in serum in RA (Poole *et al.*, 1990, 1993b; Spector *et al.*, 1992; Manincourt *et al.*, 1993). Hence, damage to cartilage in RA probably involves impairment of normal biosynthesis of matrix molecules as well as increased degradation both of which contribute to net degeneration of this tissue.

CONCLUSIONS

With the advent of much new technology our understanding of the mechanisms of cartilage matrix degradation and their regulation has progressed considerably. We are close to identifying exactly which proteinases are rate-limiting and how the synthesis and activation of these molecules are regulated. This knowledge provides a solid basis for therapeutic intervention. At the present time, potential therapeutic targets are the cysteine proteinases, plasminogen activators and metalloproteinases. However, since cysteine proteinases are primarily involved in intracellular metabolism, their inhibition would have to be selectively restricted to the extracellular environment. Moreover, since all these proteinases are also involved in normal skeletal turnover, such as osteoclast-mediated bone resorption, only partial inhibition would be advisable to restore proteinase activity to more physiological levels. In OA, regulation of proteolysis coupled to maximization of cell division (to increase the numbers of cells synthesizing matrix) and enhanced matrix and proteinase inhibitor biosynthesis would seem to be a logical approach (Fig. 15). By better understanding how the transcription and translation of these proteinases and their inhibitors is normally regulated, it is likely that our improved knowledge in this area will lead to therapeutic control of proteolysis in disease.

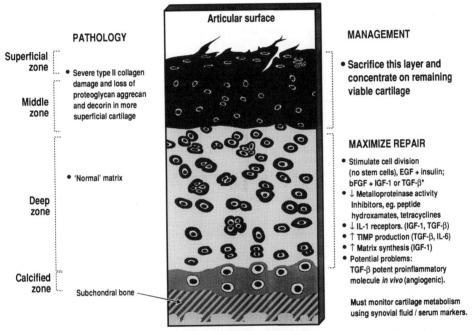

Figure 15. Important issues to be addressed when attempting to regulate cartilage damage and stimulate its repair in osteoarthritis. Increase (↑) and decreases (↓) are indicated.

ACKNOWLEDGEMENTS

The authors' studies are funded by the Shriners of North America (to ARP and MA), Medical Research Council of Canada, Pfizer Inc., Monsanto Corporation, Incyte Pharmaceuticals, Kabi Pharmacia (to ARP) and the Arthritis Society of Canada (to AH). The author expresses his sincere appreciation for the considerable creativity and stimulation offered by my students, fellows and colleagues without whom the science would not have progressed and would have been far less fun. Mark Lepik and Jane

Wishart prepared the figures. Audrey Wheeler and Michele Burman-Turner processed the manuscript.

REFERENCES

Aigner T, Bertling W, Stöss H, Weseloh G & von der Mark K (1993) Independent expression of fibril forming collagens I, II and III in chondrocytes of human osteoarthritic cartilage. *J Clin Invest* **91**: 829–837.

Akizuki S, Mow VC, Muller F, Pita JC, Howell DS & Manicourt DH (1986) Tensile properties of human knee joint cartilage. 1. Influence of ionic conditions, weight-bearing and fibrillation on the tensile properties. *J Orthop Res* **4**: 379–392.

Ala-Kokko L, Baldwin CT, Moskowitz RW & Prockop DJ (1990) Single base mutation in the type II procollagen gene (COL2A1) as a cause of primary osteoarthritis associated with a mild chondrodysplasia. *Proc Natl Acad Sci USA* **87**: 6565–6568.

Alini M, Matsui Y, Dodge GR & Poole AR (1992) The extracellular matrix of cartilage in the growth plate before and during calcification: changes in composition and degradation of type II collagen. *Calcif Tissue Int* **50**: 327–335.

Andrews HJ, Bunning RAD, Plumpton TA, Clark IM, Russell RGG & Cawston TE (1990) Inhibition of interleukin-1 induced collagenase production in human articular chrondrocytes *in vitro* by recombinant human interferon-gamma. *Arthritis Rheum* **33**: 1733–1738.

Armstrong CG & Mow VC (1982) Variations in the intrinsic mechanical properties of human articular cartilage with age, degeneration and water content. *J Bone Jt Surg Am* **64**: 88–94.

Arner EC & Pratta MA (1989) Independent effects of interleukin-1 on proteoglycan breakdown, proteoglycan synthesis and prostaglandin E_2 release from cartilage in organ culture. *Arthritis Rheum* **32**: 288–297.

Arner EC & Pratta MA (1991) Modulation of interleukin-1-induced alterations in cartilage proteoglycan metabolism by activation of protein kinase C. *Arthritis Rheum* **34**: 1006–1013.

Aruffo A, Stamenkovic I, Melnick M, Underhill CB & Seed B (1990) CD44 is the principal cell surface receptor for hyaluronate. *Cell* **61**: 1303–1313.

Bader DL, Kempson GE, Barrett AJ & Webb W (1981) The effects of leucocyte elastase on the mechanical properties of adult human articular cartilage in tension. *Biochim Biophys Acta* **677**: 103–108.

Baici A & Lang A (1990) Effect of interleukin-1β on the production of cathepsin B by rabbit articular chondrocytes. *FEBS Lett* **277**: 93–96.

Bandara G, Lin CW, Georgescu HI & Evans CH (1992) The synovial activation of chondrocytes: evidence for complex cytokine interactions involving a possible novel factor. *Biochim Biophys Acta* **1134**: 309–318.

Barry FP, Gaw JU, Young CN & Neame PJ (1992) Hyaluronan-binding region of aggrecan from pig laryngeal cartilage. Amino acid sequence, analysis of N-linked oligosaccharides and location of the keratan sulphate. *Biochem J* **286**: 761–769.

Bayliss MT & Ali SY (1978) Studies on cathepsin B in human articular cartilage. *Biochem J* **171**: 149–154.

Benton HP & Tyler JA (1988) Inhibition of cartilage proteoglycan synthesis by interleukin 1. *Biochem Biophys Res Comm* **154**: 421–428.

Biswas C & Dayer J-M (1979) Stimulation of collagenase production by collagen in mammalian cell cultures. *Cell* **18**: 1035–1041.

Brenner DA, O'Hara M, Angel P, Chojkier M & Karin M (1989) Prolonged activation of jun and collagenase genes by tumour necrosis factor-α. *Nature* **337**: 661–663.

Brinckerhoff CE, Suzuki K & Mitchell TI (1990) Rabbit procollagenase synthesized and secreted by a high yield mammalian expression vector requires stromelysin (matrix metalloproteinases-3) for maximal activation. *J Biol Chem* **265**: 22262–22269.

Bromley M & Woolley DE (1984) Chondroclasts and osteoclasts at subchondral sites of erosion in the rheumatoid joint. *Arthritis Rheum* **27**: 968–975.

Bromley M, Bertfield H, Evanson JM & Woolley DE (1985) Bidirectional erosion of cartilage in the rheumatoid knee joint. *Ann Rheum Dis* **44**: 676–681.

Brommer EJP, Dooijewaard G, Dijkmans BAC & Breedveld FC (1992) Plasminogen activators in synovial fluid and plasma from patients with arthritis. *Ann Rheum Dis* **51**: 965–968.

Brown CC, Hembry RM & Reynolds JJ (1989) Immunolocalization of metalloproteinases and their inhibition in the rabbit growth plate. *J Bone Joint Surt Am* **71**: 580–593.

Burkhardt H, Schwingel M, Menninger H, MacCartney HW & Tschesche H (1986) Oxygen radicals as effectors of cartilage destruction. Direct degradative effect on matrix components and indirect action in activation of latent collagenase from polymorphonuclear leukocytes. *Arthritis Rheum* **29**: 379–387.

Burleigh MC, Barrett AJ & Lazarus GS (1974) A lysosomal enzyme that degrades native collagen. *Biochem J* **137**: 387–398.

Burmester GR, Menche D & Merrymen P (1983) Application of monoclonal antibodies to the characterization of cells eluted from human articular cartilage. Expression of Ia antigen in certain diseases and identification of an 85-kD cell surface molecule accumulated in the pericellular matrix. *Arthritis Rheum* **26**: 1187–1195.

Buttle DJ & Saklatvala J (1992) Lysosomal cysteine endopeptidases mediate interleukin-1-stimulated cartilage proteoglycan degradation. *Biochem J* **287**: 657–661.

Buttle DJ, Saklatvala J, Tamai M & Barrett AJ (1992) Inhibition of interleukin-1 stimulated cartilage proteoglycan degradation by a lipophilic inactivator of cysteine endopeptidases. *Biochem J* **281**: 175–177.

Buttle DJ, Handley CJ, Ilic MZ, Saklatvala J, Murata M & Barrett AJ (1993) Inhibition of cartilage proteoglycan release by a specific inactivator of cathepsin B and an inhibitor of matrix metalloproteinases. Evidence for two converging-pathways of chondrocyte-mediated proteoglycan degradation. *Arthritis Rheum*, in press.

Campbell IK, Roughley PJ & Mort JS (1986) The action of human articular cartilage metalloproteinase on proteoglycan and link protein. Similarities between products of degradation *in situ* and *in vitro*. *Biochem J* **237**: 117–122.

Campbell IK, Piccoli DS, Butler DM, Singleton DK & Hamilton JA (1988) Recombinant human interleukin-1 stimulates human articular cartilage to undergo resorption and human chondrocytes to produce both tissue and urokinase-type plasminogen activator. *Biochim Biophys Acta* **967**: 183–194.

Campbell IK, Last K, Novak U, Lund LR & Hamilton JA (1991) Recombinant human interleukin-1 inhibits plasminogen activator inhibitor-1 (PAI-1) production by human articular cartilage and chondrocytes. *Biochem Biophys Res Comm* **174**: 251–257.

Case JP, Lafyatis R, Kumkumian GK, Remmers EF & Wilder RL (1990) IL-1 regulation of transin/stromelysin transcription in rheumatoid synovial fibroblasts appears to involve two antagonist transduction pathways, an inhibitory, prostaglandin-dependent pathway mediated by cAMP, and a stimulatory, protein kinase C-dependent pathway. *J Immunol* **145**: 3755–3761.

Changler GN & Wright V (1958) Deleterious effect of intra-articular hydrocortisone. *Lancet* **11**: 661–663.

Chandrasekhar S & Harvey AK (1988) Transforming growth factor-β is a potent inhibitor of IL-1 induced protease activity and cartilage proteoglycan degradation. *Biochem Biophys Res Comm* **157**: 1352–1359.

Chandrasekhar S, Harvey AK & Hrubey PS (1992) Intra-articular administration of interleukin-1 causes prolonged suppression of cartilage proteoglycan synthesis in rats. *Matrix* **11**: 1–10.

Chen J-M, Aimes RT, Ward GR, Youngleib GL & Quigley JP (1991) Isolation and characterization of a 70-kDa metalloprotease (gelatinase) that is elevated in Rous sarcoma virus-transformed chicken embryo fibroblasts. *J Biol Chem* **266**: 5113–5121.

Chin JE, Hatfield CA, Krzesicki RF & Herblin WF (1991) Interactions between interleukin-1 and basic fibroblast growth factor on articular chondrocytes. Effects on cell growth, prostanoid production and receptor modulation. *Arthritis Rheum* **34**: 314–324.

Clark IM, Powell LK, Ramsey S, Hazleman BL & Cawston TE (1993) The measurement of collagenase, tissue inhibitor of metalloproteinases (TIMP) and collagenase–TIMP complex in synovial fluids from patients with osteoarthritis and rheumatoid arthritis. *Arthritis Rheum* **36**: 372–379.

Clark SD, Kobayashi DK & Welgus HG (1978) Regulation of the expression of tissue inhibitor of metalloproteinases and collagenase by retinoids and glucocorticoids in human fibroblasts. *J Clin Invest* **80**: 1280–1288.

Collier S & Ghosh P (1988) The role of plasminogen in interleukin-1 mediated cartilage degradation. *J Rheumatol* **15**: 1129–1137.

Conca W, Kaplan PB & Krane SM (1989) Increases in levels of procollagenase messenger RNA in cultured fibroblasts induced by human recombinant interleukin 1β or serum follow c-jun expression and are dependent on new protein synthesis. *J Clin Invest* **83**: 1753–1757.

Cruwys SC, Davies DE & Pettipher ER (1990) Co-operation between interleukin-1 and the fibrinolytic system in the degradation of collagen by articular chondrocytes. *Br J Pharmacol* **100**: 631–635.

Dahlberg L, Ryd L, Heinegärd D & Lohmander LS (1992) Proteoglycan fragments in joint fluid. Influence of arthrosis and inflammation. *Acta Orthop Scand* **63**: 417–423.

Davies ME, Dingle JT, Pigott R, Power C & Sharma H (1991) Expression of intercellular adhesion molecule 1 (ICAM-1) on human articular cartilage chondrocytes. *Connect Tissue Res* **26**: 207–216.

Davies ME, Sharma H & Pigott H (1992) ICAM-1 expression on chondrocytes in rheumatoid arthritis: induction by synovial cytokines. *Mediators Infl* **1**: 71–74.

Dayer J-M, Trentham DE, David JR & Krane SM (1980) Collagens stimulate the production of mononuclear cell factor (MCF) and prostaglandins (PGE₂) by human monocytes. *Trans Ass Am Phys* **93**: 326–335.

Dayer J-M, Trentham DE & Krane SM (1982) Collagens act as ligands to stimulate human monocytes to produce mononuclear cell factor (MCF) and prostaglandins (PGE₂). *Collagen Rel Res* **2**: 523–540.

Dean DD, Muniz OE, Berman I, Pita JC, Carreno MR, Woessner JF Jr et al. (1985) Localization of collagenase in the growth plate of rachitic rats. *J Clin Invest* **76**: 716–722.

Dean DD, Martel-Pelletier J, Pelletier J-P, Howell DS & Woessner JF Jr (1989) Evidence for metalloproteinase and metalloproteinase inhibitor imbalance in human osteoarthritic cartilage. *J Clin Invest* **84**: 678–685.

Dean DD, Muniz OE, Woessner JF Jr & Howell DS (1990) Production of collagenase and tissue inhibitor of metalloproteinases by rat growth plates in culture. *Matrix* **10**: 320–330.

Dean DD, Schwartz Z, Muniz OE, Gomez R, Swain LD, Howell DS et al. (1992) Matrix vesicles are enriched in metalloproteinases that degrade proteoglycans. *Calc Tissue Int* **50**: 342–349.

Denko CW, Boja B & Moskowitz RW (1990) Growth promoting peptides in osteoarthritis: insulin, insulin-like growth factor-1, growth hormone. *J Rheumatol* **17**: 1217–1221.

Dingle JT, Horsfield P, Fell HB & Barratt MEJ (1975) Breakdown of proteoglycan collagen induced in pig articular cartilage in organ culture. *Ann Rheum Dis* **34**: 303–311.

Docherty AJP & Murphy G (1990) The tissue metalloproteinase family and the inhibitor TIMP: a study using cDNAs and recombinant proteins. *Ann Rheum Dis* **49**: 469–479.

Dodge GR & Poole AR (1989) Immunohistochemical detection and immunochemical analysis of type II collagen degradation in human, normal, rheumatoid and osteoarthritic articular cartilages and in explants of bovine articular cartilage cultured with interleukin 1. *J Clin Invest* **83**: 647–661.

Dodge GR, Pidoux I & Poole AR (1991) The degradation of type II collagen in rheumatoid arthritis: an immunoelectron microscopic study. *Matrix* **11**: 330–338.

Dubois CM, Ruscetti FW, Palaszynski EW, Falk LA, Oppenheim JJ & Keller JR (1990) Tranforming growth factor-β is a potent inhibitor of interleukin-1 (IL-1) receptor expression: proposed mechanism of inhibition of IL-1 action. *J Exp Med* **172**: 737–744.

Edwards DR, Murphy G & Reynolds JJ (1987) Transforming growth factor beta modulates the expression of collagenase and metalloproteinase inhibitor. *EMBO J* **6**: 1899–1904.

Ehrlich MG, Mankin HJ, Jones H, Wright R, Crispen C & Vigliani G (1977) Collagenase and collagenase inhibitors in osteoarthritic and normal human cartilage. *J Clin Invest* **59**: 226–233.

Ellingsworth LR, Brennan JE, Fok K, Rosen DM, Bentz H, Piez KA et al. (1986) Antibodies to the N-terminal portion of cartilage-inducting factor A and transforming growth factor β. Immunohistochemical localization and association with differentiating cells. *J Biol Chem* **261**: 12362–12367.

Eyre DR, McDevitt CA, Billingham MEJ & Muir H (1980) Biosynthesis of collagen and other matrix proteins by articular cartilage in experimental osteoarthrosis. *Biochem J* **188**: 823–837.

Eyre DR, Weis MA & Moskowitz RW (1991) Cartilage expression of a type II collagen mutation in an inherited form of osteoarthritis associated with a mild chondrodysplasia. *J Clin Invest* **87**: 357–361.

Fernandez MP, Selmin O, Martin GR, Yamada Y, Pfäffle M, Deutzmann R et al. (1988) The structure of anchorin CII, a collagen binding protein isolated from chondrocyte membrane. *J Biol Chem* **263**: 5921–5925.

Firestein GS, Paine MM & Littman BH (1991) Gene expression (collagenase, tissue inhibitor of metallo-proteinases, complement, and HLA-DR) in rheumatoid arthritis and osteoarthritis synovium. *Arthritis Rheum* **34**: 1094–1105.

Flannery CR, Lark MW & Sandy JD (1992) Identification of a stromelysin cleavage site within the interglobular domain of human aggrecan. Evidence for proteolysis at this site *in vivo* in human articular cartilage. *J Biol Chem* **267**: 1008–1014.

Forslind K, Eberhardt K, Jonsson A & Saxne T (1992) Increased serum concentrations of cartilage oligomeric protein: a prognostic marker in early rheumatoid arthritis. *Br J Rheumatol* **31**: 593–598.

Fosang AJ, Neame PJ, Hardingham TE, Murphy G & Hamilton JA (1991a) Cleavage of cartilage proteo-glycan between G1 and G2 domains by stromelysins. *J Biol Chem* **266**: 15579–15582.

Fosang AJ, Tyler JA & Hardingham TE (1991b) Effect of interleukin-1 and insulin-like growth factor-1 on the release of proteoglycan components and hyaluronan from pig articular cartilage in explant culture. *Matrix* **11**: 117–124.

Fosang AJ, Neame PJ, Last K, Hardingham TE, Murphy G & Hamilton JA (1992) The interglobular domain of cartilage aggrecan is cleaved by PUMP, gelatinases, and cathepsin B. *J Biol Chem* **267**: 19470–19474.

Franzen A, Inerot S, Bejderuf S-O & Heinegård D (1981) Variations in the composition of bovine hip articular cartilage with distance from the articular surface. *Biochem J* **195**: 535–543.

Frisch SM & Ruley HE (1987) Transcription from the stromelysin promoter is induced by interleukin-1 and repressed by dexamethasone. *J Biol Chem* **262**: 16300–16304.

Frisch SM, Reich R, Collier IE, Genrich LT, Martin G & Goldberg GI (1990) Adenovirus EIA represses protease gene expression and inhibits metastasis of human tumor cells. *Oncogene* **5**: 75–83.

Gibson GJ, Bearman CH & Flint MH (1986) The immunoperoxidase localization of type X collagen in chick cartilage and lung. *Coll Rel Res* **6**: 163–184.

Goldring MB, Sandell LJ, Stephenson ML & Krane SM (1986) Immune interferon suppresses levels of procollagen mRNA and type II collagen synthesis in cultured human articular and costal chondrocytes. *J Biol Chem* **261**: 9049–9056.

Goldring MB, Birkhead J, Sandell LJ, Kimura T & Krane SM (1988) Interleukin-1 suppresses expression of cartilage-specific types II and IX collagens and increases types I and III collagens in human chondrocytes. *J Clin Invest* **82**: 2026–2037.

Goldring MB, Birkhead J, Sandell LJ & Krane SM (1990) Synergistic regulation of collagen gene expression in human chondrocytes by tumor necrosis factor-α and interleukin-1β. *Ann NY Acad Sci* **580**: 536–539.

Gordon CV, Villanueva T, Schumacher HR & Gohel V (1984) Autopsy study correlating degree of osteoarthritis, synovitis and evidence of articular calcification. *J Rheumatol* **11**: 681–686.

Goto M, Yoshinoya S, Miyamoto T, Sasano M, Okamoto M, Nishioka K et al. (1988) Stimulation of interleukin-1α and interluekin 1-β release from human monocytes by cyanogen bromide peptides of type II collagen. *Arthritis Rheum* **31**: 1508–1514.

Gravallese EM, Darling JM, Ladd AL, Katz JN & Glimcher LH (1991) *In situ* hybridization studies of stromelysin and collagenase messenger RNA expression of rheumatoid synovium. *Arthritis Rheum* **34**: 1076–1084.

Gray ML, Pizzanelli AM, Grodzinsky AJ & Lee RC (1988) Mechanical and physiochemical determinants of the chondrocyte biosynthetic response. *J Orthop Res* **6**: 777–792.

Greenwald RA & Moy WW (1980) Effects of oxygen-derived free radicals on hyaluronic acid. *Arthritis Rheum* **23**: 455–463.

Gurr E, Shrene A, Lonnemann G & Delbrück A (1990) Increased interleukin 1β production in macrophages by proteoglycan fragments deriving from articular cartilage *in vitro*. *Agents Actions* **29**: 117–119.

Halliday DA, McNeil JD, Betts WH & Scicchitano R (1993) The substance P fragment SP-(7–11) increases prostaglandin E_2 intracellular Ca^{2+} and collagenase production in bovine articular chondrocytes. *Biochem J* **292**: 57–62.

Halliwell B & Gutteridge JMC (1986) Oxygen free radicals and iron in relation to biology in medicine: some problems and concepts. *Arch Biochem Biophys* **246**: 501–514.

Harris ED Jr, DiBona D & Krane SM (1970) A mechanism for cartilage destruction in rheumatoid arthritis. *Trans Ass Am Physicians* **83**: 267–276.

Harris ED Jr, Glauert AE & Murley A (1977) Intracellular collagen fibers at the pannus cartilage function in rheumatoid arthritis. *Arthritis Rheum* **20**: 657–665.

Harvey AK, Hrubey PS & Chandrasekhar S (1991) Transforming growth factor-β inhibition of interleukin-1 activity involves downregulation of interleukin-1 receptors on chondrocytes. *Exp Cell Res* **195**: 376–385.

Harvey AK, Stack ST & Chandrasekhar S (1993) Differential modulation of degradative and repair responses of interleukin-1-treated chondrocytes by platelet-derived growth factor. *Biochem J* **292**: 129–136.

Hasty KA, Reife RA, Kang AH & Stuart JM (1990) The role of stromelysin in the cartilage destruction that accompanies inflammatory arthritis. *Arthritis Rheum* **33**: 388–397.

Henderson B & Pettipher ER (1989) Arthritogenic actions of recombinant IL-1 and tumour necrosis factor a in the rabbit: evidence for synergistic interactions between cytokines *in vivo*. *Clin Exp Immunol* **75**: 306–310.

Henderson B, Hardingham T, Blake S & Lewthwaite J (1993) Experimental arthritis models in the study of the mechanisms of articular cartilage loss in rheumatoid arthritis. *Agents Actions* **39** (**supplement**): 15–26.

Hirose T, Patterson C, Pourmotabbed T, Mainardi CL & Hasty KA (1993) Structure–function relationship of human neutrophil collagenase: identification of regions responsible for substrate specificity and general proteinase activity. *Proc Nat Acad Sci USA* **90**: 2569–2573.

Hollander AP, Atkins RM, Eastwood DM, Dieppe PA & Elson CJ (1991) Human cartilage is degraded by rheumatoid arthritis synovial fluid but not by recombinant cytokines *in vitro*. *Clin Exp Immunol* **83**: 52–57.

Hollander AP, Heathfield TF, Webber C, Iwata Y, Bourne R, Rorabeck C et al. (1994) Incrased damage to type II collagen in osteoarthritic articular cartilage detected by a new immunoassay. *J Clin Invest* **93**: 1722–1732.

Holmes WA, Bayliss MT & Muir H (1988) Hyaluronic acid in human articular cartilage. Age related changes in content and size. *Biochem J* **250**: 435–441.

Homandberg GA, Meyers R & Xie D-L (1992) Fibronectin fragments cause chondrolysis of bovine articular cartilage slices in culture. *J Biol Chem* **267**: 3597–3604.

Howell DS & Dean DD (1992) The biology, chemistry and biochemistry of the mammalian growth plate. In Coe FL & Favus MJ (eds) *Disorders of Bone and Mineral Metabolism*, pp 313–353. New York: Raven Press.

Hughes C, Murphy G & Hardingham TE (1991) Metalloproteinase digestion of cartilage proteoglycans. Pattern of cleavage by stromelysin and susceptibility to collagenase. *Biochem J* **279**: 733–739.

Hughes CE, Caterson B, White RJ, Roughley PJ & Mort JS (1992) Monoclonal antibodies recognizing protease-generated neoepitopes from cartilage proteoglycan degradation. Application to studies of human link protein cleavage by stromelysin. *J Biol Chem* **267**: 16011–16014.

Hui-Chou CS & Lust G (1982) The type of collagen made by articular cartilage in joints of dogs with degenerative joint disease. *Coll Rel Res* **2**: 245–256.

Hutchinson NI, Lark MW, McNaul KL, Harper C, Hoerrner LA, McDonnell J et al. (1992) *In vivo* expression of stromelysin in synovium and cartilage of rabbits injected intraarticularly with interleukin-1β. *Arthritis Rheum* **35**: 1227–1233.

Ikebe T, Hirata M & Koga T (1988) Effects of human recombinant tumor necrosis factor-α and interleukin-1 on the synthesis of glycosaminoglycan and DNA in cultured rat costal chondrocytes. *J Immunol* **140**: 827–831.

Ilic MZ, Handley CJ, Robinson HC & Mok MT (1992) Mechanism of catabolism of aggrecan by articular cartilage. *Arch Biochem Biophys* **294**: 115–122.

Ishikawa H, Ohno O, Saura R, Matsubara T, Kurada T & Hirohata K (1991) Cytokine enhancement of monocyte/synovial cell attachment to the surface of cartilage: a possible trigger of pannus formation in arthritis. *Rheumatol Int* **11**: 31–36.

Ismaiel A, Atkins RM, Pease MF, Dieppe PA & Elson CJ (1992) Susceptibility of normal and arthritic human articular cartilage to degradative stimuli. *Br J Rheumatol* **31**: 369–373.

Kato Y & Iwamoto M (1990) Fibroblast growth factor is an inhibitor of chondrocyte terminal differentiation. *J Biol Chem* **265**: 5903–5909.

Kato K, Iwamoto M, Koike T, Suzuki F & Takano Y (1988) Terminal differentiation and calcification in rabbit chondrocyte cultures grown in centrifuge tubes. Regulation by transforming growth factor β and serum factors. *Proc Natl Acad Sci USA* **85**: 9552–9556.

Katsura N & Yamada K (1986) Isolation and characterization of a metalloproteinase associated with chicken epiphyseal cartilage matrix vesicles. *Bone* **7**: 137–143.

Katzenstein PL, Malemud CJ, Pathria MN, Carter JR, Sheon RP & Moskowitz RW (1990) Early-onset primary osteoarthritis and mild chondrodysplasia. Radiographic and pathologic studies with an analysis of cartilage proteoglycans. *Arthritis Rheum* **33**: 674–684.

Kempson GE (1982) Relationship between the tensile properties of articular cartilage from the human knee and age. *Ann Rheum Dis* **41**: 508–511.

Kempson GE (1991) Age-related changes in the tensile properties of human articular cartilage: a comparative study between the femoral head of the hip joint and the talus of the ankle joint. *Biochem Biophys Acta* **1075**: 223–230.

Kempson GE, Muir H, Pollard C & Tuke M (1973) The tensile properties of the cartilage of human femoral condyles related to the content of collagen and glycosaminoglycans. *Biochim Biophys Acta* **297**: 465–472.

Kerr LD, Holt JT & Matrisian LM (1988) Growth factors regulate transin gene expression by c-fos-dependent and c-fos-independent pathways. *Science* **242**: 1424–1427.

Keski-Oja J, Lohi J, Tuutila A, Tryggvason K & Vartio T (1992) Proteolytic processing of the 72,000 Da type IV collagenase by urokinase plasminogen activator. *Exp Cell Res* **202**: 471–476.

Kim S-J, Lafyatis R, Kim KY, Angel P, Fujiki H, Karin M et al. (1990) Regulation of collagenase gene expression by okadic acid, an inhibitor of protein phosphatases. *Cell Regul* **1**: 269–278.

Kimura H, Tateishi H & Ziff M (1977) Surface ultrastructure of rheumatoid articular cartilage. *Arthritis Rheum* **20**: 1085–1098.

Kobayashi I & Ziff M (1975) Electron microscopic studies of the cartilage–pannus junction in rheumatoid arthritis. *Arthritis Rheum* **18**: 475–483.

Kobayashi H, Schmitt M, Goretzki L, Chucholowski N, Calvete J, Kramer M et al. (1991) Cathepsin B efficiently activates the soluble and the tumor cell receptor-bound form of the proenzyme urokinase-type plasminogen activator (pro-uPA). *J Biol Chem* **266**: 5147–5152.

Koch AE, Polverini PJ, Kunkel SL, Harlow LA, DiPietro LA, Elner VM et al. (1992) Interleukin-8 is a macrophage-derived mediator of angiogenesis. *Science* **258**: 1798–1801.

Lafeber FPJG, van der Kraan PM, van Roy HLAM, Vitters EL, Huber-Bruning O, van den Berg W et al. (1992) Local changes in proteoglycan synthesis during culture are different for normal and osteoarthritic cartilages. *Am J Pathol* **140**: 1421–1429.

Lafyatis R, Kim SJ, Angel P, Roberts AB, Sporn MB, Karin M et al (1990) Interleukin-1 stimulates and all trans retinoic acid inhibits collagenase gene expression through its 5′-activator protein-1 binding sites. *Mol Endocrinol* **4**: 973–980.

Leboy PS, Shapiro IM, Uschmann BD, Oshima O & Lin D (1988) Gene expression in mineralizing chick epiphyseal cartilage. *J Biol Chem* **263**: 8515–8520.

Lefebvre V, Peeters-Joris C & Vaes G (1990) Modulation by interleukin-1 and tumor necrosis factor α of production of collagenase, tissue inhibitor of metalloproteinases and collagen types in differentiated and dedifferentiated articular chondrocytes. *Biochim Biophys Acta* **1052**: 366–378.

Levine JD, Clarke R, Devor M, Helms C, Moskowitz MA & Basbaum AI (1984) Intraneuronal substance P contributes to the severity of experimental arthritis. *Science* **226**: 547–549.

Lippiello L, Hall D & Mankin HJ (1977) Collagen synthesis in normal and osteoarthritic human cartilage. *J Clin Invest* **59**: 593–600.

Lohmander LS (1991) Markers of cartilage metabolism in arthrosis. A review. *Acta Orthop Scand* **62**: 623–632.

Lohmander LS, Dahlberg L, Ryd L & Heinegård D (1989) Increased levels of proteoglycan fragments in knee joint fluid after injury. *Arthritis Rheum* **32**: 1434–1442.

Lohmander LS, Hoerrner LA & Lark MW (1993) Metalloproteinases, tissue inhibitor and proteoglycan fragments in knee synovial fluid in human osteoarthritis. *Arthritis Rheum* **36**: 181–189.

Lotz M & Guerne P-A (1991) Interleukin-6 induces the synthesis of tissue inhibitor of metalloproteinases-1/erythroid potentiating activity (TIMP-1-EPA). *J Biol Chem* **266**: 2017–2020.

Lotz M, Carson DA & Vaughan JH (1987) Substance P activation of rheumatoid synoviocytes: neural pathway in pathogenesis of arthritis. *Science* **235**: 893–895.

Lotz M, Vaughan JH & Carson DH (1988) Effect of neuropeptides on production of inflammatory cytokines by human monocytes. *Science* **241**: 1218–1220.

Lotz M, Terkeltaub R & Villiger PM (1992) Cartilage and joint inflammation: regulation of IL-8 expression by human articular chondrocytes. *J Immunol* **148**: 466–473.

Loulakis P, Shrikharde A, Davis G & Maniglia CA (1992) *N*-terminal sequence of proteoglycan fragments isolated from medium of interleukin-1-treated articular-cartilage cultures. Putative site(s) of enzymic cleavage. *Biochem J* **284**: 589–593.

Luytens FP, Hascall VC, Nissley SP, Morales TI & Reddi AH (1988) Insulin-like growth factors maintain steady state metabolism of proteoglycans in bovine articular cartilage explants. *Arch Biochem Biophys* **267**: 416–425.

Makower A-M, Wroblewski J & Pawlowski A (1988) Effects of IGF-1, EGF and FGF on proteoglycans synthesized by fractionated chondrocytes of rat rib growth plate. *Exp Cell Res* **179**: 498–506.

Manincourt D-H, Triki R, Fukuda K, Devogelaer J-P, Nagant de Deuxchaisnes CN & Thonar EJ-MA (1993) Levels of circulating tumor necrosis factor α and interleukin-6 in patients with rheumatoid arthritis. Relationship to serum levels of hyaluronan and antigenic keratan sulfate. *Arthritis Rheum* **36**: 490–499.

Mankin HJ & Conger KA (1966) The acute effects of intra-articular hydrocortisone on articular cartilage in rabbits. *J Bone Joint Surg* **48A**: 1383–1388.

Mankin HJ & Lippiello L (1970) Biochemical and metabolic abnormalities in articular cartilage from osteoarthritic human hips. *J Bone Joint Surg Am* **52**: 424–434.

Marcy AI, Eiberger LL, Harrison R, Chan K, Hutchinson NI, Hagmann WK et al. (1991) Human fibroblast stromelysin catalytic domain: expression, purification and characterization of a C-terminally truncated form. *Biochemistry* **30**: 6476–6483.

Maroudas A (1976) Transport of solutes through cartilage: permeability to large molecules. *J Anat* **122**: 335–347.

Martel-Pelletier J, Cloutier JM & Pelletier JP (1990) Cathepsin B and cysteine protease inhibitors in human osteoarthritis. *J Orthop Res* **8**: 336–344.

Martel-Pelletier J, McCollum R, DiBattista J, Fawe M-P, Chin JA, Fournier S et al. (1992) The interleukin-1 receptor in normal and osteoarthritic human articular chondrocytes. Identification as the type I receptor and analysis of binding kinetics and biologic function. *Arthritis Rheum* **35**: 530–540.

Matrisian LM (1992) The matrix-degrading metalloproteinases. *Bioessays* **14**: 455–463.

McCrachen SS (1991) Expression of metalloproteinases and metalloproteinase inhibitors in human arthritic synovium. *Arthritis Rheum* **34**: 1085–1093.

McDevitt CA, Pahl JA, Ayad S, Miller RR, Uratsuji M & Andrish JT (1988) Experimental osteoarthritic articular cartilage is enriched in guanidine soluble type VI collagen. *Biochem Biophys Res Comm* **157**: 250–255.

McDonnell J, Hoerrner LA, Lark MW, Harper C, Dey T, Lobner J et al. (1992) Recombinant human interleukin-1β induced increase in levels of proteoglycans, stromelysin and leukocytes in rabbit synovial fluid. *Arthritis Rheum* **35**: 799–805.

McQuillan DJ, Handley CJ, Campbell MA, Bolis S, Milway VE & Herington AC (1986) Stimulation of proteoglycan biosynthesis by serum and insulin-like growth factor-1 in cultured bovine articular cartilage. *Biochem J* **240**: 423–430.

Menkes CJ, Renoux M, Laoussadi S, Manborgne A, Bruxelle J & Cesselin F (1993) Substance P levels in the synovium and synovial fluid from patients with rheumatoid arthritis and osteoarthritis. *J Rheum* **20**: 714–717.

Middleton JFS & Tyler JA (1992) Upregulation of insulin-like growth factor 1 gene expression in the lesions of osteoarthritic human articular cartilage. *Ann Rheum Dis* **51**: 440–447.

Miller D, Mankin H, Shaji H & D'Ambrosia R (1984) Identification of fibronectin in preparations of osteoarthritic human cartilages. *Connect Tissue Res* **12**: 267–275.

Mitchell N & Shepard N (1978) Changes in proteoglycan and collagen in rheumatoid arthritis. *J Bone Joint Surg Am* **60**: 349–354.

Mitchell PG & Cheung HS (1991) Tumor necrosis factor α and epidermal growth factor regulation of collagenase and stromelysin in adult porcine articular chondrocytes. *J Cell Physiol* **149**: 132–140.

Miyasaka N, Sato K, Goto M, Sasano M, Natsuyama M, Inoue K et al. (1988) Augmented interleukin-1 production and HLA-DR expression in the synovium of rheumatoid arthritis patients. Possible involvement of joint destruction. *Arthritis Rheum* **31**: 480–486.

Miyazaki K, Umenishi F, Funahashi K, Koshikawa N, Yasumitsu H & Umeda M (1992) Activation of TIMP-2/progelatinase A complex by stromelysin. *Biochem Biophys Res Comm* **185**: 852–859.

Mohtai M, Lane Smith R, Schurman DJ, Tsuji Y, Torti FM, Hutchinson NI et al. (1993) Expression of 92 kD type IV collagenase/gelatinase (gelatinase B) in osteoarthritic cartilage and its induction in normal human articular cartilage by interleukin-1. *J Clin Invest* **92**: 179–185.

Moll UM, Youngleib GL, Rosinski KB & Quigley JP (1990). Tumor promoter-stimulated Mr 92,000 gelatinase secreted by normal and malignant human cells: isolation and characterization of the enzyme from HT 1080 tumor cells. *Cancer Res* **50**: 6162–6170.

Morales TI & Roberts AB (1988) Transforming growth factor β regulates the metabolism of proteoglycans in bovine organ cultures. *J Biol Chem* **263**: 12828–12831.

Mörgelin M, Paulsson M, Hardingham TE, Heinegård D & Engel J (1988) Cartilage proteoglycans. Assembly with hyaluronate and link protein as studied by electron microscopy. *Biochem J* **253**: 175–185.

Mort JS, Dodge GR, Roughley PJ, Liu J, Finch SJ, Dipasquale G et al. (1993) Direct evidence for metalloproteinases mediating matrix degradation in interleukin-1 stimulated human articular cartilage. *Matrix* **13**: 95–102.

Murphy G, Cockett MI, Stephens PE, Smith BJ & Docherty AJP (1987) Stromelysin is an activator of procollagenase. A study with natural and recombinant enzymes. *Biochem J* **248**: 265–268.

Murphy G, Ward R, Hembry RM, Reynolds JJ, Kühn K & Tryggvason K (1989) Characterization of gelatinase from pig polymorphonuclear leucocytes. A metalloproteinase resembling tumour type IV collagenase. *Biochem J* **258**: 463–472.

Murphy G, Allan JS, Willenbrock F, Cockett MI, O'Connell JP & Docherty AJP (1992a) The role of the C-terminal domain in collagenase and stromelysin specificity. *J Biol Chem* **267**: 9612–9618.

Murphy G, Ward R, Gavrilovic J & Atkinson S (1992b) Physiological mechanisms for metalloproteinase activation. *Matrix* (**supplement 1**): 224–230.

Nagase H, Ogata H, Suzuki K, Enghild JJ & Salvesen G (1991) Substrate specificities and activation mechanisms of matrix metalloproteinases. *Biochem Soc Trans* **19**: 715–718.

Nakano T & Scott PG (1988) Partial purification and characterization of proteodermatan sulphate-degrading proteinases produced by human gingival fibroblasts. *Biomed Res* **9**: 269–279.

Nakata K, Ono K, Miyazaki J-I, Olsen BR, Muragaki Y, Adachi E et al. (1993) Osteoarthritis associated with mild chondrodysplasia in transgenic mice expressing α1(IX) collagen chains with a central deletion. *Proc Natl Acad Sci USA* **90**: 2870–2874.

Ng CK, Handley CJ, Preston BN & Robinson HC (1992) The extracellular processing and catabolism of hyaluronan in cultured adult articular cartilage explants. *Arch Biochem Biophys* **298**: 70–79.

Nguyen Q, Murphy G, Roughley PJ & Mort JS (1989) Degradation of proteoglycan aggregate by a cartilage metalloproteinase. Evidence for the involvement of stromelysin in the generation of link protein heterogeneity *in situ*. *Biochem J* **259**: 61–87.

Nguyen Q, Mort JS & Roughley PJ (1990) Cartilage proteoglycan aggregate is degraded more extensively by cathepsin L than by cathepsin B. *Biochem J* **266**: 519–573.

Nguyen Q, Liu J, Roughley PJ & Mort JS (1991) Link protein as a monitor *in situ* of endogenous proteolysis in adult human articular cartilages. *Biochem J* **278**: 143–147.

Nguyen Q, Mort JS & Roughley PJ (1992) Preferential mRNA expression of prostromelysin relative to procollagenase and *in situ* localization in human articular cartilage. *J Clin Invest* **89**: 1189–1197.

Nguyen Q, Murphy G, Hughes CE, Mort JS & Roughley PJ (1993) Matrix metalloproteinases cleave at two distinct sites on human cartilage link protein. *Biochem J*, in press.

Nietfeld JJ, Wilbrink B, Den Otter W, Huber J & Huber-Bruning O (1990) The effect of human interleukin 1 on proteoglycan metabolism in human and porcine cartilage explants. *J Rheumatol* **17**: 818–826.

Ogata Y, Enghild JJ & Nagase H (1992) Matrix metalloproteinase 3 (stromelysin) activates the precursor for the human matrix metalloproteinase 9. *J Biol Chem* **267**: 3581–3584.

Okada Y, Konomi H, Yada T, Kimata K & Nagase H (1989) Degradation of type IX collagen by matrix metalloproteinase 3 (stromelysin) from human rheumatoid synovial cells. *FEBS Lett* **244**: 473–476.

Okada Y, Morodomi T, Enghild JJ, Suzuki K, Yasui A, Nakanishi I et al. (1990) Matrix metalloproteinase 2 from human rheumatoid synovial fibroblasts. Purification and activation of the precursor and enzymic properties. *Eur J Biochem* **194**: 721–730.

Okada Y, Gonoji Y, Naka K, Tomita K, Nakanishi I, Iwata K et al. (1992a). Matrix metalloproteinase 9 (92 kDa gelatinase/type II collagenase) from HT1080 human fibrosarcoma cells. Purification and activation of the precursor and enzymic properties. *J Biol Chem* **267**: 21712–21719.

Okada Y, Shinmei M, Tanaka O, Nakak K, Kimura A, Nakamishi I et al. (1992b) Localization of matrix metalloproteinase (stromelysin) in osteoarthritic cartilage and synovium. *Lab Invest* **66**: 680–690.

Ollivierre F, Gubler U, Towle CA, Laurencin C & Treadwell BV (1986) Expression of IL-1 genes in human and bovine chondrocytes: a mechanism for autocrine control of cartilage matrix degradation. *Biochem Biophy Res Comm* **141**: 904–911.

Overall CM, Wrana JL & Sodek J (1989) Independent regulation of collagenase 72-kDa gelatinase and metalloproteinase inhibitor expression in human fibroblasts by transforming growth factor-β. *J Biol Chem* **264**: 1860–1869.

Page Thomas DP, King B, Stephen T & Dingle JT (1991) *In vivo* studies of cartilage regeneration after damage induced by catabolin/interleukin 1. *Ann Rheum Dis* **50**: 75–80.

Palmer RMJ, Hickery MS, Charles IG, Moncada S & Bayliss MT (1993) Induction of nitric oxide synthase in human chondrocytes. *Biochem Biophys Res Comm* **193**: 398–405.

Palmoski MJ & Brandt KD (1984) Effects of static loading and cyclic compressive loading on articular plugs *in vitro*. *Arthritis Rheum* **27**: 695–681.

Paulsson M, Mörgelin M, Wiedemann H, Beardmore-Gray M, Dunham D, Hardingham T et al. (1987) Extended and globular domains in cartilage proteoglycans. *Biochem J* **245**: 763–772.

Pelletier-J-P, Martel-Pelletier J, Howell DS, Ghandur-Mnaymneh L, Enis JE & Woessner JF Jr (1983) Collagenase and collagenolytic activity in human osteoarthritic cartilage. *Arthritis Rheum* **26**: 63–68.

Pettipher ER, Higgs GA & Henderson B (1986) Interleukin-1 induces leukocyte infiltration and cartilage proteoglycan degradation in the synovial joint. *Proc Natl Acad Sci USA* **83**: 8749–8753.

Pettipher ER, Henderson B, Hardingham T & Ratcliffe A (1989) Cartilage and proteoglycan depletion in acute and chronic antigen induced arthritis. *Arthritis Rheum* **32**: 601–607.

Pettipher ER, Edwards J, Cruwys S, Jessup E, Beesley J & Henderson B (1990) Pathogenesis of antigen-induced arthritis in mice deficient in neutrophil elastase and cathepsin G. *Am J Pathol* **137**: 1079–1082.

Pfaffle M, Ruggiero F & Hofman H (1988) Biosynthesis, secretion and extracellular localization of anchorin CII, a collagen binding protein of the calpactin family. *EMBO J* **7**: 230–242.

Phadke K (1987) Fibroblast growth factor enhances the interleukin-1 mediated chondrocyte protease release. *Biochem Biophys Res Commun* **142**: 448–453.

Poole AR (1990) Enzymatic degradation: cartilage destruction. In Brandt KD (ed) *Cartilage Changes in Osteoarthritis*, pp 63–72. Indiana University School of Medicine: Ciba-Geigy Corporation.

Poole AR (1993) The growth plate: cellular physiology cartilage assembly and mineralization. In Hall B & Newman S (eds) *Cartilage Molecular Aspects*, pp 179–211. Boca Raton: CRC Press.

Poole AR (1991) Cartilage in health and disease. In McCarty D & Koopman W (eds) *Arthritis and Allied Conditions. A Textbook of Rheumatology*, 12 edn, pp 279–333. Philadelphia: Lea and Febiger.

Poole AR & Dieppe P (1994) Biological markers in rheumatoid arthritis. *Seminars in Arthritis and Rheumatism* **23** (supplement 6): 17–31.

Poole AR (1994) Immunochemical markers of joint inflammation, skeletal damage and repair. Where are they now? *Ann Rheum Dis* **53**: 3–5.

Poole AR & Pidoux I (1989) Immunoelectron microscopic studies of type X collagen in endochondral ossification. *J Cell Biol* **109**: 2547–2554.

Poole AR, Webber C, Pidoux I, Choi H & Rosenberg LC (1986) Localization of a dermatan sulfate proteoglycan (DS-PGII) in cartilage and the presence of an immunologically related species in other tissues. *J Histochem Cytochem* **34**: 619–625.

Poole AR, Witter J, Roberts N, Piccolo F, Brandt R, Paquin J et al. (1990) Inflammation and cartilage metabolism in rheumatoid arthritis. Studies of the blood markers hyaluronic acid, orosomucoid and keratan sulfate. *Arthritis Rheum* **33**: 790–799.

Poole AR, Rizkalla G, Ionescu M, Reiner A, Brooks E, Rorabeck C et al. (1993b) Osteoarthritis in the human knee: a dynamic process of cartilage matrix degradation, synthesis and reorganization. *Agents Actions* **39** (supplement): 3–13.

Poole AR, Mort JS & Roughley PJ (1993a) Methods for evaluating mechanisms of cartilage breakdown. In Woessner JF Jr & Howell DS (eds) *Joint Cartilage Degradation. Basic and Clinical Aspects*, pp 225–260. New York: Marcel Dekker.

Poole AR, Ionescu M, Swan A and Dieppe P (1994). Changes in cartilage metabolism in arthritis are reflected by altered serum and synovial fluid levels of glycosaminoglycan epitopes on fragments of the cartilage proteopglycan aggrecan: implications for pathogenesis. *J Clin Invest* **94**: 25–33.

Prins APA, Lipman JM, McDevitt CA & Sokoloff L (1982) Effect of purified growth factors on rabbit articular chondrocytes in monolayer culture. II. Sulfated proteoglycan synthesis. *Arthritis Rheum* **25**: 1228–1238.

Pritzker KPH, Châteauvert JMD & Grynpas MD (1987) Osteoarthritic cartilage contains increased calcium, magnesium and phosphorus. *J Rheumatol* **141**: 806–810.

Quinones S, Sans J, Otani Y, Harris ED Jr & Kurkinen M (1989) Transcriptional regulation of human stromelysin. *J Biol Chem* **264**: 8339–8344.

Ratcliffe A, Fryer PR & Hardingham TE (1984) The distribution of aggregating-proteoglycans in articular cartilage: comparison of quantitative immunoelectron microscopy with radioimmunonassay and biochemical analyses. *J Histochem Cytochem* **32**: 193–201.

Ratcliffe A, Doherty M, Maini RN & Hardingham TE (1988) Increased concentrations of proteoglycan components in the synovial fluids of patients with acute but not chronic joint disease. *Ann Rheum Dis* **47**: 826–832.

Recklies AD & Golds EE (1992) Induction of synthesis and release of interleukin-8 from articular chondrocytes and cartilaged explants. *Arthritis Rheum* **35**: 1510–1519.

Rédini F, Mauviel A, Pronost S, Loyan G & Pujol J-P (1993) Transforming growth factor β exerts opposite effects from interleukin-1β on cultured rabbit articular chondrocytes through reduction of interleukin-1 receptor expression. *Arthritis Rheum* **36**: 44–50.

Rizkalla G, Reiner A, Bogoch E & Poole AR (1992) Studies of the articular cartilage proteoglycan aggrecan in health and osteoarthritis. Evidence for molecular heterogeneity and extensive molecular changes in disease. *J Clin Invest* **90**: 2268–2277.

Roberts CR, Mort JS & Roughley PJ (1987) Treatment of cartilage proteoglycan aggregate with hydrogen peroxide. Relationship between observed degradation products and those that occur naturally during ageing. *Biochem J* **247**: 349–357.

Roberts CR, Roughley PJ & Mort JS (1989) Degradation of human proteoglycan aggregate induced by hydrogen peroxide. Protein fragmentation, amino acid modification and hyaluronic acid cleavage. *Biochem J* **259**: 805–811.

Ronzière M-C, Ricard-Blum S, Tiollier J, Hartmann DJ, Garrone R & Herbage D (1990) Comparative analysis of collagens solubilized from human foetal, and normal and osteoarthritic adult articular cartilage, with emphasis on type VI collagen. *Biochim Biophys Acta* **1038**: 222–230.

Roth V & Mow VC (1980) The intrinsic tensile behaviour of the matrix of bovine articular cartilage and variation with age. *J Bone Joint Surg Am* **62**: 1102–1117.

Roughley PJ & White R (1980) Age-related changes in the structure of the proteoglycan subunits from human articular cartilage. *J Biol Chem* **255**: 217–224.

Roughley PJ, White RJ & Poole AR (1985) Identification of a hyaluronic acid-binding protein that interferes with the preparation of high-buoyant density proteoglycan aggregates from adult human articular cartilage. *Biochem J* **231**: 129–138.

Roux-Lombard P, Punzi L, Hasler F, Bas S, Todesco S, Gallati H et al. (1993) Soluble tumor necrosis factor receptors in human inflammatory synovial fluids. *Arthritis Rheum* **36**: 485–489.

Sah RL-Y, Doong J-YH & Grodzinsky AJ (1991) Effects of compression on the loss of newly synthesized proteoglycans and proteins from cartilage explants. *Arch Biochem Biophys* **286**: 20–29.

Saklatvala J (1986) Tumor necrosis factor α stimulates resorption and inhibits synthesis of proteoglycan in cartilage. *Nature* **322**: 547–549.

Saklatvala J, Pilsworth LMC & Sarsfield ST (1984) Pig catabolin is a form of interleukin-1: cartilage and bone resorb, fibroblasts make prostaglandin and collagenase and thymocyte proliferation is augmented in response to one protein. *Biochem J* **224**: 461–466.

Sandy JD, Neame PJ, Boynton RE & Flannery CR (1991a) Catabolism of aggrecan in cartilage explants. Identification of a major cleavage site within the interglobular domain. *J Biol Chem* **266**: 8683–8685.

Sandy JD, Boynton RE & Flannery CR (1991b) Analysis of the catabolism of aggrecan in cartilage explants by quantitation of peptides from the three globular domains. *J Biol Chem* **266**: 8198–8205.

Sandy JD, Flannery CR, Neme PJ & Lohmander LS (1992) The structure of aggrecan-fragments in human synovial fluid. Evidence for the involvement in osteoarthritis of a novel proteinase which cleaves the glu-373–Ala 374 bond of the interglobular domain. *J Clin Invest* **89**: 1512–1516.

Saxne T & Heinegård D (1992) Synovial fluid analysis of two groups of proteoglycan epitopes distinguishes early and late cartilage lesions. *Arthritis Rheum* **35**: 385–390.

Saxne T, Di Giovine FS, Heinegård D, Duff GW & Wollheim FA (1988) Synovial fluid concentrations of interleukin-1β and proteoglycans are inversely related. *J Autoimmunity* **1**: 373–380.

Saxne T, Glennås A, Kvien TK, Melby K & Heinegård D (1993) Release of cartilage macromolecules into the synovial fluid in patients with acute and prolonged phases of reactive arthritis. *Arthritis Rheum* **36**: 20–25.

Schalkwijk J, Joosten LAB & van den Berg WB (1989a) Insulin-like growth factor stimulation of chondrocyte proteoglycan synthesis by human synovial fluid. *Arthritis Rheum* **32**: 66–71.

Schalkwijk J, Joosten LAB & van den Berg WB (1989b) Chondrocyte non-responsiveness to insulin-like growth factor-1 in experimental arthritis. *Arthritis Rheum* **32**: 894–900.

Schneiderman R, Keret D & Maroudas A (1986) Effects of mechanical and osmotic pressure on the rate of glycosaminoglycan synthesis in the human adult femoral head cartilage. An *in vitro* study. *J Orthop Res* **4**: 393–408.

Schmid TM & Linsenmayer TF (1985) Immunohistochemical localization of short chain cartilage collagen (type X) in avian tissues. *J Cell Biol* **100**: 598–605.

Seed MP, Ismaiel S, Cheung CY, Thomson TA, Gardner CR, Atkins RM et al. (1993) Inhibition of interleukin-1β induced rat and human cartilage degradation *in vitro* by the metalloproteinase inhibitor U27391. *Ann Rheum Dis* **52**: 37–43.

Smith RJ, Justen JM, Sam LM, Rohloff NA, Ruppel PL, Brunden MN et al. (1991) Platelet-derived growth factor potentiates cellular responses of articular chondrocytes to interleukin-1. *Arthritis Rheum* **34**: 697–706.

Spector TD, Woodward L, Hall GM, Hammond A, Williams A, Butler MG et al. (1992) Keratan sulphate in rheumatoid arthritis, osteoarthritis, and inflammatory diseases. *Ann Rheum Dis* **51**: 1134–1137.

Springman EB, Angleton EL, Birkedal-Hansen H & Van Wart HE (1990) Multiple modes of activation of latent human fibroblast collagenase: evidence for the role of cys 73 active-site zinc complex in latency and a 'cysteine switch' mechanism for activation. *Proc Natl Acad Sci USA* **87**: 364–368.

Starkey P, Barrett AJ & Burleigh M (1977) The degradation of articular collagen by neutrophil proteinases. *Biochim Biophys Acta* **483**: 386–397.

Stockwell R, Billingham M & Muir H (1983) Ultrastructural changes in articular cartilage after experimental section of the anterior cruciate ligament of the dog knee. *J Anat* **136**: 425–439.

Sweet M, Thonar E, Immelman A & Solomon L (1977) Biochemical changes in progressive osteoarthrosis. *Ann Rheum Dis* **36**: 387–398.

Sweet MB, Coelho A, Schnitzler CM, Schnitzer TJ, Lenz ME, Jakim I et al. (1988) Serum keratan sulfate levels in osteoarthritic patients. *Arthritis Rheum* **31**: 648–652.

Takashima T, Kawai K, Hirohata K, Miki A, Mizogouti H & Cooke TDV (1989) Inflammatory cell changes in Haversian canals. A possible cause of osteoporosis in rheumatoid arthritis. *J Bone Joint Surg Br* **71**: 671–676.

Tateishi H (1973) Ultrastructure of synovio-cartilage junction in rheumatoid arthritis. *Kobe J Med Sch* **19**: 15–56.

Thomas JT, Cresswell CJ, Rash B, Hoyland J, Freemont AJ, Grant ME et al. (1991) The human type X gene: complete primary sequence in osteoarthritis. *Biochem Soc Trans* **19**: 804–808.

Thompson R & Oegema T (1979) Metabolic activity of articular cartilage in osteoarthritis. *J Bone Joint Surg Am* **61**: 407–416.

Thonar E, Sweet M, Immelmon A & Lyons G (1978) Hyaluronate in articular cartilage: age-related changes. *Calcif Tissue Res* **26**: 19–21.

Thonar EJ, Lenz ME, Klintworth GK, Caterson B, Pachman LM, Glickman P et al. (1985) Quantification of keratan sulfate in blood as a marker of cartilage metabolism. *Arthritis Rheum* **28**: 1367–1376.

Tiku ML, Liesch JP & Robertson FM (1990) Production of hydrogen peroxide by rabbit articular chondrocytes. Enhancement by cytokines. *J Immunol* **145**: 690–696.

Tiku K, Thakker-Varia S, Ramachandrula A & Tiku ML (1992) Articular chondrocytes secrete IL-1, express membrane IL-1 and have IL-1 inhibitory activity. *Cell Immunol* **146**: 1–20.

Tyler JA (1985a) Articular cartilage cultured with catabolin (pig interleukin 1) synthesizes a decreased number of normal proteoglycan molecules. *Biochem J* **227**: 869–878.

Tyler JA (1985b) Chondrocyte-mediated depletion of articular cartilage proteoglycans *in vitro*. *Biochem J* **225**: 493–507.

Tyler JA (1989) Insulin-like growth factor-1 can decrease degradation and promote synthesis of proteoglycan in cartilage exposed to cytokines. *Biochem J* **260**: 543–548.

Tyler JA & Benton HP (1988) Synthesis of type II collagen is decreased in cartilage cultured with interleukin-1 while the rate of extracellular degradation remains unchanged. *Coll Relat Res* **8**: 393–405.

Uhlinger E (1971) Bone changes in rheumatoid arthritis and their pathogenesis. In Muller W, Hovarth HG & Fehr K (eds) *Rheumatoid Arthritis: Pathogenetic Mechanisms and Consequences in Therapeutics*, pp 25–36. New York: Academic Press.

Urban JPG & Bayliss MT (1989) Regulation of proteoglycan synthesis rate in cartilage *in vitro*: influence of extracellular ionic composition. *Biochim Biophys Acta* **922**: 59–65.

Van Beuningen HM, Arntz OJ & van den Berg W (1991) *In vivo* effects of interleukin-1 on articular cartilage. Prolongation of proteoglycan metabolic disturbance in old mice. *Arthritis Rheum* **34**: 606–615.

Van de Loo AAJ & van den Berg WB (1990) Effects of murine recombinant interleukin 1 on synovial joints in mice: measurement of patellar cartilage metabolism and joint inflammation. *Ann Rheum Dis* **49**: 238–245.

Van de Loo FAJ, Arntz OJ, Otterness IG & van den Berg WB (1992) Protection against cartilage proteoglycan synthesis inhibition by anti-interleukin 1 antibodies in experimental arthritis. *J Rheumatol* **19**: 348–356.

Van der Kraan PM, Vitters EL & van der Berg WB (1992) Inhibition of proteoglycan synthesis by transforming growth factor β in anatomically intact cartilage of murine patellae. *Ann Rheum Dis* **51**: 643–647.

Van Kampen GPJ, Veldhuijzen JP, Kuijer R, van de Stadt RJ & Schipper CA (1985) Cartilage response to mechanical force in high-density chondrocyte cultures. *Arthritis Rheum* **28**: 419–424.

Van Wart HE & Birkedal-Hansen H (1990) The cysteine switch: a principle of regulation of metalloproteinase activity with potential applicability to the entire matrix metalloproteinase gene family. *Proc Natl Acad Sci USA* **87**: 5578–5582.

Vassali J-D, Sappino A-P & Belin D (1991) The plasminogen-activator/plasminogen system. *J Clin Invest* **88**: 1067–1072.

Venn MF & Maroudas A (1977) Chemical composition and swelling of normal and osteoarthritic femoral head cartilage. I. Chemical composition. *Am Rheum Dis* **36**: 121–129.

Vogel K & Trotter JA (1987) The effect of proteoglycans on the morphology of collagen fibrils formed *in vitro*. *Coll Rel Res* **7**: 105–114.

Von der Mark K, Kirsch T, Nerlich A, Kuss A, Weseloh G, Glückert K et al. (1992) Type X synthesis in human osteoarthritic cartilage. Indication of chondrocyte hypertrophy. *Arthritis Rheum* **35**: 806–811.

Walker GD, Fischer M, Gannon J, Thompson RC & Oegema TR Jr (1993) The expression of type X collagen in osteoarthritis. *J Orthop Res*, in press.

Walakovits LA, Moore VL, Bhardwaj N, Gallick GS & Lark MW (1992) Detection of stromelysin and collagenase in synovial fluid from patients with rheumatoid arthritis and post-traumatic knee injury. *Arthritis Rheum* **35**: 35–42.

Webber C, Glant TT, Roughley PJ & Poole AR (1987) The identification and characterization of two populations of aggregating proteoglycans of high buoyant density isolated from post-natal human articular cartilages of different ages. *Biochem J* **248**: 735–740.

Weiss C, Rosenberg L & Helfet AJ (1968) An ultrastructural study of normal young adult human articular cartilage. *J Bone Joint Surg Am* **50**: 663–674.

Weiss SJ (1989) Tissue destruction by neutrophils. *New Engl J Med* **320**: 365–376.

Weiss SJ, Peppin G, Ortiz X, Ragsdale C & Test ST (1985) Oxidative autoactivation of latent collagenase by human neutrophils. *Science* **227**: 747–749.

Werb Z, Tremble PM, Behrendtsen O, Crowley E & Domsky CH (1989) Signal transduction through the fibronectin receptor induces collagenase and stromelysin gene expression. *J Cell Biol* **109**: 877–889.

Westacott CI, Whicher JT, Barnes IC, Thompson D, Swan AJ & Dieppe PA (1990) Synovial fluid concentration of five different cytokines in rheumatic diseases. *Ann Rheum Dis* **49**: 676–681.

Wilkins E, Dieppe P, Maddison P & Evison G (1983) Osteoarthritis and articular chondrocalcinosis in the elderly. *Ann Rheum Dis* **42**: 280–284.

Witsch-Prehm P, Karbowski A, Ober B & Kresse H (1992) Influence of continuous infusion of interleukin-1α on the core protein and the core protein fragments of the small proteoglycan decorin in cartilage. *J Orthop Res* **10**: 276–284.

Witter J, Roughley PJ, Webber C, Roberts N, Keystone E & Poole AR (1987) The immunological detection and characterization of cartilage proteoglycan degradation products in synovial fluids of patients with arthritis. *Arthritis Rheum* **30**: 519–526.

Woessner JF Jr (1991) Matrix metalloproteinases and their inhibitors in connective tissue remodelling. *FASEB J* **5**: 2145–2154.

Wong SF, Halliwell B, Richmond R & Skowroneck WR (1981) The role of superoxide and hydroxyl radicals in the degradation of hyaluronic acid induced by metal ions and by ascorbic acid. *J Inorg Biochem* **14**: 127–134.

Woolley D, Crossley MJ & Evanson J (1977) Collagenase at sites of cartilage erosion in the rheumatoid joint. *Arthritis Rheum* **20**: 1231–1239.

Wu J-J, Lark M, Chun LE & Eyre DR (1991) Sites of stromelysin cleavage in collagen types II, IX and XI of cartilage. *J Biol Chem* **266**: 5625–5628.

Wurster NB & Lust G (1984) Synthesis of fibronectin in normal and osteoarthritic cartilage. *Biochem Biophys Acta* **800**: 52–58.

Yamada H, Nakagawa T, Stephens RW & Nagai Y (1987) Proteinases and their inhibitors in normal and osteoarthritic articular cartilage. *Biomed Res* **8**: 289–300.

Yoshida K, Kobayashi K, Yamagata N, Iwabuchi H, Katsura T, Sugihara S et al. (1992) Inflammatory cytokines and enzymes in synovial fluid of patients with rheumatoid arthritis and other arthritides. *Int Arch Allergy Immunol* **98**: 286–292.

10 Bone Cells and Bone Remodelling in Rheumatoid Arthritis

Tim Skerry and Maxine Gowen

INTRODUCTION

Although rheumatoid arthritis (RA) is primarily an autoimmune disease which affects the synovial joints, it has profound effects on bone growth and remodelling. The inflammatory response which is part of the disease is mediated by both local and systemic changes in expression of its activators and inhibitors. Many of these regulators of inflammation are also the controllers of normal cellular activity, so the effects of RA on bone metabolism are due to changes in the amounts, ratios and timings of their expression, rather than abnormal expression of hormones, eicosanoids or cytokines that are specific to the disease. Local changes in eicosanoid or cytokine expression have specific effects on bone cells, while the systemic effects of the acute phase response may influence bone formation or resorption because of alterations in hormone, mineral and nutrient status.

The purpose of this review is to survey briefly the normal processes involved in bone remodelling, the mechanisms by which they are controlled, and to highlight the changes induced in RA which have high impact on those processes.

CHANGES IN BONE REMODELLING IN EARLY RA

Although the primary effect of RA on remodelling is profound bone loss (Eggelmeijer *et al.*, 1993b), there are also effects on formation, which may include joint fusion or periarticular osteophyte formation (Cabral *et al.*, 1989). Both of these events may affect functional capacity; formation by physically limiting joint movement, or resorption by permitting collapse of subchondral bone, or ultimately gross pathological fracture.

Damage to the loadbearing surfaces of the joint, and collapse of the subchondral bone alters the mechanical loading of the remaining tissue, and subsequent formative events may be attempts to restore structural competence in the face of this damage. There is evidence that these attempts at repair occur when the disease is in a remission stage (Cabral *et al.*, 1989), as osteophytes are rarely seen in joints that are undergoing active destruction. Bone formation in RA therefore appears to be a reparative response to the disease, not part of its pathogenesis (Allard *et al.*, 1990).

One of the earliest features of RA is local bone loss in the vicinity of an affected joint, while over a longer period, generalized osteoporosis is also seen (Joffe and Epstein, 1991; Magaro *et al.*, 1991). Bone densitometry measurements in RA patients have shown that progressive bone loss is a feature of all rheumatoid patients who have the elevated acute phase response seen in early stages of the disease (Gough *et al.*,

1993; Eggelmeijer *et al.*, 1993a). Although loss continues after this acute stage, it is at that time that the appearance of radiologically detectable bone lesions is maximal. Bone mineral density (BMD) therefore provides an indirect but accurate indication of the progress of RA.

Periarticular bone loss in RA is due to a combination of factors. Loss of function associated with joint pain causes profound disuse-related loss, while joint effusion alters the manner of load support by the joint, and may reduce stresses in the subchondral trabeculae, with consequent effects on remodelling. As the disease progresses, bone loss may become more aggressive, leading to such severe destruction as is occasionally seen in the phalanges, which may be reduced to half their original length.

The causes of generalized bone loss in RA are harder to clarify, particularly because of difficulty of measuring whole body bone mass accurately. However, changes in the circulating levels of acute phase proteins are likely to be implicated in systemic osteoporosis. The acute phase response is associated with changes in some hormones (insulin, glucocorticoids and catecholamines) (Adami *et al.*, 1987), vitamins (Louw *et al.*, 1992), and minerals – primarily iron and zinc (Boosalis *et al.*, 1992), which have implications on regulation of bone remodelling. The acute phase response is also linked with elevated levels of circulating interleukin 1 (IL-1) and tumour necrosis factor alpha (TNFα) (Lewis, 1986; Hirokawa *et al.*, 1989; Grunfeld and Feingold, 1992; Mazlam and Hodgson, 1992), both of which have potent effects on remodelling, usually stimulating resorption. There is evidence that other cytokines such as interleukin 6 (IL-6) and interferon gamma (IFNγ) may be elevated in the acute phase response (Grunfeld and Feingold, 1992; Wegenka *et al.*, 1993), but their effects on remodelling are more equivocal.

NORMAL BONE REMODELLING

Bone remodelling is the process by which concurrent resorption and formation occur in a controlled way to replace the load-bearing extracellular matrix of the skeleton. Remodelling is often viewed as a series of steps within a cycle of events in which bone is resorbed and replaced (Fig. 1) (Baron *et al.*, 1983). In this remodelling cycle, a quiescent bone surface is covered by apparently inactive lining cells, which are thought to be of osteoblast lineage (Menton *et al.*, 1984; Miller *et al.*, 1989). Although these cells are morphologically similar, it is possible that individual cells possess specific functions such as responsiveness to and transduction of systemic or local signals, or the ability to give rise to osteoblastic precursors.

The first step of the remodelling cycle occurs after the transduction of some signal which stimulates a requirement for a resorptive event. This leads to recruitment of osteoclast precursors in the marrow, and attraction of these cells to the specific site. Activation of these cells involves differentiation, followed by fusion into activated multinucleated osteoclasts. Mononuclear osteoclast precursors cannot be identified specifically, so knowledge of much of this process is inferred (Baron *et al.*, 1986). However, it is known that osteoclast precursors originate from haematopoietic cells, probably colony-forming units of the granulocyte/macrophage lineage (CFU GM) (Orcel *et al.*, 1990). At the same time as this recruitment/activation stage occurs, the lining cells change their shape to become more rounded so that mineralized matrix is

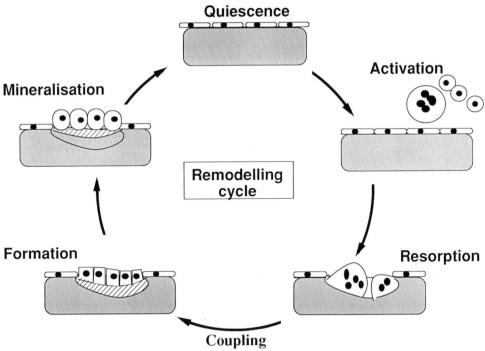

Figure 1. The remodelling cycle. Osteoclast precursors fuse and are activated to resorb a lacuna in a previously quiescent surface. These cells are replaced by osteoblasts which deposit new bone to restore the integrity of the tissue.

exposed for resorption (Ali *et al.*, 1990). Active resorption follows when the osteo-clasts bind to the bone surface by means of specific ligand receptor interactions. Recent evidence suggests that osteoclasts express integrins which are involved in cell matrix binding (Teti *et al.*, 1989; Zambonin-Zallone *et al.*, 1989). After formation of a tight sealed zone, the osteoclast removes mineral and collagen by secretion of pro-teases and hydrogen ions (Baron *et al.*, 1988). Resorption occurs until some as yet unknown signalling process inhibits osteoclastic action. It has been suggested that elevation of extracellular calcium concentration, or growth factors released from the bone matrix, may be responsible (Pfeilschifter *et al.*, 1988). A role for the osteocytes within the bone in signalling the end of resorption is also possible.

At this time, termed the reversal phase, the osteoclasts disappear and the bone surface is uncovered except for the presence of occasional mononuclear phagocytes. It is possible that these are involved in the recruitment of new osteoblast precursors, which proliferate and differentiate locally. In the reversal stage, resorption is followed by coupled formation in which mature osteoblasts deposit new osteoid – un-mineralized matrix – in the defect. Mineralization of the osteoid proceeds in a front from the existing bone surface so that the integrity of the bone is restored. At the end of the process, the lining cell population is re-established, and the surface becomes quiescent again.

Since the remodelling cycle was suggested, it has become clear that the stylized view represented in Fig. 1 is only one part of a spectrum of different possible outcomes of a remodelling event. Although it is possible that resorption could be followed by equivalent formation that fills exactly the defect created by osteoclastic resorption, it is not the inevitable consequence. Where there is a primary requirement for an increase in bone mass, as would occur in response to an increased mechanical stimulus, appositional formation occurs on a surface without previous resorption (Pead *et al.*, 1988). Conversely, it is possible to have resorption without infilling of the defect, where there is a requirement to reduce bone mass rapidly or substantially, such as in calcium deprivation or disuse (Lanyon *et al.*, 1986). Those two possibilities represent the ends of a spectrum of which the remodelling cycle is the mid point. Between the two ends are the possibilities of resorption which exceeds formation and vice versa to reduce or increase bone mass slightly.

While response to the mechanical demands of habitual activity is a primary reason for remodelling, the process is also central in calcium homeostasis. The balance between the competing demands of these two influences determines the net result of remodelling.

CELLULAR INTERACTIONS IN BONE REMODELLING

In order to understand the ways in which disease conditions affect bone remodelling, it is necessary to examine the parts of the remodelling process in greater detail, to clarify the cell types involved, their interactions, and current perceptions of the mechanisms by which they are controlled.

At each stage of the remodelling cycle, the actions of the cells responsible for resorption and formation are under tight control, which is effected by temporal and spatial expression of different cytokines. These cytokines are thought to be regulated globally by endocrine influences, and locally by paracrine and autocrine effects.

Bone lining cells are thought to receive information from two sources. Osteocytes embedded within the matrix communicate with each other and with surface cells (Doty, 1981; Curtis *et al.*, 1985), and have been suggested to provide information regarding the levels of mechanical strain experienced by the bone (Skerry *et al.*, 1989). In addition, surface cells possess receptors for both systemic and local osteotropic agents. The lining cell therefore may function to perceive and integrate the endocrine, paracrine and autocrine signals, and provide an appropriate response to initiate formation or resorption.

SYSTEMIC EFFECTS ON REMODELLING

It has been demonstrated that bone loss in RA occurs despite normal levels of parathyroid hormone (PTH) and 1,25 dihydroxyvitamin D (1,25D) – the major metabolite of vitamin D (Sambrook *et al.*, 1990). However, the importance of interactions of hormones with paracrine osteotropic agents is illustrated by the ability of prostaglandin E_2 (PGE_2) to reduce PTH receptor numbers on bone cells by over 80% (Mitchell and Goltzman, 1990). Remodelling is influenced by a number of hormones. With the exception of calcitonin (Goltzman and Tannenbaum, 1987), it is widely accepted that these agents act only indirectly on osteoclasts, binding to bone lining cells. Lining cells possess receptors for 1,25D (Boivin *et al.*, 1987), PTH (Rouleau *et al.*, 1986), thyroid hormone (Ernst and Froesch, 1987), and oestrogen (Komm *et al.*, 1988).

PTH is an 84 amino acid peptide hormone which has a major role in stimulating bone resorption and controlling calcium homeostasis. It binds to specific cell surface receptors on lining cells to stimulate recruitment of osteoclast precursor cells (Jilka, 1986), to activate these cells and to permit their access to the bone surface (Ali *et al.*, 1990). Paradoxically, it has become clear in recent years that PTH also has important functions in stimulating bone formation. The mechanism by which this occurs is unclear, but it may involve the pattern of secretion of the hormone, since studies have shown that intermittent administration enhances formation, while constant infusion of the same total amount of hormone is a potent stimulus for resorption (Hodsman and Fraher, 1990; Hock and Gera, 1992). Thyroid hormone is involved primarily in cell proliferation and therefore growth of bone, although excesses of the hormone can stimulate bone resorption (Ernst and Froesch, 1987).

As steroid hormones, both 1,25D and oestrogen both act on intranuclear rather than classical membrane receptors. While it has actions on the kidney and gut, 1,25D acts to enhance bone resorption in a similarly indirect way to PTH, by stimulating lining cell production of osteoclast activating cytokines. Sex steroids have important effects on bone growth during maturation, and oestrogen depletion, which occurs at the time of the menopause, has a high impact on bone remodelling (Kanis, 1990). While the mechanisms for the action of oestrogen are not clear (Frieri *et al.*, 1988), it has been shown that the hormone has regulatory actions on the proliferation of osteoblasts (Ernst *et al.*, 1989), and that it may alter the responsiveness of bone cells to other stimuli such as prostaglandins and mechanical loading (Cheng *et al.*, 1993).

In contrast to these agents that act indirectly to stimulate resorption, calcitonin binds specifically to osteoclasts to inhibit their action (Goltzman and Tannenbaum, 1987). Changes induced as a result of this binding include decrease in motility, retraction of cytoplasmic extensions, and possibly detachment from the bone surface.

MECHANISMS OF BONE RESORPTION

Bone resorption is accomplished by the osteoclasts which must perform two actions – removal of the hydroxyapatite mineral phase of the bone and degradation of the collagenous and non-collagenous proteins. Osteoclasts are highly polarized cells which initiate resorption by binding to the bone surface at the periphery of their zone of contact. This sealing or clear zone contains contractile proteins (Holtrop, 1975) and allows the cell to maintain specific conditions in the resorption space, which would be impossible if a tight seal was absent. Acidification of the resorption space is the result of secretion of hydrogen ions, produced by the action of carbonic anhydrase and transported across the apical 'ruffled border' membrane by a specific proton pump (Baron *et al.*, 1985). This appears to be uniquely expressed in osteoclasts and different from the classical vacuolar and potassium ATPase pumps found in other cells (Chatterjee *et al.*, 1993). A chloride/bicarbonate exchanger in the basal membrane of the cell maintains intracellular pH which would otherwise rise with acidification of the resorption space (Baron, 1989).

Degradation of matrix proteins is accomplished by enzymes such as cathepsins, which are secreted into the resorption space by exocytosis. Small vesicles manufactured in the Golgi apparatus and bound to the mannose 6-phosphate receptor are transported across the cell to the ruffled border membrane, where they fuse with it and release their contents into the resorption space (Baron, 1989).

MECHANISMS FOR CHANGES IN REMODELLING IN RA

Periarticular bone loss in RA was originally thought to be due to locally increased levels of enzymes released either directly from within the damaged joint, or from infiltrating inflammatory cells (Bowen and Fauci, 1993). However, this is not the case; bone changes are the result of alterations in paracrine regulation of remodelling, not direct action of exogenously produced enzymes. The expansion of knowledge of the control of remodelling now suggests that causes for the changes in RA are due primarily to eicosanoid and cytokine mediated influences on events of the bone remodelling cycle. Increased activation or decreased formation during the process, both of which suggest modification of the coupling process, could result in bone loss. However, both formation and resorption are elevated in RA, even during the acute phases of the disease, suggesting that intervention in the control of remodelling may occur at multiple sites in the process. Such a possibility would be consistent with the pleiotropic actions of many paracrine factors. Although knowledge of these local factors is far from complete, it has increased substantially in recent years.

LOCAL MEDIATORS OF REMODELLING

PROSTAGLANDINS

The first local regulators of bone remodelling to be discovered were the prostaglandins, which act as autocrine or paracrine agents (Raisz, 1990). The prostaglandins (PGs) are a large family of unsaturated fatty acids derived from arachidonic acid as a result of the action of cyclo-oxygenase, or prostaglandin G/H synthase (PGHS). Arachidonic acid is in turn produced as a result of action of phospholipase A2 on membrane phospholipids. Related derivatives of arachidonic acid form other members of this eicosanoid family, which includes the thromboxanes and leukotrienes. Because the enzymes which result in PG synthesis are ubiquitous, all tissues are able to synthesize PGs. Although a number of PGs including $PGF_2\alpha$ and PGI_2 have been shown to have effects on bone, PGE_2 appears to have the most potent effects. The actions of PGs on bone remodelling are complex, because they exert biphasic actions, stimulating formative and resorptive processes at different concentrations. Because it is very difficult to measure local levels of active PGs in tissues, such results are hard to interpret. However, the ability of indomethacin to inhibit bone resorption in a number of model systems suggests that the primary action of PGs in bone is to stimulate resorption (Akatsu *et al.*, 1991). The mechanisms for the effects on PGs on bone resorption are not clear. Some workers find stimulation of osteoclast formation (Akatsu *et al.*, 1989), while others have shown an increase in tartrate-resistant acid phosphatase (TRAP) positive mononuclear cells thought to be osteoclast precursors (Collins and Chambers, 1991), but a decrease in multinucleated osteoclast numbers.

The solution to such contradictory results may lie in the synergistic and antagonistic actions PGs share with many cytokines. For example, IL-1 and TNF act synergistically to induce PGE_2 release from osteoblast-like cells (Gowen *et al.*, 1990), although IL-1 and TNF induced osteoblast proliferation is inhibited by PGs (Gowen *et al.*, 1985).

Recently, it has been shown that PG synthesis by PGHS is the result of two separate enzymes, PGHS-1 and 2, which are coded for by different genes (Raisz *et al.*, 1993). In bone cells, PGHS-1 is constitutively expressed, and its mRNA expression is unaffected by osteotropic agents such as IL-1 and PTH. In contrast, PGHS-2 mRNA (and subsequent PGE_2) expression is low in normal bone cells, but is induced at high levels by IL-1 and PTH. There is also evidence that autoamplification of PGHS-2 mRNA occurs by PGE_2, although elevated prostaglandin expression in rheumatoid joints is primarily associated with the role of eicosanoids in the pain and swelling of the inflammatory response. However, since increased PGE_2 production has been connected with periarticular bone loss in RA, specific inhibitors of PGHS-2 offer new therapeutic possibilities. Inhibition of prostanoid and leukotriene synthesis is detailed in Chapter 14, this volume.

CYTOKINES

Bone remodelling is profoundly influenced by the actions of many cytokines (Goldring and Goldring, 1990), including those specifically affected by inflammatory responses. The individual actions of osteotropic cytokines have been studied extensively *in vitro* in highly specified and characterized culture systems but such experiments have led to numerous different and often contradictory results. The reasons for this are complex but they fall into three basic categories (Nathan and Sporn, 1991). Firstly, since few cytokines act alone *in vivo* the actions of individual agents may be modified by the presence of other cytokines which have synergistic or antagonistic effects. Secondly, substances which are not themselves cytokines may modify the actions of individual osteotropic cytokines. These include modifiers of receptor binding such as the soluble TNF receptor (Mohler *et al.*, 1993). In addition, there are pure receptor antagonists like the IL-1 receptor antagonist, which binds to receptors without transducing a signal (Hannum *et al.*, 1990). Finally, extracellular matrix components have the ability to modify the actions of cytokines in a number of ways. Matrix components may bind to cytokines, either to inhibit interactions with their target cells, or to potentiate their actions. This could be by presenting the cytokines to receptors in active conformation, protecting them from degradation, or sequestering them at sites of future action.

Many studies of cytokine actions are also complicated by the source of the cells and tissues used, since samples from patients at varying stages of disease conditions rarely present as homogeneous populations, and therefore can give rise to information which must be interpreted with caution.

Studies of cytokine interactions in relation to bone remodelling *in situ* are problematic in different ways, but have the advantage that the normal diverse range of cell types and other modulators of cytokine actions are present. Recent studies in both human and animal bone (Dodds *et al.*, 1993; Suva *et al.*, 1993; Fermor *et al.*, 1993) reveal that both bone formation and resorption are associated with a tightly controlled sequence of events in which gene expression for specific cytokines and matrix proteins is induced specifically, both spatially and temporally.

It is clear that the inflammatory processes in general and RA in particular influence both bone remodelling in adults (Hayward and Fiedler, 1987; Magaro *et al.*, 1991), and bone growth in juveniles (White *et al.*, 1990). Many of the normal regulatory processes in both endochondral bone formation and remodelling are associated with local expression of cytokines which are elevated by inflammatory processes (Fujita *et al.*, 1990). The following sections will review the major osteotropic cytokines which appear to be affected by inflammatory joint disease. The roles of four specific cytokines known to be altered in RA and to affect bone cell function are discussed to illustrate ways in which the disease has its effects on bone.

OSTEOTROPIC CYTOKINES IN RA

The secretion of many cytokines into synovial fluid is elevated in RA, and these will have both local and systemic effects. Many of these cytokines are those that have already been shown to have actions on bone cells. Their sources, effects on cell activity and ability to modulate bone remodelling are summarized in Table 1. The

Table 1. Cytokines implicated in bone remodelling

Cytokine	Presence in synovial fluid	Producing cell type	Osteoclast formation/ activity	Osteoblast growth/ activity	Resorption *in vivo*	Formation *in vivo*
IL-1s	+++	MC, MP, ET, AC, OB, OC?	+/+	+/−	+	+
TNFs	++	MC, MP, OB, OC	+/+	+/−	+	
IL-2	~	TH1				
IL-4	−	TH2	−/	+/−	−	
IFNγ	−	TH1, MP	−/	−/~	−	
IL-6	++++	MC > MP, AC, FB, ET, OB	+/	−/~		
IL-8	++	MC, MP, AC, FB, ET, OB		−/−		
GM-CSF	++	MC, MP, AC, FB, ET, OB	~/	+/		
TGFβ	+	MC, MP, LP, FB, ET, AC, OB, OC? PL	~/~	+/+	~	+
FGF	+	MP		~/~		
PDGF	+	MP, PL		~/−		

AC, articular chondrocytes; ET, endothelial cells; FB, synovial fibroblasts; LC, lymphocytes; MC, monocytes; MP, macrophages; OB, osteoblasts; OC, osteoclasts; PL, platelets; TH1/2, TH1/2 cells.
−, no expression/inhibition; +, positive expression/stimulation.
~, conflicting reports; space, no data.

actions of many of these agents are to enhance bone resorption, while others may have a more equivocal role. However, for some of the reasons stated in the previous section, the level of individual cytokines in synovial fluid may not be an accurate predictor of remodelling, as inhibitors and binding proteins will modulate their actions in tissues.

In order to illustrate the complexity of the interactions of osteotropic cytokines, four groups have been considered in more detail. It is clear that the circumstances surrounding the actions of all cytokines are at least as complex as this and these examples are only illustrative as a more comprehensive view is beyond the scope of this chapter.

INTERLEUKIN-1 (IL-1)

IL-1 was one of the cytokines first shown to have a positive action in stimulating bone resorption (Gowen et al., 1983). It exists in two forms (α and β), which share only limited sequence homology, but bind to the same membrane receptor (Dower et al., 1985). The mechanism of signal transduction following binding is not known, but follows internalization of the ligand–receptor complex (Shen et al., 1990), and is associated with a rapid (30 s) rise in intracellular calcium (Catherwood et al., 1983).

The effects of IL-1 on bone formation are due to effects on osteoblasts, while effects on remodelling may additionally be due to direct or indirect stimulation of recruitment and activation of osteoclasts. Osteoblast proliferation has been shown to be increased (Rickard et al., 1993) and reduced by IL-1 (Hanazawa et al., 1986). IL-1 stimulates synthesis of DNA and PGE_2, inhibiting alkaline phosphatase activity and collagen synthesis (Ikeda et al., 1988; Hurley et al., 1989). In cultured bone explants, IL-1 stimulates calcium release (Cochran and Abernathy, 1988), and increases in osteoclast number (Garrett and Mundy, 1989).

In vivo, IL-1 enhances bone resorption in both man and animals (Konig et al., 1988; Ahn et al., 1990), and is currently thought to be the cause of much of the pathological bone resorption in inflammatory diseases. In addition to enhancing osteoclast numbers, the mechanism by which bone resorption is enhanced appears to be linked with the ability of IL-1 to up-regulate expression of integrin subunits, which would have consequent effects on osteoclastic attachment and therefore the resorptive potential of those cells (Dedhar, 1989). It is interesting that bones from different regions of the skeleton respond differently to the effects of IL-1 (Cochran and Abernathy, 1988), suggesting that there is location-dependent susceptibility of skeletal cells to osteotropic influences, which could account for regional differences in growth retardation and remodelling.

TUMOUR NECROSIS FACTOR (TNF)

Although there is little structural similarity between the two cytokines, TNF shares many functions with IL-1. Like IL-1, there are two forms, $TNF\alpha$ and β, which share approximately 30% sequence homology. Two receptors exist for TNF, which bind both forms despite marked structural differences in the receptor proteins (Schall et al., 1990; Smith et al., 1990).

Bone remodelling is also profoundly affected by TNF. As with IL-1, these effects have been shown in a number of model systems ranging from cell cultures through explants, and in vivo (Konig et al., 1988). However, the effects appear to be more variable than with IL-1, as different workers have found apparently contradictory results using similar model systems. Different groups have found stimulation of proliferation of cultured bone cells (Gowen et al., 1988), no effect (Nanes et al., 1989; Shapiro et al., 1990), transient stimulation followed by inhibition (Canalis, 1987) or inhibition only (Yoshihara et al., 1990). These differences have been suggested to be due to 'postreceptor factors' (Weinberg and Larrick, 1987), which would appear to mean that other unknown influences modulate the responsiveness of cells to TNF. Such a mechanism appears to be a ubiquitous feature of most cytokines actions.

TNF and IL-1 are stated to have synergistic effects, in which suboptimal doses cause effects which are many times greater than the sum of their individual activities (Stashenko *et al.*, 1987). While such amplification can have benefits in dealing with infections (Cross *et al.*, 1989), it is clear that it also has the potential to influence profoundly bone growth and remodelling.

INTERFERON GAMMA (IFNγ)

Interferons were named because they were first discovered to interfere with viral replication (Isaacs and Lindenmann, 1957). However, as with many cytokines, it has since become clear that the actions of interferon gamma (IFNγ) are more diverse than the early discoveries suggested. Although IFNγ is produced primarily by T cells, natural killer cells and macrophages have also been suggested as sources (Trinchieri *et al.*, 1984).

In culture, IFNγ is a potent inhibitor of bone resorption. In bone explants, it inhibits osteoclast differentiation (Vignery *et al.*, 1990), and reduces the activity of existing cells in a manner similar to calcitonin (Klaushofer *et al.*, 1989). The actions of IFNγ are highly specific. It has been shown to inhibit resorption stimulated by IL-1 and TNF. The actions on resorption stimulated by PTH or 1,25D are more variable – different groups finding no effect (Gowen *et al.*, 1986) or inhibition (Fujii *et al.*, 1990; Nanes *et al.*, 1990). The mechanism of action of IFNγ is not clear, as it has been shown that it is not associated with changes in receptors for IL-1 (Shen *et al.*, 1990). It is likely that it involves the inhibition of synthesis and release of the metalloproteinases necessary for matrix degradation (Shen *et al.*, 1988). In addition, IFNγ inhibits DNA synthesis in cell cultures, an effect which is enhanced by co-incubation with TNF (Gowen *et al.*, 1988).

The action of interferon *in vivo* is in contrast with its clear ability to inhibit bone resorption *in vitro*. Although there are limited numbers of experiments to support this, Epstein's group showed a lack of effect of IFNγ on most markers of cyclosporin-induced bone loss in rats (Jacobs *et al.*, 1992). In addition, some parameters measured showed an increase in resorption. Vignery showed an increase in numbers of osteo-clasts in mice following IFNγ treatment (Vignery *et al.*, 1990), which is the opposite of the effect *in vitro* (Takahashi *et al.*, 1986).

IL-8 AND THE CHEMOKINES

Interleukin 8 (IL-8) is the best characterized member of a new class of small molecular weight (<10 000) chemotactic cytokines (Baggiolini and Sorg, 1993). Many members of this group of tissue-derived inflammatory mediators have been identified since the discovery of IL-8. The group is characterized structurally by four conserved cysteines that form two essential intrachain bonds. A structural feature has been used to define two subclasses of this group. In IL-8 and related neutrophil-activating peptides, the first two cysteines are separated by an amino acid (CXC); in monocyte chemoattract-ant protein-1 (MCP-1) and related peptides which act primarily on monocytes the two

Table 2. Members of the chemokine families

	α Subfamily	β Subfamily
Structure	C-X-C	C-C
Chemokine	IL-8/NAP-1	MCAF/MCP-1
	groα/MGSA	LD-78
	NAP-2	PAT464
	MIP-2α(groβ)	GOS19-1
	MIP-2β(groγ)	ACT-2
	PF-4	PAT744/G26
	IP-10	RANTES
		I-309
Cells acted on	Neutrophils	Monocytes
	T cells	T cells
	Keratinocytes	Macrophages
	Endothelial cells	

cysteines are adjacent (CC). Some members of the chemokine family are indicated in Table 2.

The predominant actions of this family of peptides together lead to neutrophil and monocyte infiltration into the site of production of the factors. Thus, tissue cells and peripheral blood monocytes produce chemokines when exposed to the appropriate pro-inflammatory stimulus. This stimulus can be either cytokines, such as IL-1 and TNF, bacterial products (LPS) or tumour promoters (PMA). Cells that have been reported to produce chemokines include endothelial cells, keratinocytes, melanocytes and fibroblasts.

There have been a number of reports of the production of chemokines by cells in joint tissues, particularly cartilage and bone. Monocyte chemoattractant MCP-1 is produced by human articular chondrocytes (Villiger et al., 1992) and primary human osteoblasts (Williams et al., 1992) in vitro when stimulated with IL-1. The authors suggest a role for these cells in the initiation and progression of arthritis. An MCP-1 like mouse chemokine, JE, can be produced by mouse osteoblast-like cells (MC3T3E1) in response to IL-1β, TGFβ and TNFα (Takeshita et al., 1993). Since osteoclast precursors are of the monocyte lineage it is possible that production of these factors at bony sites could lead to the recruitment and/or activation of osteoclast precursors. Indeed, LD-78 has been demonstrated to promote osteoclast-like cell differentiation in rat bone marrow cultures (Kukita et al., 1992).

The neutrophil is the predominant infiltrating cell in the rheumatoid joint and neutrophil chemoattractant and activating factors have also been shown to be produced by joint cells. Several groups have described the production of IL-8 by IL-1β-stimulated articular chondrocytes in culture (Van Damme et al., 1989; Lotz et al., 1992; Recklies and Golds, 1992) or cartilage explants (Recklies and Golds, 1992), suggesting a role in neutrophil-mediated inflammation. Similar results have been reported for primary cultures of human osteoblasts (Chaudhary et al., 1992). In an interesting study Elford and Cooper demonstrated that IL-8 stimulated neutrophil-mediated cartilage degradation by inducing neutrophil degranulation (Elford and Cooper, 1991).

These findings suggest that joint connective tissue cells such as osteoblasts and chondrocytes may act as effector cells in the induction and/or maintenance of the inflammatory response, rather than responder or bystander cells. The therapeutic potential of modulating cytokine bioactivity is reviewed in Chapter 13, this volume.

CONCLUSIONS

In this review we have attempted to summarize the control of bone remodelling in order to show areas which overlap with known changes that occur in RA. As more detailed knowledge is acquired about the specific actions of individual osteotropic agents, our ability to fit that information into a global view becomes more difficult. However, such knowledge does offer the potential for new and specific treatments of individual components of disease. Inhibition of the osteoclast proton pump, PGHS-2 synthase and cytokine synthesis are examples of logical targets for therapeutic intervention in pathological bone loss. The explosion of information generated by the now widespread use of molecular biology techniques in skeletal tissue research shows no signs of abatement. Within a short time, it is likely that the results of such work will become available to the clinician, and the effects on current perceptions of severe diseases are likely to be enormous.

REFERENCES

Adami S, Bhalla AK, Dorizzi R, Montesanti F, Rosini S, Salvagno G et al. (1987) The acute-phase response after bisphosphonate administration. *Calcif Tiss Int* **41**: 326–331.

Ahn JM, Huang CC & Abramson M (1990) Interleukin 1 causing bone destruction in middle ear cholesteatoma. *Otolaryngol Head Neck Surg* **103**: 527–536.

Akatsu T, Takahashi N, Udagawa N, Sato K, Nagata N, Moseley JM et al. (1989) Parathyroid hormone (PTH)-related protein is a potent stimulator of osteoclast-like multinucleated cell formation to the same extent as PTH in mouse marrow cultures. *Endocrinology* **125**: 20–27.

Akatsu T, Takahashi N, Udagawa N, Imamura K, Yamaguchi A, Sato K et al. (1991) Role of prostaglandins in interleukin-1-induced bone resorption in mice *in vitro*. *J Bone Miner Res* **6**: 183–190.

Ali NN, Melhuish PB, Boyde A, Bennett A & Jones SJ (1990) Parathyroid hormone, but not prostaglandin E2, changes the shape of osteoblasts maintained on bone *in vitro*. *J Bone Miner Res* **5**: 115–121.

Allard SA, Bayliss MT & Maini RN (1990) The synovium–cartilage junction of the normal human knee, implications for joint destruction and repair. *Arthritis Rheum* **33**: 1170–1179.

Baggiolini M & Sorg C (1993) *Interleukin-8 (NAP-1) and Related Cytokines*. Basel: Karger.

Baron R (1989) Polarity and membrane transport in osteoclasts. *Conn Tiss Res* **20**: 109–120.

Baron R, Vignery A & Horowitz M (1983) Lymphocytes, macrophages and the regulation of bone remodelling. In Peck WA (ed) *Bone and Mineral Research*, pp 175–243. Amsterdam: Elsevier.

Baron R, Neff L, Louvard D & Courtoy PJ (1985) Cell-mediated extracellular acidification and bone resorption: evidence for a low pH in resorbing lacunae and localization of a 100-kD lysosomal membrane protein at the osteoclast ruffled border. *J Cell Biol* **101**: 2210–2222.

Baron R, Neff L, Tran VP, Nefussi JR & Vignery A (1986) Kinetic and cytochemical identification of osteoclast precursors and their differentiation into multinucleated osteoclasts. *Am J Pathol* **122**: 363–378.

Baron R, Neff L, Brown W, Courtoy PJ, Louvard D & Farquhar MG (1988) Polarized secretion of lysosomal enzymes: co-distribution of cation-independent mannose-6-phosphate receptors and lysosomal enzymes along the osteoclast exocytic pathway. *J Cell Biol* **106**: 1863–1872.

Boivin G, Mesguich P, Pike JW, Bouillon R, Meunier PJ, Haussler MR, Dubois PM & Morel G (1987) Ultrastructural immunocytochemical localization of endogenous 1,25-dihydroxyvitamin D3 and its receptors in osteoblasts and osteocytes from neonatal mouse and rat calvaria. *Bone and Mineral* **3**: 125–136.

Boosalis MG, Gray D, Walker S, Sutliff S, Talwalker R & Mazumder A (1992) The acute phase response in autologous bone marrow transplantation. *J Med* **23**: 175–194.

Bowen BL & Fauci AS (1993) *Inflammation – Basic Principles and Clinical Correlates*, pp 877–895. New York: Raven Press.

Cabral AR, Loya BL & AlarconSegovia D (1989) Bone remodeling and osteophyte formation after remission of rheumatoid arthritis. *J Rheumatol* **16**: 1421–1427.

Canalis E (1987) Effects of tumour necrosis factor on bone formation *in vitro*. *Endocrinology* **121**: 1596–1604.

Catherwood BD, Onishi T & Deftos LJ (1983) Effect of estrogens and phosphorus depletion on plasma calcitonin in the rat. *Calcif Tiss Int* **35**: 502–507.

Chatterjee D, Neff L, Chakraborty M, Fabricant C & Baron R (1993) Sensitivity to nitrate and other oxyanions further distinguishes the vanadate-sensitive osteoclast proton pump from other vacuolar H^+-ATPases. *Biochemistry (USA)* **32**: 2808–2812.

Chaudhary LR, Spelsberg TC & Riggs BL (1992) Production of various cytokines by normal human osteoblast-like cells in response to interleukin-1beta and tumor necrosis factor-alpha: lack of regulation by 17beta-estradiol. *Endocrinology* **130**: 2528–2534.

Cheng MZ, Zaman G & Lanyon LE (1993) Estrogen enhances the osteogenic effects of mechanical loading and exogenous prostacyclin, but not prostaglandin-E2. *J Bone Miner Res* **8**: 151.

Cochran DL & Abernathy CK (1988) Modulation of bone resorption by glycosaminoglycans: effects of parathyroid hormone and interleukin-1. *Bone* **9**: 331–335.

Collins DA and Chambers TJ (1991) Effect of prostaglandins E1, E2, and F2alpha on osteoclast formation in mouse bone marrow cultures. *J Bone Miner Res* **6**: 157–164.

Cross AS, Sadoff JC, Kelly N, Bernton E & Gemski P (1989) Pretreatment with recombinant murine tumor necrosis factor alpha/cachectin and murine interleukin 1 alpha protects mice from lethal bacterial infection. *J Exp Med* **169**: 2021–2027.

Curtis TA, Ashrafi SH & Weber DF (1985) Canalicular communications in the cortices of human long bones. *Anat Rec* **212**: 336–344.

Dedhar A (1989) Regulation of expression of the cell adhesion receptors, integrins, by recombinant human interleukin-1 beta in human osteosarcoma cells: inhibition of cell proliferation and stimulation of alkaline phosphatase activity. *J Cell Physiol* **138**: 291–299.

Dodds RA, Merry KH, Littlewood AJ & Gowen M (1994) The expression of mRNA for IL-1β, IL-6, and TGFβ1 in developing human bone and cartilage. *J Histochem Cytochem* **42**: 599–606.

Doty SB (1981) Morphological evidence of gap junctions between bone cells. *Calcif Tiss Int* **33**: 509–512.

Dower SK, Kronheim SR, March CJ, Conlon PJ, Hopp TP, Gillis S & Urdal DL (1985) Detection and characterization of high affinity plasma membrane receptors for human interleukin 1. *J Exp Med* **162**: 501–515.

Eggelmeijer F, Camps JAJ, Valkema R, Papapoulos SE, Pauwels EKJ, Dijkmans BAC & Breedveld FC (1993a) Bone mineral density in ambulant, non-steroid treated female patients with rheumatoid arthritis. *Clin Exp Rheumatol* **11**: 381–385.

Eggelmeijer F, Papapoulos SE, Westedt ML, Van P, Dijkmans BAC & Breedveld FC (1993b) Bone metabolism in rheumatoid arthritis: relation to disease activity. *Br J Rheumatol* **32**: 387–391.

Elford PR & Cooper PH (1991) Induction of neutrophil-mediated cartilage degradation by interleukin-8. *Arthritis Rheum* **34**: 325–332.

Ernst M & Froesch ER (1987) Triiodothyronine stimulates proliferation of osteoblast-like cells in serum-free culture. *FEBS Letters* **220**: 163–166.

Ernst M, Heath JK & Rodan GA (1989) Estradiol effects on proliferation, messenger ribonucleic acid for collagen and insulin-like growth factor-I, and parathyroid hormone-stimulated adenylate cyclase activity in osteoblastic cells from calvariae and long bones. *Endocrinology* **125**: 825–833.

Fermor B, Mason DJ, Gowen M & Skerry TM (1994) Differences in gene expression in growing bone. *Bone*, in press.

Frieri M, Snyder B, Edwards WT, Hayes WC, Gilsanz V, Roe T et al. (1988) Local and systemic factors in the pathogenesis of osteoporosis. *N Eng J Med* **319**: 793–795.

Fujii Y, Sato K, Kasono K, Satoh T, Fujii T & Shizume K (1990) Prolonged and ubiquitous inhibition by interferon gamma of bone resorption induced by parathyroid hormone-related protein, 1,25-dihydroxy-vitamin D3, and interleukin 1 in fetal mouse forearm bones. *Calcif Tiss Int* **47**: 178–182.

Fujita T, Matsui T, Nakao Y, Shiozawa S & Imai Y (1990) Cytokines and osteoporosis. *Ann NY Acad Sci* **587**: 371–375.

Garrett IR & Mundy GR (1989) Relationship between interleukin-1 and prostaglandins in resorbing neonatal calvaria. *J Bone Miner Res* **4**: 789–794.

Goldring MB & Goldring SR (1990) Skeletal tissue response to cytokines. *Clin Orthop Rel Res* **285**: 245–278.

Goltzman D & Tannenbaum GS (1987) Induction of hypocalcemia by intracerebroventricular injection of calcitonin: evidence for control of blood calcium by the nervous system. *Brain Research* **416**: 1–6.

Gough A, Lilley J, Eyre S & Emery P (1993) Rapid bone loss in early rheumatoid arthritis, due to disease activity. *Proceedings Fourth International Conference on Osteoporosis*, 175–176.

Gowen M, Wood DD, Ihrie EJ, McGuire MKB & Russell RGG (1983) An interleukin 1-like factor stimulates bone resorption *in vitro*. *Nature* **306**: 378–380.

Gowen M, Wood DD & Russell RG (1985) Stimulation of the proliferation of human bone cells *in vitro* by human monocyte products with interleukin-1 activity. *J Clin Invest* **75**: 1223–1229.

Gowen M, Nedwin GE & Mundy GR (1986) Preferential inhibition of cytokine-stimulated bone resorption by recombinant interferon gamma. *J Bone Miner Res* **1**: 469–474.

Gowen M, MacDonald BR & Russell RG (1988) Actions of recombinant human gamma-interferon and tumor necrosis factor alpha on the proliferation and osteoblastic characteristics of human trabecular bone cells *in vitro*. *Arthritis Rheum* 31: 1500–1507.

Gowen M, Chapman K, Littlewood AJ, Hughes D, Evans DB & Russell G (1990) Production of tumor necrosis factor by human osteoblasts is modulated by other cytokines, but not by osteotropic hormones. *Endocrinology* 126: 1250–1255.

Grunfeld C & Feingold KR (1992) Tumor necrosis factor, interleukin, and interferon induced changes in lipid metabolism as part of host defense. *Proc Soc Exp Biol Med* 200: 224–227.

Hanazawa S, Ohmori Y, Amano S, Hirose K, Miyoshi T, Kumegawa M & Kitano S (1986) Human purified interleukin-1 inhibits DNA synthesis and cell growth of osteoblastic cell line (MC3T3-E1), but enhances alkaline phosphatase activity in the cells. *FEBS Letts* 203: 279–284.

Hannum CH et al. (1990) Interleukin-1 receptor antagonist activity of a human interleukin-1 inhibitor. *Nature* 343: 336–340.

Hayward M & Fiedler NC (1987) Mechanisms of bone loss: rheumatoid arthritis, periodontal disease and osteoporosis. *Agents Actions* 22: 251–254.

Hirokawa M, Takatsu H, Niitsu H, Nishinari T, Nimura T, Itoh T et al (1989) Serum tumor necrosis factor-alpha levels in allogeneic bone marrow transplant recipients with acute leukemia. *Tohoku J Exp Med* 159: 237–244.

Hock JM & Gera I (1992) Effects of continuous and intermittent administration and inhibition of resorption on the anabolic response of bone to parathyroid hormone. *J Bone Miner Res* 7: 65–72.

Hodsman AB & Fraher LJ (1990) Biochemical responses to sequential human parathyroid hormone (1–38) and calcitonin in osteoporotic patients. *Bone and Mineral* 9: 137–152.

Holtrop ME (1975) The ultrastructure of bone. *Ann Clin Lab Sci* 5: 264–271.

Hurley MM, Fall P, Harrison JR, Petersen DN, Kream BE & Raisz LG (1989) Effects of transforming growth factor alpha and interleukin-1 on DNA synthesis, collagen synthesis, procollagen mRNA levels, and prostaglandin E2 production in cultured fetal rat calvaria. *J Bone Miner Res* 4: 731–736.

Ikeda E, Kusaka M, Hakeda Y, Yokota K, Kumegawa M & Yamamoto S (1988) Effect of interleukin 1 beta on osteoblastic clone MC3T3-E1 cells. *Calcif Tiss Int* 43: 162–166.

Isaacs A & Lindenmann J (1957) Virus interference I: the interferon. *Proc Royal Soc Lond* 147: 258–250.

Jacobs TW, Joffe II, Katz IA, Stein B, Li MK, Ke HZ et al. (1992) Interferon gamma fails to prevent cyclosporine A induced osteopenia in the rat. *Bone and Mineral* 17S: 202.

Jilka RL (1986) Parathyroid hormone-stimulated development of osteoclasts in cultures of cells from neonatal murine calvaria. *Bone* 7: 29–40.

Joffe I & Epstein S (1991) Osteoporosis associated with rheumatoid arthritis: pathogenesis and management. *Semin Arthritis Rheum* 20: 256–272.

Kanis JA (1990) Osteoporosis and osteopenia. *J Bone Miner Res* 5: 209–211.

Klaushofer K, Horandner H, Hoffmann O, Czerwenka E, Konig U, Koller K & Peterlik M (1989) Interferon gamma and calcitonin induce differential changes in cellular kinetics and morphology of osteoclasts in cultured neonatal mouse calvaria. *J Bone Miner Res* 4: 585–606.

Komm BS, Terpening CM, Benz DJ, Graeme KA, Gallegos A, Korc M et al (1988) Estrogen binding, receptor mRNA, and biologic response in osteoblast-like osteosarcoma cells. *Science* 241: 81–84.

Konig A, Muhlbauer RC & Fleisch H (1988) Tumor necrosis factor alpha and interleukin-1 stimulate bone resorption *in vivo* as measured by urinary [3H]tetracycline excretion from prelabeled mice. *J Bone Miner Res* 3: 621–627.

Kukita T, Nakao J, Hamada F, Kukita A, Inai T, Kurisu K & Nomiyama H (1992) Recombinant LD78 protein, a member of the small cytokine family, enhances osteoclast differentiation in rat bone marrow culture system. *Bone and Mineral* 19: 215–223.

Lanyon LE, Rubin CT & Baust G (1986) Modulation of bone loss during calcium insufficiency by controlled dynamic loading. *Calcif Tiss Int* 38: 209–216.

Lewis GP (1986) *Mediators of Inflammation*, pp 36–43. Bristol: Wright.

Lotz M, Terkeltaub R & Villiger PM (1992) Cartilage and joint inflammation: regulation of IL-8 expression by human articular chondrocytes. *J Immunol* 148: 466–473.

Louw JA, Werbeck A, Louw MEJ, Kotze TJVW, Cooper R & Labadarios D (1992) Blood vitamin concentrations during the acute-phase response. *Critical Care Medicine* 20: 934–941.

Magaro M, Tricerri A, Piane D, Zoli A, Serra F, Altomonte L & Mirone L (1991) Generalized osteoporosis in non-steroid treated rheumatoid arthritis. *Rheumatol Int* 11: 73–76.

Mazlam MZ & Hodgson HJF (1992) Peripheral blood monocyte cytokine production and acute phase response in inflammatory bowel disease. *Gut* 33: 773–778.

Menton DN, Simmons DJ, Chang S & Orr BY (1984) From bone lining cell to osteocyte an SEM study. *Anat Rec* 209: 29–39.

Miller SC, Bowman BM & Jee WS (1989) Bone lining cells: structure and function. *Scanning Microsc* 3: 953–960.

Mitchell J & Goltzman D (1990) Mechanisms of homologous and heterologous regulation of parathyroid hormone receptors in the rat osteosarcoma cell line UMR-106. *Endocrinology* **126**: 2650–2660.

Mohler KM, Torrance DS, Smith CA, Goodwin RG, Stremler KE, Fung VP et al (1993) Soluble tumor necrosis factor (TNF) receptors are effective therapeutic agents in lethal endotoxemia and function simultaneously as both TNF carriers and TNF antagonists. *J Immunol* **151**: 1548–1561.

Nanes MS, McKoy WM & Marx SJ (1989) Inhibitory effects of tumor necrosis factor-alpha and interferon-gamma on deoxyribonucleic acid and collagen synthesis by rat osteosarcoma cells (ROS 17/2.8). *Endocrinology* **124**: 339–345.

Nanes MS, Rubin J, Titus L, Hendy GN & Catherwood BD (1990) Interferon-gamma inhibits 1,25-dihydroxyvitamin D3-stimulated synthesis of bone GLA protein in rat osteosarcoma cells by a pretranslational mechanism. *Endrocrinology* **127**: 588–594.

Nathan CF & Sporn MB (1991) Cytokines in context. *J Cell Biol* **113**: 981–986.

Orcel P, Bielakoff J & de VM (1990) Formation of multinucleated cells with osteoclast precursor features in human cord monocytes cultures. *Anat Rec* **226**: 1–9.

Pead MJ, Skerry TM & Lanyon LE (1988) Direct transformation from quiescence to bone formation in the adult periosteum following a single brief period of bone loading. *J Bone Miner Res* **3**: 647–656.

Pfeilschifter JP, Seyechin S & Mundy GR (1988) Transforming growth factor beta inhibits bone resorption in fetal rat long bones. *J Clin Invest* **82**: 680–685.

Raisz LG (1990) The role of prostaglandins in the local regulation of bone remodelling. *Prog Clin Biol Res* **332**: 195–203.

Raisz LG, Vosnesensky OS, Alander CB, Kawaguchi H & Pilbeam CC (1993) Auto-amplification of inducible prostaglandin G/H synthase in osteoblastic MC3T3-E1 and PY1A cells. *J Bone Miner Res* **8**: S161.

Recklies AD & Golds EE (1992) Induction of synthesis and release of interleukin-8 from human articular chondrocytes and cartilage explants. *Arthritis Rheum* **35**: 1510–1519.

Rickard DJ, Gowen M & MacDonald BR (1993) Proliferative responses to estradiol, IL-1alpha and TGFβ by cells expressing alkaline phosphatase in human osteoblast-like cell cultures. *Calcif Tiss Int* **52**: 227–233.

Rouleau MF, Warshawsky H & Goltzman D (1986) Parathyroid hormone binding *in vivo* to renal, hepatic, and skeletal tissues of the rat using a radioautographic approach. *Endocrinology* **118**: 919–931.

Sambrook PN, Shawe D, Hesp R, Zanelli JM, Mitchell R, Katz D et al (1990) Rapid periarticular bone loss in rheumatoid arthritis. Possible promotion by normal circulating concentrations of parathyroid hormone or calcitriol (1,25 dihydroxyvitamin D3). *Arthritis Rheum* **33**: 615–622.

Schall TJ, Lewis M, Koller KJ, Lee A, Rice GC, Wong GHW et al. (1990) Molecular cloning and expression of a receptor for human tumor necrosis factor. *Cell* **61**: 361–370.

Shapiro S, Tatakis DN & Dziak R (1990) Effects of tumor necrosis factor alpha on parathyroid hormone-induced increases in osteoblastic cell cyclic AMP. *Calcif Tiss Int* **46**: 60–62.

Shen V, Kohler G, Jeffrey JJ & Peck WA (1988) Bone-resorbing agents promote and interferon-gamma inhibits bone cell collagenase production. *J Bone Miner Res* **3**: 657–666.

Shen V, Cheng SL, Kohler NG & Peck WA (1990) Characterization and hormonal modulation of IL-1 binding in neonatal mouse osteoblastlike cells. *J Bone Miner Res* **5**: 507–515.

Skerry TM, Bitensky L, Chayen J & Lanyon LE (1989) Early strain-related changes in enzyme activity in osteocytes following bone loading *in vivo*. *J Bone Miner Res* **4**: 783–788.

Smith CA, Davis T, Anderson DC, Solam L, Beckmann MP, Jerzy R et al (1990) A receptor for tumor necrosis factor defines an unusual family of cellular and viral proteins. *Science* **248**: 1019–1025.

Stashenko P, Dewhirst FE, Peros WJ, Kent RL & Ago JM (1987) Synergistic interactions between interleukin 1, tumor necrosis factor, and lymphotoxin in bone resorption. *J Immunol* **138**: 1464–1468.

Suva LJ, Seedor JG, Endo N, Quartuccio HA, Thompson DD, Bab I et al. (1993) Pattern of gene expression during bone formation following rat tibial marrow ablation. *J Bone Miner Res* **83**: 379–388.

Takahashi N, Mundy GR & Roodman GD (1986) Recombinant human interferon-gamma inhibits formation of human osteoclast-like cells. *J Immunol* **137**: 3544–3549.

Takeshita A, Hanazawa S, Amano S, Matumoto T & Kitano S (1993) IL-1 induces expression of monocyte chemoattractant JE in clonal mouse osteoblastic cell line MC3T3-E1. *J Immunol* **150**: 1554–1562.

Teti A, Grano M, Carano A, Colucci S & Zambonin-Zallone A (1989) Immunolocalization of beta 3 subunit of integrins in osteoclast membrane. *Boll Soc Ital Biol Sper* **65**: 1031–1037.

Trinchieri G, Matsumoto-Kobayashi M, Clark SV, London L & Perussia B (1984) Response of human peripheral blood natural killer cells to interleukin-2. *J Exp Med* **160**: 1140–1147.

Van Damme J, Schaafsma MR, Conings R, Lenaerts JP, Put W, Billiau A et al. (1989) Interleukin 1 induces different cytokines in human fibroblasts. Lymphokine Research **8**: 289–292.

Vignery A, Niven FT & Shepard MH (1990) Recombinant murine interferon-gamma inhibits the fusion of mouse alveolar macrophages *in vitro* but stimulates the formation of osteoclastlike cells on implanted syngeneic bone particles in mice *in vivo*. *J Bone Miner Res* **5**: 637–644.

Villiger PM, Terkeltaub R & Lotz M (1992) Monocyte chemoattractant protein-1 (MCP-1) expression in human articular cartilage induction by peptide regulatory factors and differential effects of dexamethasone and retinoic acid. *J Clin Invest* **90**: 488–496.

Wegenka UM, Buschmann J, Lutticken C, Heinrich PC & Horn F (1993) Acute-phase response factor, a nuclear factor binding to acute-phase response elements, is rapidly activated by interleukin-6 at the posttranslational level. *Mol Cell Biology* **13**: 276–288.

Weinberg JB & Larrick JW (1987) Receptor-mediated monocytoid differentiation of human promyelocytic cells by tumor necrosis factor: synergistic actions with interferon-gamma and 1,25-dihydroxyvitamin D3. *Blood* **70**: 994–1002.

White PH, Vreugdenhil G, Lowenberg B, Van E & Swaak AJG (1990) Growth abnormalities in children with juvenile rheumatoid arthritis. Anaemia of chronic disease in rheumatoid arthritis: raised serum interleukin-6 (IL-6) levels and effects of IL-6 and anti-IL-6 on *in vitro* erythropoiesis. *Clin Orthop Rel Res* **10**: 127–130.

Williams SR, Jiang Y, Cochran D, Dorsam G & Graves DT (1992) Regulated expression of monocyte chemoattractant protein-1 in normal human osteoblastic cells. *Am J Physiol–Cell Physiol* **263**: C194–C199.

Yoshihara R, Shiozawa S, Imai Y & Fujita T (1990) Tumor necrosis factor alpha and interferon gamma inhibit proliferation and alkaline phosphatase activity of human osteoblastic SaOS-2 cell line. *Lymphokine Res* **9**: 59–66.

Zambonin-Zallone A, Teti A, Grano M, Rubinacci A, Abbadini M, Gaboli M et al (1989) Immunocytochemical distribution of extracellular matrix receptors in human osteoclasts: a beta 3 integrin is colocalized with vinculin and talin in the podosomes of osteoclastoma giant cells. *Exp Cell Res* **182**: 645–652.

11 Leukocyte Adhesion and Leukocyte Traffic in Rheumatoid Arthritis

Nancy Oppenheimer-Marks and Peter E. Lipsky

INTRODUCTION

Cell adhesion plays an integral role in the development and progression of a variety of chronic inflammatory diseases. Such adhesive events involve cellular interactions between infiltrating and resident tissue cells or between both cell types and components of extracellular matrices (ECM). Cellular adhesive events mediate the extravasation of inflammatory cells from the blood stream, the maintenance of vascular integrity, the localization of cells within the tissue and the propagation of local inflammatory and immune responses. Each adhesive event involves the utilization of specific cell surface receptors that mediate the cell–cell or cell–ECM interactions. Expression and activity of these receptor–counterreceptor pairs are tightly regulated, providing a dynamic system that controls the various events at inflammatory sites.

Chronic inflammatory diseases, such as rheumatoid arthritis (RA), are characterized by persistent immunologic activity within the affected tissue (reviewed in Chapters 2–4, this volume). Although the etiologic stimulus that initiates the extravasation of cells into rheumatoid synovial tissue remains unclear, it appears that the continuous influx of inflammatory cells into the synovium and their activity within the tissue play a role in the persistent expression of cell adhesive mechanisms that sustain the chronic inflammation. This may result from the local secretion of mediators that increase the expression of adhesion receptors by vascular endothelium, through which inflammatory cells migrate to enter the synovial tissue. Additionally, inflammatory mediators may stimulate the selected chemotaxis of specific cell populations into the tissue and act directly on the migrated cells to stimulate their trafficking within the tissue. Finally, adhesive mechanisms maintain infiltrated cells in specific microenvironments, and mediate their activation within these extravascular sites as well. Developing a more complete understanding of the identity and roles of specific adhesion receptor–counterreceptor pairs during the pathogenesis of chronic inflammation should provide clues concerning a means to control chronic synovial inflammation more effectively.

HISTOLOGICAL FEATURES OF RHEUMATOID SYNOVIUM

The rheumatoid synovium is a multicompartment tissue with differences in the nature of cells that accumulate in the various locations. This implies that unique adhesive mechanisms are operative within the same inflammatory site to account for this non-uniform cellular distribution. The synovial membrane lines all intracapsular structures

Mechanisms and Models in Rheumatoid Arthritis
ISBN 0–12–340440–1

except for the articular cartilage surfaces. It normally consists of a relatively uniform layer of Type A and Type B lining cells, which progressively hypertrophies during the course of RA. Thus, the lining cells increase in number resulting in a thickened appearance upon histological examination (see Chapter 8, this volume). Normally, the collagen matrix that supports the lining layer contains only small numbers of dendritic-like cells, mast cells and sparse leukocytes. During synovitis, however, the matrix becomes profoundly infiltrated with inflammatory cells, which apparently extravasate into the tissue through the numerous blood vessels that appear throughout the tissue. All normal synovial joint spaces contain a small amount of fluid which covers the surfaces of the synovium and cartilage. During disease, the volume of fluid increases and in addition to the normal nutrients and metabolic waste products present, the fluid becomes enriched with inflammatory cells and products released during the immune reactions occurring within the tissue. Thus, the rheumatoid synovial tissue and fluid compartments are sites of intense cellular trafficking and activity.

The rheumatoid synovial membrane is richly infiltrated with mononuclear cells, the most abundant being the T lymphocyte. However, also quite evident are B lymphocytes, plasma cells, dendritic cells and cells of the monocyte/macrophage lineage. Several studies have indentified the phenotype of the T cells that accumulate in rheumatoid synovial tissue. Thus, *in situ* studies have demonstrated the appearance of CD4$^+$ and CD8$^+$ T cells in lymphocyte aggregates, although their pattern of organization appears to be related to the progressive nature of the disease (Kurosaka and Ziff, 1983; Yanni *et al.*, 1993). Analysis of T cells isolated directly from synovial tissue reveals a greater total number of CD4$^+$ than CD8$^+$ T cells (Cush and Lipsky, 1988). These synovial tissue T cells appear to be activated since the density of CD4 and CD3 is reduced, in comparison to RA peripheral blood T cells, and they express CD69, HLA-DR, very late antigen (VLA)-1 (CD49a/CD29) and decreased amounts of L-selectin (Table 1) (Klareskog *et al.*, 1981; Forre *et al.*, 1982a; Poulter *et al.*, 1985;

Table 1. Phenotype of synovial tissue lymphocytes

Differentiation markers	Activation markers	Adhesion receptors
CD4$^+$	CD69$^+$	LFA-1^{bright}
CD45RO$^+$	HLA-DR$^+$	CD44^{bright}
CD45RA$^-$	VLA-1$^+$	LFA-3^{bright}
CD45RB^{dim}	CD4^{dim}	ICAM-1$^+$
CD7^{dim}	CD3^{dim}	VLA-4$^+$
CD29^{bright}		VLA-5$^+$
		α4/β7$^+$
		L-selectin$^-$

Hemler *et al.*, 1986; Burmester *et al.*, 1987; Goto *et al.*, 1987; Cush and Lipsky, 1988). Nearly all of the synovial tissue CD4$^+$ T cells are of the memory subset since they are CD29^{bright}, CD7^{dim}, CD45RO$^+$ and CD45RA^{dim} (Pitzalis *et al.*, 1987; Cush and Lipsky, 1988; Nakao *et al.*, 1989). By contrast, rheumatoid synovium is nearly devoid of naive CD4$^+$/CD45RA^{bright} T cells. Whether the T cells that accumulate in the synovium relate to a selective migration of a particular population of activated T cells into the tissue or the local activation of a subset of resting memory T cells with an enhanced migratory capacity is a matter of intense investigation.

Rheumatoid synovial fluids also contain large numbers of leukocytes, including lymphocytes and neutrophils. The remaining cells in joint fluid include monocytes, occasional macrophages, dendritic cells and synovial lining cells (Zvaifler, 1973; see also Freemont, Chapter 5, this volume). The appearance of these cell populations in the fluid is indicative of their trafficking through the tissue to accumulate within this compartment. Unlike synovial tissue, there is a greater number of $CD8^+$ and fewer $CD4^+$ T cells in synovial fluid (Fox et al., 1982; Reme et al., 1990; Smith and Roberts Thomson, 1990). The reasons for the differences in the distribution of these cells are not known. It is presumed that cells enter the synovium by migrating through post-capillary venules to the synovial tissue and then enter the synovial fluid from which they exit the joint via lymphatics. However, the exact pathway of tissue trafficking in the synovium has not been resolved. It is possible that the abundance of $CD8^+$ T cells and neutrophils in the synovial fluid relates to their greater intrinsic motility permit-ting their more rapid movement out of the tissue. Alternatively, there may be mech-anisms that specifically retain $CD4^+$ T cells in the tissue or direct or retain $CD8^+$ T cells and neutrophils in the fluid. The trafficking of neutrophils through the tissue may play a critical role in the perpetuation of chronic inflammation, perhaps by the elabor-ation of mediators that affect the subsequent infiltration into tissue of specific T cell subsets. For example, in a rat model, in which neutrophils were selectively depleted by specific anti-neutrophil mAb, $CD4^+$ T cells were inhibited from infiltrating into tissue sites into which the chemotactic factor IL-8 was introduced (Kudo et al., 1991). Infiltration of $CD8^+$ T cells was not similarly inhibited, suggesting that neutrophils elaborate a factor(s) that specifically recruits $CD4^+$ T cells into tissue.

THE VASCULATURE IN RHEUMATOID SYNOVIUM

In the early acute phase of RA, damaged vasculature may provide an important route for the infiltration of inflammatory cells into the affected tissue. However, as the inflammation becomes chronic, the extravasation of cells into the tissue appears to result from receptor-mediated events between specific cell surface adhesion molecules on the migrating cells and their counterreceptors on endothelial cells (EC). Thus, synovial tissue EC express cell surface adhesion receptors that bind leukocytes. More-over, the EC of rheumatoid synovium express increased adhesiveness for peripheral blood mononuclear cells (Oppenheimer-Marks and Ziff, 1986; Jalkanen et al., 1986). During the course of RA, changes occur in many of the EC of postcapillary venules, presumably in response to cytokines and other factors in their environment, which tend to alter their phenotypic and functional characteristics, enhancing their capacity to mediate transendothelial migration of inflammatory cells. In this regard, the high endothelial venules (HEV), which are specialized postcapillary venules of lymphoid tissue, develop in response to immunologic activity and lymphocyte trafficking in the tissue (Freemont, 1987; Freemont et al., 1983; Iguchi and Ziff, 1986; Yannie et al., 1993; see Freemont, Chapter 5, this volume). The EC in synovia from patients with active, untreated disease exhibit an HEV-like morphology especially in regions near lymphocyte aggregates (Yanni et al., 1993). In contrast, tissue samples from patients whose disease had been modified by treatment exhibited relatively flatter endothelium. Only when lymphocyte aggregates were observed were tall HEV present, suggesting that in these instances, the morphologic change may have developed in response to the local immunologic activity. Moreover, trafficking into tissue may be restricted and confined to these focal areas. The development of HEV-like blood vessels has been examined in sites of delayed type hypersensitivity reactions in the skin of primates, and depends on the exposure to proinflammatory cytokines. Thus, concomitant stimulation with TNFα and IFNγ induced the appearance of HEV as well as the adhesion and extravasation of inflammatory cells (Munro et al., 1989). Maintenance of the HEV morphology, therefore, depends on the trafficking of cells in the tissue and their production of cytokines.

MECHANISMS OF CELL ADHESION DURING THE INFILTRATION OF INFLAMMATORY CELLS INTO RHEUMATOID SYNOVIUM

A number of specific adhesive mechanisms appear to play a role in the accumulation of inflammatory cells in the rheumatoid synovium. Specific recognition mechanisms that mediate the initial binding and transendothelial migration of leukocytes into sites of chronic inflammation have been identified and these processes are profoundly modulated by proinflammatory mediators. Central to these mechanisms are the activities of specific cell surface adhesion receptors. Adhesion receptors are responsible for the initial stabilized binding of leukocytes to the blood vessel wall and their subsequent transendothelial migration into perivascular tissue, whether it be during normal recirculation through lymphoid tissue or into sites of inflammation, including rheumatoid synovium. Not only does the binding of adhesion receptors to specific counterreceptors facilitate adhesion and transendothelial migration, but ligation of adhesion receptors is also likely to deliver intracellular signals as well. Thus, adhesion receptors, such as lymphocyte function associated antigen-1 (LFA-1) and VLA-4, deliver costimulatory signals to inflammatory cells when they are engaged by their counterreceptors, intercellular adhesion molecule-1 (ICAM-1) and vascular cell adhesion molecule-1 (VCAM-1), or the extracellular matrix molecule fibronectin, respectively (Altmann et al., 1989; Davis et al., 1990; Shimizu et al., 1990a; van Seventer et al., 1990, 1991; Damle and Aruffo, 1991).

Tables 2–4 list the adhesion receptors that are likely to facilitate the infiltration of leukocytes into sites of inflammation. Adhesion receptors that are members of the immunoglobulin, selectin, and integrin superfamilies mediate much of the adhesive interactions that occur during the infiltration of leukocytes into sites of inflammation. With the exception of LFA-3 (CD58), all of the adhesion receptors are transmembrane proteins and are members of supergene families of adhesion receptor molecules. LFA-3 exists as either a transmembrane protein or as a glycophosphatidylinositol-linked molecule, both of which are involved in adhesive interactions (Springer, 1990).

The expression of adhesion receptors on EC is regulated by the actions of proinflammatory mediators and endotoxin. Each receptor binds at least one counterreceptor expressed by leukocytes, many of which are also functionally regulated by activation stimuli. Thus, for example, VLA-4, -5, -6, LFA-1 and Mac-1, which are constitutively expressed by cells, require an activation step for them to bind their ligands. Their functional activation occurs without changes in the level of expression of the integrin adhesion molecules (Shimizu et al., 1990b; Springer, 1990). Thus,

Table 2. Members of the immunoglobulin family of adhesion receptors that mediate leukocyte interactions with EC

Receptor	Counter-receptor	Distribution	Regulation
ICAM-1 (CD54)	LFA-1 (CD11a/CD18) Mac-1 (CD11b/CD18) Leukosialin (CD43)	Endothelial cells, synovial fibroblasts, synovial macrophages, epithelial cells, germinal centre dendritic cells, activated lymphocytes	Increased by IL-1, TNFα, IFNγ, endotoxin
ICAM-2 (CD102)	LFA-1 (CD11a/CD18)	Endothelial cells, haematopoietic cell lines	Constitutive
VCAM-1 (CD106)	VLA-4 CD49d/CD29) α4/β7	Endothelial cells, synovial lining cells, germinal centre dendritic cells, synovial macrophages, bone marrow fibroblasts	Induced by IL-1, TNFα, Il-4
LFA-3 (CD58)	CD2	Endothelial cells, leukocytes, epithelial cells, some T cells	?
PECAM-1 (CD31)	?	Endothelial cells, platelets, leukocytes, smooth muscle cells	?
MAdCAM-1	α4β7	Endothelial cells of mucosal tissue	Induced by TNFα IL-1β

Table 3. Members of the selectin family of adhesion receptors that mediate leukocyte interactions with EC

Receptor	Counter-receptor	Distribution	Regulation
E-selectin	Sialyl Lewis X, L-selectin, CLA sialyl Lewis A, LFA-1	Activated endothelial cells	Induced by IL-1, TNFα
L-selectin	E-selectin, P-selectin PNAd, CD34, GLYCAM-1 MAdCAM-1, charged oligosaccharides	Resting leukocytes	Decreased by activation stimuli
P-selectin	Sialyl Lewis X, L-selectin, CD15	Activated platelets, activated endothelial cells	Induced by thrombin, histamine

stimulation of T cells with protein kinase C activating phorbol esters or by engaging the CD3 molecular complex induces the ability of the T cells to utilize beta$_1$ and beta$_2$ integrins to bind extracellular matrix molecules and cellular counterreceptors (Dustin and Springer, 1989; Shimizu *et al.*, 1990b). Additionally, ligation of CD31 on a subset of T cells leads to the functional activation of VLA-4 (Tanaka *et al.*, 1992). In contrast to this there are adhesion receptors, such as L-selectin, CD2 and CD44, that are constitutively active, and thus do not require an activation step for them to bind their counterreceptors.

ADHESION MOLECULE EXPRESSION IN RHEUMATOID SYNOVITIS

The role of specific adhesion receptors during the extravasation of inflammatory cells into rheumatoid synovium has not been completely delineated. The EC of rheumatoid

Table 4. Members of the integrin family of adhesion receptors that mediate adhesive interactions of leukocytes

Sub-family	Receptor	Counter-receptor	Distribution	Regulation
Beta$_1$ (CD29)	VLA-1 (CD49a/CD29)	Laminin, collagen	Activated T cells, fibroblasts, liver sinusoids, mesangial cells, some cell lines	Induced by mitogen, antigen
	VLA-2 (CD49b/CD29)	Collagen, laminin	Activated T cells, platelets, endothelial cells	Increased by mitogen, antigen
	VLA-4 (CD49d/CD29)	VCAM-1, fibronectin	Lymphocytes, monocytes, thymus cells, eosinophils, haematopoietic cell lines	Functional activation by antigen
	VLA-5 (CD49e/CD29)	Fibronectin	Lymphocytes, monocytes, thymus cells, endothelial cells, fibroblasts	Functional activation by antigen
	VLA-6 (CD49f/CD29)	Laminin	Lymphocytes, platelets, endothelial cells, fibroblasts	Functional activation by antigen
Beta$_2$ (CD18)	LFA-1 (CD11a/CD18)	ICAM-1, ICAM-2, ICAM-3 E-selectin	All haematopoietic cells except red blood cells	Functional activation, increased expression by various mitogenic stimuli
	Mac-1 (CD11b/CD18)	ICAM-1, fibrinogen, endotoxin, Factor X, iC3b	Monocytes, granulocytes, macrophages, large granular lymphocytes, some B cells, some T cells	Increased expression by chemotactic factors
	p150/95 (CD11c/CD18)	Fibrinogen, iC3b	Monocytes, granulocytes, macrophages, large granular lymphocytes, some B cells, hairy cell leukemia cells	Increased by TNFα
Beta$_7$	α4/β7	MAdCAM-1, VCAM-1, fibronectin	B and T cells, macrophages	?
	α^E/β7	?	Intestinal intraepithelial lymphocytes	Increased by TGFβ$_1$

synovium express a variety of adhesion receptors that bind leukocytes. This is most likely a direct result of the activities of proinflammatory cytokines, such as IL-1β and TNFα, that are elaborated within the tissue, and which among their other activities, induce or up-regulate the expression of adhesion receptors by EC. Thus, several reports have indicated that the EC of rheumatoid synovium express ICAM-1, VCAM-1, E-selectin, and P-selectin (Hale *et al.*, 1989; Koch *et al.*, 1991; Morales-Ducret *et al.*, 1991; Grober *et al.*, 1993). The most intensely and broadly expressed EC adhesion receptor is ICAM-1, which is present on venules, capillaries and arterioles. E-selectin is also expressed on nearly all vessels, while VCAM-1 is expressed by EC to a lesser degree (Koch *et al.*, 1991; Veale *et al.*, 1993). Until recently, P-selectin activity was restricted to binding neutrophils. However, P-selectin may also bind lymphocytes (McEver, 1992). P-selectin expressed by EC in synovial tissue was recently shown to bind peripheral blood monocytes, and thus may be important in facilitating the entry of this cell population into the tissue (Grober *et al.*, 1993). However, the assay utilized frozen sections of tissue, and thus the physiologic role of P-selectin in monocyte extravasation requires further delineation. VCAM-1 expressed by synovial tissue EC has been demonstrated to mediate the binding of synovial T cells. Recent data also suggest a role for ICAM-1 in mediating the entrance of lymphocytes into synovial tissue. Thus, an anti-ICAM-1 monoclonal antibody (mAb) inhibited the transendo-thelial migration of lymphocytes *in vitro* (Oppenheimer-Marks *et al.*, 1991). Further-more, administration of this mAb to RA patients with early and active disease had a marked modifying effect on disease activity, presumably by altering lymphocyte traf-ficking into tissue (Kavanaugh *et al.*, 1994). Thus, it is likely that ICAM-1 serves an important role in lymphocyte infiltration into tissue.

A subset of circulating T cells from RA patients is spontaneously competent to bind ICAM-1. This has been demonstrated by measuring interactions of RA or normal peripheral blood T cells with substrates that have been precoated with purified ICAM-1 (Oppenheimer-Marks and Lipsky, unpublished observation). These results imply that this subset of circulating T cells in patients with RA expresses LFA-1 in an activated form and, therefore, is directly competent to bind ICAM-1. Expression of an activated form of LFA-1 may be a feature related to an overall increased activation state of circulating T cells in RA patients, and may contribute to their increased accumulation within rheumatoid synovium by mediating their transendothelial mi-gration into the tissue. Subsets of synovial tissue and fluid T cells also express acti-vated VLA-4 as evidenced by their ability to bind to fibronectin-coated substrates (Laffon *et al.*, 1991). The nature of this subset, however, has not been identified. The data indicate that subsets of circulating T cells as well as those found at inflammatory sites in RA express activated integrins that can facilitate their entry into synovial tissue.

In chronic RA, neutrophils traffic out of the tissue and accumulate in the synovial fluid compartment. The reasons for this are not certain at this time, but may be related to the lack of expression of most beta$_1$ integrins by neutrophils (Hemler, 1990). Neutrophils only express $\alpha6/\beta1$ (Rieu *et al.*, 1993). As a result, adhesive mechanisms, which would mediate neutrophil binding to ECM components other than laminin, are absent and neutrophils would, therefore, be subjected to modest adhesive restraints within the tissue. In contrast, strong chemotactic signals, by for example IL-8 and the activated complement component, C5a, emanating from the fluid compartment might stimulate the migration of neutrophils out of the tissue. Once in the fluid, neutrophils assume their characteristic agranular, vacuolated appearance and may remain in this compartment.

REGULATION OF TRANSENDOTHELIAL MIGRATION OF INFLAMMATORY CELLS

In general, leukocyte extravasation involves the concerted activities of a variety of adhesion receptors. The migration of leukocytes into perivascular tissue is a multistep adhesive process that involves the induction or activation of cell surface adhesion receptors to mediate stable leukocyte binding to EC, which is followed by the migration of the bound cells through the EC layer. Essential to this process is that extravasating cells possess an intrinsic migratory capacity.

Table 5. Adhesion receptors utilized during neutrophil interactions with EC

	Neutrophils	Endothelial cells
Early	L-selectin, sialyl Lewis X, CD15	P-selectin
	PECAM-1 (CD31)	?
	?	PECAM-1 (CD31)
Intermediate	L-selectin, sialyl Lewis X or A, LFA-1	E-selectin
Late	LFA-1 (CD11a/CD18)	ICAM-1 (CD54), ICAM-2, E-selectin
	Mac-1 (CD11b/CD18)	ICAM-1 (CD54), Fibrinogen
	p150/95 (CD11c/CD18)	Fibrinogen

Normally, neutrophils roll along the surface of the endothelium (Lawrence and Springer, 1991; Butcher, 1991). At sites of inflammation, where E-selectin and P-selectin are expressed by EC, this process has been shown to be mediated by either of these molecules binding to L-selectin (Picker *et al.*, 1991a; Butcher, 1991) (Table 5). This type of adhesive interaction is not stable and by itself does not lead to the transendothelial migration of neutrophils. Rather, stable interactions occur as a result of the formation of additional adhesions between integrins on neutrophils and ICAM-1 on EC. This stabilized binding and transendothelial migration of neutrophils occurs as a response of neutrophils to the activities of inflammatory mediators. Thus, leukotrienes, complement components, and chemokines such as IL-8, activate neutrophils and induce changes in the adhesiveness of the cells (Kishimoto *et al.*, 1989; Huber *et al.*, 1991). In this series of events, L-selectin expression is down-regulated and concomitantly, there is an increased expression and activation of Mac-1, which by binding to ICAM-1 strengthens neutrophil interactions with EC. These mediators most likely also activate LFA-1, on neutrophils since both LFA-1 and Mac-1 have been suggested to mediate the transendothelial migration of neutrophils (Smith *et al.*, 1988, 1989). Recently, it was suggested that CD31 (PECAM-1) also plays a role in the transendothelial migration of neutrophils (Muller *et al.*, 1993).

The precise mechanisms involved in the establishment of stabilized lymphocyte binding to EC have not been delineated. There is a redundancy in the number of receptor–counterreceptor pairs that are capable of supporting adhesive interactions between lymphocytes and EC (Fig. 1). L-selectin, which does not require an activation step, has been reported to mediate lymphocyte binding to TNFα-activated EC in addition to binding GlyCAM-1, a mucin-like adhesion molecule expressed by peripheral lymph node EC (Kansas *et al.*, 1991; Lasky *et al.*, 1992). Thus, the ligation of L-selectin may initiate intracellular signalling events that lead to stabilized T cell–EC binding. Normally, VLA-4 and LFA-1 both require an activation step to become competent to bind their counterreceptors. This does not involve increased expression of these molecules by lymphocytes, but appears to relate to conformational changes in their structure. For activated peripheral blood T cells, the requirement for an activation step for integrins appears to be unnecessary. Both VLA-4 and LFA-1 mediate lymphocyte adhesion to EC, although all of the binding cannot be accounted for by the activities of these two molecules. VLA-4 recognition of VCAM-1 is most important in binding T cells to cytokine-activated EC. On the other hand, LFA-1 functions

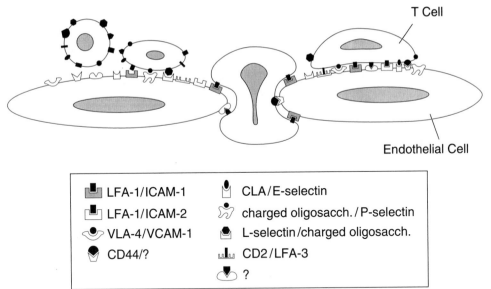

T Cell

Endothelial Cell

▣ LFA-1/ICAM-1	◕ CLA/E-selectin
▣ LFA-1/ICAM-2	🐟 charged oligosacch./P-selectin
☙ VLA-4/VCAM-1	◕ L-selectin/charged oligosacch.
◕ CD44/?	⊔⊔ CD2/LFA-3
	▽ ?

Figure 1. T lymphocytes express a repertoire of adhesion receptors that mediate adhesive interactions with endothelial cells at sites of inflammation. Binding of T cells to EC occurs by the interaction of a variety of adhesion receptors with their specific counterreceptors. At sites of inflammation, initial adhesive interactions may result from the binding of L-selectin to charged oligosaccharide groups on cytokine activated EC. Similarly, early interactions may also be mediated by charged oligosaccharides on T cells interacting with P-selectin on activated EC. Thus, interactions between LFA-1/ICAM-1, LFA-1/ICAM-2, VLA-4/VCAM-1, CD2/LFA-3, CLA/E-selectin, CD44 and its unidentified counterreceptor, as well as between other as yet unidentified receptor pairs, could then account for the stabilized adhesion of T cells to EC at sites of inflammation. The transendothelial migration of T cells is mediated by a variety of adhesion receptors, including LFA-1/ICAM-1, CD44 and its unidentified counter-receptor, as well as other as yet unidentified receptor pairs. Once the T cells have migrated into the perivascular tissue, additional adhesive interactions occur between the T cells and components of extracellular matrices as well as with other cells present within the tissue.

during adhesion of resting or activated T cells to unstimulated EC by binding to both ICAM-1 and ICAM-2. Both, E-selectin and P-selectin, which are expressed by activated EC, also appear to be involved in lymphocyte binding (Picker *et al.*, 1991a; McEver, 1992). A subset of memory T cells adheres to E-selectin, and for many of these T cells this is mediated by cutaneous lymphocyte antigen (CLA) (Picker *et al.*, 1991b). Whether CLA requires an activation step to bind to E-selectin has not yet been reported. In addition, LFA-1 was recently shown to bind to E-selectin through its carbohydrate moieties (Kotovuori *et al.*, 1993). The nature of the lymphocyte counterreceptor that binds P-selectin has not been reported, but it most likely is related to sialylated forms of blood group antigens, Lewis X and Lewis A, as all members of the selectin family specifically recognize charged forms of these oligosaccharides (Foxall *et al.*, 1992; Nelson *et al.*, 1993).

In contrast to the process of T cell–EC binding, there is a limited number of adhesion receptors that have been identified to mediate the transendothelial migration of lymphocytes (Fig. 1). To date, the receptor pair, LFA-1/ICAM-1, and the homing receptor CD44, have been implicated in the transendothelial migration of lymphocytes (Oppenheimer-Marks *et al.*, 1990, 1991). MAb blocking experiments conducted *in vitro* have demonstrated that the transendothelial migration of T cells bound to EC is inhibited by anti-LFA-1 or anti-ICAM-1 mAb, but not by mAb against VLA-4, VCAM-1, LFA-3 or E-selectin (Oppenheimer-Marks *et al.*, 1991). Thus, although a number of adhesion receptors mediate initial adhesive events between T cells and EC, they do not necessarily serve a similar function during transendothelial migration.

Under conditions whereby both T cells and EC have been exposed to activation stimuli, part of the transendothelial migration of the activated lymphocytes is mediated by CD44 (Oppenheimer-Marks *et al.*, 1990). CD44 is not related to the integrin, immunoglobulin or selectin superfamilies. Rather, CD44 is more closely related to proteoglycan link protein, and has a number of different ligand specificities, including the ECM components, hyaluronic acid and collagen, as well as a receptor expressed by mucosal tissue EC (Haynes *et al.*, 1989). It is likely, therefore, that both lymphocyte–EC binding and transendothelial migration utilize a multiplicity of receptors. This redundancy may be necessary for a succession of adhesive interactions between lymphocytes and the endothelium that facilitate lymphocyte entry into tissue.

CHEMOKINES

Soluble mediators emerging from the tissue are involved in the signalling events controlling the adhesiveness of leukocytes. Aside from cytokines influencing adhesion receptor expression by EC, low molecular weight (6–10 kDa) cytokines, referred to as chemokines, that act as chemoattractants also play a role. Chemokines are related by primary structure, particularly by conservation of a 4 cysteine motif (Miller and Krangel, 1992). Based on the spacing of the cysteines, chemokines can be classified into two groups, C-X-C (also called α) and C-C (also called β), depending on whether the first two cysteines are adjacent or are separated by an intervening amino acid residue. Among the members of the C-X-C chemokines are interleukin-8 (IL-8) (also referred to as neutrophil activating protein-1, neutrophil activating factor, NAF, and monocyte-derived neutrophil chemotactic factor, MDNCF, as well as others), melanocyte growth-stimulatory activity (MGSA), neutrophil-activating peptide 2, and a neutrophil-activating protein derived from epithelial cells (ENA-78) (Table 6). In general, C-X-C chemokines are potent chemoattractants and activators of neutrophils but not of monocytes. On the other hand, members of the C-C chemokines, including human monocyte chemotactic protein-1 (MCP-1), *R*egulated upon *A*ctivation, *N*ormal *T* *E*xpressed, and *S*ecreted (RANTES), and the macrophage inflammatory proteins 1α and 1β (MIP-1α, MIP-1β) are chemoattractants for monocytes but not neutrophils. In addition, IL-8, RANTES, MIP-1α and MIP-1β are also chemotactic for lymphocytes (Miller and Krangel, 1992).

IL-8 is present in synovial fluid, and is produced by a variety of cell types, including synovial tissue macrophages, EC, fibroblasts, keratinocytes, and T cells. Cells have been shown to secrete both long and short forms of IL-8 that are 77 and 72 amino acids long, respectively (Hebert *et al.*, 1990). The predominant form secreted by EC is the long form, whereas T cells and macrophages secrete predominantly the shorter form. Thrombin has been shown to convert the long form into the shorter one, which is several times more potent in functional assays *in vitro*. *In vivo* the two forms appear

Table 6. Chemokines that may have a facilitatory role in the accumulation of leukocytes in the cellular compartments of rheumatoid synovial tissue

Group	Chemokine	Source	Target cell
C-X-C	IL-8	Endothelial cells, monocytes, neutrophils, synovial tissue macrophages, fibroblasts, keratinocytes, hepatocytes, chondrocytes, mesothelial cells, T cells	Neutrophils, T cells, melanoma cells, basophils
C-C	RANTES	T cells	Memory T cell subsets, monocytes, eosinophils
	MIP-1α	Monocytes, macrophages, T and B cells	T-cell subsets, B cells, eosinophils
	MIP-1β	Monocytes, macrophages, T and B cells	T-cell subsets
	MCP-1	Endothelial cells, fibroblasts, monocytes, vascular smooth muscle	Monocytes, basophils

to behave similarly, indicating that processing of the long form may occur by physiologic mechanisms (Hebert *et al.*, 1990; Hechtman *et al.*, 1991; Nourshargh *et al.*, 1992). IL-8 is abundant in synovial fluids from RA and non-RA arthritides, including gout, osteoarthritis, and psoriatic arthritis (Brennan *et al.*, 1990). Its concentration in these synovial fluids has been reported to range from 1 to 9 ng/ml. RANTES appears to be produced by antigen or mitogen activated T lymphocytes (Schall *et al.*, 1990). On the other hand, MIP-1α and MIP-1β are produced by many cell types including B and T lymphocytes (Lipes *et al.*, 1988).

In addition to the direct effects IL-8 has on lymphocytes *in vitro* (Larsen *et al.*, 1989; Barker *et al.*, 1991), recent *in vivo* recirculation studies have suggested that IL-8 may actually indirectly recruit lymphocytes into extravascular sites. This was recently demonstrated by Kudo *et al.* (1991) who selectively depleted neutrophils, *in vivo*, and as a result they eliminated the ability of IL-8 to induce the accumulation of CD4[+], but not CD8[+] lymphocytes. These results imply that neutrophil trafficking through tissue is necessary for the subsequent transendothelial migration of specific populations of lymphocytes by the elaboration of a factor(s) that specifically recruits CD4[+] T cells into tissue.

It is uncertain whether the net effect of IL-8 is pro- or anti-inflammatory. On the one hand, treatment of neutrophils with IL-8 inhibited their subsequent binding to EC *in vitro* (Gimbrone *et al.*, 1989). Moreover, intravenous administration of IL-8 inhibited the transendothelial migration of neutrophils into sites of acute inflammation, and inhibited neutrophil responses to local subcutaneous injection of IL-8, FMLP, C5a and TNFα (Hechtman *et al.*, 1991). In contrast, subcutaneous injection of IL-8 has been shown to induce neutrophil accumulation *in vivo*, and *in vitro* studies have demonstrated that IL-8 produced by cytokine-activated EC is secreted directionally from the basal surface of cultured EC (Kudo *et al.*, 1991; Huber *et al.*, 1991). The EC-derived IL-8 has chemotactic activity for neutrophils, and also activated neutrophils to decrease the expression of L-selectin and up-regulate the beta$_2$ integrins (Huber *et al.*, 1991). This suggests that in certain circumstances IL-8 might facilitate acute inflammatory responses. Thus, in various models IL-8 may exert pro- or anti-inflammatory effects. The net effect *in vivo* remains to be determined, and may differ in various kinds of inflammation. Moreover, the compartment in which IL-8 is located may determine its ability to exert chemotactic activity.

RANTES has been demonstrated to be chemotactic for monocytes and a subpopulation of $CD4^+$ memory T cells (Schall *et al.*, 1990; Taub *et al.*, 1993). RANTES induces the chemotaxis of lymphocytes at 200-fold lower concentrations than the optimal concentration for monocytes (Schall *et al.*, 1990). Thus, RANTES may selectively recruit the migration of specific subpopulations of lymphocytes into tissue. Both MIP-1α and MIP-1β chemoattract specific populations of lymphocytes, although the nature of the subpopulations is a matter of debate. For example, MIP-1α was recently shown to chemoattract either $CD4^+$ T cells (Taub *et al.*, 1993) or $CD8^+$ (Tanaka *et al.*, 1993) T cells specifically. These differences may be related to the concentrations of chemokine used and the assay situation, as a recent report by Schall *et al.* (1993) demonstrated the ability of MIP-1α and MIP-1β to induce the chemotaxis of different lymphocyte populations in a concentration-dependent fashion. Nevertheless, the data support the conclusion that chemokines play an important role in facilitating the extravasation of cells into inflammatory sites. Moreover, chemokines may exert profound effects on the trafficking of inflammatory cells within tissue, and thus direct cells to different cellular compartments.

THE MIGRATION OF SPECIFIC POPULATIONS OF T CELLS INTO RHEUMATOID SYNOVIUM

There is an enrichment in RA synovial tissue of $CD4^+$ memory T cells (see Chapters 2 and 4, this volume). There are a number of possibilities that could explain this finding. Suggestions have been made that synovial tissue EC might express unique vascular addressins that recruit only those T cell subsets that bear the appropriate counter-receptors, and in an analogous manner that EC of peripheral and mucosal lymphoid tissue express addressins that bind T cells bearing appropriate counterreceptors (Butcher, 1990). In this regard, synovial fluid T cells can bind to HEV of mucosal lymphoid tissue, and T cell clones have been identified that uniquely bind to EC in synovial tissue (Kadioglu and Sheldon, 1992; Salmi *et al.*, 1992). Thus, synovial fluid T cells clearly express counterreceptors for mucosal HEV suggesting that synovial and mucosal EC may express similar addressins. The nature of the vascular addressin of synovial tissue EC has, however, not been identified, although vascular adhesion protein-1 (VAP-1), a recently described lymphocyte adhesion protein, is expressed by synovial EC and, to a lesser extent, by EC of peripheral lymph node (Salmi and Jalkanen, 1992). Recently it was shown that the mucosal addressin, MAdCAM-1, binds a beta7 integrin, α4/β7 (Berlin *et al.*, 1993). However, it is doubtful that synovial fluid cells utilize α4/β7 for binding MAdCAM-1, since they express only very low levels of this molecule (A.I. Lazarovits, pers. commun.). The infiltration into tissue of $CD4^+$ T cells may also result from the action of specific chemotactic factors, such as RANTES or MIP-1α or 1β, that might selectively stimulate the migration of memory T cells into the synovium. It has also been suggested that specific antigen, within the synovial tissue, might influence the nature of the T cell that accumulates in the tissue. In support of this possibility are findings that EC are capable of presenting antigen to T cells, and could, therefore, recruit into tissue only T cells that are responsive to a particular antigen (Geppert and Lipsky, 1989). Moreover, *in vitro* analyses have indicated that HLA-DR positive EC support T-cell binding more effectively than HLA-DR negative T cells, implying that specific recognition by T cells of HLA-DR bound endogenous peptides may play a role in their migration (Masuyama *et al.*, 1986). Since EC in the rheumatoid synovium are known to express HLA-DR, albeit modestly, these molecules could contribute to selective recruitment of T cells into the tissue.

Analysis of T cells isolated directly from synovial tissue reveals a greater total number of CD4$^+$ than CD8$^+$ T cells (Cush and Lipsky, 1988). These synovial tissue T cells appear to be activated since the density of CD4 and CD3 is reduced, in comparison to RA peripheral blood T cells, and they express CD69, HLA-DR, very late activation (VLA)-1 antigen (CD49a/CD29), and decreased amounts of L-selectin (Klareskog *et al.*, 1981; Forre *et al.*, 1982a; Poulter *et al.*, 1985; Hemler *et al.*, 1986; Burmester *et al.*, 1987; Goto *et al.*, 1987; Cush and Lipsky, 1988). Nearly all of the synovial tissue CD4$^+$ T cells are of the memory subset since they are CD29^{bright}, CD7^{dim}, CD45RO$^+$ and CD45RA^{dim} (Pitzalis *et al.*, 1987; Cush and Lipsky, 1988; Nakao *et al.*, 1989). By contrast, rheumatoid synovium is nearly devoid of naive CD4$^+$/CD45RA^{bright} T cells. Recent *in vivo* and *in vitro* studies indicate that it is unlikely that these T cells migrate into the tissue as CD45RA$^+$, naive T cells and then differentiate within the tissue into CD45RA$^-$/CD45RO$^+$ memory T cells. Rather the data suggest that memory, and not naive, CD4$^+$ T cells exhibit a greater intrinsic transendothelial migratory capacity, and therefore preferentially migrate into extra-lymphoid tissue sites (Pietschmann *et al.*, 1992). This conclusion is supported by the *in vivo* observation that CD4$^+$/CD45RO$^+$ T cells preferentially migrate into delayed type hypersensitivity lesions *in vivo* in humans (Pitzalis *et al.*, 1991). Moreover, memory CD4$^+$ T cells are more able to bind to EC than naive T cells (Damle and Doyle, 1990). Thus, mechanisms other than those utilized during normal lymphocyte recirculation are likely to facilitate the infiltration of memory cells into these inflammatory sites. Related to this are the findings that activated memory T cells also elaborate factors which could autoregulate their extravasation. Thus, once activated in the tissue, memory T cells could increase the permeability properties of EC, and also induce the expression of adhesion receptors by EC (Damle and Doyle, 1990; Damle *et al.*, 1991). The immunohistochemistry of T cells in rheumatoid synovia is reviewed by Edwards and Wilkinson in Chapter 7, this volume.

The relationship of the phenotype of T cells to their migratory capacity has been addressed by *in vitro* studies. Phenotypic analyses of T cells that are recovered following their transendothelial migration into collagen gels, indicate that the predominant migrating CD4$^+$ T cell is also CD45RO$^+$ (Pietschmann *et al.*, 1992). Not all of the CD45RO$^+$ T cells are migratory, however, since many do not migrate. This suggests that only a subset of memory T cells in the peripheral circulation exhibits a transendothelial migratory capacity. Flow cytometric analyses have been conducted to delineate further the identity of the CD4$^+$ memory T cells in the migrated population. These T cells are also CD29^{bright}/L-selectin^{low}/CD7^{dim}. This phenotype parallels that of CD4$^+$ T cells present in rheumatoid synovium (Cush and Lipsky, 1991). Particularly noteworthy is that IL-1 or IFNγ activation of the EC did not affect the phenotype of the migrating CD4$^+$ T cells, even though the absolute number of migrating T cells increased. Thus, the regulatory effect on transendothelial migration by these cytokines may be primarily to expand the degree to which a particular memory T cell subset that possesses an intrinsic migratory capacity infiltrates into a particular tissue, rather than inducing the migration of different T-cell subsets. Other studies have extended these observations and shown that there are minimal differences in the T-cell populations found in normal and RA patient peripheral blood that exhibit a capacity for transendothelial migration (Cush *et al.*, 1993). Although more activated T cells are found in the peripheral blood of RA patients, and many of these cells exhibit a migratory capacity, there were no other reported differences in their cell surface phenotype. Thus, the capacity of T cells to infiltrate into synovial tissue appears to be an intrinsic behaviour of specific T-cell populations. Based on the observations that RA peripheral blood T cells express activated integrin adhesion receptors, it seems likely that the activated T-cell population of RA peripheral blood that exhibits a migratory capacity may be that which expresses the activated form of LFA-1. Thus, whether a particular T cell extravasates into tissue will depend not only on its ability to migrate, but requires the expression of appropriate functionality active adhesion receptors such that its transmigration through the vascular endothelium is facilitated.

THERAPEUTIC STRATEGIES TARGETING ADHESION RECEPTORS FOR THE CONTROL OF RA

New strategies to control chronic RA could involve targeting of the molecules involved in entry of inflammatory cells into the synovium. One rationale behind these involves the prevention of leukocyte infiltration into synovial tissue by blocking specific cell surface adhesion receptors that mediate interactions between leukocytes and EC (see Panayi, Chapter 4, this volume). Moreover, anti-adhesion receptor therapy might also block the local activation of cells that results from the ligation of specific adhesion receptors. Members of the beta$_2$ (CD18) integrins (LFA-1 and Mac-1) play a pivotal role in leukocyte adhesion to EC and subsequent transendothelial migration into perivascular connective tissue. Therefore, studies have been conducted to examine the role of these molecules in the development of chronic synovitis in the Glynn Dumonde model of antigen-induced arthritis in the rabbit (Jasin *et al.*, 1992). Intra-articular injection of antigen induces an acute inflammatory response which resolves, followed by a chronic persistent arthritis in the injected joint. The chronic phase, which has certain similarities with RA, is a widely used example of chronic arthritis with an immune pathogenesis (reviewed in detail in Chapter 24, this volume). The chronic synovitis in this model is characterized by the presence of dense cellular infiltrates composed of macrophages, lymphocytes and plasma cells with a tendency to form lympoid follicles, yielding a histologic picture similar to RA (Jasin, 1988).

Administration of anti-CD18 mAb during the acute phase of this model prevented the development of the chronic phase. The mechanism of action is related to prevention of the entry of neutrophils during the acute Arthus reaction. It is likely that blocking neutrophil trafficking through the tissue prevents the subsequent development of the lymphocyte-mediated chronic arthritis to develop. The striking decrease in the number and proportion of neutrophils in the inflammatory synovial fluid underscores the importance of beta$_2$ integrins in the processes of adhesion and transendothelial migration of these inflammatory cells. Although local production of antibodies and accumulation of immune complexes in cartilage occurred during the chronic phase in the anti-CD18 treated animals, they were insufficient to sustain chronic synovitis in the absence of antecedent PMN-mediated acute inflammation.

Other studies have utilized mAb against ICAM-1 in adjuvant arthritis in rats (Iigo *et al.*, 1991). Adjuvant arthritis is prevented when mAb to ICAM-1 is given at the time of immunization with adjuvant presumably by inhibiting the immunization process. Administration of mAb to ICAM-1 to animals in whom adjuvant arthritis was induced by adaptive transfer of primed cells also diminished arthritis suggesting that entry of inflammatory cells into target tissue was also blocked. Also particularly noteworthy is that administration of mAb against ICAM-1 to RA patients with active disease had a marked modifying effect on disease activity (Kavanaugh *et al.*, 1993). Thus, among its effects, the anti-ICAM-1 mAb altered lymphocyte trafficking into tissue as evidenced by a marked lymphocytosis in the patients and suppression of the patient's delayed type hypersensitivity response to recall antigen as well. These results support the conclusion that interference with adhesion receptor activity, in particular ICAM-1 and beta$_2$ integrins, might have therapeutic potential in inflammatory arthritis.

CONCLUSIONS

The activities of a variety of adhesion receptors play central roles in the pathogenesis of RA. Adhesion molecules exert pleiotropic effects during inflammatory conditions, including the mediation of inflammatory cell interactions with EC and ECM molecules, transendothelial migration, as well as the delivery of costimulatory signals to these cells. Chemotactic signals emerging from tissue may profoundly influence the adhesion receptor mediated trafficking of inflammatory cells into and within the tissue, and thus control the multicellular compartmentalization of rheumatoid synovial tissue and fluid. Finally, approaches to modify the expression or utilization of adhesion molecules promise to provide new therapeutic intervention to control rheumatoid inflammation.

REFERENCES

Altmann DM, Hogg N, Trowsdale J & Wilkinson D (1989) Cotransfection of ICAM-1 and HLA-DR reconstitutes human antigen-presenting cell function in mouse L cells. *Nature* **338**: 512–514.

Barker JNWN, Jones ML, Mitra RS, Crockett-Torabe E, Fantone JC, Kunkel SL et al. (1991) Modulation of keratinocyte-derived interleukin-8 which is chemotactic for neutrophils and T lymphocytes. *Am J Path* **139**: 869–876.

Berlin C, Berg EL, Briskin MJ, Andrew DP, Kilshaw PJ, Holzmann B et al. (1993) α4β7 integrin mediates lymphocyte binding to the mucosal vascular addressin MAdCAM-1. *Cell* **74**: 185–195.

Brennan FM, Zachariae COC, Chantry D, Larsen CG, Turner M, Maini RN et al. (1990) Detection of interleukin-8 biological activity in synovial fluids from patients with rheumatoid arthritis and production of interleukin-8 mRNA by isolated synovial cells. *Eur J Immunol* **20**: 2141–2144.

Burmester GR, Jahn B, Rohwer P, Zacher J, Winchester RJ & Kalden JR (1987) Differential expression of Ia antigens by rheumatoid synovial lining cells. *J Clin Invest* **80**: 595–604.

Butcher EC (1990) Cellular and molecular mechanisms that direct leukocyte traffic. *Am J Pathol* **136**: 3–11.

Butcher EC (1991) Leukocyte–endothelial cell recognition: three (or more) steps for specificity and diversity. *Cell* **67**: 1033–1036.

Cush JJ & Lipsky PE (1988) Phenotypic analysis of synovial tissue and peripheral blood lymphocytes isolated from patients with rheumatoid arthritis. *Arthritis Rheum* **31**: 1230–1238.

Cush JJ & Lipsky PE (1991) Cellular basis for rheumatoid inflammation. *Clin Orthop* **265**: 9–22.

Cush JJ, Pietschmann P, Oppenheimer-Marks N & Lipsky PE (1993) The intrinsic migratory capacity of memory T cells contributes to their accumulation in the rheumatoid synovium. *Arthritis Rheum* **35**: 1434–1444.

Damle NK & Aruffo A (1991) Vascular cell adhesion molecule 1 induces T-cell antigen receptor-dependent activation of CD4[+] T lymphocytes. *Proc Natl Acad Sci* **88**: 6403–6407.

Damle NK & Doyle LV (1990) Ability of human T lymphocytes to adhere to vascular endothelial cells and to augment endothelial permeability to macromolecules is linked to their state of pot-thymic maturation. *J Immunol* **144**: 1233–1240.

Damle NK, Eberhardt C & Van der Vieren M (1991) Direct interaction with primed CD4[+] CD45RO[+] memory T lymphocytes induces expression of endothelial leukocyte adhesion molecule-1 and vascular cell adhesion molecule-1 on the surface of vascular endothelial cells. *Eur J Immunol* **21**: 2915–2923.

Davis LS, Oppenheimer-Marks N, Bednarczyk JL, McIntyre BW & Lipsky PE (1990) Fibronectin promotes proliferation of naive and memory T cells by signaling through both the VLA-4 and VLA-5 integrin molecules. *J Immunol* **145**: 785–793.

Dustin ML & Springer TA (1989) T-cell receptor cross-linking transiently stimulates adhesiveness through LFA-1. *Nature* **341**: 619–623.

Forre O, Dobloug JH & Natvig JB (1982a) Augmented numbers of HLA-DR-positive T lymphocytes in the synovial fluid and synovial tissue of patients with rheumatoid arthritis and juvenile rheumatoid arthritis. *Scand J Immunol* **15**: 227–231.

Forre O, Thoen J, Lea T, Dobloug JH, Mellbye OJ, Natvig JB et al. (1982b) *In situ* characterization of mononuclear cells in rheumatoid tissues, using monoclonal antibodies. No reduction of T8-positive cells or augmentation in T4-positive cells. *Scand J Immunol* **16**: 315–319.

Fox RI, Fong S, Sabharwal N, Carstens SA, Kung PC & Vaughan JH (1982) Synovial fluid lymphocytes differ from peripheral blood lymphocytes in patients with rheumatoid arthritis. *J Immunol* **128**: 351–354.

Foxall C, Watson SR, Dowbenko D, Fennie C, Lasky LA, Kiso M et al. (1992) The three members of the selectin receptor family recognize a common carbohydrate epitope, the sialyly lewis[x] oligosaccharide. *J Cell Biol* **117**: 895–902.

Freemont AJ (1987) Molecules controlling lymphocyte-endothelial interactions in lymph nodes are produced in vessels in inflamed synovium. *Ann Rheum Dis* **4**: 924–928.

Freemont AJ, Jones CJP, Bromley M & Andrews P (1983) Changes in vascular endothelium related to lymphocyte collections in diseased synovia. *Arthritis Rheum* **26**: 1427–1433.

Geppert TD & Lipsky PE (1989) Antigen presentation by cells that are not of bone marrow origin. *Reg Immunol* **2**: 60–71.

Gimbrone MA Jr, Obin MS, Brock AF, Luis EA, Hass PE, Hebert CA et al. (1989) Endothelial interleukin-8: a novel inhibitor of leukocyte–endothelial interactions. *Science* **246**: 1601–1604.

Goto M, Miyamoto T, Nishioka K & Uchida S (1987) T cytotoxic and helper cells are markedly increased, and T suppressor and inducer cells are markedly decreased, in rheumatoid synovial fluids. *Arthritis Rheum* **30**: 737–743.

Grober JS, Bowen BL, Ebling H, Athey B, Thompson CB, Fox DA et al. (1993) Monocyte–endothelial adhesion in chronic rheumatoid arthritis. *In situ* detection of selectin and integrin dependent interactions. *J Clin Invest* **91**: 2609–2619.

Hale LP, Martin ME, McCollum DE, Nunley JA, Springer TA, Singer KH et al. (1989) Immunohistologic analysis of the distribution of cell adhesion molecules within the inflammatory synovial microenvironment. *Arthritis Rheum* **32**: 22–30.

Haynes BF, Telen MJ, Hale LP & Denning SM (1989) CD44[−] A molecule involved in leukocyte adherence and T cell activation. *Immunol Today* **10**: 423–428.

Hebert CA, Luscinskas FW, Kiely J-M, Luis E, Darbonne WC, Bennett GL et al. (1990) Endothelial and leukocyte form of IL-8: conversion by thrombin and interactions with neutrophils. *J Immunol* **145**: 3033–3040.

Hechtman DH, Cybulsky MI, Fuchs HJ, Baker JP & Gimbrone MA Jr (1991) Intravascular IL-8. Inhibitor of polymorphonuclear leukocyte accumulation at sites of acute inflammation. *J Immunol* **147**: 883–892.

Hemler ME (1990) VLA proteins in the integrin family. Structures, functions and their role on leukocytes. *Ann Rev Immunol* **8**: 365–400.

Hemler ME, Glass D, Coblyn JS & Jacobson JG (1986) Very late activation antigens on rheumatoid synovial fluid T lymphocytes. Association with stages of T cell activation. *J Clin Invest* **78**: 696–702.

Huber AR, Kunkel SL, Todd III RF & Weiss SJ (1991) Regulation of transendothelial neutrophil migration by endogenous interleukin-8. *Science* **254**: 99–102.

Iguchi T & Ziff M (1986) Electron microscopic study of rheumatoid synovial vasculature. *J Clin Invest* **77**: 355–361.

Iigo Y, Takashi T, Tamatani T, Miyasaka M, Higashida T, Yagita H et al. (1991) ICAM-1 dependent pathway is critically involved in the pathogenesis of adjuvant arthritis in rats. *J Immunol* **147**: 4167–4171.

Jalkanen S, Steere AC, Fox RI & Butcher EC (1986) A distinct endothelial cell recognition system that controls lymphocyte traffic into inflamed synovium. *Science* **233**: 556–558.

Jasin HE (1988) Chronic arthritis in rabbits. *Meth Enzymol* **162**: 379–385.

Jasin HE, Lightfoot E, Davis LS, Rothlein R, Faanes RB & Lipsky PE (1992) Amelioration of antigen-induced arthritis in rabbits treated with monoclonal antibodies to leukocyte adhesion molecules. *Arthritis Rheum* **35**: 541–549.

Kadioglu A & Sheldon P (1992) Adhesion of rheumatoid peripheral blood and synovial fluid mononuclear cells to high endothelial venules of gut mucosa. *Ann Rheum Dis* **51**: 126–127.

Kansas GS, Spertini O, Stoolman LM & Tedder TF (1991) Molecular mapping of functional domains of the leukocyte receptor for endothelium, LAM-1. *J Cell Biol* **114**: 351–358.

Kavanaugh AF, Nichols L & Lipsky PE (1992) Treatment of refractory rheumatoid arthritis with a monoclonal antibody to intercellular adhesion molecule-1 (ICAM-1). *Arthritis Rheum* **37**: 992–999.

Kishimoto TK, Jutila MA, Berg EL & Butcher EC (1989) Neutrophil Mac-1 and MEL-14 adhesion proteins inversely regulated by chemotactic factors. *Science* **245**: 1238–1241.

Klareskog L, Forsum U, Tjernlund UM, Kabelitz D & Wigren A (1981) Appearance of anti-HLA-DR-reactive cells in normal and rheumatoid synovial tissue. *Scand J Immunol* **14**: 183–192.

Koch AE, Burrows JC, Haines GK, Carlos TM, Harlan JM & Leibovich SJ (1991) Immunolocalization of endothelial and leukocyte adhesion molecules in human rheumatoid and osteoarthritic synovial tissue. *Lab Invest* **64**: 313–320.

Kotovuori P, Tontti E, Pigott R, Shepard M, Kiso M, Hasegawa A et al. (1993) The vascular E-selectin binds to the leukocyte integrins CD11/CD18. *Glycobiology* **3**: 131–136.

Kudo C, Araki A, Matsushima K & Sendo F (1991) Inhibition of IL-8 induced W3/25$^+$ (CD4$^+$) T lymphocyte recruitment into subcutaneous tissues of rats by selective depletion of *in vivo* neutrophils with a monoclonal antibody. *J Immunol* **147**: 2196–2201.

Kurosaka M & Ziff M (1983) Immunoelectron microscopic study of the distribution of T cell subsets in rheumatoid synovium. *J Exp Med* **158**: 1191–1210.

Laffon A, Garcia-Vicuna R, Humbria A, Postigo AA, Corbi AL, de Landazuri MO et al. (1991) Upregulated expression and function of VLA-4 fibronectin receptors on human activated T cells in rheumatoid arthritis. *J Clin Invest* **88**: 546–552.

Larsen CG, Anderson AO, Appella E, Oppenheim JJ & Matsushima K (1989) The neutrophil-activating protein (NAP-1) is also chemotactic for lymphocytes. *Science* **243**: 1464–1466.

Lawrence MB & Springer TA (1991) Leukocytes roll on a selectin at physiologic flow rates: Distinction from and prerequisite for adhesion through integrins. *Cell* **65**: 859–873.

Lipes MA, Napolitano M, Jeang K-T, Chang NT & Leonard WJ (1988) Identification, cloning, and characterization of an immune activation gene. *Proc Natl Acad Sci USA* **85**: 9704–9708.

Masuyama J-I, Minato N & Kano S (1986) Mechanisms of lymphocyte adhesion to human vascular endothelial cells in culture. T lymphocyte adhesion to endothelial cells through HLA-DR antigens induced by gamma interferon. J Clin Invest **77**: 1596–1605.

McEver RP (1992) Leukocyte interactions mediated by P-selectin. In Smith CW, Kishimoto TK, Lipsky PE, Rothlein R & Rosenthal AS (eds) *The Structure and Function of Molecules Involved in Leukocyte Adhesion II*, pp 135–150. New York: Springer-Verlag.

Miller MD & Krangel MS (1992) Biology and biochemistry of the chemokines: a family of chemotactic and inflammatory cytokines. *Crit Rev Immunol* **12**: 17–46.

Morales-Ducret CRJ, Wayner E & Firestein GS (1991) Vascular cell adhesion molecule-1 expression and regulation in synovial tissue and fibroblast-like synoviocytes. *Arthritis Rheum* **34**: s155.

Muller WA, Weigel SA, Deng X & Phillips DM (1993) PECAM-1 is required for transendothelial migration of leukocytes. *J Exp Med* **178**: 449–460.

Munro JM, Pober JS & Cotran RS (1989) Tumor necrosis factor and interferon-γ induce distinct patterns of endothelial activation and associated leukocyte accumulation in skin of *Papio anubis. Am J Path* **135**: 121–133.

Nakao H, Eguchi K, Kawakami A, Migita K, Otsubo T, Ueki Y et al. (1989) Increment of Ta1 positive cells in peripheral blood from patients with rheumatoid arthritis. *J Rheumatol* **16**: 907–910.

Nelson RM, Dolich S, Aruffo A, Cecconi O & Bevilacqua (1993) Higher-affinity oligosaccharide ligands for E-selectin. *J Clin Invest* **91**: 1157–1166.

Nourshargh S, Perkins JA, Showell HJ, Matsushima K, Williams TJ & Collins PD (1992) A comparative study of the neutrophil stimulatory activity *in vitro* and pro-inflammatory propertis *in vivo* of 72 amino acid and 77 amino acid IL-8. *J Immunol* **148**: 106–111.

Oppenheimer-Marks N & Ziff M (1986) Binding of normal human mononuclear cells to blood vessels in rheumatoid synovial membrane. *Arthritis Rheum* **29**: 789–792.

Oppenheimer-Marks N, Davis LS & Lipsky PE (1990) Human T lymphocyte adhesion to endothelial cells and transendothelial migration. Alteration of receptor use relates to the activation status of both the T cell and the endothelial cell. *J Immunol* **145**: 140–148.

Oppenheimer-Marks N, Davis LS, Bogue DT, Ramberg J & Lipsky PE (1991) Differential utilization of ICAM-1 and VCAM-1 during the adhesion and transendothelial migration of human T lymphocytes. *J Immunol* **147**: 2913–2921.

Picker LJ, Warnock RA, Burns AR, Doerschuk CM, Berg EL & Butcher EC (1991a) The neutrophil selectin LECAM-1 presents carbohydrate ligands to the vascular selectins ELAM-1 and GMP-140. *Cell* **66**: 921–933.

Picker LJ, Kishimoto TK, Smith WC, Warnock RA & Butcher EC (1991b) ELAM-1 is an adhesion molecule for skin homing T cells. *Nature* **349**: 796–799.

Pietschmann P, Cush JJ, Lipsky PE & Oppenheimer-Marks N (1992) Identification of subsets of human T cells capable of enhanced transendothelial migration. *J Immunol* **149**: 1170–1178.

Pitzalis C, Kingsley G, Murphy J & Panayi G (1987) Abnormal distribution of the helper–inducer and suppressor–inducer T-lymphocyte subsets in the rheumatoid joint. *Clin Immunol Immunpathol* **45**: 252–258.

Pitzalis C, Kingsley GH, Covelli M, Meliconi R, Markey A & Panayi GS (1991) Selective migration of the human helper–inducer memory T cell subset: confirmation by *in vivo* cellular kinetic studies. *Eur J Immunol* **21**: 369–376.

Poulter LW, Duke O, Panayi GS, Hobbs S, Raftery MJ & Janossy G (1985) Activated T lmphocytes of the synovial membrane in rheumatoid arthritis and other arthropathies. *Scand J Immunol* **22**: 683–690.

Reme T, Portier M, Frayssinoux F, Combe B, Miossec P, Favier F & Sany J (1990) T cell receptor expression and activation of synovial lymphocyte subsets in patients with rheumatoid arthritis. Phenotyping of multiple synovial sites. *Arthritis Rheum* **33**: 485–492.

Rieu P, Lasavre P & Halbwachs-Mecarelli L (1993) Evidence for integrins other than $\beta2$ on polymorphonuclear neutrophils: expression of $\alpha6\beta1$ heterodimer. *J Leuk Biol* **53**: 576–582.

Salmi M & Jalkanen S (1992) A 90-kilodalton endothelial cell molecule mediating lymphocyte binding in humans. *Science* **257**: 1407–1409.

Salmi M, Granfors K, Leirisalo-Repo M, Hamalainen M, MacDermott R, Leino R et al. (1992) Selective endothelial binding of interleukin-2-dependent human T-cell lines derived from different tissues. *Proc Natl Acad Sci* **89**: 11436–11440.

Schall TJ, Jongstra J, Dyer BJ, Jorgensen J, Clayberger C, Davis MM et al. (1988) A human T cell-specific molecule is a member of a new gene family. *J Immunol* **141**: 1018–1025.

Schall TJ, Bacon K, Toy KJ & Goeddel DV (1990) Selective attraction of monocytes and T lymphocytes of the memory phenotype by cytokine RANTES. *Nature* **347**: 669–671.

Schall, TJ, Bacon K, Camp RDR, Kaspari JW & Goeddel DV (1993) Human macrophage inflammatory protein α (MIP-1α) and MIP-1β chemokines attract distinct populations of lymphocytes. *J Exp Med* **177**: 1821–1825.

Shimizu Y, van Seventer GA, Horgan KJ & Shaw S (1990a) Costimulation of proliferative responses of resting CD4$^+$ T cells by the interaction of VLA-4 and VLA-5 with fibronectin or VLA-6 with laminin. *J Immunol* **145**: 59–67.

Shimizu Y, van Seventer GA, Horgan KJ & Shaw S (1990b) Regulated expression and binding of three VLA ($\beta1$) integrin receptors on T cells. *Nature* **345**: 250–253.

Smith CW, Rothlein R, Hughes BJ, Mariscalco MM, Rudloff HE, Schmalsteig FC et al. (1988) Recognition of an endothelial determinant for CD18-dependent human neutrophil adherence and transendothelial migration. *J Clin Invest* **82**: 1746–1756.

Smith CW, Marlin SD, Rothlein R, Toman C & Anderson DC (1989) Cooperative interactions of LFA-1 and Mac-1 with intercellular adhesion molecule-1 in facilitating adherence and transendothelial migration of human neutrophils *in vitro*. *J Clin Invest* **83**: 2008–2017.

Smith MD & Roberts-Thompson PJ (1990) Lymphocyte surface marker expression in rheumatic diseases: Evidence for prior activation of lymphocytes *in vivo*. *Ann Rheum Dis* **49**: 81–87.

Springer TA (1990) Adhesion receptors of the immune system. *Nature* **346**: 425–434.

Taub DD, Conlon K, Lloyd AR, Oppenheim JJ & Kelvin DJ (1993) Preferential migration of activated CD4$^+$ and CD8$^+$ T cells in response to MIP-1α and MIP-1β. *Science* **260**: 355–358.

Tanaka Y, Albelda SM, Horgan KJ, van Seventer GA, Shimizu Y, Newman W et al. (1992) CD31 expressed on distinctive T cell subsets is a preferred amplifier of $\beta1$ integrin-mediated adhesion. *J Exp Med* **176**: 245–253.

Tanaka Y, Adams DH, Hubscher S, Hirano H, Siebenlist U & Shaw S (1993) T-cell adhesion induced by proteoglycan-immobilized cytokine MIP-1β. *Nature* **361**: 79–82.

van Seventer, GA, Shimizu Y, Horgan KJ & Shaw S (1990) The LFA-1 ligand ICAM-1 provides an important costimulatory signal for T cell receptor-mediated activation of resting T cells. *J Immunol* **144**: 4579–4586.

van Seventer GA, Newman W, Shimizu Y, Nutman TB, Tanaka Y, Horgan KJ et al. (1991) Analysis of T cell stimulation by superantigen plus major histocompatability complex class II molecules or by CD3 monoclonal antibody: Costimulation by purified adhesion ligands VCAM-1, ICAM-1, but not ELAM-1. *J Exp Med* **174**: 901–913.

Veale D, Yanni G, Rogers S, Barnes L, Bresnihan B & Fitzgerald O (1993) Reduced synovial membrane macrophage numbers, ELAM-1 expression, and lining layer hyperplasia in psoriatic arthritis as compared with rheumatoid arthritis. *Arthritis Rheum* **36**: 893–899.

Yanni G, Whelan A, Feighery C, Fitzgerald O & Bresnihan B (1993) Morphometric analysis of synovial membrane blood vessels in rheumatoid arthritis: Associations with the immunohistologic features, synovial fluid, cytokine levels and the clinical course. *J Rheumatol* **20**: 634–638.

Zvaifler N (1973) The immunopathology of joint inflammation in rheumatoid arthritis. *Adv Immunol* **16**: 265–336.

Humoral Mediators in
Rheumatoid Arthritis

12 Growth Factors in the Pathogenesis of Rheumatoid Arthritis

John Zagorski and Sharon M. Wahl

INTRODUCTION

Rheumatoid arthritis (RA) is a progressive degenerative disease of the extremities that is characterized by inflammation of the joint synovial lining, massive accumulation of T lymphocytes and mononuclear phagocytes, proliferation of synovial cells and erosive destruction of bone and cartilage (Poole, 1993; Poole *et al.*, 1993; see also Poole *et al.*, Chapter 9, this volume). While the etiology of RA remains elusive, it is generally believed that a foreign infectious agent, either bacteria or virus, may initiate a host inflammatory response in the joints which develops into an autoimmune disease and then progresses into a chronic inflammatory state (Harris, 1988; Firestein, 1991; McCulloch *et al.*, 1993). This point is reviewed in Chapters 3 and 22, this volume.

Even though the causative agent(s) of RA is unknown, the mechanisms involved in the subsequent host response leading to the chronic disease are becoming clearer. Since RA is an on-going disease, host-derived soluble factors must be present not only during the initiation of inflammation in the affected sites, but must also be continuously replenished during the progression of the disease. These soluble factors should *a priori* supply the biological activities necessary to explain the observed pathology of RA and this obvious fact helps us to make predictions concerning their identities. For the purpose of discussion, it is perhaps useful to consider the multistep nature of RA as the sum of many individual steps or actions. To reach the stage of flagrant RA, the inflammatory response has to be initiated, leukocytes recruited into the joints and activated, and synovial lining cells induced to proliferate. Consequently, host molecules that regulate these activities, such as the polypeptide growth factors, are of interest to the rheumatologist.

Numerous studies have been published that implicate growth factors in the pathogenesis of RA; however, most of the evidence is circumstantial in nature. In particular, much effort has been expended to characterize the phenotypes of isolated synovial cells or cell populations and their responses to exogenously added growth factors *in vitro*. While these studies may be used to extrapolate physiological actions *in vivo*, they do not directly address the question of how important a given molecule is in the disease process. Very few definitive experiments have been done that specifically ask whether a particular growth factor is either necessary or sufficient for the development of RA symptoms *in vivo* using animal models. While this chapter summarizes data correlating growth factor expression with disease pathology, it also attempts to emphasize the data that directly test growth factor requirements in RA and to interpret these results with respect to the known activities of the molecules. It also focuses

Mechanisms and Models in Rheumatoid Arthritis   Copyright © 1995 Academic Press Ltd
ISBN 0–12–340440–1   All rights of reproduction in any form reserved

primarily on polypeptide growth factors since cytokines have been covered in other chapters of this volume (2, 9, 10, 11, 13, 26).

MESENCHYMAL-CELL GROWTH FACTORS

One striking characteristic of RA is the excessive proliferation of synovial fibroblasts in inflamed joints. See Chapter 8, this volume, for a discussion of the kinetics of fibroblast division in the rheumatoid synovium. Since this process is presumably driven by growth factors for these cells, platelet-derived growth factor (PDGF) and the members of the fibroblast growth factor (FGF) family of peptides have become obvious candidates in the pathogenesis of RA. PDGF is a 30 kDa heterodimeric glycoprotein and is the major growth factor released during platelet activation (see Ross *et al.* (1986) for a comprehensive review). Seven members of the FGF family have been described (Burgess and Maciag, 1989; Goddard, 1992). By far the best characterized of these proteins are the two that were first purified and designated acidic FGF (aFGF) and basic FGF (bFGF) for their acidic and basic isoelectric points. Both aFGF and bFGF are growth factors for fibroblasts and endothelial cells as well as angiogenic factors (Folkman and Klagsbrun, 1987), activities which are consistent with processes that are on-going in arthrogenesis, namely, synovial hyperproliferation and angiogenesis. More recently, five additional proteins have been identified with activities similar to those of aFGF and bFGF. Since each of these molecules has been independently reported by several groups, nomenclatures have varied. Recently, the members of the FGF family have been assigned the designations FGFs 1 through 7 (Goddard, 1992), although FGF-1 and FGF-2 are still more commonly referred to by their historic names, aFGF and bFGF.

Both PDGF and aFGF have been identified within synovial tissues removed from RA patients. Using immunohistochemistry to identify the protein, Sano *et al.* (1990) demonstrated intense aFGF staining of RA synovia that was much less prominent in osteoarthritis (OA) samples; normal samples were not examined. Furthermore, the aFGF staining correlated with the degree of monocytic cell infiltrate determined by morphology (H&E staining). These results have been extended to show that PDGF immunostaining is also significantly greater in RA than OA samples. However, normal samples were not examined (Remmers *et al.*, 1991a). In this study, PDGF immunostaining correlated with the extent of mononuclear cell infiltration and with aFGF immunostaining although recent studies suggest that there is a novel PDGF-like molecule which is not PDGF (Bradham *et al.*, 1991). aFGF expression in a rat model of chronic inflammation has also been examined and found to be positive in synovia of euthymic Lewis rats but not athymic animals (Sano *et al.*, 1990 and see discussion below). Further studies examined the potential biological activity of aFGF and PDGF in arthritic tissues and demonstrated that phosphotyrosine-containing proteins co-localized with these growth factors in tissue sections (Sano *et al.*, 1993). Since the receptors for both aFGF and PDGF are protein tyrosine kinases, these data suggest that aFGF and PDGF were actively signalling in the RA tissues.

Considerable attention has been focused on synovial lining cells as a source of growth factors. Eguchi *et al.* (1992) have demonstrated that when fibroblastic synovial cells (synovioblasts), as well as umbilical vein endothelial cells, were wounded *in vitro* they released a growth-promoting activity for synovial cells and, to a lesser extent, endothelial cells. The activity produced by wounded endothelial cells was inhibitable by a blocking monoclonal antibody against bFGF. These results suggest that cell trauma or other stimuli in the rheumatoid joint may release growth factors that feed an autocrine proliferative loop. This hypothesis is consistent with the observations that vascular injury is observed early in the development of RA (Schumacher and Kitridou, 1972) and that cultured synoviocytes synthesize bFGF, express high affinity FGF receptors and proliferate *in vitro* in response to exogenous bFGF (Melnyk *et al.*, 1990). Curiously, the cDNA sequences of aFGF and bFGF, like those for IL-1α and IL-1β (Auron *et al.*, 1984; March *et al.*, 1985), do not code for traditional secretory signal sequences, making extracellular release problematic (Jaye *et al.*, 1986; Abraham *et al.*, 1986). Passive release of intracellular FGFs via cell damage may be an alternative to active secretion, allowing their rapid availability in response to a specific stimulus: trauma.

Autocrine growth factor expression is certainly not a novel phenomenon in proliferative disorders and it has been suggested that in this respect RA resembles a localized neoplasm (Fassbender, 1985). However, others have reported that although RA synovial cells constitutively make up to 10 times the amount of bFGF as normal synovial cells in culture, RA synovial cell growth *in vitro* is not significantly inhibited by anti-bFGF antibodies (Goddard *et al.*, 1992). In this study, expression of FGF-5 and FGF-7 was also detected in synovial cells using RT-PCR. It is possible that the failure of the anti-bFGF antibodies to inhibit RA synovial cell growth was caused by the presence of FGF-5 and FGF-7 activities that were not blocked. In support of this, multiple protein species were detected by the bFGF antibodies on western blots of RA synovial cell lysates, but their identities were not precisely determined (Goddard *et al.*, 1992).

In a survey of the effects of various growth factors on synovial cell proliferation, Remmers *et al.* demonstrated that PDGF, aFGF and bFGF but not EGF, TGFβ, IL-1α, TNFα nor IFNγ stimulated ^{3}H-thymidine incorporation into RA synovioblasts, consistent with the results of others (Butler *et al.*, 1989; Kumkumian *et al.*, 1989; Remmers *et al.*, 1990). These three factors also supported long-term growth of synovioblasts in serum-free media, an effect which was inhibited by TGFβ$_1$ and TFGβ$_2$. Synovial fluids from patients with RA also stimulated ^{3}H-thymidine incorporation into synovioblasts in a dose-dependent manner, but this effect was inhibited up to 82% by antibodies against PDGF. Explanted synovial tissues cultured *in vitro* also express a mitogen for synovioblasts that is inhibitable by antibodies against PDGF (Remmers *et al.*, 1991b).

COLONY-STIMULATING FACTORS: G-CSF, GM-CSF, M-CSF

Four haematopoietic growth factors, initially characterized by their abilities to induce growth of specific cell lineages in soft agar culture, have collectively been designated 'colony-stimulating factors' (CSFs; see Dexter *et al.* (1990) for a comprehensive treatise on these proteins). Granulocyte-macrophage CSF (GM-CSF) induces the proliferation of progenitor cells of these two lineages while macrophage colony stimulating factor (M-CSF) specifically supports cells of the monocyte/macrophage lineage and granulocyte colony stimulating factor (G-CSF) primarily supports granulocytes. The fourth molecule, IL-3 (multi-CSF, mast-cell growth factor), is highly pleiotropic and may help support the development of many types of haematopoietic progenitors. A role for IL-3 in the pathogenesis of RA is unlikely, however, since it has not been observed in arthritic synovia (Firestein *et al.*, 1988).

Although the CSFs were first located (and named) on the basis of their proliferative activities on immature leukocytes (reviewed in Metcalf, 1989), they have multiple additional activities. In fact, the activities of these proteins are nearly reversed when assayed on mature rather than progenitor target cells, becoming activation factors rather than differentiation and proliferative ones (Hamilton *et al.*, 1980; Weisbart *et al.*, 1985; Fleischmann *et al.*, 1986). Since the accumulation and activation of macrophages is a hallmark of RA, it has been of obvious interest to examine the association between CSFs and chronic joint inflammation.

Considerable circumstantial evidence exists implicating CSFs in the pathogenesis of RA. However, as related above for PDGF and the FGFs, much of this evidence is based either on observations that synovial cells in culture express CSFs constitutively or in response to pro-inflammatory stimuli, or that the proteins have been detected in primary synovial samples. Both IL-1 and TNF have been shown to induce GM-CSF and G-CSF in cultured synovioblasts *in vitro* (Leizer *et al.*, 1990; Alvaro-Gracia *et al.*, 1990). In the latter study, the effect of TNF, but not IL-1, was suppressed when IFNγ was co-administered. Similar results were obtained in an independent study although IFNγ was found to suppress both TNF and IL-1 induced expression (Hamilton *et al.*, 1992). GM-CSF and G-CSF expression in response to IL-1α was also suppressed by dexamethasone but enhanced by bFGF which, as related above, has been identified in RA synovia. In stark contrast to these results, IFNγ has been shown to increase three-fold the constitutive expression of M-CSF in synovioblasts (Hamilton *et al.*, 1993). Even more surprising, dexamethasome also increased both constitutive and IL-1-induced M-CSF expression in these cells, an effect opposite to its actions on GM-CSF and G-CSF expression.

The data concerning the antagonistic role of IFNγ in G-CSF and GM-CSF expression are in agreement with the observation that IFNγ is consistently found to be absent in RA synovia (Firestein and Zvaifler, 1987). However, since IFNγ is a major inducer of class II expression on macrophages (Nathan and Yoshida, 1987), this deficiency creates the separate problem of explaining the high levels of MHC class II antigen expression on RA macrophages. GM-CSF is also active in inducing MHC class II antigens on macrophages and is abundant in RA synovia, suggesting that it may be the primary mediator of class II expression in arthritis (Alvaro-Gracia *et al.*, 1989). A direct experimental demonstration of an inhibitory role for IFNγ in RA has been obtained using a streptococcal cell-wall induced arthritis model in rats in which exogenously administered IFNγ suppressed arthritic lesions (Allen *et al.*, 1991; Wahl *et al.*, 1991 and see below), consistent with its limited efficacy in human RA (Lemmel *et al.*, 1987; Cannon *et al.*, 1988; Veys *et al.*, 1988).

GM-CSF has been shown to be constitutively expressed by synovial macrophages and to stimulate their growth *in vitro* (Alvaro-Gracia *et al.*, 1991; Haworth *et al.*, 1991). Constitutive GM-CSF expression was evident with freshly isolated cells, but after 9 days in culture, stimulation with IL-1 or TNF was required (Alvaro-Gracia *et al.*, 1991). The transient, constitutive GM-CSF expression by the inflammatory macrophages was most likely dependent on autocrine expression of TNFα since antibodies against TNFα inhibited GM-CSF production when included in the culture medium (Haworth *et al.*, 1991). Further support for a TNFα autocrine loop is provided by the observation that RA mononuclear cells express higher levels of TNF receptors relative to normal cells, thus making them more sensitive to this cytokine (Brennan *et al.*, 1992). Surprisingly, growth stimulatory activity for M-CSF on synovial macrophages has also been tested and been found to be lacking (Yamamoto *et al.*, 1991).

Unfortunately, there have been relatively few studies in which the expression of the various CSFs has been examined on primary synovial samples (synovial fluids and tissue). In one early report, Firestein *et al.* (1988) detected M-CSF activity in RA synovial fluid and mRNA in tissue. However, the analysis of message expression was done on dispersed cells cultured *in vitro* for 3 days and so may not reflect accurately the situation *in vivo*. In follow-up experiments, *in situ* hybridization was used to assess the expression of cytokines including GM-CSF in synovial fluid and tissue-derived cells. A significant percentage of RA synovial tissue cells, but not RA synovial fluid cells, was positive for mRNA for GM-CSF as well as for IL-6, IL-1β, TNFα and TGFβ (Firestein *et al.*, 1990). Significantly, IFNγ message was not detected. Colony-stimulating activity has also been detected directly in the synovial fluids of patients with RA although the assays employed could not establish the identities of the proteins (Williamson *et al.*, 1988). In a more convincing study, Chu *et al.* (1992) compared the expression of several cytokines at the cartilage/pannus junction (CPJ) in RA and normal tissues. Using antibodies raised against recombinant human proteins and immunohistochemical analyses, both GM-CSF and TGFβ (as well as IL-1α, TNFα and IL-6) were found to be abundant in RA samples but absent from normal controls.

In a recent study, Kotake *et al.* (1992) reported increased numbers of myeloid precursor cells (colony-forming units) in the marrow of tibial bones adjacent to sites of arthritis in RA patients. Since active haematopoiesis does not normally occur at this site in humans (Hashimoto, 1962), these data suggest that haematopoietic growth factors present in the arthritic lesion may be stimulating leukocyte development inappropriately (see Chapter 10 for further discussion). Local *de novo* maturation of leukocytes by growth factors present at the arthritic site may exacerbate the inflammation caused by cells recruited from the circulation.

Direct evidence for CSF involvement in RA *in vivo* is, unfortunately, meagre. However, administration of M-CSF has been shown to worsen the severity and extend the chronic phase of inflammation in a *Streptococcus agalactiae* model of RA (Abd *et al.*, 1991). Treatment of Wistar rats with 50 000 U of M-CSF at the time of injection of *S. agalactiae* sonicate and for the subsequent 3 days resulted in a persistent arthritic response (>25 days). In contrast, joint inflammation in control animals receiving only streptococcal sonicate peaked at 10–15 days and subsided to near normal after 25 days. The fact that continuous infusion of M-CSF was not necessary suggests that M-CSF can act early in the disease process.

Two somewhat anecdotal studies on humans have also been reported, both involving treatment of patients with recombinant GM-CSF. In one instance, in which GM-CSF was used during cancer chemotherapy on a patient with RA, the cytokine treatment was reported to exacerbate the arthritis (De Vries *et al.*, 1991). This effect was gradually reduced after the GM-CSF was discontinued. In another patient with Felty's syndrome, GM-CSF was used to treat the granulocytopenia associated with the disease but this treatment also aggravated the arthritis. This effect was associated with a massive increase in circulating neutrophils and eosinophils and elevated levels of IL-6 and acute-phase response proteins (Hazenberg *et al.*, 1989).

In another interesting report, the anti-arthritic gold compound auranofin was tested for its ability to inhibit TNF- and GM-CSF-mediated neutrofil degranulation (Richter, 1990). Although the mechanism of action of auranofin is unknown, previous studies have demonstrated several inhibitory activities towards neutrophils (Dimartino and Walz, 1977; Hafström *et al.*, 1983; Herlin *et al.*, 1989). Pre-incubation of neutrophils with concentrations of auranofin achieved *in vivo* during treatment of arthritis made cells refractory to TNF- and GM-CSF-inducd lactoferrin and myeloperoxidase secretion. This result suggests that the mechanism by which auranofin exerts its anti-arthritic effects may, at least in part, be via desensitization of leukocytes to the activities of cytokines and growth factors within the arthritic joint.

Although the presence of growth factors such as PDGF, FGF and the CSFs in RA synovial fluids and tissues suggests that these proteins play a role in the pathogenesis of the disease process, it is difficult and premature to infer their relative contributions. Cultured synovial cells, often used as targets to evaluate the activities of protein factors *in vitro*, presumably lose their *in vivo* phenotypes during culture. Also, a recent study has emphatically demonstrated that cultures of synovial cells obtained from individual RA patients differ in their *in vitro* synthesis of growth factors (Bucala *et al.*, 1991). Thus, properties of cells and proteins seen *in vitro* may not be an accurate reproduction of their contributions to the maintenance of chronic inflammation *in vivo*. Further, it is clear from the results described above that multiple inflammatory mediators with overlapping activities are found in the arthritic joint. Analysis of the activities of individual molecules on cells *in vitro* certainly provides important clues to *in vivo* processes but does not prove involvement *in vivo*.

TRANSFORMING GROWTH FACTOR β

The transforming growth factor-βs (TGFβ) are a family of three mammalian 25-kDa proteins, TGFβ$_1$, TGFβ$_2$, TGFβ$_3$ (for recent comprehensive reviews see Roberts and Sporn, 1990; Wahl, 1992: McCartney-Francis and Wahl, 1994). Of these proteins, TGFβ$_1$ and TGFβ$_2$ have been the best characterized and appear to have many inter-changeable activities. Both of these molecules have a bewildering array of pro- and anti-inflammatory activities on numerous cell types and in fact, virtually every cell type tested expresses TGFβ receptors (reviewed in Segarini, 1991). Expression of TGFβ activity is complicated and involves transcriptional, translational and post-translational mechanisms. The latter is a particularly important point to consider since TGFβ is secreted in an inactive, latent form, and many studies have been limited to showing its presence without demonstrating that it is functionally active.

Three receptors for the TGFβs have been identified and cloned. The type I and type II receptors are glycoproteins with native molecular weights of 65 kDa and 85–100 kDa, respectively. However, the type III receptor is a proteoglycan of approximate mass of 250–350 kDa. Since the three TGFβ receptors share limited primary sequence homology, it seems likely that they are functionally non-equivalent. This has certainly been demonstrated for the type III receptor, which does not signal in response to ligand binding. Recent evidence indicates that its function is to 'present' ligand to the other TGFβ receptors expressed on the cell surface (López-Casillas *et al.*, 1993). Receptor regulation is complex and on monocytes, TGFβ has been shown to regulate expression of its own receptors. This is an important observation since it provides for a negative feedback mechanism (Brandes *et al.*, 1991b,c; Brandes *et al.*, unpublished).

Although the primary activities of TGFβ can best be summarized as immunosuppressive, TGFβ is also the most potent leukocyte chemoattractant known (Wahl *et al.*, 1987; Adams *et al.*, 1991; Brandes *et al.*, 1991b), clearly a proinflammatory property. When injected intra-articularly into rats, TGFβ has been shown to elicit rapid recruitment of neutrophils and monocytes into the joints (Allen *et al.*, 1990; Fava *et al.*, 1991). However, TGFβ is also capable of 'deactivating' peritoneal macrophages by making them refractory to the normally activating effect of phorbol myristic acetate (PMA) (Tsunawaki *et al.*, 1988). Also, although TGFβ induces the expression of IL-1β in isolated peripheral blood monocytes, this expression subsequently feeds back to induce expression of IL-1 receptor-antagonist which limits the pro-inflammatory response (Wahl *et al.*, 1993c). Thus, the presence of TGFβ at a particular site may promote or suppress the inflammatory response depending on the local circumstances. Supportive evidence for the biphasic functions for TGFβ *in vivo* is provided by studies utilizing a rat model of chronic inflammation (see below).

As is the situation with other cytokines mentioned above, TGFβ levels are elevated in the synovial fluids of RA patients and animals with experimentally induced RA-like chronic inflammation (Wahl *et al.*, 1988a; Lotz *et al.*, 1990; Miossec *et al.*, 1990; Thorbecke *et al.*, 1992). However, the use of correlative studies to assess the role of TGFβ in RA has been quite confusing. Brennan *et al.* (1990) compared the levels of active and latent TGFβ in synovial fluids from patients with RA and non-RA joint inflammation. Both forms of TGFβ were detected in each group of patients but more was detected in the non-RA group than in the RA group, suggesting an inverse relationship between TGF-β levels and severity of joint disease. However, it has also been reported that RA but not OA synovial cells proliferate under serum-free conditions *in vitro* and that this growth is inhibited by anti-TGFβ antibodies (Goddard *et al.*, 1992). These data, suggesting an autocrine proliferative loop, are more consistent with a direct relationship between TGFβ expression and RA pathogenesis.

As with most complex pathologies, the *in vitro* study of individual cell types and molecules cannot possibly reproduce the interacting networks of cellular and molecular pathways operating *in vivo*. Animal models of human disease are thus a necessity for the elaboration of the mechanisms involved in disease progression. In the case of RA, a particularly successful model has been the streptococcal cell wall model. A single injection of streptococcal cell wall (SCW) fragments into the peritoneal cavities of genetically susceptible Lewis rats results in biphasic inflammation in the joints which resembles RA (Cromartie *et al.*, 1977; Imamichi *et al.*, 1993). Approximately 3 days after SCW injection, an acute inflammation develops in the joints which partially subsides after 1 week. Following a delay period, joint inflammation resumes and within 3 weeks becomes chronic. In addition to the joint inflammation, massive mononuclear cell influx into the liver and spleen results in hepatic granuloma formation and spleen cell dysfunction during the chronic phase of the joint inflammation (Wahl, 1988; Manthey *et al.*, 1990). The acute phase of the disease is relatively insensitive to rat strain or sex, but the chronic phase is dependent on several factors including strain, sex and age and is also T-cell dependent (Hines *et al.*, 1993 and see below). Bacterial cell-wall induced arthritis is discussed in Chapter 22, this volume.

High levels of TGFβ are found in the inflamed joints of rats injected with SCW suggesting a positive correlation with the disease process (Fava *et al.*, 1989; Lafyatis *et al.*, 1989; Wahl, 1991). This is supported by experiments in which direct injection of TGFβ into the joints of Lewis rats results in acute arthritic swelling (Allen *et al.*, 1990; Fava *et al.*, 1991). Consistent with these results, injection of a blocking antibody against TGFβ into the joints of rats receiving SCW intraperitoneally inhibits the chronic phase of inflammation (Wahl *et al.*, 1993a). Thus, it seems clear that local expression of TGFβ in the joint favours a pro-inflammatory state and that inhibition of local TGFβ is therapeutic. Paradoxically, intraperitoneal injection of TGFβ into rats results in resistance to SCW-initiated inflammation even when the TGFβ is administered 10 days after the SCW injections and after the acute phase subsides (Brandes *et al.*, 1991a). This latter result may in part be explained by the ability of TGFβ to inhibit leukocytosis (Brandes *et al.*, 1991a), the requisite chemotactic gradient, and the adhesiveness of endothelial cells for neutrophils and some lymphocytes (Gamble and Vadas, 1988, 1991). Specifically, TGFβ has recently been shown to inhibit both basal and TNFα-induced expression of E-selectin on endothelial cells (Gamble *et al.*, 1993). Since E-selectin is thought to participate in the initial binding of circulating leukocytes to vascular endothelial cells at inflammatory sites (Butcher, 1991; reviewed in detail in Chapter 11, this volume), E-selectin down-regulation *in vivo* would presumably be immunosuppressive.

Results very similar to those obtained with the SCW-rat model have been reported in another animal model. When injected into genetically susceptible mice, type-II collagen also induces a chronic joint inflammation that resembles arthritis (Trentham *et al.*, 1977; Stuart *et al.*, 1982; see Chapters 19 and 23, this volume). Using this model, Kuruvilla *et al.* (1991) and Thorbecke *et al.* (1992) demonstrated that when injected intraperitoneally, TGFβ significantly reduces both the incidence and severity of joint inflammation. TGFβ treatment was most efficacious when administered immediately prior to the onset of the disease or at the time of onset and continuing during the progressive phase. However, at higher doses, some protection was obtained when administered soon after collagen immunization, fully 4 weeks before arthritic incidence. Conversely, systemic injection of anti-TGFβ antibodies by this same route aggravates the arthritis by accelerating the onset of inflammation, but has little effect on the severity of joint swelling. The deleterious effect of the antibody was presumably caused by inhibition of the immunosuppressive activity of endogenous TGFβ. In related studies, direct injection of TGFβ into the joints of collagen-immunized mice was shown to increase dramatically both the incidence and severity of arthritis (Cooper *et al.*, 1992). Similar treatment of normal rabbits also produces an arthritis-like inflammation (Elford *et al.*, 1992).

Collectively, the data obtained with the SCW-rats and type-II collagen mice point to a model in which systemic presence of TGFβ may be immunosuppressive due to its ability to interfere with chemotaxis of circulating monocytes, inhibit endothelial adhesiveness, and act as an IL-1 antagonist (Wahl *et al.*, 1988b, 1990; Harvey *et al.*, 1991) while local expression of TGFβ is pro-inflammatory due to its chemotactic and proliferative activities (DeLarco and Todaro, 1978; McCartney-Francis *et al.*, 1990). In addition, the TGFβ results obtained with the animal models highlight the limitations of *in vitro* studies which, by their nature, cannot reproduce the natural cell–cell and cell–cytokine interactions found *in vivo*.

T LYMPHOCYTE GROWTH FACTORS

T-cell accumulation in inflamed joints is a characteristic of arthritis, but the role of T-cell populations in chronic RA is controversial. For example, SCW-induced arthritis does not occur in nude (athymic) Lewis rats as it does in euthymic animals (Ridge *et al.*, 1985; Allen *et al.*, 1985). Also, administration of cyclosporin A, an inhibitor of T-lymphocyte activation, dramatically reduces joint inflammation in Lewis rats injected with SCW (Yocum *et al.*, 1986). While these data strongly implicate T cells in the development of chronic arthritis, the products of activated T cells such as TNFβ, IL-2 (T-cell growth factor), IL-3 (multi-CSF), IL-4 and IFNγ are conspicuously absent from synovial fluids (Firestein and Zvaifler, 1987; Firestein *et al.*, 1988; Saxne *et al.*, 1988; Miossec *et al.*, 1990; see Chapter 13, this volume) and T cells in human RA are morphologically quiescent (Nykanen *et al.*, 1986; Lalor *et al.*, 1987). It is possible that the difficulty in observing soluble T-cell products in RA may be due to their transient expression by 'activated' T cells early in the disease process.

Not only are the products of activated T lymphocytes absent from arthritic synovia, numerous attempts to demonstrate oligoclonal expansion of T cells at these sites have been inconsistent at best (e.g. Savill *et al.*, 1987; Stamenkovic *et al.*, 1988; Duby *et al.*, 1989). While these results suggest that synovial T lymphocytes are not responding to any specific antigen, it is also possible that RA T cells are subject to local conditions favouring anergy (Nossal and Pike, 1980; Miller and Morahan, 1992). Regardless of the mechanisms involved, the apparent heterogeneity of T-cell receptors on RA lymphocytes suggests that the requirement for T cells in RA does not include extensive clonal expansion. The contradictory observations of T-cell dependence and questionable T-cell activation in arthritis continue unresolved. More detailed discussion of this subject is found in Chapters 2, 3, 19 and 22, this volume.

The importance of the observations that IL-4 and IFNγ are absent from RA samples is heightened by the demonstrations that both molecules suppress SCW-induced arthritis in Lewis rats when supplied exogenously (Allen *et al.*, 1991, 1993; Wahl *et al.*, 1991). The protective effect of IL-4 is most likely explained by the well-established immunosuppressive activity of IL-4 on monocytes (Wong *et al.*, 1992; Allen *et al.*, 1993 and references therein) suggesting that the absence of IL-4 from arthritic joints contributes to the overall pro-inflammatory state of the RA synovium. However, since monocyte activation is normally enhanced by IFNγ (Nathan and Yoshida, 1987), it is more difficult to explain the suppressive effect of IFNγ in the rat SCW arthritis model. This paradox may have been somewhat diminished by the demonstration that IFNγ down-regulates the receptor for the chemotactic peptide C5a (Katona *et al.*, 1991; Wahl *et al.*, 1991), resulting in a reduced chemotactic response (Wahl *et al.*, 1991), and by the observations that IFNγ inhibits constitutive production of IL-1β (Ruschen *et al.*, 1989) and cytokine-induced CSF expression (Leizer *et al.*, 1990; Alvaro-Gracia *et al.*, 1990; Hamilton *et al.*, 1992) by RA synovial macrophages. Thus, IFNγ may exert opposite immunomodulatory activities depending upon when or where it is expressed, results which are reminiscent of TGFβ.

PROTEASES AND SYNOVIAL DEGRADATION

Despite the excessive proliferation of synovioblasts and recruitment of leukocytes at sites of chronic joint inflammation, RA is as much a disease of degeneration as growth. An important component of late-stage RA is the severe joint destruction that results from degradation of articular cartilage and resorption of bone, presumably caused by secretion of proteases by synovial cells (see Chapters 6, 9, 10 and 17, this volume). The accumulation of phagocytic macrophages and neutrophils within the synovium would alone provide an ample reservoir for proteolytic activity (Muirden, 1972), but the proliferation of synovial fibroblasts adds additional capacity for tissue destruction. In agreement with this scenario, high levels of several proteases have been observed in arthritic synovial fluids compared to normal synovial fluids (Krane, 1975; Breedveld *et al.*, 1987; Walakovits *et al.*, 1992). Although specific protease inhibitors have also been detected in arthritis synovial fluid (Cawston *et al.*, 1984; McCachren, 1991), it has been suggested that an imbalance in the levels of proteases and their inhibitors may exist in arthritic diseases which could produce a net pro-proteolytic environment (Dean *et al.*, 1987 and Chapters 9 and 17, this volume).

Since TGFβ is normally associated with extracellular matrix deposition and wound repair, it might not be considered an obvious candidate as a mediator of cartilage destruction in arthritis. In fact, TGFβ has been demonstrated to induce synthesis of plasminogen activator inhibitor-1 (PAI-1), the natural inhibitor of urokinase-type plasminogen activator (UPA) in a human fibrosarcoma cell line (Laiho *et al.*, 1987) and TIMP (tissue inhibitor of metalloproteinases; Wright *et al.*, 1991). UPA, like the related protein tissue-type plasminogen activator (TPA), is responsible for cleaving plasminogen into its active form of plasmin. Plasmin in turn has the capacity to activate proteolytically many other proenzymes, thus perpetuating protease cascades. TGFβ has also been shown to suppress epidermal growth factor (EGF) and bFGF-induced collagenase and stromelysin expression in the human MRC-5 fibroblast cell line (Edwards *et al.*, 1987).

However, some evidence is emerging that TGFβ may actually enhance proteolytic degradation in RA. For example, TGFβ has been shown to induce UPA activity in human synovioblasts (Hamilton *et al.*, 1991) and type IV collagenase secretion in human peripheral blood monocytes (Wahl *et al.*, 1993b). Although type IV collagen is not a constituent of cartilage and bone, expression of type IV collagenase in inflamed synovia may lead to degradation of synovial microvascular basement membranes, thus allowing easier access of circulating leukocytes to the synovial spaces. It is interesting that the presence in synovia of these two enzymes, also strongly implicated in the invasive phenotype of metastatic neoplasms (Aznavoorian *et al.*, 1993), again provides an association between these two proliferative disorders.

CONCLUSIONS AND FUTURE PROSPECTS

It is certainly not surprising that the immunopathogenesis of RA is complex and probably dependent on numerous pro-inflammatory mediators. Within the inflammatory and immunological milieu of the RA synovium, the coexpression of redundant and pleiotropic proteins presumably creates cytokine networks capable of self-perpetuation under appropriate circumstances. A representation of such a network is

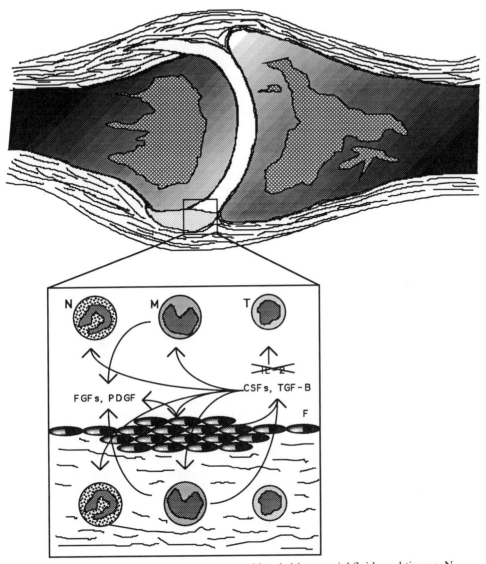

Figure 1. Growth factor networks in rheumatoid arthritis synovial fluids and tissues. N, Neutrophils; M, macrophages; T, T lymphocytes; F, synovial fibroblast.

given in Fig. 1. The portion of the diagram enclosed by the smaller insert represents a region of synovial inflammation and extensive proliferation of synovial fibroblasts (stippled area). In the enlarged insert, the normal monolayer organization of synovial lining fibroblasts is shown in the early stages of what is ostensibly 'focus' formation. Continued proliferation of synovioblasts results in the intrusion of a cellular mass into the joint space.

It is becoming quite clear that because of the redundancy and pleiotropy of the RA cytokine network (see Arend and Dayer (1990) for a brief review), data obtained from the *in vitro* study of individual molecules involved in the RA cytokine network should mainly be used as a guide for further *in vivo* studies. In fact, direct examination of growth factor requirements using *in vivo* models of RA must occur if promising therapeutic targets are to be identified. Using the SCW- and type II collagen-induced animal arthropathies, it is now certain that TGFβ is essential for the development of RA-like symptoms and that its antagonism at the local level is beneficial. Therefore, even though the complex mix of activities found within the RA joint portends a pharmaceutical challenge, as demonstrated *in vivo* for TGFβ, it is clear that interruption of a cytokine network can lead to its dissolution.

REFERENCES

Abd AHA, Savage NW, Halliday WJ & Hume DA (1991) The role of macrophages in experimental arthritis induced by *Streptococcus agalactiae* sonicate: Actions of macrophage colony stimulating factor (CSF-1) and other macrophage modulating agents. *Lymphokine Cytokine Res* 10: 43–50.

Abraham JA, Whang JL, Tumolo A, Meria A, Friedman J, Gospodarowicz D et al. (1986) Human basic fibroblast growth factor: Nucleotide sequence and genomic organization. *EMBO J* 5: 2523–2528.

Adams DH, Hathaway M, Shaw J, Burnett D, Elias E & Strain AJ (1991) Transforming growth factor-β induces human T-lymphocyte migration *in vitro*. *J Immunol* 147: 609–612.

Allen JB, Malone DG, Wahl SM, Calandra GB & Wilder RL (1985) Role of the thumus in streptococcal cell wall-induced arthritis and hepatic granuloma formation: Comparative studies of the pathology and cell wall distribution in athymic and euthymic rats. *J Clin Invest* 76: 1042–1056.

Allen JB, Manthey CL, Hand AR, Ohura K, Ellingsworth L & Wahl SM (1990) Rapid onset synovial inflammation and hyperplasia induced by transforming growth factor β. *J Exp Med* 171: 231–247.

Allen JB, Bansal G, Feldman GM, Hand AO, Wahl LM & Wahl SM (1991) Suppression of bacterial cell wall-induced polyarthritis by recombinant gamma interferon. *Cytokine* 3: 98–106.

Allen JB, Wong HL, Costa GL, Bienkowski MJ & Wahl SM (1993) Suppression of monocyte function and differential regulation of IL-1 and IL-1ra by IL-4 contribute to resolution of experimental arthritis. *J Immunol*, in press.

Alvaro-Gracia JM, Zvaifler NJ & Firestein GS (1989) Cytokines in chronic inflammatory arthritis. IV. Granulocyte/macrophage colony-stimulating factor-mediated induction of class II MHC antigen on human monocytes: a possible role in rheumatoid arthritis. *J Exp Med* 170: 865–875.

Alvaro-Gracia JM, Zvaifler NJ & Firestein GS (1990) Cytokines in chronic inflammatory arthritis. V. Mutual antagonism between interferon-gamma and tumor necrosis factor-alpha on HLA-DR expression, proliferation, collagenase production, and granulocyte macrophage colony-stimulating factor production by rheumatoid arthritis synoviocytes. *J Clin Invest* 86: 1790–1798.

Alvaro-Gracia JM, Zvaifler NJ, Brown CB, Kaushansky K & Firestein GS (1991) Cytokines in chronic inflammatory arthritis. VI. Analysis of the synovial cells involved in granulocyte-macrophage colony-stimulating factor production and gene expression in rheumatoid arthritis and its regulation by IL-1 and tumor necrosis factor-α. *J Immunol* 146: 3365–3371.

Arend WP & Dayer J-M (1990) Cytokines and cytokine inhibitors or antagonists in rheumatoid arthritis. *Arthritis Rheum* 33: 305–315.

Auron PE, Webb AC, Rosenwasser LJ, Mucci SF, Rich A, Wolff SM et al. (1984) Nucelotide sequence of human monocyte interleukin 1 precursor cDNA. *Proc Natl Acad Sci USA* 81: 7907–7911.

Aznavoorian S, Murphy AN, Stetler-Stevenson WG & Liotta LA (1993) Molecular aspects of tumor cell invasion and metastasis. *Cancer* 71: 1368–1383.

Bradham DM, Igarashi A, Potter RL & Grotendorst GR (1991) Connective tissue growth factor: a cysteine-rich mitogen secreted by human vascular endothelial cells is related to the SRC-induced immediate early gene product CEF-10. *J Cell Biol* 114: 1285–1294.

Brandes ME, Allen JB, Ogawa Y & Wahl SM (1991a) Transforming growth factor β1 suppresses acute and chronic arthritis in experimental animals. *J Clin Invest* 87: 1108–1113.

Brandes ME, Mai UEH, Ohura K & Wahl SM (1991b) Human neutrophils express type I TGF-β receptors and chemotax to TGF-β. *J Immunol* 147: 1600–1606.

Brandes ME, Wakefield LM & Wahl SM (1991c) Modulation of monocyte type I transforming growth factor-β receptors by inflammatory stimuli. *J Biol Chem* 266: 19697–19703.

Breedveld FC, Lafeber GJM, Seigert CEH, Vlemming L-J & Cats A (1987) Elastase and collagenase activities in synovial fluid of patients with arthritis. *J Rheumatol* 14: 1008–1012.

Brennan FM, Chantry D, Turner M, Foxwell B, Maini R & Feldmann M (1990) Detection of transforming growth factor-beta in rheumatoid arthritis synovial tissue: lack of effect on spontaneous cytokine production in joint cell cultures. *Clin Exp Immunol* 81: 278–285.

Brennan FM, Gibbons DL, Mitchell T, Cope AP, Maini RN & Feldmann M (1992) Enhanced expression of tumor necrosis factor receptor mRNA and protein in mononuclear cells isolated from rheumatoid arthritis synovial joints. *Eur J Immunol* **22**: 1907–1912.

Bucala R, Ritchlin C, Winchester R & Cerami A (1991) Constitutive production of inflammatory and mitogenic cytokines by rheumatoid synovial fibroblasts. *J Exp Med* **173**: 569–574.

Burgess WH & Maciag T (1989) The heparin-binding (fibroblast) growth factor family of proteins. *Annu Rev Biochem* **58**: 575–606.

Butcher EC (1991) Leukocyte–endothelial cell recognition: Three (or more) steps to specificity and diversity. *Cell* **67**: 1033–1036.

Butler DM, Leizer T & Hamilton JA (1989) Stimulation of human synovial fibroblast DNA synthesis by platelet-derived growth factor and fibroblast growth factor: Differences to the activation by IL-1. *J Immunol* **142**: 3098–3103.

Cannon GW, Pincus SH, Emkey RD, Denes A, Cohen SA, Wolfe A et al. (1988) Double-blind trial of recombinant γ-interferon versus placebo in the treatment of rheumatoid arthritis. *Arthritis Rheum* **32**: 964–973.

Cawston TE, Mercer E, De Silva M & Hazleman BL (1984) Metalloproteinases and collagenase inhibitors in rheumatoid synovial fluid. *Arthritis Rheum* **27**: 285–290.

Chu CQ, Field M, Allard S, Abney E, Feldman M & Maini RN (1992) Detection of cytokines at the cartilage/pannus junction in patients with rheumatoid arthritis: implications for the role of cytokines in cartilage destruction and repair. *Br J Rheumatol* **31**: 653–661.

Cooper WO, Fava RA, Gates CA, Cremer MA & Townes AS (1992) Acceleration of the onset of collagen-induced arthritis by intra-articular injection of tumor necrosis factor or transforming growth factor-beta. *Clin Exp Immunol* **89**: 244–250.

Cromartie WJ, Craddock JG, Schwab JM, Anderle SK & Yang C-H (1977) Arthritis in rats after systemic injection of streptococcal cells or cell walls. *J Exp Med* **146**: 1585–1602.

Dean DD, Azzo W, Martel-Pelletier J, Pelletier J-P & Woessner JF (1987) Levels of metalloproteinases and tissue inhibitor of metalloproteinases in human osteoarathritic cartilage. *J Rheumatol* **14** (**supplement**): 43–44.

DeLarco JE & Todaro GJ (1978) Growth factors from murine sarcoma virus-transformed cells. *Proc Natl Acad Sci USA* **75**: 4001–4005.

De Vries DGE, Willemse PHB, Biesma B, Stern AC, Limburg PC & Vallenga E (1991) Flare-up of rheumatoid arthritis during GM-CSF treatment after chemotherapy. *Lancet* **338**: 517–518.

Dexter TM, Garland JM & Testa NG (eds) (1990) *Colony Stimulating Factors: Molecular and Cellular Biology.* New York: Marcel Dekker.

Dimartino MJ & Walz DT (1977) Inhibition of lysosomal enzyme release from rat leukocytes by auranofin. *Inflammation* **2**: 131–142.

Duby AD, Sinclair AK, Osnorne-Lawrence SL, Zeldes W, Kan L & Fox DA (1989) Clonal heterogeneity of synovial fluid T lymphocytes from patients with rheumatoid arthritis. *Proc Natl Acad Sci USA* **86**: 6206–6210.

Edwards DR, Murphy G, Reynolds JJ, Whitham SE, Docherty AJP, Angel P et al. (1987) Transforming growth factor beta modulates the expression of collagenase and metalloproteinase inhibitor. *EMBO J* **6**: 1899–1904.

Eguchi K, Migita K, Nakashima M, Ida H, Terada K, Sakai M et al. (1992) Fibroblast growth factors released by wounded endothelial cells stimulate proliferation of synovial cells. *J Rheumatol* **19**: 1925–1932.

Elford PR, Graeber M, Ohtsu H, Aeberhard M, Legendre B, Wishart WL et al. (1992) Induction of swelling, synovial hyperplasia and cartilage proteoglycan loss upon intra-articular injection of transforming growth factor β-2 in the rabbit. *Cytokine* **4**: 232–238.

Fassbender HG (1985) The disease picture in rheumatoid arthritis as a result of different pathomechanisms. *Z Rheumatol* **44**: 33–46.

Fava R, Olsen N, Keski-Oja J, Moses H & Pincus T (1989) Active and latent forms of transforming growth factor β activity in synovial effusions. *J Exp Med* **169**: 291–296.

Fava RA, Olsen NJ, Postlethwaite AE, Broadley KN, Davidson JM, Nanney LB et al. (1991) Transforming growth factor β1 (TGF-β1) induced neutrophil recruitment to synovial tissues: implications for TGF-β-driven synovial inflammation and hyperplasia. *J Exp Med* **173**: 1121–1132.

Firestein GS (1991) The immunopathogenesis of rheumatoid arthritis. *Curr Opinion Rheumatol* **3**: 398–406.

Firestein GS & Zvaifler NJ (1987) Peripheral blood and synovial fluid monocyte activation in inflammatory arthritis. II. Low levels of synovial fluid and synovial tissue interferon suggest that gamma-interferon is not the primary macrophage activating factor. *Arthritis Rheum* **30**: 864–871.

Firestein GS, Xu W-D, Townsend K, Broide D, Alvaro-Gracia J, Glasebrook A et al. (1988) Cytokines in chronic inflammatory arthritis. I. Failure to detect T cell lymphokines (interleukin 2 and interleukin 3) and presence of macrophage colony-stimulating factor (CSF-1) and a novel mast cell growth factor in rheumatoid synovitis. *J Exp Med* **168**: 1573–1586.

Firestein GS, Alvaro-Gracia JM & Maki R (1990) Quantitative analysis of cytokine gene expression in rheumatoid arthritis. *J Immunol* **144**: 3347–3353.

Fleischmann S, Golde DW, Weisbart RH & Gasson JC (1986) Granulocyte-macrophage colony-stimulating factor enhances phagocytosis of bacteria by human neutrophils. *Blood* **68**: 708–711.

Folkman J & Klagsbrun M (1987) Angiogenic factors. *Science* **235**: 442–447.

Gamble JR & Vadas MA (1988) Endothelial adhesiveness for blood neutrophils is inhibited by transforming growth factor-β. *Science* **242**: 97–99.

Gamble JR & Vadas MA (1991) Endothelial adhesiveness for human T-lymphocytes is inhibited by TGF-β. *J Immunol* **146**: 1149–1154.

Gamble JR, Khew-Goodall Y & Vadas MA (1993) Transforming growth factor-β inhibits E-selectin expression on human endothelial cells. *J Immunol* **150**: 4494–4503.

Goddard DH (1992) Regulation of synovial cell growth by polypeptide growth factors. *DNA Cell Biol* **11**: 259–263.

Goddard DH, Grossman SL, Williams WV, Weiner DB, Gross JL, Eidsvoog K & Dasch JR (1992) Regulation of synovial cell growth: coexpression of transforming growth factor β and basic fibroblast growth factor by cultured synovial cells. *Arthritis Rheum* **35**: 1296–1303.

Hafström I, Uden AM & Palmblad J (1983) Modulation of neutrophil functions by auranofin. *Scand J Rheumatol* **12**: 97–105.

Hamilton JA, Stanley ER, Burgess AW & Shadduck R (1980) Stimulation of macrophage plasminogen activator by colony stimulating factors. *J Cell Physiol* **103**: 435–445.

Hamilton JA, Piccoli DS, Leizer T, Butler DM, Croatto M & Royston AKM (1991) Transforming growth factor β stimulates urokinase-type plasminogen activator and DNA synthesis, but not prostaglandin E_2 production, in human synovial fibroblasts. *Proc Natl Acad Sci USA* **88**: 7180–7184.

Hamilton JA, Piccoli DS, Cebon J, Layton JE, Rathanaswani P, McColl SR & Leizer T (1992) Cytokine regulation of colony-stimulating factor (CSF) production in cultured human synovial fibroblasts. II. Similarities and differences in the control of interleukin-1 induction of granulocyte-macrophage CSF and granulocyte-CSF production. *Blood* **79**: 1413–1419.

Hamilton JA, Filonzi EL & Ianches G (1993) Regulation of macrophage colony stimulating factor (M-CSF) production in cultured human synovial fibroblasts. *Growth Factors* **9**: 157–165.

Harris ED (1988) Pathogenesis of rheumatoid arthritis: a disorder associated with dysfunctional immuno-regulation. In Gallin JI, Goldstein IM & Snyderman R (eds) *Inflammation: Basic Principles and Clinical Correlates*, pp 751–773. New York: Raven.

Harvey AK, Hrubey PS & Chandrasekhar S (1991) Transforming growth factor-β inhibition of interleukin-1 activity involves down-regulation of interleukin-1 receptors on chondrocytes. *Exp Cell Res* **195**: 376–385.

Hashimoto M (1962) Pathology of bone marrow. *Acta Haematol* **27**: 193–216.

Haworth C, Brennan FM, Chantry D, Turner M, Maini RN & Feldmann M (1991) Expression of granulo-cyte-macrophage colony-stimulating factor in rheumatoid arthritis: regulation by tumor necrosis factor-α. *Eur J Immunol* **21**: 2575–2579.

Hazenberg BPC, van Leeuwen MA, van Rijswijk MH, Stern AC & Vellenga E (1989) Correction of granulocytopenia in Felty's syndrome by granulocyte-macrophage colony-stimulating factor: Simultaneous induction of interleukin-6 release and flare-up of the arthritis. *Blood* **74**: 2769–2770.

Herlin T, Fogh K, Christiansen NO & Kragbaille K (1989) Effect of auranofin on eicosanoids and protein kinase C in human neutrophils. *Agents Actions* **28**: 121–129.

Hines KL, Christ M & Wahl SM (1993) Cytokine regulation of the immune response: an *in vivo* model. *Immunomethods*, in press.

Imamichi T, Uchida I, Wahl SM & McCartney-Francis N (1993) Expression and cloning of migration inhibitory factor-related protein (MRP) 8 and MRP14 in arthritis-susceptible rats. *Biochem Biophys Res Commun* **194**: 819–825.

Jaye M, Howk R, Burgess W, Ricca GA, Chiu I-M, Ravera MW et al (1986) Human endothelial cell growth factor: cloning, nucleotide sequence, and chromosome localization. *Science* **233**: 541–545.

Katona IM, Ohura K, Allen JB, Wahl LM, Chenoweth DE & Wahl SM (1991) Modulation of monocyte chemotactic function in inflammatory lesions: role of inflammatory mediators. *J Immunol* **146**: 708–714.

Kotake S, Higaki M, Sato K, Himeno S, Morita H, Kim KJ et al. (1992) Detection of myeloid precursors (granulocyte/macrophage colony forming units) in the bone marrow adjacent to rheumatoid arthritis joints. *J Rheumatol* **19**: 1511–1516.

Krane SM (1975) Collagenase production by human synovial tissues. *Ann NY Acad Sci* **256**: 289–303.

Kumkumian GK, Lafyatis R, Remmers EF, Case JP, Kim S-J & Wilder RL (1989) Platelet-derived growth factor and IL-1 interactions in rheumatoid arthritis: regulation of synoviocyte proliferation, prostaglandin production, and collagenase transcription. *J Immunol* **143**: 833–837.

Kuruvilla AP, Shah R, Hochwald GM, Liggitt HD, Palladino MA & Thorbecke GJ (1991) Protective effect of transforming growth factor β1 on experimental autoimmune diseases in mice. *Proc Natl Acad Sci USA* **88**: 2918–2921.

Laiho M, Saksela O & Keski-Oja J (1987) Transforming growth factor-β induction of type-1 plasminogen activator inhibitor: pericellular deposition and sensitivity to exogenous urokinase. *J Biol Chem* **262**: 17467–17474.

Lafyatis R, Thompson NL, Remmers EF, Flanders KC, Roche NS, Kim S-J et al. (1989) Transforming growth factor-β production by synovial tissues from rheumatoid patients and streptococcal cell wall arthritic rats. *J Immunol* **143**: 1142–1148.

Lalor PA, Mapp PI, Hall PA & Revell PA (1987) Proliferative activity of cells in the synovium as demonstrated by a monoclonal antibody. *Rheumatol Int* **7**: 183–186.

Leizer T, Cebon J, Layton JE & Hamilton JA (1990) Cytokine regulation of colony-stimulating factor production in cultured human synovial fibroblasts: I. Induction of GM-CSF and G-CSF production by interleukin-1 and tumor necrosis factor. *Blood* **76**: 1989–1996.

Lemmel EM, Brackertz D, Franke M, Gaus W, Hartl PW, Machalke K et al. (1987) Results of a multicenter placebo-controlled double-blind randomized phase III clinical study of the treatment of rheumatoid arthritis with interferon-gamma. *Rheumatol Int* **8**: 87–93.

López-Casillas F, Wrana JL & Massagué J (1993) Betaglycan presents ligand to the TGFβ signaling receptor. *Cell* **73**: 1435–1444.

Lotz M, Kekow J & Carson DA (1990) Transforming growth factor-β and cellular immune responses in synovial fluids. *J Immunol* **144**: 4189–4194.

Manthey CL, Allen JB, Ellingsworth LR & Wahl SM (1990) *In situ* expression of transforming growth factor beta in Streptococcal cell wall-induced granulomatous inflammation and hepatic fibrosis. *Growth Factors* **4**: 17–26.

March CJ, Mosley B, Larsen A, Cerretti DP, Braedt G, Price V et al. (1985) Cloning, sequence and expression of two distinct human interleukin-1 complementary DNAs. *Nature* **315**: 641–647.

McCachren SS (1991) Expression of metalloproteinases and metalloproteinase inhibitor in human arthritic synovium. *Arthritis Rheum* **34**: 1085–1092.

McCartney-Francis N & Wahl SM (1994) TFGβ: a matter of life and death. *J Leuk Biol* **55**: 401–409.

McCartney-Francis N, Mizel D, Wong H, Wahl L & Wahl SM (1990) TGF-β regulates production of growth factors and TGF-β by human peripheral blood monocytes. *Growth Factors* **4**: 27–35.

McCulloch J, Lydyard PM & Rook GAW (1993) Rheumatoid arthritis: how well do the theories fit the evidence? *Clin Exp Immunol* **92**: 1–6.

Melnyk VM, Shipley GD, Sternfeld MD, Sherman L & Rosenbaum JT (1990) Synoviocytes synthesize, bind, and respond to basic fibroblast growth factor. *Arthritis Rheum* **33**: 493–500.

Metcalf D (1989) The molecular control of cell division, differentiation commitment and maturation in haemopoietic cells. *Nature* **339**: 27–30.

Miller JFAP & Morahan G (1992) Peripheral T cell tolerance. *Ann Rev Immunol* **10**: 51–69.

Miossec P, Naviliat M, D'Angeac AD, Sany J & Banchereau J (1990) Low levels of interleukin-4 and high levels of transforming growth factor β in rheumatoid synovitis. *Arthritis Rheum* **33**: 1180–1187.

Muirden KD (1972) Lysosomal enzymes in synovial membrane in rheumatoid arthritis. *Ann Rheum Dis* **31**: 265–271.

Nathan C & Yoshida R (1987) Cytokines: interferon-γ. In Gallin JI, Goldstein IM & Snyderman R (eds) *Inflammation: Basic Principles and Clinical Correlates*, pp 229–251. New York: Raven.

Nossal GJV & Pike BL (1980) Clonal anergy: persistence in tolerant mice of antigen-binding B lymphocytes incapable of responding to antigen or mitogen. *Proc Natl Acad Sci USA* **77**: 1602–1606.

Nykanen P, Bergroth V, Raunio P, Nordstrom D & Konttinen YT (1986) Phenotypic characterization of ^{3}H-thymidine incorporating cells in rheumatoid arthritis synovial membrane. *Rheumatol Int* **6**: 269–271.

Poole AR (1993) Cartilage in health and disease. In McCarty DJ & Koopman WJ (eds) *Arthritis and Allied Conditions*, pp 279–333. Philadelphia: Lea and Febiger.

Poole AR, Mort JS & Roughley PJ (1993) Methods for evaluating mechanisms of cartilage breakdown. In: Woessner JF & Howell DS (eds) *Joint Cartilage Degradation: Basic and Clinical Aspects*, pp 225–260. New York: Marcel Dekker.

Remmers EF, Lafyatis R, Kumkumian GK, Case JP, Roberts AB, Sporn MB et al. (1990) Cytokines and growth regulation of synoviocytes from patients with rheumatoid arthritis and rats with streptococcal cell wall arthritis. *Growth Factors* **2**: 179–188.

Remmers EF, Sano H, Lafyatis R, Case JP, Kumkuman GK, Hla T et al. (1991a) Production of platelet derived growth factor B chain (PDGF-B/c-sis) mRNA and immunoreactive PDGF B-like polypeptide by rheumatoid synovium: coexpression with heparin binding acidic fibroblast growth factor-1. *J Rheumatol* **18**: 7–13.

Remmers EF, Sano H & Wilder RL (1991b) Platelet-derived growth factors and heparin-binding (fibroblast) growth factors in the synovial tissue pathology of rheumatoid arthritis. *Semin Arthritis Rheum* **21**: 191–199.

Richter J (1990) Effect of auranofin on cytokine induced secretion of granule proteins from adherent human neutrophils. *Ann Rheum Dis* **50**: 372–375.

Ridge SC, Zabriske JB, Oronsky AL & Kerwar SS (1985) Streptococcal cell wall arthritis: studies with nude (athymic) inbred Lewis rats. *Cell Immunol* **96**: 231–234.

Roberts AB & Sporn MB (1990) The transforming growth factor-betas. In Sporn MB & Roberts AB (eds) *Peptide Growth Factors and Their Receptors: Handbook of Experimental Pharmacology*, pp 419–458. Heidelberg: Springer-Verlag.

Ross R, Raines EW & Bowen-Pope DF (1986) The biology of platelet-derived growth factor. *Cell* **46**: 155–169.

Ruschen S, Lemm G & Warnatz H (1989) Spontaneous and LPS-stimulated production of intracellular IL-1β by synovial macrophages in rheumatoid arthritis is inhibited by IFN-γ. *Clin Exp Immunol* **76**: 246–251.

Sano H, Forough R, Maier JAM, Case JP, Jackson A, Engleka K et al. (1990) Detection of high levels of heparin binding growth factor-1 (acidic fibroblast growth factor) in inflammatory arthritic joints. *J Cell Biol* **110**: 1417–1426.

Sano H, Engleka K, Mathern P, Hla T, Crofford LJ, Remmers EF et al. (1993) Coexpression of phospho-tyrosine-containing proteins, platelet-derived growth factor-B, and fibroblast growth factor-1 *in situ* in synovial tissues of patients with rheumatoid arthritis and Lewis rats with adjuvant or streptococcal cell wall arthritis. *J Clin Invest* **91**: 553–565.

Savill CM, Delves PJ, Kioussis D, Walker P, Lydyard PM, Colaco B et al. (1987) A minority of patients with rheumatoid arthritis show a dominant rearrangement of T-cell receptor β-chain genes in synovial lymphocytes. *Scand J Immunol* **25**: 629–635.

Saxne T, Palladino MA, Heinegård D, Talal N & Wollheim FA (1988) Detection of tumor necrosis factor α but not tumor necrosis factor β in rheumatoid arthritis synovial fluid and serum. *Arthritis Rheum* **31**: 1041–1045.

Schumacher HR & Kitridou RC (1972) Synovitis of recent onset: a clinicopathologic study during the first month of the disease. *Arthritis Rheum* **15**: 465–485.

Segarini PR (1991) TGF-β receptors. In Bock GR & Marsh J (eds) *Clinical Applications of TGF-β*, pp 29–50. New York: Wiley.

Stamenkovic I, Stegagno M, Wright KA, Krane SM, Amento EP, Colvin RB et al. (1988) Clonal dominance among T lymphocyte infiltrates in arthritis. *Proc Natl Acad Sci USA* **85**: 1179–1183.

Stuart JM, Townes AS & Kang AH (1982) The role of collagen autoimmunity in animal models and human disease. *J Invest Derm* **79**: 121s–127s.

Thorbecke GJ, Shah R, Leu CH, Kuruvilla AP, Hardison AM & Palladino MA (1992) Involvement of endogenous tumor necrosis factor α and transforming growth factor β during induction of collagen type II arthritis in mice. *Proc Natl Acad Sci USA* **89**: 7375–7379.

Trentham DE, Townes AS & Kang AH (1977) Autoimmunity to type II collagen: an experimental model of arthritis. *J Exp Med* **146**: 857–868.

Tsunawaki S, Sporn M, Ding A & Nathan C (1988) Deactivation of macrophages by transforming growth factor-β. *Nature* **334**: 260–262.

Veys EM, Mielants H, Verbruggen G, Grosclaude JP, Meyer W, Galazka AR et al. (1988) Recombinant interferon-gamma in rheumatoid arthritis. A double-blind study comparing human recombinant interferon-gamma with placebo. *J Rheumatol* **15**: 570–574.

Wahl SM (1988) Fibrosis: bacterial-cell-wall-induced hepatic granulomas. In Gallin JI, Goldstein IM & Snyderman R (eds) *Inflammation: Basic Principles and Clinical Correlates*, pp 841–860. New York: Raven.

Wahl SM (1991) Cellular and molecular interactions in the induction of inflammation in rheumatic diseases. In Kresina TF (ed) *Monoclonal Antibodies, Cytokines and Arthritis: Mediators of Inflammation and Therapy*, pp 101–132. New York: Marcel Dekker.

Wahl SM (1992) Transforming growth factor beta (TGF-β) in inflammation: a cause and a cure. *J Clin Immunol* **12**: 61–74.

Wahl SM, Hunt DA, Wakefield LM, McCartney-Francis N, Wahl LM, Roberts AB et al. (1987) Transforming growth factor (TGF-beta) induces chemotaxis and growth factor production. *Proc Natl Acad Sci USA* **84**: 5788–5792.

Wahl SM, Hunt DA, Bansal G, McCartney-Francis N, Ellingsworth L & Allen JB (1988a) Bacterial cell wall-induced immunosuppression: role of transforming growth factor β. *J Exp Med* **168**: 1403–1417.

Wahl SM, Hunt DA, Wong HL, Dougherty S, McCartney-Francis N, Wahl LM et al. (1988b) Transforming growth factor-β is a potent immunosuppressive agent that inhibits IL-1 dependent lymphocyte proliferation. *J Immunol* **140**: 3026–3032.

Wahl SM, Allen JB, Wong HL, Dougherty SF & Ellingsworth LR (1990) Antagonistic and agonistic effects of transforming growth factor-β and IL-1 in rheumatoid synovium. *J Immunol* **145**: 2514–2519.

Wahl SM, Allen JB, Ohura K, Chenoweth DE & Hand AR (1991). IFN-γ inhibits inflammatory cell recruitment and the evolution of bacterial cell wall-induced arthritis. *J Immunol* **146**: 95–100.

Wahl SM, Allen JB, Costa GL, Wong HL & Dasch JR (1993a) Reversal of acute and chronic synovial inflammation by anti-transforming growth factor β. *J Exp Med* **177**: 225–230.

Wahl SM, Allen JB, Weeks BS, Wong HL & Klotman PE (1993b) Transforming growth factor β enhances integrin expression and type IV collagenase secretion in human monocytes. *Proc Natl Acad Sci USA* **90**: 4577–4581.

Wahl SM, Costa GL, Corcoran M, Wahl LM & Berger AE (1993c) Transforming growth factor-β mediates IL-1-dependent induction of IL-1 receptor antagonist. *J Immunol* **150**: 3553–3560.

Walakovits LA, Moore VL, Bhardwaj N, Gallick GS & Lark MW (1992) Detection of stromelysin and collagenase in synovial fluid from patients with rheumatoid arthritis and post-traumatic injury. *Arthritis Rheum* **35**: 35–42.

Weisbart RH, Golde DW, Clark SC, Wong GG & Gasson JC (1985) Human granulocyte-macrophage colony-stimulating factor is a neutrophil activator. *Nature* **314**: 361–363.

Williamson DJ, Begley CG, Vadas MA & Metcalf D (1988) The detection and initial characterization of colony-stimulating factors in synovial fluid. *Clin Exp Immunol* **72**: 67–73.

Wong HL, Lotze MT, Wahl LM & Wahl SM (1992) Administration of recombinant IL-4 to humans regulates gene expression, phenotype, and function in circulating monocytes. *J Immunol* **148**: 2118–2125.

Wright JK, Cawston TE & Hazleman BL (1991) Transforming growth factor beta stimulates the production of the tissue inhibitor of metalloproteinases (TIMP) by human synovial and skin fibroblasts. *Biochem Biophys Acta* **1094**: 207–210.

Yamamoto M, Yasuda M, Shiokawa S & Nobunaga M (1991) Effects of colony-stimulating factors on proliferation and activation of synovial cells. *Clin Rheumatol* **10**: 277–282.

Yocum DE, Allen JB, Wahl SM, Calandra GB & Wilder RL (1986) Inhibition by cyclosporin A of streptococcal cell wall-induced arthritis and hepatic granulomas in rats. *Arthritis Rheum* **29**: 262–273.

13 Naturally Occurring Cytokine Inhibitors in Rheumatoid Arthritis

Gary S. Firestein

INTRODUCTION

Cytokines play a central role in the perpetuation of rheumatoid arthritis (RA). Their ability to induce cellular proliferation, metalloproteinase and prostaglandin production, expression of adhesion molecules, and secretion of other cytokines contributes to synovial inflammation and tissue destruction. The cytokine profile of synovitis has been carefully mapped, resulting in a detailed understanding of complex paracrine and autocrine networks in arthritis (Firestein and Zvaifler, 1990; Arend and Dayer, 1990). Although the inflamed joint contains a broad range of cytokines, the profile is not random since most of the factors detected are derived from macrophages and fibroblasts, including IL-1, IL-6, TNFα, colony-stimulating factors (e.g. GM-CSF), and chemokines (e.g. IL-8) (Firestein and Zvaifler, 1990). In contrast, T-cell derived products like IFNγ, IL-2, or TNFβ are difficult or impossible to detect. Although the relative absence lymphokines from T cells might simply reflect our inability to measure minute amounts in the synovial microenvironment, this observation has engendered a lively debate on the role of T cells in RA (Panayi *et al.*, 1992; also Chapters 2 and 4, this volume).

Positive cytokine feedback loops that amplify cellular responses are normally opposed by negative circuits that attempt to re-establish homeostasis. For instance, the natural IL-1 antagonist, IL-1ra, is produced *in vivo* in response to endotoxin exposure in humans and probably serves to modulate the devastating effects of septic shock (Ulich *et al.*, 1992). These negative feedback systems also appear to operate in RA in an attempt to re-establish synovial homeostasis. Clearly, defective or inadequate production of these factors could contribute to the perpetuation of chronic synovitis. In this chapter, some of these naturally occurring cytokine inhibitors will be discussed, with an emphasis on cytokines known to be important in synovitis. (The role of cytokines in the pathology of RA is also discussed in Chapters 2, 9, 10, 11, 12, 26 and 27, this volume).

INTERLEUKIN 1 ANTAGONISTS

The interleukin 1 system is essential to homeostasis and normal immune responses. IL-1α and -β comprise the agonist arm of this family (Dinarello, 1991). Both are synthesized as 31-kDa precursor peptides; the precursor for IL-1α is biologically active, but unprocessed IL-1β is inactive. Precursor-IL-1β is cleaved to the active 17-kDa protein and released into the extracellular space after the cell is stimulated (e.g. by endotoxin or other cytokines) or in other specialized situations, including apoptosis (programmed cell death) (Mosley *et al.*, 1987; Dinarello, 1991; Hogquist *et al.*, 1991). At least two high affinity surface receptors for IL-1 exist and bind to IL-1α and -β. The type I IL-1 receptor (IL-1R) is expressed on a variety of cells, including T cells, synoviocytes, chondrocytes, and fibroblasts, while the type II receptor is expressed on B cells and macrophages (Dinarello, 1991). The functional role of the type II receptor is not clear, since it possesses only a very short cytosolic domain (29 amino acids compared to 213 amino acids for the type I receptor). A competitive antagonist that binds to both IL-1Rs known as the IL-1 receptor antagonist has also recently been identified (see below).

IL-1 is critically involved in the pathogenesis of arthritis (Firestein and Zvaifler, 1990; Arend and Dayer, 1990). In addition to its role in antigen presentation to T cells, it also has profound effects on synovial cells. For instance, IL-1 stimulates fibroblast-like synoviocytes to proliferate, secrete cytokines like GM-CSF and IL-8, and produce metalloproteinases that can digest the extracellular matrix (Balavoine *et al.*, 1986; Alvaro-Gracia *et al.*, 1990; see Chapters 8 and 9, this volume). Injection of IL-1 directly into joints causes synovitis and parenteral administration markedly exacerbates experimental antigen-induced arthritis (Henderson and Pettipher, 1989; Chandrasekhar *et al.*, 1990). Immunoreactive and biologically active IL-1 are present in RA synovial effusions, although the actual concentrations that have been reported vary considerably depending on the type of assay used (Miossec *et al.*, 1986; Symons *et al.*, 1989; Rooney *et al.*, 1990). About 10% of rheumatoid synovial cells contain detectable levels of IL-1β mRNA (Firestein *et al.*, 1990). The vast majority of cells expressing the IL-1β gene are macrophages. IL-1 protein is also found in these synovial macrophages. IL-1 positive cells in the synovium are interspersed throughout the intimal lining and sublining perivascular mononuclear cell aggregates and appear to be particularly abundant near the cartilage–pannus junction (Miossec *et al.*, 1986; Koch *et al.*, 1992). In light of the purported importance of IL-1, recent descriptions of specific inhibitors in the joints of patients with RA are surprising.

IL-1 RECEPTOR ANTAGONIST (IL-1ra)

Biology of IL-1ra

IL-1ra is a naturally occurring IL-1 inhibitor that was described in the supernatants of human monocytes as well as in the urine of febrile patients (Arend *et al.*, 1985, 1991). IL-1ra binds directly to type I and II IL-1 receptors (IL-1R) and competes with IL-1 for the ligand binding site (Carter *et al.*, 1990; Hannum *et al.*, 1990; Dripps *et al.*, 1991b). It is a pure antagonist; that is, no detectable signal is transduced and the receptor–ligand complex is not internalized after it binds to the IL-1R (Dripps *et al.*, 1991a). This is distinctly different from the IL-1:IL-1R complex, which enters the cell and migrates to the nucleus. Although IL-1ra binds to the IL-1 receptor with the same affinity as IL-1α and IL-1β, it is a relatively weak inhibitor because IL-1 activates cells even if only a small percentage of receptors are occupied. Hence, a large excess of the inhibitor is needed to saturate the receptor and block IL-1-mediated stimulation (Arend *et al.*, 1990; Smith *et al.*, 1991). Typically, the concentration of IL-1ra *in vitro* must be 10- to 100-fold higher than IL-1 to achieve significant inhibition (see Fig. 1). Recombinant IL-1ra inhibits a variety of IL-1-mediated events in cultured cells

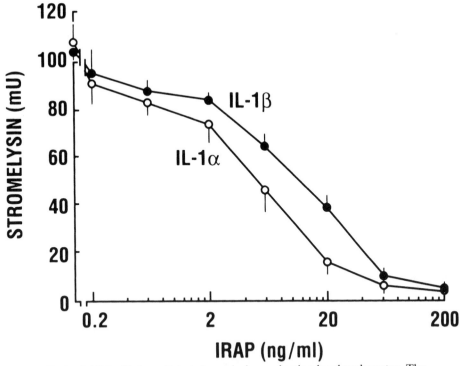

Figure 1. IL-1ra inhibits IL-1 mediated stromelysin production by chondrocytes. The concentration of IL-1 used in these experiments was 0.3 ng/ml. Over a 100-fold excess of IL-1ra was needed to block IL-1 biological activity. IRAP, IL-1 receptor antagonist protein. From Smith *et al.* (1991).

derived from the joint, including the induction of metalloproteinase and prostaglandin production by chondrocytes and synoviocytes.

Two structural variants of IL-1ra have been described: (a) secretory IL-1ra, or sIL-1ra, which is synthesized with a signal peptide that allows it to be transported out of cells (Carter *et al.*, 1990; Eisenberg *et al.*, 1990); and (b) intracellular IL-1ra, or icIL-1ra, which lacks a leader peptide due to alternative splicing of mRNA and therefore remains intracellular (Haskill *et al.*, 1991). sIL-1ra is a major product of mononuclear phagocytes, particularly mature tissue macrophages, while icIL-1ra is produced by keratinocytes and other epithelial cells (Haskill *et al.*, 1991; Bigler *et al.*, 1992). Both forms may be produced simultaneously by fibroblasts and alveolar macrophages (Chan *et al.*, 1993; Quay *et al.*, 1993). The role of icIL-1ra in the immune response is not established. It might represent a homeostatic mechanism in the skin, where icIL-1ra in keratinocytes could be released after tissue injury or necrosis. Alternatively, localized apoptosis might release intracellular proteins like icIL-1ra into the micro-environment.

While IL-1 and IL-1ra production are, in many circumstances, closely linked, they clearly have distinct regulatory controls (Janson *et al.*, 1991). The relative balance between IL-1 and IL-1ra expression *in vitro* depends on a variety of factors. Cell maturity is one important variable, and IL-1 predominates in immature monocytes while IL-1ra is more prevalent in mature macrophages. Cytokines also regulate the production of IL-1ra, since IL-4 and GM-CSF increase secretion of IL-1ra by mono-cytes. In some cases, both the agonist and antagonist are simultaneously produced by the same cell (Roux-Lombard *et al.*, 1989; Janson *et al.*, 1991).

IL-1ra in rheumatoid arthritis

Because of the importance of IL-1 in RA, the discovery of IL-1ra led to the obvious hypothesis that IL-1ra deficiency contributes to the disease. Yet, unexpectedly high concentrations of the protein (up to 50 ng/ml) are present in rheumatoid synovial effusions as measured with a sensitive and specific immunoassay (Malyak *et al.*, 1994). Furthermore, immunohistochemical studies of rheumatoid synovium reveal large amounts of IL-1ra protein in rheumatoid synovial tissue, particularly in perivascular mononuclear cells and the synovial intimal lining (Deleuran *et al.*, 1992a; Koch *et al.*, 1992; Firestein *et al.*, 1992). IL-1ra protein is especially abundant in and about regions containing IL-1 protein. The presence of IL-1ra in synovium is not specific to RA, since it is also present in osteoarthritis synovial tissue, albeit in lesser amounts. Normal synovium is completely devoid of immunoreactive IL-1ra.

Single and double label immunohistochemistry studies show that macrophages are the primary source of IL-1ra in the sublining region (Firestein *et al.*, 1992). Both macrophages and a population of non-macrophages (presumably fibroblast-like syno-viocytes) in the intimal lining contain immunoreactive IL-1ra. One potential limi-tation of immunohistochemistry is that it cannot determine whether a protein is produced by the labelled cell or whether the protein is secreted elsewhere and sub-sequently internalized or bound by the cell. To address this question, molecular biology techniques have been used to study synovial gene expression. Northern blot analysis of whole tissue RNA extracts demonstrate abundant IL-1ra mRNA, confirm-ing local gene transcription (Firestein *et al.*, 1992). *In situ* hybridization studies reveal that the distribution of IL-1ra mRNA correlates with IL-1ra protein. Further evidence of synovial IL-1ra production is provided by the demonstration of glycosylated IL-1ra in the supernatants of cultured synovial tissue cells by western blot analysis (see Fig 2). Bioassays of these supernatants indicate that synovial IL-1ra is biologically active.

How can these data be reconciled with the notion that IL-1ra deficiency might contribute to synovitis? The answer might lie in the fact that the biological importance of IL-1 as a pro-inflammatory mediator depends on a variety of influences, especially the balance between IL-1 and its various inhibitors. Hence, the absolute amount of IL-1ra and other inhibitors is not as important as their concentrations relative to IL-1. While is is impossible to measure the amount of IL-1 and IL-1ra directly in the synovial microenvironment, accurate assays have determined the relative amounts of each produced by cultured synovial tissue cells. These studies show that the ratio of IL-1ra to IL-1 is relatively low (from 1:1 in cell lysates to 4:1 in culture supernatants) compared to the 10- to 100-fold excess of IL-1ra needed to block IL-1-mediated metalloproteinase and prostaglandin synthesis by mesenchymal cells (Arend *et al.*, 1990; Smith *et al.*, 1991; Firestein *et al.*, 1994).

The reason for low synovial IL-1ra production is complex and appears to involve at least two distinct processes. First, fibroblast-like synoviocytes, which account for much of the immunoreactive IL-1ra in the synovial intimal lining, selectively produce

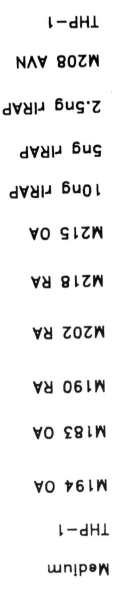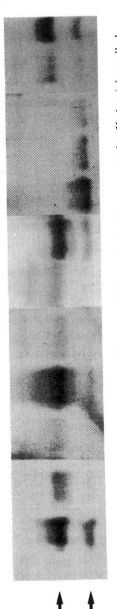

Figure 2. IL-1ra production by synovial cells. Western blot analysis demonstrated immunoreactive IL-1ra (also called IRAP, or IL-1 receptor antagonists protein) secretion by freshly isolated synovial tissue cells. Samples of 2-day culture supernatants of rheumatoid arthritis (RA), osteoarthritis (OA), and avascular necrosis (AVN) were assayed. Recombinant hIL-1ra and supernatants from phorbol ester activated THP-1 cells were included as positive control for non-glycosylated and glycosylated forms of the protein, respectively. The majority of IL-1ra secreted by synovial cells appeared to be the higher molecular weight glycosylated form. Other studies showed that the IL-1ra was biologically active. From Firestein *et al.* (1992) with permission.

the intracellular form of the IL-1ra. Evidence for this conclusion is derived from two observations: (a) supernatants of cultured fibroblast-like synoviocytes contain little IL-1ra, while cell lysates contain large amounts; and (b) quantitative reverse transcriptase–polymerase chain reaction (RT-PCR) studies demonstrate that the vast majority of IL-1ra mRNA is the alternatively spliced icIL-1ra form in the fibroblast-like cells (Firestein *et al.*, 1994). Therefore, most, if not all, of the IL-1ra produced by these cells remains intracellular and is not normally secreted into the extracellular space. However, icIL-1ra might be released from synoviocytes *in vivo* by alternative routes, such as apoptosis. A variety of stimuli can induce apoptosis, such as metabolic poisons (e.g. actinomycin D) or oxygen radicals. One characteristic finding in apoptotic cells is degradation of DNA into discrete nucleosomes that can be visualized using agarose gel electrophoresis. Of interest, this pattern has been observed in DNA isolated directly from arthritic synovium as well as from cultured synovial cells (Firestein, unpublished data). It is possible, therefore, that low levels of programmed cell death occur *in situ* and contribute to IL-1ra release.

A second reason for low synovial IL-1ra production is a relative defect in IL-1ra production by synovial tissue macrophages. Macrophages isolated from other sites, such as alveolar macrophages or monocyte-derived macrophages, are highly efficient IL-1ra producers (Moore *et al.*, 1992). Although purified synovial macrophages produce IL-1ra, they only secrete about 1% as much as macrophages isolated from other sites (Tsai *et al.*, 1992; Firestein *et al.*, 1994). Low IL-1ra secretion by synovial macrophages might result, in part, from excess alternative splicing to the intracellular form.

One rather puzzling aspect of these studies is the relatively high concentration of IL-1ra reported in RA synovial fluid compared to the small amounts produced by synovial tissue. For most cytokines, the synovium is the primary site of gene expression, and fresh synovial fluid mononuclear cells usually contain only limited amounts of cytokine mRNA (Firestein *et al.*, 1990). Although the evidence is indirect, IL-1ra might be an exception to this paradigm since it appears to be synthesized by neutrophils, which selectively accumulate in the intra-articular cavity. The concentrations of IL-1ra in rheumatoid effusions correlate with the number of neutrophils in the synovial fluid, and IL-1ra is perhaps the most abundant new protein synthesized by recently activated neutrophils (McColl *et al.*, 1992). Moreover, recent data show that synovial fluid neutrophils in RA contain IL-1ra protein, and that these cells secrete increased amounts if they are treated with GM-CSF, which is known to be present in synovial fluid (Xu *et al.*, 1989; Malyak *et al.*, 1994). Therefore, neutrophils might be an important source of IL-1ra in joint effusions. If true, this would provide an explanation for the apparent discrepancy between the relative amounts of IL-1ra found in these two joint compartments (i.e. synovial fluid and synovium), since granulocytes usually do not reside in the synovial membrane (Firestein *et al.*, 1987).

The presence of an IL-1ra defect in arthritis implies that administration of pharmacologic doses of IL-1ra would be beneficial, and clinical studies to test this hypothesis are in progress. Preliminary data indicate that the recombinant protein is well tolerated in humans and has a pharmacokinetic profile that is amenable to long-term therapy (even though very large doses would be needed). Unfortunately, a beneficial effect of IL-1ra in some animal models of arthritis has been somewhat difficult to demonstrate. This might reflect the fact that IL-1ra functions primarily as an anti-inflammatory agent and does not inhibit cell-mediated immune responses that might be important in arthritis (Nicod *et al.*, 1992). In some contrived models, such as the direct injection of IL-1 into the joint, benefit has been reported (Henderson *et al.*, 1991). Also, a physiologic role of IL-1ra in the resolution of synovitis is supported by the correlation between synovial fluid IL-1ra concentrations and clinical improvement in the acute arthritis of Lyme disease (Miller *et al.*, 1993). It is important to remember that the relevance of animal models or Lyme disease to RA is unclear, and the only way to test the efficacy is to perform a controlled clinical study. See Chapters 2 and 26, this volume, for descriptions of the inhibition of other cytokines in RA and models of RA.

ANTAGONISTIC CYTOKINES

A second mechanism of cytokine inhibition in RA is the local production of a second cytokine that antagonizes the function of the first. While many antagonistic cytokines have been described, perhaps the best characterized in RA is transforming growth factor-beta (TGFβ). TGFβ is a complex growth factor with multiple isoforms whose actions *in vitro* depend on culture conditions, the cells used, and the concentrations of the protein (see Chapter 12, this volume). Overall, TGFβ is a potent inhibitor of IL-1 biological activity. For instance, incubation of chondrocytes with IL-1β leads to a marked decrease in proteoglycan and collagen biosynthesis, and much of this effect is abolished if cells are pretreated with TGFβ. While the mechanism is not fully established, down-regulation of IL-1R expression might account for some of the inhibition since TGFβ decreases the number of surface receptors by nearly 50% (Harvey *et al.*, 1991; Rédini *et al.*, 1993). The affinity of the IL-1R for its ligand is unchanged, however. TGFβ can also indirectly contribute to IL-1 inhibition by inducing IL-1ra production.

The role of TGFβ in arthritis is also complex. It can serve as an autocrine growth factor for cultured fibroblast-like synoviocytes (Goddard *et al.*, 1990, 1992) and inhibits metalloproteinase production by synoviocytes and fibroblasts from a variety of sources (Raghu *et al.*, 1989; Overall *et al.*, 1989). This effect appears to be mediated at the level of gene expression, since TGFβ decreases collagenase mRNA synthesis. TGFβ-mediated matrix preservation is also enhanced by an increase in production of tissue inhibitors of metalloproteinases (TIMPs), a family of proteins that bind to metalloproteinases and inhibit their action. Furthermore, synthesis of matrix proteins like collagen is increased. The combination of decreased proteolysis and increased collagen production has led to the suggestion that TGFβ plays an important role in wound healing.

Although large amounts of TGFβ protein are present within the joints of rodents with experimental inflammatory arthritis, its specific role in the pathogenesis of synovitis is very confusing: depending on the model used and the timing of administration, exogenous TGFβ can either exacerbate or ameliorate experimental models of arthritis (Brandes *et al.*, 1991; Cooper *et al.*, 1992; Elford *et al*, 1992; Wahl *et al.*, 1993). For example, parenteral treatment with recombinant TGFβ₁ decreases the severity of polyarthritis in streptococcal cell wall arthritis. The benefit is observed if therapy is initiated either before immunization or after the onset of acute arthritis. In contrast, antibodies that neutralize TGFβ decrease synovial inflammation in other models of arthritis. Also, direct intra-articular injections with TGFβ$_1$ or TGFβ$_2$ cause acute synovitis with synovial lining hyperplasia. Intra-articular TGFβ also accelerates collagen-induced arthritis.

As with streptococcal cell wall arthritis, immunoreactive TGFβ is abundant in RA synovium. High concentrations of the peptide are also found in synovial effusions (Lafyatis et al., 1989; Fava et al., 1989; Miossec et al., 1990c; Brennan et al., 1990; Lotz et al., 1990; Chu et al., 1991). The majority of synovial fluid TGFβ is present in an inactive latent form, and mild acid treatment can convert it to the biologically active protein in vitro. While only a fraction of TGFβ is active in synovial fluid, levels of the active protein are certainly high enough to be biologically meaningful. In fact, TGFβ probably accounts for much of the IL-1 inhibitory activity in synovial fluid as measured by a thymocyte proliferation assay (Wahl et al., 1990). Hence, TGFβ, like IL-1ra, appears to be a particularly important inhibitor of IL-1 activity in synovial effusions. Its function in synovial tissue is not established, but the diverse effects in animal models suggest that a clear cut role of TGFβ as either pro- or anti-inflammatory in RA is far from understood. Moreover, the animal data imply that systemic TGFβ might have a beneficial immunoregulatory effect, while the presence of the cytokine in the joint cavity might even be deleterious. The roles of TGFβ in arthritis are also discussed in Chapters 9 and 12, this volume.

SOLUBLE IL-1 BINDING PROTEINS

Soluble cytokine receptors or soluble binding proteins can absorb free cytokines and prevent them from engaging functional receptors on cells. While these obviously could inhibit cytokine action, it should be kept in mind that they might also function as carrier proteins that protect cytokines from degradation and deliver them directly to cells. However, the role of the soluble IL-1R in normal immunity or as a negative feedback mechanism in inflammation has not been established. A therapeutic potential for soluble IL-1R is possible, since recombinant IL-1R protects against synovitis induced by direct injection of IL-1 into joints.

A novel soluble IL-1 binding protein has been identified in supernatants of a human B cell line and in RA synovial fluid and has recently joined the panoply of IL-1 inhibitors present in the rheumatoid joint (Symons et al., 1990, 1991). This 47-kDa protein is proteolytically cleaved from the cell surface by serine proteases and binds specifically to IL-1β, but not to IL-1ra or IL-1α. Both the biologically active 17-kDa form of IL-1β as well as the inactive 31-kDa precursor bind to the protein. The purified binding protein is able to absorb only IL-1β from culture supernatants and, hence, prevents IL-1β from engaging cell surface IL-1 receptors. Therefore, it exhibits several characteristics that distinguish it from the type I IL-1R. Recent studies suggest that the binding protein might be a soluble form of the type II IL-1R (although both IL-1α and IL-1ra should bind to the protein if this is true).

ANTI-IL-1α ANTIBODIES

Specific antibodies that bind to and neutralize cytokines can also inhibit cytokine activity. Very little is known about natural anticytokine antibodies in vivo, although one might anticipate their presence in diseases with marked B cell hyperreactivity. In this regard, it is notable that neutralizing anti-IL-1α antibodies are found in the blood of about 16% of RA patients and only 5% of normal individuals (Suzuki *et al.*, 1991). Similar studies have not been performed on synovial fluid, although it would be surprising if it were devoid of anti-IL-1α activity since plasma proteins generally are also present in synovial effusions, albeit at lower concentrations. Many pertinent questions arise concerning this autoantibody. For instance, is it truly directed against IL-1α, or does it result from molecular mimicry? Does the antibody simply block IL-1α activity or does it serve other functions, like delivering the cytokine to Fc-receptor bearing cells? Where is the site of antibody production (synovium versus peripheral lymphoid organs)? Is this antibody unique, or are antibodies that bind cytokines a general feature of RA? The use of specific cytokine-neutralizing antibodies in the study of the pathology of experimental arthritis is reviewed by Otterness *et al.* (Chapter 26, this volume). The administration of anti-TNF antibodies to RA patients is described by Maini *et al.* (Chapter 2, this volume).

TNF-α ANTAGONISTS

TNF BIOLOGY

TNFα, like IL-1, has been implicated in the pathogenesis of RA (Firestein and Zvaifler, 1990, reviewed in Chapter 2, this volume). TNF (originally so-designated because of its ability to cause haemorrhagic necrosis of a murine sarcoma), is synthesized by a variety of cells (including macrophages, fibroblasts, and T lymphocytes) as a 26-kDa precursor peptide (Kunkel *et al.*, 1989; Vilcek and Lee, 1991). It exists in solution as an active homotrimer with three 17-kDa subunits. The TNFα gene (as well as the closely related lymphocyte protein, TNFβ) is located in the major histocompatibility region of human chromosome 6. Like many cytokines, its expression is regulated, in part, by posttranscriptional events, and the rate of mRNA degradation is tightly controlled by an endogenous ribonuclease(s) that recognizes an AU-rich tail in the 3' untranslated region.

TNFα shares many biological functions with IL-1, including the ability to stimulate metalloproteinase production, cytokine synthesis, and proliferation of synoviocytes (Alvaro-Gracia *et al.*, 1990). IL-1 and TNFα are usually additive or synergistic in biological assays. TNFα is readily detected in most rheumatoid synovial fluids using immunoassays, although biological activity is difficult to demonstrate (perhaps due to the presence of inhibitors (see below)) (Saxne *et al.*, 1988; Miossec *et al.*, 1990c; Westacott *et al.*, 1990). Immunoreactive TNFα is found in RA synovial tissue, particularly in the lining and in perivascular lymphoid aggregates (Deleuran *et al.*, 1992b), and TNFα mRNA is primarily localized to synovial macrophages (Firestein *et al.*, 1990).

SOLUBLE RECEPTORS

Two types of TNFα receptors have been characterized (Hohmann *et al.*, 1989; Brockhaw *et al.*, 1990; Hohmann *et al.*, 1990; Schoenfeld *et al.*, 1991). A 55-kDa receptor (415 amino acids) has lower affinity for TNFα and exhibits a high degree of homology with the nerve growth factor receptor. A 75-kDa TNF-R (461 amino acids) binds to TNFα with about 5- to 10-fold greater affinity than does the 55-kDa TNF-R. The relative levels of surface expression of each receptor vary depending on the cell type, and distinct functions appear to be subserved by each (Browning and Ribolini, 1989; Hohmann *et al.*, 1990). TNFβ also binds to both TNF-Rs.

A naturally occurring inhibitor of TNF activity was first identified in the urine of febrile patients (Seckinger *et al.*, 1988). Purification of this material revealed that it was a solubilized form of the TNF-Rs (Engelmann *et al.*, 1989; Seckinger *et al.*, 1990). Additional studies have since shown that the extracellular domain of both the 55-kDa and 75-kDa receptors are shed from cell surfaces (Nophar *et al.*, 1990; Porteu *et al.*, 1991) and that proteolytic cleavage is responsible for release of the soluble receptors. The soluble receptors can form stable complexes with TNFα and thereby inhibit biological activity. Significant amounts of soluble p55 and p75 TNF-R (>1 ng/ml) are present in the plasma of normal individuals and likely represent an important homeostatic mechanism (Novick *et al.*, 1989). Very high levels of both soluble TNF-Rs are released into the blood of patients with inflammatory diseases, including RA, and in rheumatoid synovial fluid where levels can exceed 50 ng/ml (see Fig. 3). This is considerably higher than the concentration of TNFα in the blood or synovial fluid (10–100 pg/ml) and represents a formidable inhibitor. The concentrations of both p55 and p75 in synovial effusions probably explain why biologically active TNF is difficult to detect in RA synovial fluid despite the presence of immunoreactive protein (Roux-Lombard and Dayer, 1991; Cope *et al.*, 1992; Heilig *et al.*, 1992; Roux-Lombard *et al.*, 1993). Quantitative studies of sTNF-R levels in synovial fluid show a positive correlation between the concentrations of p75 and p55, although there is a modest preponderance of the latter. There is no correlation between the cell count or the number of neutrophils in synovial effusions.

While little is known about the regulation of receptor shedding in the joint, synovial tissue mononuclear cells do have increased surface expression and mRNA levels for both TNF-Rs compared to osteoarthritis synovial cells or peripheral blood cells (Brennan *et al.*, 1992). Cultured fibroblast-like synoviocytes express the lower affinity 55-kDa TNF-R and continuously shed this receptor into culture supernatants (Alvaro-Gracia *et al.*, 1993) (see Table 1). IFNγ, which markedly enhances surface expression of HLA-DR on synoviocytes, modestly increases expression of the lower affinity TNF-R without changing the affinity or the rate of receptor shedding.

The functional significance of soluble TNF-R obviously depends on the relative amounts of agonist and antagonist. As noted above, concentrations of the soluble TNF-Rs are quite high compared to TNFα levels in the blood and in synovial effusions, where TNFα levels are typically 10 to 100 pg/ml. As with IL-1 antagonists, the balance between agonist and antagonist appears to be shifted towards the antagonist in the synovial fluid compartment. Studies designed to examine critically this ratio in the synovial membrane have not yet been performed for TNF-R, but the presumed importance of TNFα in the rheumatoid cytokine network suggests that the agonist probably prevails within the synovial microenvironment.

ANTAGONISTIC CYTOKINES

Cytokines that antagonize TNFα biological activity have also been described. IFNγ appears to be an important TNFα antagonist, as it inhibits TNFα-mediated synovio-

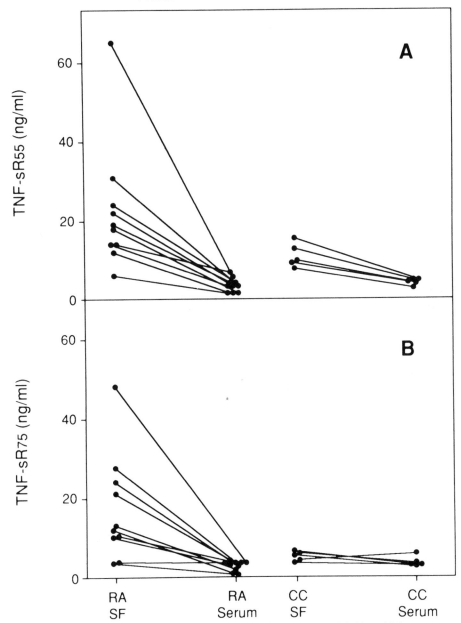

Figure 3. Soluble TNF-R concentrations in serum and synovial fluid. Very high concentrations of both the p55 (A) and p75 (B) soluble TNF-Rs are present in RA synovial fluid, particularly when compared to matched serum samples. However, serum samples still contain much more TNF-R than TNFα. Note that while chondrocalcinosis (CC) samples contain soluble TNF-Rs, RA samples are quite a bit higher. From Roux-Lombard *et al.* (1993).

cyte proliferation, GM-CSF secretion, and collagenase production (Alvaro-Gracia *et al.*, 1990). Early data suggested that the inhibition was specific for TNFα, but additional studies indicate that IFNγ also blocks some IL-1-mediated activities (Johnson

Table 1. TNFα receptor expression on fibroblast-like synoviocytes

Condition	Receptors/cell	kDa	Soluble 55 kDa TNF-R*
Medium	2800	7.4×10^{-10} M	112 ± 48
IFNγ (100 U/ml)	3400	7.0×10^{-10} M	128 ± 50

* pg/ml/10^5 cells.
IFNγ modestly increases TNF-R expression without changing either the affinity or the rate of receptor shedding. Cells were incubated in medium or 100 U/ml of IFNγ for 24 h prior to receptor analysis. TNF-R assays were performed by Scatchard analysis using I^{125}-TNFα. Soluble 55-kDa receptors were assayed by ELISA. Adapted from Alvaro-Gracia et al. (1993).

et al., 1989; Hamilton et al., 1992). The relationship between TNFα and IFNγ is of particular interest because TNFα also antagonizes some actions of IFNγ on synovio-cytes, such as induction of HLA-DR expression. The ability of these cytokines to inhibit each others' stimulating action on synoviocytes has been termed 'mutual antag-onism' (Alvaro-Gracia et al., 1990). This relationship is fairly specific to synoviocytes, since these two cytokines are generally additive or synergistic on other cell types (Zuber et al., 1988; Elias et al., 1988; Scharffetter et al., 1989). Originally, mutual antagonism between TNFα and IFNγ on synoviocytes was thought to be true for all actions of these cytokines. However, more recent data demonstrate that both induce adhesion molecules like ICAM-1 and VCAM-1 on synoviocytes and their effects are additive or synergistic (Chin et al., 1990; Morales-Ducret et al., 1992). Therefore, TNFα/IFNγ mutual antagonism is selective and depends on the specific function examined.

Studies of TNFα/IFNγ antagonism have not yet elucidated the mechanism. One potential explanation is that they down-regulate the expression of each others' surface receptors. However, Scatchard analyses using iodinated cytokines indicate IFNγ actually increases TNF-R display (Alvaro-Gracia et al., 1993). TNFα also paradoxi-cally increases IFNγ receptor surface expression. The interaction between the two cytokines appears to have effects at the level of gene expression since IFNγ inhibits the accumulation of G-CSF and GM-CSF mRNA in TNFα/IL-1 treated synoviocytes.

Antagonism between IFNγ and TNFα (as well as IL-1) raises the interesting hy-pothesis that IFNγ deficiency contributes to rheumatoid synovitis. This notion is actually antithetical to early paradigms of RA, which purported that IFNγ was a critical pro-inflammatory factor that regulated HLA-DR expression and antigen pres-entation in the joint. In fact, RA peripheral blood T cells have a specific defect in IFNγ production (Hasler et al., 1983; Combe et al., 1985) and only very low levels of IFNγ have been detected in synovial fluid (Firestein and Zvaifler, 1987; Miossec et al., 1990c). Furthermore, GM-CSF, not IFNγ, has been identified as the major HLA-DR-inducing factor in supernatants of RA synovial cells (Alvaro-Gracia et al., 1989). These data suggest that IFNγ might be an anti-inflammatory cytokine that normally helps maintain synovial homeostasis and that the absence of IFNγ in the joint contrib-utes to unopposed TNFα- and IL-1-mediated stimulation.

This hypothesis implies that 'replacement' therapy with pharmacologic doses of IFNγ might correct this defect and decrease joint inflammation. In fact, clinical trials have demonstrated modest improvement in RA patients treated with IFNγ (Cannon et al., 1989). Perhaps the complexity and redundancy of cytokine networks prevents a single agent like IFNγ from being more effective. For example, the relative absence of other suppressive cytokines, like IL-4, might also contribute to disease. This notion is supported by *in vitro* studies of synovial tissue explants showing that exogenous IL-4 decreases production of metalloproteinases and immunoglobulins (Miossec *et al.*, 1992). This raises the possibility that combinations of cytokines that antagonize pro-inflammatory factors might be more effective than single agents.

INTERLEUKIN 2

INTERLEUKIN 2 IN ARTHRITIS

In contrast to IL-1 and TNFα, the role of IL-2 in chronic RA is less well established. Early studies suggested that significant amounts of this T-cell growth factor are in synovial effusions, but recent data indicate that little, if any, IL-2 is present (Firestein *et al.*, 1988; Miossec *et al.*, 1990c). However, IL-2 mRNA has been detected in synovial tissue (Buchan *et al.*, 1988); this apparent paradox might be due to the induction of tolerance in synovial T cells, since a similar phenotype can be produced in tolerant T cells *in vitro* (i.e. high mRNA, low protein production) (Schall *et al.*, 1992). Although small amounts of IL-2 could potentially be produced in the synovial microenvironment, its role in established disease is undefined.

SOLUBLE RECEPTORS

The soluble IL-2 receptor (IL-2R) is one of the best characterized and most extensively studied soluble cytokine receptors in RA. Surface IL-2Rs are displayed on a many cells types, including monocytes, B cells, and activated T cells. It is normally expressed by a small percentage of resting peripheral blood T cells (about 1–2%), and activation by antigen or mitogen rapidly increases both the percentage of cells expressing the IL-2R as well as the surface density on the positive cells. The receptor is comprised of two membrane polypeptides (p55 and p75); high affinity IL-2 binding occurs when both are present and in physical contact with each other (Hatakeyama *et al.*, 1989). The low affinity binding protein, p55 (also called Tac), consists of a 251 amino acid polypeptide with extracellular, transmembrane, and short cytosolic domains encoded by a single structural gene on chromosome 10 in humans. The full length Tac protein undergoes extensive N- and O-linked glycosylation. Activated IL-2 bearing cells spontaneously shed the extracellular domain of the p55 IL-2R (about 191 amino acids) after proteolytic cleavage (Robb and Kutny, 1987). The resultant soluble receptor binds to IL-2, albeit with low affinity. The soluble IL-2R/IL-2 complex is unstable and has a short half-life. Soluble IL-2R cannot compete with high affinity receptors on cell membranes for IL-2 binding (Miossec *et al.*, 1990b). Hence, soluble IL-2Rs appear to be inefficient inhibitors of IL-2 biological activity and might have limited capacity for absorbing excess IL-2 or serving as carrier proteins. However, other studies suggest that soluble IL-2Rs do have some immunoregulatory potential (Kondo *et al.*, 1988).

The percentage of cells in the rheumatoid synovium that express the IL-2R is similar to that of resting peripheral blood lymphocytes (Cush and Lipsky, 1988). However, the percentage of synovial fluid T cells that are IL-2R positive is much higher (Lafton *et al.*, 1989). Elevated concentrations of soluble IL-2R are present in serum and synovial effusions of patients with RA, and the levels of IL-2R correlate with disease activity (Keystone *et al.*, 1988; Symons *et al.*, 1988; Miossec *et al.*, 1990a) (see Fig. 4). While it is assumed that activated T cells are the source of soluble IL-2R,

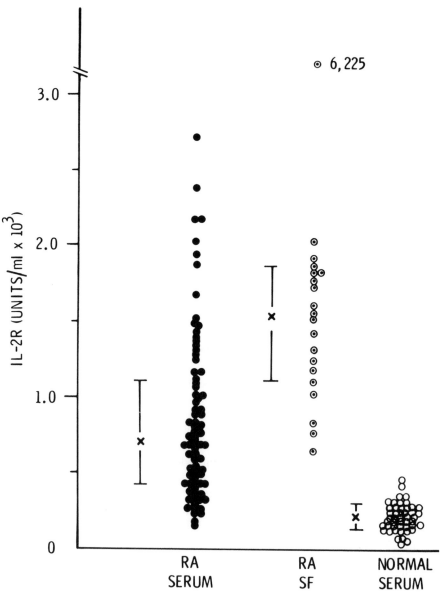

Figure 4. Elevated soluble IL-2 receptors in rheumatoid arthritis. Levels of soluble IL-2R were measured in sera and synovial fluids (SF) from patients with RA and in sera from healthy controls. High levels were present in most rheumatoid samples. Evaluation of paired samples indicated that soluble IL-2R concentrations in synovial fluid were higher in serum suggesting local shedding of receptors (not shown). From Keystone *et al.* (1988).

this has not been confirmed, and many other cells that express the IL-2R, like mono-cytes and B cells, are also potential sources. Osteoarthritis synovial effusions also contain low concentrations of soluble IL-2R.

Because RA synovial fluids inhibit IL-2-mediated cell proliferation *in vitro*, it is only natural to assume that this activity is due to soluble IL-2R. This appears to be supported by the observation that IL-2 inhibitory activity correlates with the concen-tration of soluble IL-2R in synovial effusions (Symons *et al.*, 1988; Miossec *et al.*, 1990b). Column chromatography of synovial fluid reveals a fraction that putatively corresponds to the receptor/IL-2 complex (Symons *et al.*, 1988). However, the short half-life of the intact complex makes copurification very difficult to confirm, and this fraction might actually contain a different inhibitor. This, along with the observation that soluble IL-2Rs are inefficient inhibitors of IL-2-mediated activation of T cells, suggest that the correlation between the inhibitory activity and sIL-2R levels might be coincidental.

HIGH MOLECULAR WEIGHT IL-2 INHIBITORY ACTIVITY

Although soluble IL-2Rs in synovial fluid do not appear to function as effective inhibitors of IL-2 biological activity, other factor(s) in RA SF do exhibit this property. While non-specific toxic effects (e.g. from hyaluronic acid) can potentially contribute to inhibition of IL-2-mediated cell proliferation, Miossec and colleagues have also demonstrated a high molecular weight inhibitor (Kashiwado *et al.*, 1987). The gel purified factor, which is not an antibody, inhibits IL-2-mediated proliferation of mitogen-stimulated human peripheral blood T cells.

GM-CSF

A variety of GM-CSF-mediated actions are likely important in RA, including the activation of granulocytes and induction of class II major histocompatibility antigens on macrophages (Alvaro-Gracia *et al.*, 1989). Studies of GM-CSF inhibitors in RA are scant, although there is some evidence from bioassays that synovial fluid contains a factor(s) that inhibits GM-CSF induction of colony-formation by stem cells in the peripheral blood or bone marrow (Xu *et al.*, 1989). While the nature of the inhibitory activity is unknown, recent studies describing a soluble GM-CSF receptor suggest that this is a possible candidate (Raines *et al.*, 1991; Sasaki *et al.*, 1992). This topic is reviewed in detail in Chapter 12, this volume.

EXTRACELLULAR MATRIX AND CYTOKINE INTERACTIONS

Originally thought to be an inert tissue framework for cells, the extracellular matrix is now known to play an important role in the regulation of cellular adhesion and activation. For instance, fibronectin stimulates synoviocyte metalloproteinase produc-tion by crosslinking surface fibronectin receptors (Werb *et al.*, 1989). Within hours after the receptors are crosslinked, stromelysin and collagenase account for as much as 5% of proteins secreted by cultured synovial fibroblasts. The response is specific, since gelatinase and inhibitors of metalloproteinases like TIMP are not affected by fibronectin receptor engagement. The matrix can also indirectly participate in synovitis by activating cytokines like fibroblast growth factor (FGF). FGF function is greatly enhanced when it associates with matrix molecules containing negatively charged proteoglycans like heparan sulphate (Yayon *et al.*, 1991). In contrast, some macromolecules inhibit cytokine activity by absorbing them from the extracellular milieu and preventing receptor engagement. The interaction of TGFβ with decorin is an example of this phenomenon (Border *et al.*, 1992). Decorin associates with type I collagen fibrils and contains large numbers of leucine residues. It inhibits TGFβ biological activity by reversibly binding to the growth factor. The biological import-ance of this type of interaction has been demonstrated in animal models of glomerulo-nephritis where TGFβ plays a pathogenic role. Administration of decorin in these circumstances significantly retards renal damage. Other cytokines, including GM-CSF, can also bind to matrix macromolecules. It is unclear whether this process primarily serves to inhibit local cytokine function or acts as a reservoir to maintain a supply of growth factor that can be released later into the extracellular milieu long after the cell that produced it has migrated away or been down-regulated.

ROLE OF CYTOKINE ANTAGONISTS IN SYNOVITIS

The rheumatoid synovial membrane and synovial fluid are teeming with pro- and anti-inflammatory factors. One can conclude *a priori* that the net balance in RA must be towards the former or else the disease would be self-limited. However, this balance is probably tenuous, and subtle shifts in cytokine levels could potentially have major effects that contribute to the waxing and waning nature of the disease. Local differ-ences in the agonist:antagonist ratios might vary depending on the cellular compo-sition of each compartment. For example, synovial tissue and synovial fluid neutrophil contents are very different, and this might contribute to regional variations in IL-1ra concentrations. The synovium also exhibits a significant preponderance of $CD4^+$ memory T cells while $CD8^+$ T cells are more prevalent in synovial effusions (reviewed in Chapter 11, this volume). Compartmentalization is apparent within the synovial membrane itself, with regional variations in metalloproteinase and complement pro-tein gene expression within lining and sublining regions (Firestein *et al.*, 1991). Hence, the joint is an organized structure with each separate compartment demonstrating a distinct cell mix and cytokine milieu.

Most current data suggest that cytokine antagonists are dominant in synovial fluid: TNFα biological activity is difficult or impossible to detect in effusions and other inhibitors like TGFβ and IL-1ra are abundant. The net result is an environment in which cell proliferation and activation are very much blunted. This might account for defective synovial fluid T-cell function, including decreased proliferation and cytokine production. The situation might be reversed in the synovium, which is probably a more relevant compartment for understanding the pathogenesis of RA. In this region, the balance between IL-1 and IL-1ra appears to favour IL-1. Also, the sequelae of TNF-α biological activity can be demonstrated in synovium despite persistent shed-ding of inhibitors like TNF-R. For instance, addition of anti-TNFα antibodies to synovial cell cultures inhibits production of IL-1α and GM-CSF suggesting that bio-logically active TNFα plays a pivotal role (Haworth *et al.*, 1991). The reasons for the differences between the tissue and fluid phase of the joint are not clear; perhaps cytokine antagonists are less effective (or agonists more effective) within the three-dimensional framework of the synovium where the extracellular matrix can present cytokines or their antagonists in a tightly controlled evironment. This contrasts with synovial effusion, where cytokine gradients and high levels in a microenvironment are inherently much more difficult to achieve due to the nature of a fluid compartment.

Overall, despite abundant evidence of very effective cytokine antagonists in the joint, it is clear that amounts of the inhibitors are insufficient to counteract pro-inflammatory factors. Perhaps the inhibitors are not present in high enough concentrations, or perhaps they are not synthesized in the right location or at the correct time. The functions of cytokines in the initiation and perpetuation of RA is well established, and the possibility that the relative amounts of cytokine antagonists are too low is now being tested in clinical studies using pharmacologic doses of inhibitors like IL-1ra or antibodies to TNFα (Chapter 2, this volume). However, we must be cautious not to overinterpret the results of such trials, since the comlexity and redundancy of the cytokine networks suggest that combinations of inhibitors will be needed. For instance, inhibition of IL-1 without addressing the effects of TNFα might have minimal benefit. Another issue that will ultimately have to be faced is the difficulty and expense of using parenteral recombinant proteins to treat chronic diseases like RA. A small molecule approach (i.e. organic molecules that inhibit cytokine production or action) will have significant advantages, although this might lack the exquisite specificity characteristic of antibody or recombinant protein therapy.

REFERENCES

Alvaro-Gracia JM, Zvaifler NJ & Firestein GS (1989) Cytokines in chronic inflammatory arthritis. IV. Granulocyte/macrophage colony-stimulating factor-mediated induction of class II MHC antigen on human monocytes: a possible role in rheumatoid arthritis. *J Exp Med* **170**: 865–875.

Alvaro-Gracia JM, Zvaifler NJ & Firestein GS (1990) Cytokines in chronic inflammatory arthritis. V. Mutual antagonism between interferon-gamma and tumor necrosis factor-alpha on HLA-DR expression, proliferation, collagenase production, and granulocyte macrophage colony-stimulating factor production by rheumatoid arthritis synoviocytes. *J Clin Invest* **86**: 1790–1798.

Alvaro-Gracia JM, Yu C, Zvaifler NJ & Firestein GS (1993) Mutual antagonism between IFN-gamma and TNF-alpha on fibroblast-like synoviocytes: paradoxical induction of IFN-gamma and TNF-alpha receptor expression. *J Clin Immunol* **13**: 212–218.

Arend WP (1991) Interleukin 1 receptor antagonist. A new member of the interleukin 1 family. *J Clin Invest* **88**: 1445–1451.

Arend WP & Dayer J-M (1990) Cytokine and cytokine inhibitors or antagonists in rheumatoid arthritis. *Arthritis Rheum* **33**: 305–315.

Arend WP, Joslin JG & Massoni RJ (1985) Effects of immune complexes on production by human monocytes of interleukin 1 or an interleukin 1 inhibitor. *J Immunol* **134**: 3868–3875.

Arend WP, Welgus HG, Thompson RC & Eisenberg SP (1990) Biological properties of recombinant human monocyte-derived interleukin 1 receptor antagonist. *J Clin Invest* **85**: 1694–1697.

Balavoine J-F, deRochemontiex B, Williamson K, Seckinger P, Cruchaud A & Dayer J-M (1986) Prostaglandin E2 and collagenase production by fibroblasts and synovial cells is regulated by urine-derived human interleukin 1 and inhibitor(s). *J Clin Invest* **78**: 1120–1124.

Bigler CF, Norris DA, Weston WL & Arend WP (1992) Interleukin-1 receptor antagonist production by human keratinocytes. *J Invest Dermatol* **98**: 38–44.

Border WA, Noble NA, Yamamoto T, Harper JR, Yamaguchi Y, Pierschbacher MD et al. (1992) Natural inhibitor of transforming growth factor-beta protects against scarring in experimental kidney disease. *Nature* **360**: 361–364.

Brandes ME, Allen JB, Ogawa Y & Wahl SM (1991) Transforming growth factor beta 1 suppresses acute and chronic arthritis in experimental animals. *J Clin Invest* **87**: 1108–1113.

Brennan FM, Chantry D, Turner M, Foxwell B, Maini R & Feldmann M (1990) Detection of transforming growth factor-beta in rheumatoid arthritis synovial tissue: lack of effect on spontaneous cytokine production in joint cell cultures. *Clin Exp Immunol* **81**: 278–285.

Brennan FM, Gibbons DL, Mitchell T, Cope AP, Maini RN & Feldmann M (1992) Enhanced expression of tumor necrosis factor receptor mRNA and protein in mononuclear cells isolated from rheumatoid arthritis synovial joints. *Eur J Immunol* **22**: 1907–1912.

Brockhaw M, Schoenfeld H-J, Schlaeger E-J, Hunziker W, Lesslauer W & Loetscher H (1990) Identification of two types of tumor necrosis factor receptors on human cell lines by monoclonal antibodies. *Proc Natl Acad Sci USA* **87**: 3127–3131.

Browning J & Ribolini A (1989) Studies on the differing effects of tumor necrosis factor and lymphotoxin on the growth of several human tumor lines. *J Immunol* **143**: 1859–1867.

Buchan G, Barrett K, Fujita T, Taniguchi T, Maini R & Feldmann M (1988) Detection of activated T cell products in the rheumatoid joint using cDNA probes to Interleukin-2 (IL-2) IL-2 receptor and IFN-gamma. *Clin Exp Immunol* **71**: 295–301.

Cannon GW, Pincus SH, Emkey RD, Denes A, Cohen SA, Wolfe F et al. (1989) Double-blind trial of recombinant gamma-interferon versus placebo in the treatment of rheumatoid arthritis. *Arthritis Rheum* **32**: 964–973.

Carter DB, Deibel MR Jr, Dunn CJ, Tomich CS, Laborde AL, Slightom JL et al. (1990) Purification, cloning, expression and biological characterization of an interleukin-1 receptor antagonist protein. *Nature* **344**: 633–638.

Chan LS, Hammerberg C, Kang K, Sabb P, Tavakkol A & Cooper KD (1992) Human dermal fibroblast interleukin-1 receptor antagonist (IL-1ra) and interleukin-1 beta (IL-1 beta) mRNA and protein are co-stimulated by phorbol ester; implication for a homeostatic mechanism. *J Invest Dermatol* **99**: 315–322.

Chandrasekhar S, Harvey AK, Hrubey PS & Bendele AM (1990) Arthritis induced by interleukin-1 is dependent on the site and frequency of intraarticular injection. *Clin Immunol Immunopathol* **55**: 382–394.

Chin JE, Winterrowd GE, Krzesicki RF & Sanders ME (1990) Role of cytokines in inflammatory synovitis. The coordinate regulation of intercellular adhesion molecule 1 and HLA class I and class II antigens in rheumatoid synovial fibroblasts. *Arthritis Rheum* **33**: 1776–1786.

Chu CQ, Field M, Abney E, Zheng RQ, Allard S, Feldmann M & Maini RN (1991) Transforming growth factor-beta 1 in rheumatoid synovial membrane and cartilage/pannus junction. *Clin Exp Immunol* **86**: 380–386.

Combe B, Pope RM, Fischbach M, Darnell B, Baron S & Talal N (1985) Interleukin-2 in rheumatoid arthritis. Production of and response to interleukin-2 in rheumatoid synovial fluid, synovial tissue and peripheral blood. *Clin Exp Immunol* **59**: 520–528.

Cooper WO, Fava RA, Gates CA, Cremer MA & Townes AS (1992) Acceleration of onset of collagen-induced arthritis by intra-articular injection of tumour necrosis factor or transforming growth factor-beta. *Clin Exp Immunol* **89**: 244–250.

Cope AP, Aderka D, Doherty M, Engelmann H, Gibbons D, Jones AC et al. (1992) Increased levels of soluble tumor necrosis factor receptors in the sera and synovial fluid of patients with rheumatic diseases. *Arthritis Rheum* **35**: 1160–1169.

Cush JJ & Lipsky PE (1988) Phenotypic analysis of synovial tissue and peripheral blood lymphocytes isolated from patients with rheumatoid arthritis. *Arthritis Rheum* **31**: 1230–1238.

Deleuran BW, Chu CQ, Field M, Brennan FM, Katsikis P, Feldmann M et al. (1992a) Localization of interleukin-1 alpha, type 1 interleukin-1 receptor and interleukin-1 receptor antagonist in the synovial membrane and cartilage/pannus junction in rheumatoid arthritis. *Br J Rheumatol* **31**: 801–809.

Deleuran BW, Chu CQ, Field M, Brennan FM, Mitchell T, Feldmann M et al. (1992b) Localization of tumor necrosis factor receptors in the synovial tissue and cartilage–pannus junction in patients with rheumatoid arthritis. Implications for local actions of tumor necrosis factor alpha. *Arthritis Rheum* **35**: 1170–1178.

Dinarello CA (1991) Interleukin-1 and interleukin-1 antagonism. *Blood* **77**: 1827–1852.

Dripps DJ, Brandhuber BJ, Thompson RC & Eisenberg SP (1991a) Interleukin-1 (IL-1) receptor antagonist binds to the 80-kDa IL-1 receptor but does not initiate IL-1 signal transduction. *J Biol Chem* **266**: 10331–10336.

Dripps DJ, Verderber E, Ng RK, Thompson RC & Eisenberg SP (1991b) Interleukin-1 receptor antagonist binds to the type II interleukin-1 receptor on B cells and neutrophils. *J Biol Chem* **266**: 20311–20315.

Eisenberg SP, Evans RJ, Arend WP, Verderber E, Brewer MT, Hannum CH et al. (1990) Primary structure and functional expression from complementary DNA of a human interleukin-1 receptor antagonist. *Nature* **343**: 341–346.

Elford PR, Graeber M, Ohtsu H, Aeberhard M, Legendre B, Wishart WL et al. (1992) Induction of swelling, synovial hyperplasia and cartilage proteoglycan loss upon intra-articular injection of transforming growth factor beta-2 in the rabbit. *Cytokine* **4**: 232–238.

Elias JA, Krol RC, Freundlich B & Sampson PM (1988) Regulation of human lung fibroblast glycosaminoglycan production by recombinant interferons, tumor necrosis factor and lymphotoxin. *J Clin Invest* **81**: 325–333.

Engelmann H, Aderka D, Rubinstein M, Rotman D & Wallach D (1989) A tumor necrosis factor-binding protein purified to homogeneity from human urine protects cells from tumor necrosis factor toxicity. *J Biol Chem* **264**: 11974–11980.

Fava R, Olsen N, Keski-Oja J, Moses H & Pincus T (1989) Active and latent forms of transforming growth factor beta activity in synovial effusions. *J Exp Med* **169**: 291–296.

Firestein GS & Zvaifler NJ (1987) Peripheral blood and synovial fluid monocyte activation in inflammatory arthritis II. Low levels of synovial fluid and synovial tissue interferon suggest that gamma interferon is not the primary macrophage activating factor. *Arthritis Rheum* **30**: 864–871.

Firestein GS & Zvaifler NJ (1990) How important are T cells in chronic rheumatoid synovitis? *Arthritis Rheum* **33**: 768–773.

Firestein GS, Tsai V & Zvaifler NJ (1987) Cellular immunity in the joints of patients with rheumatoid arthritis and other forms of chronic synovitis. *Rheumatic Diseases Clinics of North America* **13**: 191–213.

Firestein GS, Xu WD, Townsend K et al. (1988) Cytokines in chronic inflammatory arthritis. I. Failure to detect T cell lymphokines (IL-2 and IL-3) and presence of macrophage colony-stimulating factor (CSF-1) and a novel mast cell growth factor in rheumatoid synovitis. *J Exp Med* **168**: 1573–1586.

Firestein GS, Alvaro-Gracia JM & Maki R (1990) Quantitative analysis of cytokine gene expression in rheumatoid arthritis. *J Immunol* **144**: 3347–3353.

Firestein GS, Paine MM & Littman BH (1991) Gene expression (collagenase, tissue inhibitor of metallo-proteinases, complement, and HLA-DR) in rheumatoid arthritis and osteoarthritis synovium: quantitative analysis and effect of intraarticular corticosteroids. *Arthritis Rheum* **34**: 1094–1105.

Firestein GS, Berger AE, Tracey DE, Chosay JG, Chapman DL, Paine MM et al. (1992) IL-1 receptor antagonist protein production and gene expression in rheumatoid arthritis and osteoarthritis synovium. *J Immunol* **149**: 1054–1062.

Firestein GS, Boyle D, Yu C, Paine MM, Zvaifler NJ & Arend WP (1994) Synovial IL-1ra and IL-1 balance in rheumatoid arthritis. *Arthritis Rheum* **37**: 644–652.

Goddard DH, Grossman SL & Moore ME (1990) Autocrine regulation of rheumatoid arthritis synovial cell growth *in vitro*. *Cytokine* **2**: 149–155.

Goddard DH, Grossman SL, Williams WV, Weiner DB, Gross JL, Eidsvoog K & Dasch JR (1992) Regulation of synovial cell growth. Coexpression of transforming growth factor beta and basic fibroblast growth factor by cultured synovial cells. *Arthritis Rheum* **35**: 1296–1303.

Hamilton JA, Piccoli DS, Cebon J, Layton JE, Rathanaswani P, McColl SR et al. (1992) Cytokine regulation of colony-stimulating factor (CSF) production in cultured human synovial fibroblasts. II. Similarities and differences in the control of interleukin-1 induction of granulocyte-macrophage CSF and granulocyte-CSF production. *Blood* **79**: 1413–1419.

Hannum CH, Wilcox CJ, Arend WP, Joslin FG, Dripps DJ, Heimdal PL et al. (1990) Interleukin-1 receptor antagonist activity of a human interleukin-1 inhibitor. *Nature* **343**: 336–340.

Harvey AK, Hrubey PS & Chandrasekhar S (1991) Transforming growth factor-beta inhibition of interleukin-1 activity involves down-regulation of interleukin-1 receptors on chondrocytes. *Exp Cell Res* **195**: 376–385.

Haskill S, Martin G, Van Le L, Morris J, Peace A, Biegler CF et al. (1991) cDNA cloning of an intracellular form of the human interleukin 1 receptor antagonist associated with epithelium. *Proc Natl Acad Sci USA* **88**: 3681–3685.

Hasler F, Bluestein HG, Zvaifler NJ & Epstein LB (1983) Analysis of the defects responsible for the impaired regulation of EBV-induced B cell proliferation by rheumatoid arthritis lymphocytes. *J Immunol* **131**: 768–772.

Hatakeyama M, Tsudo M, Minamoto S, Kono T, Doi T, Miyata T et al. (1989) Interleukin-2 receptor beta chain gene: generation of three receptor forms by cloned human alpha and beta chain cDNAs. *Science* **244**: 551–556.

Haworth C, Brennan FM, Chantry D, Turner M, Maini RN & Feldmann M (1991) Expression of granulocyte-macrophage colony-stimulating factor in rheumatoid arthritis: regulation by tumor necrosis factor-alpha. *Eur J Immunol* **21**: 2575–2579.

Heilig B, Wermann M, Gallati H, Brockhaus M, Berke B, Egen O et al. (1992) Elevated TNF receptor plasma concentrations in patients with rheumatoid arthritis. *Clin Invest* **70**: 22–27.

Henderson B & Pettipher ER (1989) Arthritogenic actions of recombinant IL-1 and tumour necrosis factor alpha in the rabbit evidence for synergistic interactions between cytokines *in vivo*. *Clin Exp Immunol* **75**: 306–310.

Henderson B, Thompson RC, Hardingham T & Lewthwaite J (1991) Inhibition of interleukin-1-induced synovitis and articular cartilage proteoglycan loss in the rabbit knee by recombinant human interleukin-1 receptor antagonist. *Cytokine* **3**: 246–249.

Hogquist KA, Nett MA, Unanue ER & Chaplin DD (1991) Interleukin 1 is processed and released during apoptosis. *Proc Natl Acad Sci USA* **88**: 8485–8489.

Hohmann, H-P, Remy R, Brockhaus M & van Loon APGM (1989) Two different call types have different major receptors for human tumor necrosis factor (TNFα). *J Biol Chem* **264**: 14927–14934.

Hohmann H-P, Brockhaus M, Baeuerle PA, Remy R, Kolbeck R & van Loon APGM (1990) Expression of the types A and B tumor necrosis factor (TNF) receptor is independently regulated, and both receptor mediate activation of the transcription factor NF-kB. TNFα is not needed for induction of a biological effect via TNF receptors. *J Biol Chem* **265**: 22409–22417.

Janson RW, Hance KR & Arend WP (1991) Production of IL-1 receptor antagonist by human *in vitro*-derived macrophages. Effects of lipopolysaccharide and granulocyte-macrophage colony-stimulating factor. *J Immunol* **147**: 4218–4223.

Johnson WJ, Kelley A, Connor JR, Dalton BJ & Meunier PC (1989) Inhibition of interferon-gamma-induced Ia antigen expression on synovial fibroblasts by IL-1. *J Immunol* **143**: 1614–1618.

Kashiwado T, Miossec P, Oppenheimer-Marks N & Ziff M (1987) Inhibitor of interleukin-2 synthesis and response in rheumatoid synovial fluid. *Arthritis Rheum* **30**: 1339–1347.

Keystone EC, Snow KM, Bombardier C, Chang CH, Nelson DL & Rubin LA (1988) Elevated soluble interleukin-2 receptor levels in the sera and synovial fluids of patients with rheumatoid arthritis. *Arthritis Rheum* **31**: 844–849.

Koch AE, Kunkel SL, Chensue SW, Haines GK & Strieter RM (1992) Expression of interleukin-1 and interleukin-1 receptor antagonist by human rheumatoid synovial tissue macrophages. *Clin Immunol Immunopathol* **65**: 23–27.

Kondo N, Kondo S, Shimizu A, Honjo T & Hamuro J (1988) A soluble 'Anchorminus' interleukin 2 receptor suppresses *in vitro* interleukin 2-mediated immune responses. *Immunol Lett* **19**: 299–308.

Kunkel SL, Remick DG, Strieter RM & Larrick JW (1989) Mechanisms that regulate the production and effects of tumor necrosis factor-α. *Crit Rev Immunol* **9**: 93–117.

Lafton A, Sanchez-Madrid F, Ortiz de Landazuri M, Jimenez Cuesta A, Ariza A, Ossorio C & Sabando P (1989) Very late activation antigen on synovial fluid T cells from patients with rheumatoid arthritis and other rheumatic diseases. *Arthritis Rheum* **32**: 386–392.

Lafyatis R, Thompson NL, Remmers EF, Flanders KC, Roche NS, Kim SJ et al. (1989) Transforming growth factor-beta production by synovial tissues from rheumatoid patients and streptococcal cell wall arthritic rats. Studies on secretion by synovial fibroblast-like cells and immunohistologic localization. *J Immunol* **143**: 1142–1148.

Lotz M, Kekow J & Carson DA (1990) Transforming growth factor-beta and cellular immune responses in synovial fluids. *J Immunol* **144**: 4189–4194.

Malyak M, Swaney RE & Arend WP (1994) Synovial fluid interleukin-1 receptor antagonist (IL-1ra) levels in rheumatoid arthritis and other arthropathies: potential contribution from synovial fluid neutrophils. *Arthritis Rheum*, in press.

McColl SR, Paquin R, Menard C & Beaulieu AD (1992) Human neutrophils produce high levels of the interleukin 1 receptor antagonist in response to granulocyte/macrophage colony-stimulating factor and tumor necrosis factor alpha. *J Exp Med* **176**: 593–598.

Miller LC, Lynch EA, Isa S, Logan JW, Dinarello CD & Steere AC (1993) Balance of synovial fluid 1L-1β and IL-1 receptor antagonist and recovery from Lyme arthritis. *Lancet* **341**: 146–148.

Miossec P, Dinarello CA & Ziff M (1986) Interleukin-1 lymphocyte chemotactic activity in rheumatoid arthritis synovial fluid. *Arthritis Rheum* **29**: 461–470.

Miossec P, Elhamiani M, Chichehian B, D'Angeac AD, Sany J & Hirn M (1990a) Interleukin 2 (IL 2) inhibitor in rheumatoid synovial fluid: correlation with prognosis and soluble IL 2 receptor levels. *J Clin Immunol* **10**: 115–120.

Miossec P, Elhamiani M, Edmonds-Alt X, Sany J & Hirn M (1990b) Functional studies of soluble low-affinity interleukin-2 receptors in rheumatoid synovial fluid. *Arthritis Rheum* **33**: 1688–1694.

Miossec P, Naviliat M, Dupuy d'Angeac A, Sany J & Banchereau J (1990c) Low levels of interleukin-4 and high levels of transforming growth factor beta in rheumatoid synovitis. *Arthritis Rheum* **33**: 1180–1187.

Miossec P, Briolay J, Dechanet J, Wijdenes J, Martinez-Valdez H & Banchereau J (1992) Inhibition of the production of proinflammatory cytokines and immunoglobulins by interleukin-4 in an *ex vivo* model of rheumatoid synovitis. *Arthritis Rheum* **35**: 874–883.

Moore SA, Strieter RM, Rolfe MW, Standiford TJ, Burdick MD & Kunkel SL (1992) Expression and regulation of human alveolar macrophage-derived interleukin-1 receptor antagonist. *Am J Resp Cell Mol Biol* **6**: 569–575.

Morales-Ducret J, Wayner E, Elices MJ, Alvaro-Gracia JM, Zvaifler NJ & Firestein GS (1992) Alpha 4/beta 1 integrin (VLA-4) ligands in arthritis. Vascular cell adhesion molecule-1 expression in synovium and on fibroblast-like synoviocytes. *J Immunol* **149**: 1424–1431.

Mosley B, Urdal DL, Prickett KS, Larsen A, Cosman D, Conlon PJ et al. (1987) The interleukin-1 receptor binds the human interleukin-1 alpha precursor but not the interleukin-1 beta precursor. *J Biol Chem* **262**: 2941–2944.

Nicod LP, el Habre F & Dayer JM (1992) Natural and recombinant interleukin 1 receptor antagonist does not inhibit human T-cell proliferation induced by mitogens, soluble antigens or allogeneic determinants. *Cytokine* **4**: 29–35.

Nophar Y, Kemper O, Brakebusch C, Engelmann H, Zwang R, Aderka D et al. (1990) Soluble forms of tumor necrosis factor receptors (TNF-Rs). The cDNA for the type I TNF-R, cloned using amino acid sequence data of its soluble form, encodes both the cell surface and a soluble form of the receptor. *EMBO J* **9**: 3269–3278.

Novick D, Engelmann H, Wallach D & Rubinstein M (1989) Soluble cytokine receptors are present in normal human urine. *J Exp Med* **170**: 1409–1414.

Overall CM, Wrana JL & Sodek J (1989) Independent regulation of collagenase, 72-kDa progelatinase, and metalloendoproteinase inhibitor expression in human fibroblasts by transforming growth factor-beta. *J Biol Chem* **264**: 1860–1869.

Panayi GS, Lanchbury JS & Kingsley GH (1992) The importance of the T cell in initiating and maintaining the chronic synovitis of rheumatoid arthritis [editorial]. *Arthritis Rheum* **35**: 729–735.

Porteu F, Brockhaus M, Wallach D, Engelmann H & Nathan CF (1991) Human neutrophil elastase releases a ligand-binding fragment from the 75-kDa tumor necrosis factor (TNF) receptor. Comparison with the proteolytic activity responsible for shedding of TNF receptors from stimulated neutrophils. *J Biol Chem* **266**: 18846–18853.

Quay J, Arend WP & Becker S (1993) IL-1 and IL-1 receptor antagonist production in human alveolar macrophages infected with respiratory syncytial virus. *J Inf Dis*, in press.

Raghu G, Masta S, Meyers D & Narayanan AS (1989) Collagen synthesis by normal and fibrotic human lung fibroblasts and the effect of transforming growth factor-beta. *Am Rev Resp Dis*, **140**: 95–100.

Raines MA, Liu L, Quan SG, Joe V, diPersio JF & Golde DW (1991) Identification and molecular cloning of a soluble human granulocyte-macrophage colony-stimulating factor receptor. *Proc Natl Acad Sci USA* **88**: 8203–8207.

Rédini F, Mauviel A, Pronost S, Loyau G & Pujol J-P (1993) Transforming growth factor β exerts opposite effects from interleukin-1β on cultured rabbit articular chondrocytes through reduction of interleukin-1 receptor expression. *Arthritis Rheum* **36**: 44–50.

Robb RJ & Kutny RM (1987) Structure-function relationships for the IL 2-receptor system IV. Analysis of the sequence and ligand-binding properties of soluble tac protein. *J Immunol* **139**: 855–862.

Rooney M, Symons JA & Duff GW (1990) Interleukin 1 beta in synovial fluid is related to local disease activity in rheumatoid arthritis. *Rheumatol Int* **10**: 217–219.

Roux-Lombard P & Dayer JM (1991) Soluble tumor necrosis factor (TNF) receptors in human inflammatory synovial fluids (SF). *Arthritis Rheum* **34**: S47.

Roux-Lombard P, Modoux C & Dayer JM (1989) Production of interleukin-1 (IL-1) and a specific IL-1 inhibitor during human monocyte-macrophage differentiation: influence of GM-CSF. *Cytokine* **1**: 45–51.

Roux-Lombard P, Punzi L, Hasler F, Bas S, Todesco S, Gallati H et al. (1993) Soluble tumor necrosis factor receptors in human inflammatory synovial fluids. *Arthritis Rheum* **36**: 985–989.

Sasaki K, Chiba S, Mano H, Yazaki Y & Hirai H (1992) Identification of a soluble GM-CSF binding protein in the supernatant of a human choriocarcinoma cell line. *Biochem Biophys Res Comm* **183**: 252–257.

Saxne T, Palladino MA Jr, Heinegard D, Talal N & Wollheim FA (1988) Detection of tumor necrosis factor alpha but not tumor necrosis factor beta in rheumatoid arthritis synovial fluid and serum. *Arthritis Rheum* **31**: 1041–1045.

Schall TJ, O'Hehir RE, Goeddel DV & Lamb JR (1992) Uncoupling of cytokine mRNA expression and protein secretion during the induction phase of T cell anergy. *J Immunol* **148**: 381–387.

Scharffetter K, Heckmann M, Hatamochi A, Mauch C, Stein B, Riethmuller G et al. (1989) Synergistic effect of tumor necrosis factor and interferon-gamma on collagen synthesis of human skin fibroblasts *in vitro*. *Exp Cell Res* **181**: 409–419.

Schoenfeld H-J, Poeschi B, Frey JR, Loetscher H, Hunziker W, Lustig A et al. (1991) Efficient purification of recombinant human tumor necrosis factor β from *Escherichia coli* yields biologically active protein with a trimeric structure that binds to both tumor necrosis factor receptors. *J Biol Chem* **266**: 3863–3869.

Seckinger P, Isaaz S & Dayer JM (1988) A human inhibitor of tumor necrosis factor α. *J Exp Med* **167**: 1511–1516.

Seckinger P, Zhang JH & Hauptmann B (1990) Characterization of a tumor necrosis factor α (TNF-α) inhibitor: evidence of immunological cross-reactivity with the TNF receptor. *Proc Natl Acad Sci USA* **87**: 5188–5192.

Smith RJ, Chin JE, Sam LM & Justen JM (1991) Biologic effects of an interleukin-1 receptor antagonist protein on interleukin-1 stimulated cartilage erosion and chondrocyte responsiveness. *Arthritis Rheum* **34**: 78–83.

Suzuki H, Ayabe T, Kamimura J & Kashiwagi H (1991) Anti-IL-1 alpha autoantibodies in patients with rheumatic diseases and in healthy subjects. *Clin Exp Immunol* **85**: 407–412.

Symons JA, Wood NC, Di Giovine FS & Duff GW (1988) Soluble IL-2 receptor in rheumatoid arthritis: correlation with disease activity, IL-1 and IL-2 inhibition. *J Immunol* **141**: 2612–2618.

Symons JA, McDowell TL, di Giovine FS, Wood NC, Capper SJ & Duff GW (1989) Interleukin 1 in rheumatoid arthritis: potentiation of immune responses within the joint. *Lymphokine Research* **8**: 365–372.

Symons JA, Eastgate JA & Duff GW (1990) A soluble binding protein specific for interleukin 1 beta is produced by activated mononuclear cells. *Cytokine* **2**: 190–198.

Symons JA, Eastgate JA & Duff GW (1991) Purification and characterization of a novel soluble receptor for interleukin 1. *J Exp Med* **174**: 1251–1254.

Thompson RC, Dripps DJ & Eisenberg SP (1992) Interleukin-1 receptor antagonist (IL-1ra) as a probe and as a treatment for IL-1 mediated disease. *Int J Immunopharmacol* **14**: 475–480.

Tsai V, Firestein GS, Arend W & Zvaifler NJ (1992) Cytokine induced differentiation of cultured non-adherent macrophages. *Cell Immunol* **144**: 203–216.

Ulich TR, Guo K, Yin S, del Castillo J, Yi ES, Thompson RC et al. (1992) Endotoxin-induced cytokine gene expression *in vivo*. IV. Expression of interleukin-1 alpha/beta and interleukin-1 receptor antagonist mRNA during endotoxemia and during endotoxin-initiated local acute inflammation. *Am J Pathol* **141**: 61–68.

Vilcek J & Lee TH (1991) Tumor necrosis factor. *J Biol Chem* **266**: 7313–7316.

Wahl SM, Allen JB, Wong HL, Dougherty SF & Ellingsworth LR (1990) Antagonistic and agonistic effects of transforming growth factor-beta and IL-1 in rheumatoid synovium. *J Immunol* **145**: 2514–2519.

Wahl SM, Allen JB, Costa GL, Wong HL & Dasch JR (1993) Reversal of acute and chronic synovial inflammation by anti-transforming growth factor beta. *J Exp Med* **177**: 225–230.

Werb Z, Tremble PM, Behrendtsen O, Crowley E & Damsky CH (1989) Signal transduction through the fibronectin receptor induces collagenase and stromelysin gene expression. *J Cell Biol* **109**: 877–889.

Westacott CI, Whicher JT, Barnes IC *et al.* (1990) Synovial fluid concentration of five different cytokines in rheumatic diseases. *Ann Rheum Dis* **49**: 676–681.

Xu WD, Firestein GS, Taetle R, Kaushansky K & Zvaifler NJ (1989) Cytokines in chronic inflammatory arthritis: II. Granulocyte-macrophage colony stimulating factor in rheumatoid synovial effusions. *J Clin Invest* **83**: 876–882.

Yayon A, Klagsbrun M, Esko JD, Leder P & Ornitz DM (1991) Cell surface, heparin-like molecules are required for binding of basic fibroblast growth factor to its high affinity receptor. *Cell* **64**: 841–848.

Zuber P, Acolla RS, Carel S, Diserens AC & de Tribolet N (1988) Effects of recombinant human tumor necrosis factor-alpha on the surface phenotype and the growth of human malignant glioma cell lines. *Int J Cancer* **42**: 780–786.

14 Approaches to Novel Anti-arthritic Drugs by Modulation of the Arachidonic Acid Cascade

Rodger M. McMillan, Stephen J. Foster and John S. Shaw

INTRODUCTION

Arachidonic acid metabolism via cyclo-oxygenase and 5-lipoxygenase leads to formation of pro-inflammatory prostanoids and leukotrienes respectively. Non steroidal anti-inflammatory drugs (NSAIDs), which represent the major symptomatic therapy in theumatic diseases, exert their effects by blocking cyclo-oxygenase. This accounts for their therapeutic efficacy but, since prostanoids are responsible for maintaining gastrointestinal integrity, the mechanism also explains their major side-effects.

In this chapter several potential approaches for novel therapies, based on modulation of the arachidonic acid metabolites, are discussed. Two approaches for discovering drugs with the efficacy, but not the side-effects, of NSAIDs are described based on the developing knowledge of isoforms of cyclo-oxygenase and prostanoid receptor subtypes. The potential for anti-inflammatory therapies by inhibition of the 5-lipoxygenase pathway is reviewed and the status of several classes of leukotriene synthesis inhibitors is summarized. Finally, recent findings on the effects of combinations of cyclo-oxygenase and lipoxygenase inhibitors are presented. These data indicate the possibility of improved efficacy and safety from drugs that inhibit leukotriene and prostanoid synthesis by blocking a novel cytoplasmic form of phospholipase A2.

NOVEL APPROACHES TO MODULATION OF CYCLO-OXYGENASE PRODUCTS

PROSTANOIDS IN INFLAMMATION AND PAIN

Since the NSAIDs inhibit prostanoid synthesis, they provide the best tools with which to understand the contribution of the prostanoids to the symptoms of rheumatoid arthritis (RA). The ability of NSAIDs to reduce the primary symptoms of arthritis (inflammation and pain/hyperalgesia) is established beyond doubt, as is the ability of these agents to produce unwanted, and sometimes serious, gastrointestinal side-effects. It follows that prostanoids play a major role as mediators of inflammation and the accompanying pain and hyperalgesia. They are also essential for the maintenance of gastrointestinal integrity. Despite enormous efforts over the past two decades, an NSAID which is free from gastrointestinal toxicity has yet to be developed.

Mechanisms and Models in Rheumatoid Arthritis   Copyright © 1995 Academic Press Ltd
ISBN 0–12–340440–1

Measurement of the prostanoids produced in rheumatoid joints has been employed to determine the importance of different cyclo-oxygenase products. The levels of PGE_2, $PGF_{2\alpha}$, TXB_2, PGD_2 and 6-keto $PGF_{1\alpha}$ are all reported to be elevated in synovial fluid from RA patients with PGE_2 concentrations the highest of those measured (Trang et al., 1977; Brodie et al., 1980; Egg, 1984; Daymond and Rowell, 1988; Atik, 1990). In vitro studies using cultured synovial cells from RA patients have revealed that these cells produce large amounts of PGE_2, with smaller amounts of TXB_2, $PGF_{2\alpha}$ and 6-keto-$PGF_{1\alpha}$ (Robinson et al., 1979; Seppala, 1978; Moilanen et al., 1989).

The peripheral actions of prostanoids are well documented. When injected into the skin of human volunteers both PGE_1 and PGE_2 produce a long-lasting erythema. PGD_2 produces similar effects but at higher doses (Flower et al., 1976). PGE_2 also induces hyperalgesia (Sciberras et al., 1987). Similar effects of the E-prostaglandins are found in the rat, although PGI_2 is considerably more potent (Higgs et al., 1978; Ferreira et al., 1978) and $PGF_{2\alpha}$ is inactive (Crunkhorn and Willis, 1971). Both PGE_2 and PGI_2, when injected into a joint, can mimic many of the symptoms of RA. In a series of elegant studies by Schaible and co-workers, both PGE_2 and PGI_2 were found to sensitize a proportion of cat knee joint nociceptive nerones to mechanical stimuli (Heppelmann et al., 1986; Schaible and Schmidt, 1988; Schepelmann et al., 1992). PGI_2 is the more effective of the two. Similar conclusions were reached by Iggo and colleagues using a rat ankle joint preparation (Grubb et al., 1991; Birrell et al., 1991; McQueen et al., 1991). Thus, in the periphery, both PGE_2 and PGI_2 are involved in the sensitization to pain of inflamed joints. Whilst exogenously applied PGI_2 is the more potent of the two, PGE_2 is present in higher concentrations in inflamed joints.

In addition to the peripheral roles of prostanoids, studies in the last few years have demonstrated that they also have a central role. PGs are synthesized in the spinal cord in response to noxious stimuli with PGE_2 and PGD_2 the major products (Coderre et al., 1990). Injection of prostanoids into the spinal cord induces hyperalgesia. Taiwo and Levine (1986) showed that intrathecally administered PGE_2 reduced the mechanical pain threshold in the paw pressure test in the rat. The minimum effective dose of PGE_2 was 10 ng/rat. Even at the higher dose of 100 ng/rat, PGE_2 had no effect when administered intracerebroventricularly, thus ruling out the possibility that the intrathecally administered prostanoid produced its effect by diffusing into the brain. More recently (Uda et al., 1990) it has been shown that intrathecal administration of PGE_2 or PGD_2 to mice caused a significant reduction in hot plate (55°C) latency, and increased the writhing response induced by 0.6% acetic acid. The lowest effective doses of PGE_2 and PGD_2 were 0.001 ng and 0.5 ng respectively.

Further support for a role of prostanoids in spinal hyperalgesia comes from studies with cyclo-oxygenase inhibitors. For example, intrathecal administration of aspirin caused a significant inhibition of nociceptive C-fibre activation induced by electrical stimulation of the sural nerve (Jurna et al., 1992). More recently, evidence has been obtained in the rat formalin test. The basis of this assay is that intradermal injection of formalin in volunteers gives rise to an intense burning pain of short duration. This subsides and is replaced after several minutes by a more prolonged, but less intense pain. In rats, the injection of formalin causes scratching and licking of the injection site. The response is again biphasic with an early intense phase being followed by a prolonged response of lower intensity. Dickenson and Sullivan (1987) have shown that the second phase of the response is a direct consequence of the initial afferent barrage, and is due to changes in the sensitivity of spinal cord neurones; that is, the first phase of the response represents a spinal hyperalgesia.

Systemically administered NSAIDs are known to inhibit only the second phase of the formalin response (Dray and Dickenson, 1991). Malmberg and Yaksh (1992a,b) have reported that NSAIDs also attenuate the second phase of the formalin response when applied locally to the spinal cord. Recently these same authors have shown that whilst antagonists at the tachykinin NK1 receptor or the glutamate NMDA receptor can attentuate the second phase of the response, they are only effective if administered before the formalin injection. In contrast, the NSAIDs were effective even if administered after the first phase of the response was complete. They also inhibited the effects of substance P and NMDA. This suggests that whilst glutamate and substance P can initiate the changes leading to spinal hyperalgesia, a cyclo-oxygenase product is essential to maintain the response.

ANTAGONISM OF PROSTANOID RECEPTORS

In addition to the gastrointestinal toxicity of NSAIDs, a consistent finding in clinical trials is that the relief produced by these drugs is less than complete. At normal therapeutic doses, NSAIDs typically reduce by between 35 and 50% the number of swollen or tender joints, and are only slightly more effective at reducing the duration of morning stiffness (Grennan et al., 1983; Vasey et al., 1987; Atkinson et al., 1988; Kolodny, 1988). One interpretation of these findings is that the limited improvement produced by NSAID therapy reflects the extent of the contribution of prostanoids to the symptoms of RA. An alternative explanation, given the toxicity of these compounds, is that the use of NSAIDs in the clinic is restricted by side-effects to doses which are submaximally effective.

Cyclo-oxygenase inhibitors inhibit the synthesis of all prostanoids. It is perhaps not surprising that drugs with such a wide-ranging action produce unwanted side-effects. It is unlikely that all the prostanoids contribute to pain and inflammation. It is equally difficult to imagine that the symptoms of arthritis require activation of all types of prostanoid receptors. By identifying the relevant cyclo-oxygenase products, and the receptors through which they act to produce the symptoms of arthritis, it may be possible to devise more selective, and less toxic therapies.

The classification of prostanoid receptors has been hampered by a lack of truly selective agonists and antagonists. A comprehensive nomenclature system for prostanoid receptors has been proposed by Coleman and Kennedy (Coleman et al., 1980; Coleman and Kennedy, 1985; Kennedy et al., 1983). These authors suggested a system based on the relative potencies of the natural prostanoids in a range of isolated tissue systems. In tissues where PGE_2 was the most potent agonist, the receptors were deemed to be of the EP-type. Where PGD_2, $PGF_{2\alpha}$, TXA_2 or PGI_2 were the most potent, the receptors were named DP, FP, TP or IP respectively.

More recently it has become evident that the effects of PGE_2 involve more than one type of receptor. Consequently, the EP receptor has been further divided into subtypes designated EP_1, EP_2 and EP_3 (Coleman et al., 1987). In addition, the presence of a fourth (EP_4) subtype has recently been proposed (Louttit et al., 1992). This classification relies on the relative agonist potencies of a range of natural and synthetic

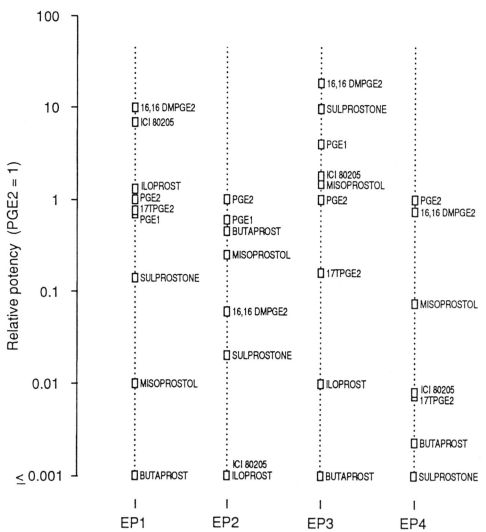

Figure 1. Schematic representation of the potencies of prostanoids at the four EP receptor subtypes. Data summarized from Dong *et al.* (1986), Coleman *et al.* (1987), Eglen and Whiting (1989), Lawrence *et al.* (1992), Lawrence and Jones (1992), Louttit *et al.* (1992) and Brown, Harding and Shaw (unpublished). 16,16,DMPGE2: 16,16,dimethyl PGE_2; ICI 80205: ω-tetranor-16-*p*-chlorophenoxy PGE_2; 17PTPGE2: 17-phenyl-trinor-PGE_2.

prostanoids (Fig. 1). It is almost certain that further prostaglandin receptor subtypes will be characterized in the future. There is already evidence that the TP receptor on the platelet differs from that on vascular smooth muscle (Furci *et al.*, 1991), and the existence of IP-receptor subtypes has also been proposed (Armstrong *et al.*, 1989).

An important lesson from receptor classification studies is that none of the naturally occurring prostanoids, and few of the synthetic agonists, are totally selective for a single receptor type or subtype. Of particular relevance are the findings that PGI_2 is a potent agonist at the EP_1 site (Eglen and Whiting, 1988) and that PGE_1, but not PGE_2

has high affinity for the prostacyclin (IP) receptor (Carroll and Shaw, 1989). Classically, receptor classification is best achieved using antagonists. In the case of EP_1, a number of selective antagonists have been reported. Thus, compounds from Searle (SC19220, SC25469) and Glaxo (AH-6809) (Sanner et al., 1973; Coleman et al., 1985; Drower et al., 1987) have been shown to antagonize the EP_1 receptor subtype without significant activity at other prostanoid receptors. These compounds have modest potency and poor in vivo activity. To date no selective antagonists at either EP_2, EP_3 or IP receptor have been reported.

As was discussed above, the cyclo-oxygenase products most widely implicted in causing inflammation and pain/hyperalgesia are PGE_2 and PGI_2. The receptors responsible for the actions of PGE_2 must be one of the EP subtypes, whilst PGI_2 could act at either IP or EP_1 sites. The nature of the EP-receptor subtype involved in pain and hyperalgesia is not entirely clear. The selective EP_1 receptor antagonists SC-19220 and SC-25469 were effective in a number of rodent analgesia assays (Ferreira et al., 1978; Drower et al., 1987). These findings are supported by an in vitro study where the response of nociceptive afferent neurones to noxious agents in the perfused rabbit ear preparation was enhanced by PGE_1 and this effect was abolished by SC-19220 (Juan and Seewann, 1980). In addition, another EP_1 antagonist, AH6809, abolished the hyperalgesia induced by intrathecal administration of PGE_2 (Uda et al., 1990) which implicates EP_1 receptors in the spinal actions of PGE_2.

Studies with synthetic agonists suggest that receptors other than EP_1 may also be important. Thus, Birrell et al. (1991) showed that the IP-receptor agonist, cicaprost, which lacks significant activity at the EP_1 receptor, directly excites a large proportion of nociceptive neurones in the rat ankle joint and sensitizes them to mechanical stimulation. In a similar study in the cat knee, Schepelmann et al. (1992) reported that a higher proportion of neurones were sensitive to PGI_2 than PGE_2. Both sets of data suggest a role for IP receptors. In addition, EP_3 receptors may be involved in some situations since Kumazawa et al. (1992) found that a relatively selective EP_3 agonist M&B 28767 was more potent than PGE_2 at enhancing bradykinin-induced nociceptor activation in dog testes in vitro.

The current data do not permit a definitive conclusion about the potential for development of safer analgesic/anti-inflammatory agents by modulating prostanoid receptors. Some EP_1 antagonists have anti-hyperalgesic actions but proof of the hypothesis requires the development of improved EP_1 antagonists and selective antagonists of IP and other EP receptors.

INHIBITION OF CYCLO-OXYGENASE ISOFORMS

Until recently, most evidence pointed to the existence of a single cyclo-oxygenase (PGH synthase) enzyme as the rate-limiting step in the synthesis of prostanoids. However, since 1991 it has become clear that there are at least two forms of the cyclo-oxygenase enzyme that are encoded by distinct genes. Cyclo-oxygenase I (COX-I) is the 'classical' form which is constitutively expressed in a wide range of cells and tissues. COX-II is a more recently discovered form, which is expressed following cell activation with agents such as cytokines and mitogens (Kujubu and Herschman, 1992; Masferrer et al., 1992; Lee et al., 1992). The two forms of the enzyme share approximately 62% homology and have similar catalytic properties. The enhanced synthesis of prostanoids following exposure of macrophages to lipopolysaccharide appears to be entirely due to induction of COX-II (Lee *et al.*, 1992; O'Sullivan *et al.*, 1992). The mitogen-induced expression of COX-II is inhibited by dexamethasone, whereas the activity of the type I enzyme was unaffected (Lee *et al.*, 1992; Kujubu *et al.*, 1993), and it has been proposed that glucocorticoids play a physiological role in suppressing the synthesis of this enzyme (Masferrer *et al.*, 1992).

The precise role of the two isoforms is the subject of considerable research activity. COX-I is likely to be the key enzyme responsible for producing PGs in tissues where they have physiological roles, for example the gastrointestinal tract. Since COX-II is induced by inflammatory cytokines, a specific inhibitor of this isoform could be anti-inflammatory without inhibiting gastroprotective prostanoids. No truly specific inhibitors of either isoform are available but recent studies by Smith and co-workers lend some support to this hypothesis (Meade *et al.*, 1993). They demonstrated that most conventional anti-inflammatory agents were either equipotent against both isoforms (e.g. piroxicam, indomethacin) or exhibited some selectivity for COX-I (e.g. flurbiprofen, meclofenamic acid). In contrast 6-methoxy-2-naphthyl acetic acid, the active metabolite of nabumetone, was approximately 10 times more potent as an inhibitor of COX-II than COX-I. Since nabumetone is reported to have a reduced incidence of gastrointestinal side-effects, these data will stimulate research activity to discover more specific inhibitors of the inducible enzyme.

MODULATION OF 5-LIPOXYGENASE PRODUCTS

5-LIPOXYGENASE AND LEUKOTRIENES

The 5-lipoxygenase pathway is the source of a potent group of inflammatory mediators, the leukotrienes. Arachidonic acid is converted in a two-stage process, catalysed by 5-lipoxygenase, to an unstable epoxide, leukotriene A_4 (LTA_4), which occupies a pivotal point in the enzymatic cascade. Enzymic hydrolysis of LTA_4 leads to formation of dihydroxy acid, leukotriene B_4 (LTB_4). Alternatively, LTA_4 can be metabolized, via a specific glutathione transferase, to form a group of peptide-containing leukotrienes: LTC_4, LTD_4 and LTE_4.

Both classes of leukotrienes may contribute to inflammatory reactions. Peptidyl-LTs were originally described as slow-reacting substances of anaphylaxis, by virtue of their prolonged contractile activity on airway and intestinal smooth muscle. It is now believed that they are key mediators of allergic inflammation. By enhancing vascular permeability, stimulating mucus secretion and inducing eosinophilia, peptido-LTs have a major role in certain pulmonary inflammatory diseases, such as asthma and allergic rhinitis. Potent selective antagonists of peptido-LT receptors have been developed. Some, some as Accolate (ICI204,219; Zeneca), have shown clinical efficacy in trials in human asthma and have considerable potential as novel anti-inflammatory therapies in asthma. However, since these drugs have not been evaluated in arthritides they are beyond the scope of this review.

Of more interest in inflammatory joint diseases has been LTB_4, which is a potent leukocyte chemotactic agent. LTB_4 is chemotactic for neutrophils, monocytes and eosinophils. LTB_4 elevates cytosolic calcium concentrations and this leads to stimulation of a variety of leukocyte responses such as chemokinesis, chemotaxis, aggregation and degranulation. *In vivo* administration of LTB_4 also activates leukocytes. Intradermal injection of LTB_4 in several species, notably rabbit and man, causes marked accumulation of neutrophils in the skin. Intravenous injection causes transient neutropenia (Bray *et al.*, 1981) whilst LTB_4 administration in the hamster cheek pouch stimulates adhesion of neutrophils to the microvasculature (characterized by a change from 'rolling' to 'sticking' neutrophils) and subsequently diapadesis (Dahlen, 1982).

Neutrophil activation is associated with induction of inflammation. LTB_4 enhances vascular permeability in rabbit skin and co-administration with a vasodilator prostanoid results in plasma exudation (Wedmore and Williams, 1981). In this system, LTB_4 and PGE_2 act synergistically to produce oedema and similar effects are observed with other chemotactic agents or other vasodilators. Oedema induced in rabbits by mixtures of LTB_4 and PGE_2 is dependent on circulating neutrophils since mixtures of these eicosanoids fail to induce oedema in neutropenic animals (Wedmore and Williams, 1981). In man, LTC_4, LTD_4 and LTE_4 elicited erythema and wheal formation whereas LTB_4 produced a transient wheal with subsequent induration characterized by a neutrophil infiltrate (Soter *et al.*, 1983). Synergy between LTB_4 and PGE_2 or PGD_2 has also been demonstrated in human skin (Lewis *et al.*, 1981; Archer *et al.*, 1987).

Two classes of LTB_4 receptors have been identified. A high affinity receptor appears to mediate chemokinesis and a lower affinity receptor is responsible for stimulating degranulation and oxidative burst. Selective LTB_4 antagonists have been reported to be anti-inflammatory in preclinical models but there are no published data on their clinical efficacy. A recent review (Djurik *et al.*, 1992) summarizes the status of LTB_4 antagonists.

5-Lipoxygenase is located primarily in leukocytes. A number of groups have purified the enzyme from natural sources and the rat and human variants have been cloned. Both are 78-kDa proteins and they exhibit 93% amino acid identity (Dixon *et al.*, 1988; Balcarek *et al.*, 1988). In common with other lipoxygenases, the mechanism of 5-lipoxygenase appears to involve an iron-catalysed redox cycle (see McMillan and Walker, 1992). However, there are features that distinguish the enzyme from other lipoxygenases. Catalytic activity is dependent on calcium and membrane translocation of 5-lipoxygenase is required for leukotriene synthesis in intact leukocytes. An 18-kDa membrane protein (5-lipoxygenase activating protein; FLAP) was discovered in pioneering studies by researchers at Merck, who demonstrated that expression of both 5-lipoxygenase and FLAP was necessary for leukotriene synthesis (Dixon *et al.*, 1990). Originally it was believed that FLAP could represent the membrane docking site for 5-lipoxygenase but no direct interaction of the two proteins has been observed. It now appears that FLAP binds arachidonic acid and its role may be to present substrate to the enzyme in a suitable form for catalysis (Kargman *et al.*, 1993). A third protein, the docking site for 5-lipoxygenase, is presumed to exist but has not been identified.

CLASSIFICATION OF LEUKOTRIENE SYNTHESIS INHIBITORS

Based on the proposed mechanism of 5-lipoxygenase and the requirement for membrane translocation in initiating leukotriene synthesis, inhibitors of leukotriene synthesis are conveniently considered in four classes.

Redox-based Inhibitors

The vast majority of patents on lipoxygenase inhibitors cover agents which have the potential to participate in redox processes. The common experience of pharmaceutical scientists in this area was that such inhibitors are readily discovered; indeed nonspecific anti-oxidants such as NDGA show potent lipoxygenase inhibitory properties. The major disadvantage of such inhibitors is that they interfere with a wide range of other redox-based enzymes. For example, an early prototype inhibitor, BW755C, inhibited both 5-lipoxygenase and cyclo-oxygenase which complicated the analysis of its biological actions. More selective redox-based inhibitors were developed at Zeneca (formerly ICI Pharmaceuticals) based on indazolinones which have much weaker redox properties than BW755C. An example from this class, ICI207968, was 300-fold more potent as an inhibitor of leukotriene biosynthesis compared to prostaglandin synthesis (Foster *et al.*, 1990). The compound was also orally active as an inhibitor of leukotriene biosynthesis but ICI207968 was not developed since it caused species-dependent induction of methaemoglobin formation. In a range of analogues, induction of methaemoglobin was directly related to redox potential although 5-lipoxygenase inhibition was not. Further studies led to the discovery of carboxamido analogues that had comparable lipoxygenase inhibitory potency to ICI207968 *in vitro* but did not induce methaemoglobin (Bruneau *et al.*, 1991). However no analogue combined adequate oral potency with freedom from methaemoglobinaemia. Similar problems have been encountered by other companies with redox inhibitors and agents in this class must be regarded as imperfect pharmacological tools. The generation and control of free radicals is reviewed in detail in Chapter 16, this volume.

Iron Ligand Inhibitors

In view of the role of iron at the active site of lipoxygenases, agents which have the capacity to ligand iron have been designed as 5-lipoxygenase inhibitors. A series of aceto-hydroxamates were reported by Wellcome and these included BWA4C (Tateson *et al.*, 1988). In common with the redox agents described above, these compounds had limited selectivity for 5-lipoxygenase compared to cyclo-oxygenase. BWA4C was orally active as an inhibitor of leukotriene synthesis in animals and in human volunteers. Further clinical development was precluded by the accumulation of high levels of metabolites of the compound.

A related structural class, N-hydroxy ureas, were discovered at Abbott. These have similar iron-liganding properties to hydroxamates and not surprisingly the lipoxygenase inhibitory profiles of the two classes of agent are similar. For example, the lead compound, zileuton (A-64077), has similar modest selectivity for 5-lipoxygenase compared to cyclo-oxygenase (approximately 15-fold). Zileuton is orally active as an inhibitor of leukotriene synthesis (Carter *et al.*, 1991) and inhibits leukotriene synthesis in human volunteers (Rubin *et al.*, 1991) but its short half-life necessitates frequent administration: 24-h suppression of leukotriene synthesis requires dosing of zileuton at 600 mg q.i.d. Another N-hydroxy urea has been developed by Abbott, A78773. This is more potent and more selective than zileuton and studies in human volunteers demonstrate that 24-h suppression is possible with once daily administration (Rubin *et al.*, 1992).

Non-redox Inhibitors

The aforementioned inhibitors have the potential to interact with other iron-dependent redox enzymes and it is notable that agents from both classes inhibit cyclo-oxygenase at concentrations of only 10–100 times those that inhibit 5-lipoxygenase. This contrasts with the very high selectivity of cyclo-oxygenase inhibitors, which essentially are devoid of lipoxygenase inhibitory activity. Another feature observed with cyclo-oxygenase inhibitors is enantioselectivity. With optically active cyclo-oxygenase inhibitors, enzyme inhibiton predominates in one enantiomer and this usually translates to anti-inflammatory activity. In contrast optically active 5-lipoxygenase inhibitors of the Redox or Iron Ligand classes generally fail to show enantioselectivity. These observations led to a focus at Zeneca/ICI on non-redox approaches to lipoxygenase inhibition.

A series of 5-lipoxygenase inhibitors, which were devoid of redox or iron ligand properties were discovered – methoxyalkyl thiazoles. This series demonstrated marked structure activity relationships: small changes in structure were associated with large changes in lipoxygense inhibitory potency (Bird et al., 1991). This was a feature that was notably absent in the Redox and Iron Ligand inhibitors. In addition, using an optically active analogue, ICI216800, evidence was obtained for enantioselectivity in lipoxygenase inhibition (McMillan et al., 1990). These data implied that methoxyalkyl thiazoles, uniquely amongst published lipoxygenase inhibitors, showed a chiral interaction with enzyme. Whilst the methoxyalkyl thiazoles are valuable pharmacological tools for in vitro studies, their in vivo utility is limited by poor oral absorption and short half-lives. Structural modification resulted in the discovery of more potent inhibitors with improved oral activity, methoxyalkyl tetrahydropyrans (Crawley et al., 1992). These are exemplified by Zeneca ZD2138 (formerly ICID2138), which potently inhibits 5-lipoxygenase with more than 25 000-fold selectivity with respect to cyclo-oxygenase (McMillan et al., 1992). Although, ZD2138 is achiral, related optically active analogues exhibit enantioselective inhibition. Once daily administration of ZD2138 suppresses leukotriene synthesis in man (Yates et al., 1992).

FLAP Antagonists

Another class of leukotriene synthesis inhibitors, which act by binding to FLAP and preventing the membrane translocation of 5-lipoxygenase, has been described. The first such compound, MK886, was discovered at Merck Frosst and was characterized by potent, selective inhibition of leukotriene synthesis in intact leukocytes and blood without a direct inhibition of 5-lipoxygenase in cell-free assays (Gillard et al., 1989). This compound, and related analogues, were employed in the studies, described above, which led to the identification of FLAP. MK886 exhibited potent, prolonged oral activity as an inhibitor of leukotriene synthesis in experimental animals. However clinical development was limited by a short half-life in man (approx. 2 h).

A group of quinoline-containing compounds have also been shown to act as FLAP antagonists. Two examples, Revlon REV-5901 (now PF-5901; Purdue Frederick) and WY50,296 (Wyeth), selectively inhibited leukotriene synthesis in vitro and WY50,295 also showed potent oral activity (Coutts et al., 1985; Musser and Kreft, 1990). However both compounds exhibited species differences in their inhibitory potency, with approximately 10-fold less potency in human compared to rodent blood (Proudman *et al.*, 1991). Thus, it is not surprising that neither compound inhibited leukotriene synthesis following oral administration in humans. Another quinoline-containing inhibitor, Bay-x1005 (Bayer) has been reported to inhibit leukotriene synthesis selectively *in vitro* and *in vivo* and also inhibits leukotriene synthesis following oral administration in volunteers.

Merck Frosst have reported a third group of FLAP antagonists, quindoles, which represent hybrid molecules containing structural features from both quinoline and MK886. A representative from this series, MK591, had a similar preclinical pharmacological profile to MK886 (Brideau *et al.*, 1992) but showed improved human pharmacokinetics. A single oral dose of MK591 suppressed leukotriene synthesis in blood and urinary leukotriene excretion for at least 24 h in volunteers and asthmatic subjects.

ANTI-INFLAMMATORY EFFECTS OF LEUKOTRIENE SYNTHESIS INHIBITORS

Evaluation of the anti-inflammatory effects of leukotriene synthesis inhibitors has been a controversial area, particularly in relation to arthritis. As discussed above, LTB_4 may act as an endogenous amplifier of leukocyte recruitment in arthritides but several factors complicated evaluation of this hypothesis. For example, there are no animal models of arthritis that mimic the chronic elevation of synovial fluid neutrophils which characterizes RA. Also many 'traditional' models of arthritis have been developed in the past to evaluate non-steroidal anti-inflammatory drugs and are thus highly dependent on cyclo-oxygenase products. Finally many studies are carried out in the rat, a species that is refractory to the chemotactic activity of LTB_4 due to the absence in that species of its high affinity receptor.

Another factor that has hindered these studies has been the inadequacies of previous 5-lipoxygenase inhibitors such as BW755C which lacked selectivity for 5-lipoxygenase. Thus, when comparative anti-inflammatory studies were reported with BW755C and the cyclo-oxygenase inhibitor, indomethacin, additional activity observed with BW755C were presumed to be due to lipoxygenase inhibition (Higgs *et al.*, 1979). However, subsequent investigations demonstrated that the original anti-inflammatory activity of BW755C in rats could be accounted for entirely by inhibition of cyclo-oxygenase (Foster *et al.*, 1985).

Indazolinones such as ICI207968 are weak redox inhibitors which exhibited sufficient selectivity for 5-lipoxygenase to exclude any contribution of cyclo-oxygenase inhibition to their *in vivo* biological actions. Anti-inflammatory effects were evaluated in topical models of inflammation induced by arachidonic acid. Application of high doses of arachidonic acid to mouse ear (Young *et al.*, 1984) or rabbit skin (Aked *et al.*, 1986) induces a rapid onset of inflammatory oedema associated with neutrophil infiltration. Oxidation products of arachidonic acid metabolism, including prostaglandins and leukotrienes, have been implicated as mediators of the inflammatory response induced by arachidonic acid in these species (Opas *et al.*, 1985; Aked and Foster, 1987) and in the rabbit model the inflammatory reactions were shown to be dependent on circulating leukocytes. ICI207968 was active in the rabbit skin model when dosed either orally or topically. In the topical studies the compound produced parallel inhibition of neutrophil accumulation and plasma exudation. In addition the anti-inflammatory potency of a range indazolinone analogues was correlated with their lipoxygenase inhibitory potency (Foster *et al.*, 1990).

The data with indazolinones suggested that anti-inflammatory activity in the series was a consequence of inhibition of leukotriene synthesis but a contribution from an indirect redox mechanism could not be excluded. In the rabbit skin model, non-redox inhibitors of 5-lipoxygenae (methoxyalkyl thiazoles and methoxy tetrahydropyrans) caused inhibition of plasma exudation. As in the case of the indazolinones, anti-inflammatory activity correlated with lipoxygenase inhibitory potency and most convincingly inhibition of plasma exudation by an optically active methoxy alkylthiazole, ICI216800, was enantioselective: only the lipoxygenase inhibitory enantiomer was anti-inflammatory (McMillan *et al.*, 1990). Further studies with the more potent non-redox inhibitor, ZD2138, confirmed the anti-inflammatory activity of lipoxygenase inhibitors in arachidonic acid models (McMillan *et al.*, 1992) and as described below there is also evidence of a synergistic interaction between lipoxygenase and cyclo-oxygenase inhibitors.

CLINICAL STUDIES WITH INHIBITORS OF LEUKOTRIENE SYNTHESIS

A number of leukotriene synthesis inhibitors have been evaluated in man. There are no reports of redox inhibitors in clinical development but examples of the other inhibitor classes are under clinical evaluation. The drug which is at the most advanced stage of development is zileuton, which has been evaluated in a Phase II study in RA. Treatment with zileuton was associated with a significant improvement in swollen and painful joints in patients who flared following withdrawal of conventional non-steroidal anti-inflammatory drugs (Weinblatt *et al.*, 1992). However, there was also a significant improvement in the placebo group and the overall assessment was that zileuton produced a trend towards clinical benefit. The treatment regimen used for this study (800 mg b.i.d.) produces only intermittent lipoxygenase inhibition because of the short half-life of zileuton (2.3 h). A definitive study in RA would require more frequent administration of zileuton or use of a lipoxygenase inhibitor with a longer half-life. In this regard studies in RA with ZD2138 and A78773, which produce sustained lipoxygenase inhibition with once-daily dosing, will be critical. Zileuton has been evaluated in other inflammatory diseases. Clinical improvement has been reported in ulcerative colitis using the same dosing regimen as in RA (Collawn *et al.*, 1989). More frequent dosing to suppress leukotriene synthesis might be expected to produce a more pronounced effect. Using a regimen that caused maintenance of lipoxygenase inhibition (600 mg, q.i.d.), it has been demonstrated that zileuton improves airway function and symptoms in asthma (Israel *et al.*, 1993).

Clearly, studies with zileuton in chronic inflammatory diseases can be compromised by the need to use frequent, high doses of the drug. The development of a second generation of leukotriene synthesis inhibitors with improved potency and larger half-lives (viz. ZD2138, A-78773, MK591, Bay-X-1005) offers the potential for agents with improved anti-inflammatory efficacy.

INTERACTIONS BETWEEN CYCLO-OXYGENASE AND 5-LIPOXYGENASE INHIBITORS

ANTI-INFLAMMATORY EFFECTS OF COMBINATIONS OF CYCLO-OXYGENASE AND 5-LIPOXYGENASE INHIBITORS

As discussed above, prostaglandins and leukotrienes act independently and in some cases synergistically to induce inflammatory reactions. Therefore, inhibition of both prostaglandin and leukotriene production might be expected to produce greater anti-inflammatory efficacy than inhibition of individual mediators. Any improvement in efficacy would be beneficial in the treatment of inflammatory conditions. This hypothesis has been explored at Zeneca Pharmaceuticals.

In order to investigate the hypothesis it was important to utilize an animal model in which both protaglandins and leukotrienes contribute to the inflammatory process. We used the arachidonic acid-induced mouse ear oedema model to investigate the anti-inflammatory efficacy of cyclo-oxygenase and 5-lipoxygenase inhibitors. In our hands orally administered cyclo-oxygenase inhibitors were either inactive or weakly active in this model whereas 5-lipoxgenase inhibitors were moderately active. This is demonstrated by the experiment shown in Fig. 2 in which indomethacin, flurbiprofen

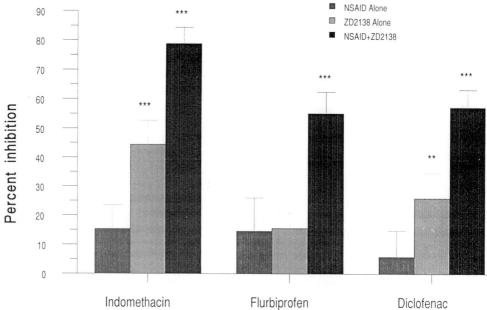

Figure 2. Synergistic anti-inflammatory activity of ICI D2138 and NSAIDs on arachidonic-acid induced mouse ear oedema. Groups of 10 mice were dosed with the indicated NSAID (3 mg/kg p.o., open bars) or ICI D2138 (10 mg/kg p.o., crosshatched bars) alone or in combination (filled bars). Control groups of 20 mice received vehicle alone. Values shown are means ± SEM per cent inhibition of inflammatory oedema. Oedema weights of the ear punch discs from the control vehicle-dosed animals were 7.2 ± 0.4, 9.6 ± 0.5 and 10.0 ± 0.5 mg for the indomethacin, flurbiprofen and diclofenac experiments respectively. ** = $P < 0.01$ and *** = $P < 0.001$ with respect to the control group. The experiment is typical of three.

and diclofenac (3 mg/kg p.o.) were inactive whereas the selective 5-lipoxygenase inhibitor ZD2138 (McMillan *et al.*, 1992) produced moderate inhibition of the oedema. It is striking that the combined administration of ZD2138 with each of the NSAIDs produced a synergistic anti-inflammatory effect. We have also shown that oral administration of MK886 (30 mg/kg), a novel selective inhibitor of leukotriene synthesis (Gillard *et al.*, 1989), caused 25% inhibition of arachidonic-acid induced oedema, but when MK886 was co-administered with indomethacin (10 mg/kg p.o.) a synergistic anti-inflammatory effect of 70% was achieved. Since co-administration of leukotrienes and prostaglandins to certain experimental animals and man produce synergistic inflammatory effects, it is reasonable to speculate, based on these data, that the synergistic anti-inflammatory activity is a consequence of inhibiton of both classes of eicosanoid. In fact Higgs *et al.* (1979) suggested that dual inhibitors of arachidonate cyclo-oxygenase and lipoxygenase would have a more comprehensive anti-inflammatory effect than cyclo-oxygenase inhibitors. Although the discovery of a safe, orally effective mixed inhibitor in a single molecule has proved elusive to date, such mixed inhibition can be achieved by co-administration of a selective 5-lipoxygenase inhibitor and NSAID. With the recent discovery of orally active, potent selective 5-lipoxygenase inhibitors this hypothesis can now be evaluated in the clinic.

LEUKOTRIENES, PROSTANOIDS AND THE GASTROINTESTINAL TRACT

Gastrointestinal toxicity is a major side-effect associated with NSAIDs. The ulcerogenic properties of NSAIDs are, in part, a consequence of their ability to inhibit the synthesis of the cytoprotective prostanoids (Whittle and Vane, 1984). Although reduced mucosal blood flow has been suggested to play a role, the precise mechanism of mucosal ulceration is unclear. Recently, however, Asako *et al.* (1992a,b) observed that superfusion of rat mesenteric venules with aspirin or indomethacin caused the adherence of leukocytes to the venule endothelium. Salicylate, which lacks ulcerogenic and cyclo-oxygenase activity, failed to induce leukocyte adherence. A role for neutrophils in the pathogenesis of NSAID-induced gastropathy in the rat is supported by the observation that depletion of circulating neutrophils with an antineutrophil antiserum prevented the production of ulcers by NSAIDs (Wallace *et al.*, 1990). This has been further supported by the demonstration that pretreating animals with antibodies against the β-subunit (CD18) of the adhesion complex CD11b/CD18 prevented indomethacin-induced ulceration (Wallace *et al.*, 1991). Neutrophils may contribute to the ulceration process by occluding the microcirculation, reducing blood flow and thus producing local ischaemia and predisposition to injury by the gastric components. Additionally, neutrophils may contribute to local tissue damage by producing destructive proteinases and reactive oxygen or nitrogen metabolites.

Studies to date suggest that gastrointestinal toxicity is not a concern with 5-lipoxygenase inhibitors. On the contrary, because of the pathological effects of the leukotrienes, 5-lipoxygenase inhibitors may have utility for the treatment of NSAID-induced gastropathy and other gastrointestinal disturbances. Thus, LTB_4, by stimulating neutrophil chemotaxis and activation, could be implicated in some of the damage associated with NSAID toxicity. Also, the peptidoleukotrienes may exert damaging effects on gastric function through stimulation of pepsin secretion, reduced mucosal blood flow, interference with gastric emptying and exacerbation of mucosal injuries by damaging factors such as ethanol and hydrochloric acid (Guslandi, 1987).

Animal experiments have been carried out to investigate the hypothesis that 5-lipoxygenase inhibitors reduce NSAID toxicity. Administration of indomethacin (30 mg/kg s.c.) to the rat induces ulceration of the gastric mucosa within 5 h and this can be inhibited by pre-administration of lipoxygenase inhibitors such as BW755C and ICI2078968 (Foster *et al.*, 1989). These studies do not unequivocally support a role for leukotrienes in the pathogenesis of NSAID-induced gastric ulceration since these lipoxygenase inhibitors are redox agents and may, therefore, interfere with redox processes which may play a critical role in ulcer formation. However, Zeneca ZM230487 (formerly ICI230487) an orally active, non-redox 5-lipoxygenase inhibitor (Crawley *et al.*, 1992) produced a dose-related inhibition of indomethacin-induced gastric ulceration in the rat as shown in Fig. 3. We have also shown that oral adminis-

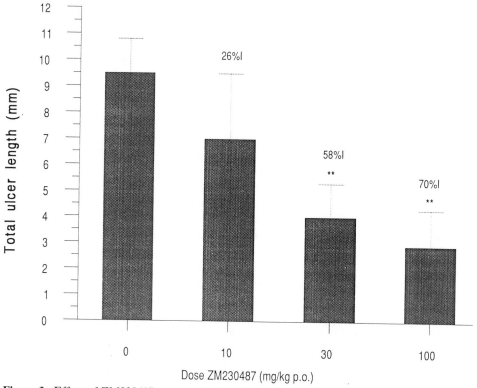

Figure 3. Effect of ZM230487 on acute indomethacin-induced gastric ulceration in the rat. Groups of 10 rats were dosed orally with ZM230487 or vehicle (0.5% hydroxypropylmethyl-cellulose in 0.1% polysorbate 80) and 15 min later they were injected subcutaneously with indomethacin (30 mg/kg). Five hours later the animals were killed, the stomachs excised and gastric ulceration quantitated macroscopically. ** = $P < 0.01$ with respect to the control group. Per cent inhibition of gastric ulcers is indicated above the SEM bars.

tration of ZM230487 or ZD2138 (10 mg/kg b.i.d.), to rat, inhibits gastrointestinal toxicity (assessed histologically), increase in acute phase protein (α1-acid glycoprotein) and weight loss induced by subacute administration of indomethacin (4.5 mg/kg/day for 5 days).

In addition, Peskar (1988) showed that the peptidyl-leukotriene receptor antagonists L-660,711 and L649,923 protected rats against indomethacin-induced gastric lesions. Other studies have investigated inhibitors of leukotriene synthesis in similar models. Vaananen *et al.* (1992) showed that several inhibitors of 5-L0 and FLAP reduced gastrointestinal damage induced by indomethacin. In that study the potency of the compounds as protective agents was correlated with their inhibition of gastric leukotriene synthesis. The studies employed structurally diverse agents including some that were devoid of anti-oxidant effects. Thus, the authors were able to exclude a redox mechanism. In a separate study, Asako *et al.* (1992a) showed that the stimulation of leukocyte adherence by aspirin or indomethacin could be prevented by treatment with either the FLAP antagonist MK886 (L663,536) or an LTB_4 antagonist, SC41930.

Taken together, these results support a role for leukotrienes in the gastrointestinal toxicity associated with NSAIDs and suggest that treatment of inflammatory conditions with 5-lipoxygenase inhibitor/NSAID combinations would be expected to be much less toxic to the gastrointestinal tract than NSAIDs alone. Further support for this concept comes from preclinical studies with dual inhibitors of cyclo-oxygenase and 5-lipoxygenase. Researchers from Warner Lambert successfully combined hydroxamates with a variety of NSAIDs and demonstrated that the resulting dual inhibitors, in contrast to the parent NSAID, failed to induce gastric ulceration in stressed rats (Flynn *et al.*, 1990). Interestingly, an inverse correlation of cyclo-oxygenase/5-lipoxygenase selectivity and induction of ulcers were observed. Thus as more 5-lipoxygenase inhibitory activity was introduced into the NSAID pharmacophore, a commensurate decrease in ulceration occurred.

CYTOSOLIC PHOSPHOLIPASE A2 INHIBITION

The release of arachidonic acid from membrane phospholipids is the rate-limiting step in the biosynthesis of the prostaglandins and leukotrienes. Arachidonic acid is found at the sn2 position of most glycerophospholipids, which include the precursors of platelet activating factor (PAF). In most cell types arachidonic acid release is dependent on the activation of phospholipase A2.

Several phospholipases A2 have been identified. The majority of these enzymes have been relatively small proteins with molecular weights of about 14 kDa. They are calcium-dependent enzymes: optimal activity requires concentrations of calcium in the millimolar range, which are only likely to be found extracellularly. These enzymes also show marked preference for classes of phospholipid containing certain basic head groups but show no preference for liberation of arachidonic acid compared to other fatty acids at the sn2 position of these phospholipids.

Recently the cDNA sequence has been reported for another type of phospholipase A2 found in the cytosol of the human cell line U937 (Clark *et al.*, 1991). This enzyme has a predicted molecular weight of 85.2 kDa and shows no sequence homology with the secretory phospholipases A2. Unlike the secretory enzymes, the cytosolic phospholipase A2 (cPLA) is stimulated by concentrations of calcium found in activated cells. In addition to calcium-dependence of catalytic activity, the enzyme undergoes a calcium-dependent translocation from cytosol to membrane (Clark *et al.*, 1990; Channan *et al.*, 1990). Crucially, the cPLA2 shows marked preference for hydrolysing arachidonic acid instead of other fatty acids from the sn2 position of glycerophospholipids but the enzyme exhibits no preference for phospholipid type (Leslie *et al.*, 1988).

The human cPLA2 has greater than 95% amino acid sequence homology with a similar enzyme from mouse RAW 264.7 cells. Similar enzymes have been identified in other leukocyte cell lines, human THP1 and moust J774, and in mouse spleen and rat kidney. This degree of species homology is usually reserved for proteins which have a fundamental role within the cell. All of the cell types in which this cPLA2 has been identified have the capacity to produce either leukotrienes or prostaglandins. These data suggest that this cPLA2 is the enzyme responsible for initiating the biosynthesis of leukotrienes, prostaglandins and possibly PAF.

Given that this cytosolic phospholipase may be the most important form which generates arachidonic acid and eicosanoid mediators it is potentially a novel target for a new class of anti-inflammatory agent. Such agents would be expected to have the combined efficacy of an NSAID and 5-lipoxygense inhibitor and possibly a PAF antagonist without the gastrointestinal toxicity side-effects associated with NSAIDs. There are currently no literature reports of selective cPLA2 inhibitors, but it is likely to be the focus of intense activity by the pharmaceutical industry during the next few years.

CONCLUSIONS

Recent developments in our knowledge of arachidonic acid metabolism have highlighted a number of novel pharmacological approaches for development of anti-inflammatory drugs. The discovery of subtypes of prostanoid receptors and cyclo-oxygenase isoforms has led to a search for specific prostanoid receptor antagonists and COX-II inhibitors which may provide the anti-inflammatory/analgesic efficacy of NSAIDs with improved gastrointestinal safety.

The pro-inflammatory actions of leukotrienes stimulated the search for inhibitors of 5-lipoxygenase inhibitors. Examples from several structural classes are undergoing clinical development. Preclinical data indicate that co-administration of 5-lipoxygenase inhibitors with cyclo-oxygense inhibitors results in enhanced anti-inflammatory efficacy and reduced gastrointestinal toxicity. Clinical studies are required to determine whether these observations translate to humans. However, such data have stimulated interest in drugs that block synthesis of both classes of eicosanoids. Inhibition of release of arachidonic acid, the precursor for prostanoids and leukotrienes, is a rational approach to such drugs. The recent demonstration that cytosolic PLA2 exhibits specificity for arachidonic acid and liberation from phospholipids, make it an attractive target for designs of improved anti-inflammatory agents.

REFERENCES

Aked DM & Foster SJ (1987) *Br J Pharmacol* **92**: 545–552.
Aked D, Foster SJ, Howarth A, McCormick ME & Potts HC (1986) *Br J Pharmacol* **89**: 431–438.
Archer CB, Page CP, Juhlin L, Morley J & MacDonald DM (1987) *Prostaglandins* **33**: 799–805.
Armstrong RA, Lawrence RA, Jones RL, Willson NH & Collier A (1989) *Br J Pharmacol* **97**: 657–668.
Asako H, Kubes P, Wallace J, Gaginella T, Wolf RE & Granger DN (1992a) *Am J Physiol* **262**: G903–G908.
Asako H, Kubes P, Wallace J, Wolfe RE & Granger DN (1992b) *Gastroenterology* **103**: 146–152.

Atik OS (1990) *Prostaglandins Leukot Essent Fatty Acids* **39**: 253–254.

Atkinson M, Germain G & Lee P (1988) *J Rheumatol* **15**: 1001–1004.

Balcarek JM et al. (1988) *J Biol Chem* **263**: 13937–13941.

Bird TGC, Bruneau P, Crawley GC, Edwards MP, Foster SJ, Girodeau et al. (1991) *J Med Chem* **34**: 2176–2186.

Birrell GJ, McQueen DS, Iggo A, Coleman RA & Grubb BD (1991) *Neurosci Lett* **124**: 5–8.

Bray MA, Cunningham FM, Ford-Hutchinson AW & Smith MJH (1981) *Br J Pharmacol* **72**: 483–486.

Brideau C, Chan C, Charleson S, Denis D, Evans JF, Ford-Hutchinson AW et al. (1992) *Can J Pharmacol* **70**: 799–807.

Brodie MJ, Hensby CN, Parke A & Gordon D (1980) *Life Sci* **27**: 603–608.

Bruneau P, Delvare C, Edwards MP & McMillan RM (1991) *J Med Chem* **34**: 1028–1036.

Carroll JA & Shaw JS (1989) *Br J Pharmacol* **98** (**supplement**): 925P.

Carter GW, Young PR, Albert DH, Bousha J, Dyer R, Bell RL et al. (1991) *J Pharmacol Exp Ther* **256**: 929–937.

Channon JY & Leslie CC (1990) *J Biol Chem* **265**: 5409–5413.

Clark JD, Milona N & Knopf JL (1990) *Proc Natl Acad Sci* **87**: 7708–7712.

Clark JD, Lin L-L, Kriz RW, Ramesha CS, Sultzman LA, Lin AY et al. (1991) *Cell* **65**: 1043–1051.

Coderre TJ, Gonzales R, Goldyne ME, West J & Levine JD (1990) *Neurosci Lett* **115**: 253–258.

Coleman RA & Kennedy I (1980) *Br J Pharmacol* **68**: 533–539.

Coleman RA & Kennedy I (1985) *Prostaglandins* **29**: 363–375.

Coleman RA, Humphrey PPA, Kennedy I, Levy GP & Lumley P (1980) *Br J Pharmacol* **69**: 225P–266P.

Coleman RA, Kennedy I & Sheldrich RLG (1985) *Br J Pharmacol* **85**: 273P.

Coleman RA, Kennedy I & Sheldrick RLG (1987) *Adv Prostaglandin, Thromboxane Leukotriene Res* **17**: 467–470.

Coutts SM, Khandwala A, Van Inwegen R, Chakraborty V, Musser J, Bruens J et al. In Bailey JM (ed) *Prostaglandins, Leukotrienes and Lipoxins*, pp 627–637. New York: Plenum.

Crawley GC, Bird TGC, Bruneau P, Dowell RI, Edwards PN, Foster SJ et al. (1992) *J Lipid Mediators* **6**: 249–257.

Crunkhorn P & Willis AL (1971) *Br J Pharmacol* **41**: 507–512.

Dahlen SE et al. (1981) *Proc Natl Acad Sci USA* **78**: 3887–3891.

Daymond TJ & Rowell FJ (1988) *Drugs* **35** (**supplement 1**): 4–8.

Dickenson AH & Sullivan AF (1987) *Pain* **30**: 349–360.

Dixon RAF et al. (1988) *Proc Natl Acad Sci USA* **85**: 416–420.

Dixon RAF et al. (1990) **323**: 282–284.

Djuirck SW, Fretland DJ & Penning TD (1992) *Drugs of the Future* **17**: 819–830.

Dong YJ, Jones RL & Wilson NH (1986) *Br J Pharmacol* **87**: 97–107.

Dray A & Dickenson AT (1991) *Pain* **47**: 79–83.

Drower EJ, Stapelfeld A, Mueller RA & Hammond DL (1987) *Eur J Pharmacol* **133**: 249–256.

Egg D (1984) *Z Rheumatol* **43**: 89–96.

Eglen RM & Whiting RL (1988) *Br J Pharmacol* **94**: 591–601.

Eglen RM & Whiting RL (1989) *Br J Pharmacol* **98**: 1335–1343.

Ferreira SH, Nakamura M & Abreu Castro MS (1978) *Prostaglandins* **16**: 31–37.

Flower RJ, Harvey EA & Kingston WP (1976) *Br J Pharmacol* **56**: 229–233.

Flynn DL, Caparis T, Cetenko WJ, Connor DT, Dyer RD, Kostlan CR et al. (1990) *J Med Chem* **33**: 2070–2072.

Foster SJ, McCormick ME, Howarth A & Aked D (1985) *Biochem Pharmacol* **35**: 1709–1717.

Foster SJ, Aked DM, McCormick & Potts HC (1989) *Br J Pharmacol* **96**: 38P.

Foster SJ, Bruneau P, Walker ER & McMillan RM (1990) *Br J Pharmacol* **99**: 113–118.

Furci L, Fitzgerald DL & Fitzgerald GA (1991) *J Pharmacol Exp Ther* **258**: 74–81; *Gastroenterology* **103**: 146–152.

Gillard JA et al. (1989) *Can J Physiol Pharmacol* **67**: 456–464.

Grennan DM, Aarons L, Siddiqui M, Richards M, Thompson R & Higham C (1983) *Br J Clin Pharmacol* **15**: 311–316.

Grub BD, Birrell GJ, McQueen DS & Iggo A (1991) *Exp Brain Res* **84**: 383–392.

Guslandi M (1987) *Prostaglandins, Leukotrienes and Medicine* **26**: 203–208.

Heppelmann B, Pfeffer A, Schaible H-G & Schmidt RF (1986) *Pain* **26**: 337–351.

Higgs EA, Moncada S & Vane JR (1978) *Prostaglandins* **16**: 153–162.

Higgs GA, Flower RJ & Vane JR (1979) *Biochem Pharmacol* **28**: 1959–1961.

Israel E, Rubin P, Kemp JP, Grossman J, Pierson W, Siegel SC et al. (1993) *Am Internal Medicine* **119**: 1059–1066.

Juan H & Seewann S (1980) *Eur J Pharmacol* **65**: 267–278.

Jurna I, Spohrer B & Bock R (1992) *Pain* **49**: 249–256.

Kennedy I, Coleman RA, Humphrey PPA & Lumley P (1983) *Adv Prostaglandin Thromboxane Leuko-triene Res* **11**: 327–332.

Kolodny AL (1988) *J Rheumatol* **15**: 1205–1211.

Kujubu DA & Herschman HR (1992) *J Biol Chem* **267**: 7991–7994.

Kujubu DA, Reddy ST, Fletcher BS & Herschman HR (1993) *J Biol Chem* **268**: 5425–5430.

Kumazawa T, Minagawa M, Narumiya S & Namba T (1992) *Soc Neurosci Abstracts*, p 200.

Lawrence RA & Jones RL (1992) *Br J Pharmacol* **105**: 817–824.

Lawrence RA, Jones RL & Wilson NH (1992) *Br J Pharmacol* **105**: 271–278.

Lee SH, Soyoola E, Chanmugam P, Sun W, Zhong H, Liou S et al. (1992) *J Biol Chem* **267**: 25934–25938.

Leslie CC et al. (1988) *Biochim Biophy Acta* **963**: 476–492.

Lewis RA, Soter NA, Corey EJ & Austen KF (1981) *Clinical Res* **29**: 492A.

Louttit JB, Head SA & Coleman RA (1992) *8th International Conference on Prostaglandins and Related Compounds, July 26–31, 1992*, Montreal, Canada, p 68.

Malmberg AB & Yaksh TL (1992a) *J Pharmacol Exp Ther* **263**: 136–146.

Malmberg AB & Yaksh TL (1992b) *Science* **257**: 1276–1279.

Masferrer JL, Seibert K, Zweifel B & Needleman P (1992) *Proc Natl Acad Sci* **89**: 3917–3921.

McMillan RM & Walker ERH (1992) *Trends Pharmacol Sci* **13**: 323–330.

McMillan RM, Girodeau J-M & Foster SJ (1990) *Br J Pharmacol* **101**: 501–503.

McMillan RM, Spruce KE, Crawley GC, Walker ERH & Foster SJ (1992) *Br J Pharmacol* **107**: 1042–1047.

McQueen DS, Iggo A, Birrel GJ & Grubb BD (1991) *Br J Pharmacol* **104**: 178–182.

Meade EA, Smith WL & DeWitt DL (1993) *J Biol Chem* **268**: 6610–6614.

Moilanen E, Alanko J, Nissila M, Hamalainen M, Isomaki H & Vapaatalo H (1989) *Agents Actions* **28**: 290–297.

Musser JH & Kreft AF (1990) *Drugs of the Future* **15**: 73–80.

Newton J Jr & Hanna N (1991) *Biochem Pharmacol* **42**: 825–831.

O'Sullivan MG, Chilton FH, Huggins EM & McCall CE (1992) *J Biol Chem* **267**: 14547–14550.

Opas EE, Bonney RJ & Humes JL (1985) *J Invest Derm* **84**: 253–256.

Peskar B (1988) *Gastroenterology* **94**: A351.

Proudman KE, Moores SM & McMillan RM (1991) *Br J Pharmacol* **102**: B64P.

Robinson DR, Dayer JM & Krane SM (1979) *Ann NY Acad Sci* **332**: 279–294.

Rubin P, Dube L, Braeckman R, Swanson L, Hansen R, Albert D et al. (1991) *Progress in Inflammation Res and Therapy*, 103–112.

Rubin P et al. (1992) *Proc 8th Int. Conf. Prostaglandins and Related Compounds*, abstr. 154.

Sanner JH, Mueller RA & Schulzw RH (1973) *Adv Biosci* **9**: 139–148.

Schaible H-G & Schmidt RF (1988) *J Physiol (Lond)* **60**: 2180–2195.

Schepelmann K, Messlinger K, Schaible H-G & Schmidt RF (1992) *Neuroscience* **50**: 237–247.

Sciberras DG, Goldenberg MM, Bolognese JA, James I & Baber NS (1987) *Br J Clin Pharmacol* **24**: 753–761.

Seppala E (1987) *Clin Rheumatol* **6**: 170–176.

Soter NA, Lewis RA, Corey EJ & Austen KF (1983) *J Invest Dermatol* **80**: 115–119.

Taiwo YO & Levine JD (1986) *Brain Res* **373**: 81–84.

Tateson JE et al. (1988) *Br J Pharmacol* **94**: 528–539.

Trang LE, Granstrom E & Lovgren O (1977) *Scand J Rheumatol* **6**: 151–154.

Uda R et al. (1990) *Brain Res* **510**: 26–32.

Vaananen PM, Keenan CM, Grisham MB & Wallace JL (1992) *Inflammation* **16**: 227–240.

Vasey FB, Germain BF, Espinoza LR, Box P, Bockow BI, Lipani JA et al. (1987) *Am J Med* **83** (supplement 4B): 55–59.

Wallace JL, Keenan CM & Granger DN (1990) *Am J Physiol* **259**: G462–467.

Wallace JL, Arfors K-E & McKnight GW (1991) *Gastroenterology* **100**: 878–883.

Wedmore CV & Williams TJ (1981) *Nature* **289**: 646–650.

Weinblatt ME, Kremer JM, Coblyn JS, Helfgott S, Maier AL, Petrillo G et al. (1992) *J Rheumatol* **19**: 1537–1541.

Whittle BJR & Vane JR (1984) *Arch Toxicol* **7**: 315–322.

Yates RA et al. (1992) *Am Rev Resp Dis* **145**: A745.

Young JM, Spires DA, Bedford CJ, Wagner B, Ballaran SJ & Young LM (1984) *J Invest Derm* **82**: 367–371.

15 Free Radicals and Rheumatoid Disease

Barry Halliwell

INTRODUCTION

Interest in the role of free radicals and other oxygen-derived species in human rheumatoid disease stems from the seminal work of McCord (1974), who pointed to the decreased viscosity of synovial fluid from the joints of patients with rheumatoid arthritis (RA) and showed that a similar decrease in viscosity could be produced by exposing synovial fluid, or solutions of hyaluronic acid (the glycosaminoglycan responsible for most of the synovial fluid viscosity) to a system generating the superoxide radical, $O_2^{\cdot-}$. McCord's observations led to a flurry of interest in the use of intra-articular injections of the antioxidant enzyme superoxide dismutase (SOD) as a treatment in RA. However, the clinical data presented never succeeded in convincing many rheumatologists (reviewed by Greenwald, 1991) and even the original proponents of this treatment now admit that it is unlikely to be very helpful (Flohe, 1988). What is the current situation? Simply that we do not know the real importance of free radicals in inflammatory joint disease, because the question has never been investigated properly. Before expanding on this point, I will clarify a few basic principles.

BASIC DEFINITIONS

Electrons in atoms occupy regions of space known as orbitals. Each orbital can hold a maximum of two electrons. A free radical is simply defined as any species capable of independent existence that contains one or more unpaired electrons, an unpaired electron being one that is alone in an orbital. Table 1 gives examples of biologically relevant free radicals. Most biological molecules are non-radicals, containing only paired electrons. A superscript dot is used to denote free radical species.

Radicals can react with other molecules in a number of ways (reviewed by Halliwell and Gutteridge, 1989). Thus, if two radicals meet, they can combine their unpaired electrons and join to form a covalent bond (a shared pair of electrons):

$$A^{\cdot} + A^{\cdot} \rightarrow A\text{--}A \tag{1}$$

An example is the very fast reaction of superoxide radical ($O_2^{\cdot-}$) with nitric oxide radical ($NO^{\cdot}$) to form the non-radical peroxynitrite (Saran *et al.*, 1990; Huie and Padmaja, 1993):

$$O_2^{\cdot-} + NO^{\cdot} \rightarrow ONOO^{-} \tag{2}$$

A radical might donate its unpaired electron to another molecule. Thus $O_2^{\cdot-}$ reduces

Mechanisms and Models in Rheumatoid Arthritis
ISBN 0–12–340440–1

Table 1. Examples of free radicals

Name	Formula	Comments
Hydrogen atom	H$\cdot$	The simplest free radical known
Trichloromethyl	CCl$_3\cdot$	A carbon-centred radical (i.e. the unpaired electron residues on carbon). CCl$_3\cdot$ is formed during metabolism of CCl$_4$ in the liver and contributes to the toxic effects of this solvent
Superoxide	O$_2\cdot^-$	An oxygen-centred radical
Hydroxyl	OH$\cdot$	An oxygen-centred radical. The most highly-reactive oxygen radical known
Thiyl	RS$\cdot$	General name for a group of radicals with an unpaired electron residing on sulphur
Peroxyl, alkoxyl	RO$_2\cdot$, RO$_2\cdot$	Oxygen-centred radicals formed during the breakdown of organic peroxides
Oxides of nitrogen	NO$\cdot$, NO$_2\cdot$	Both are free radicals. NO$\cdot$ is formed *in vivo* from the amino acid L-arginine. NO$_2\cdot$ is made when NO$\cdot$ reacts with O$_2$ and is found in polluted air and smoke from burning organic materials, e.g. cigarette smoke

ferric (Fe^{3+}) cytochrome c to ferrous (Fe^{2+}) cytochrome c, a reaction often used to assay O$_2\cdot^-$ production by activated phagocytes:

$$\text{cyt c (Fe}^{3+}) + O_2\cdot^- \rightarrow \text{cyt c (Fe}^{2+}) + O_2 \tag{3}$$

A radical might take an electron from another molecule in order to pair. For example, O$_2\cdot^-$ oxidizes ascorbic acid, a process which may occur in the inflamed rheumatoid joint (Blake *et al.*, 1981a):

$$\text{Ascorbate} + O_2\cdot^- + H^+ \rightarrow \text{Ascorbate radical} + H_2O_2 \tag{4}$$

Left to itself, O$_2\cdot^-$ undergoes the dismutation reaction:

$$O_2\cdot^- + O_2\cdot^- + 2H^+ \rightarrow H_2O_2 + O_2 \tag{5}$$

Hydrogen peroxide, H$_2$O$_2$, does not contain unpaired electrons and thus is not a free radical. The term 'reactive oxygen species' is often used to encompass the oxygen free radicals (O$_2\cdot^-$ and OH$\cdot$) and important non-radical derivative of oxygen such as H$_2$O$_2$ and hypochlorous acid (HOCl).

RADICALS *IN VIVO*

The chemical reactivity of oxygen free radicals varies. The most reactive is hydroxyl radical (OH$\cdot$). Exposure of living organisms to ionizing radiation causes homolytic fission of O–H bonds in water (living organisms are at least 70% water) to give H$\cdot$ and OH$\cdot$. Hydroxyl radical reacts at a diffusion-controlled rate with almost all molecules in living cells. Hence, when OH$\cdot$ is formed *in vivo*, it damages whatever it is generated next to; it cannot migrate any significant distance within the cell. The harmful effects of excess exposure to ionizing radiation upon living organisms are thought to be largely initiated by attack of OH· upon proteins, DNA and lipids (reviewed by von Sonntag, 1987).

Whereas OH· is probably always harmful, other (less-reactive) free radicals may be useful *in vivo*. Free radicals are known to be produced metabolically in living organisms. Thus, nitric oxide radical (NO·) is synthesized from the amino acid L-arginine by vascular endothelial cells, phagocytes and many other cell types. However, although human phagocytes can make NO·, it is not yet clear how often they do so *in vivo* (Carreras *et al.* 1994). Nitric oxide produced by endothelium helps to regulate vascular tone, and NO· may also be involved in neurotransmission (Moncada, 1992). Human chondrocytes have the capacity to make NO· (Palmer *et al.* 1993). Superoxide radical ($O_2^{·-}$), the one-electron reduction product of oxygen, is produced by phagocytic cells and helps them to kill bacteria (Curnutte and Babior, 1987). There are reports that vascular endothelial cells can produce $O_2^{·-}$ (Arroyo *et al.*, 1990; Babbs *et al.*, 1991).

Another killing mechanism used by neutrophils (but not by macrophages) is the enzyme myeloperoxidase (Weiss, 1989). It uses H_2O_2 produced from $O_2^{·-}$ to oxidize chloride ions into hypochlorous acid, HOCl, a powerful antibacterial agent (many household bleaches are solutions of the sodium salt of hypochlorous acid, NaOCl):

$$H_2O_2 + Cl^- \rightarrow HOCl + OH^- \tag{6}$$

Evidence is accumulating to suggest that smaller amounts of extracellular $O_2^{·-}$ may be generated, perhaps as an intercellular signal molecule, by several other cell types, including not only endothelial cells but also lymphocytes and fibroblasts. Thus, Meier *et al.* (1990) reported that treatment of human fibroblasts with synovial fluid from RA patients causes $O_2^{·-}$ secretion by these cells.

In addition to this metabolic generation of $O_2^{·-}$, some $O_2^{·-}$ is produced within cells by mitochondria and endoplasmic reticulum; this is usually thought to be an unavoidable consequence of the 'leakage' of electrons onto O_2 from their correct paths in electron transfer chains and of chemical 'autoxidation' reactions, in which substances are oxidized directly by O_2 to make $O_2^{·-}$ and H_2O_2 (Fridovich, 1983).

The metabolic significance of the production by $O_2^{·-}$ by endothelial cells is uncertain at present. One possibility is that $O_2^{·-}$ and NO· antagonize each other (Moncada, 1992) and that controlled variations in the production of NO· and $O_2^{·-}$ by endothelium provide one mechanism for regulation of vascular tone (Halliwell, 1989). Inappropriate antagonism of NO· by $O_2^{·-}$ has been suggested to contribute to impaired endothelium-mediated vasodilation in some pathological states, for example, in hypertension and vasoconstriction (Laurindo *et al.*, 1991; Nakazano *et al.*, 1991).

Another suggestion is that the interaction of $O_2^{·-}$ and NO· is not merely antagonistic, but also dangerous (Beckman *et al.*, 1991). The product, peroxynitrite (Eq. 2) may be directly toxic to cells. It may also decompose, after protonation, to form a wide variety of toxic products, possibly including some OH· (Beckman *et al.*, 1991, 1994; Van der Vliet *et al.*, 1994). Evidence consistent with $O_2^{·-}$/NO· interactions *in vivo* has been presented (Beckman *et al.*, 1991, 1994; Kaur and Halliwell, 1994).

TRANSITION METALS

Many transition metals have variable oxidation numbers, for example iron as Fe^{2+} or Fe^{3+} and copper as Cu^+ or Cu^{2+}. Changing between oxidation states involves accepting and donating single electrons, for example:

$$Fe^{3+} + e^- \rightleftharpoons Fe^{2+} \tag{7}$$

$$Cu^{2+} + e^- \rightleftharpoons Cu^+ \tag{8}$$

Thus transition metal ions are remarkably good promoters of free radical reactions. For example, they react with hydrogen peroxide (H_2O_2) to form $OH^{\cdot}$ radicals. In the past 20 years, there have been repeated suggestions that the reactive species produced in reactions (9) and (10) is not $OH^{\cdot}$, but none has received experimental support (reviewed by Halliwell and Gutteridge, 1992):

$$Cu^+ + H_2O_2 \rightarrow Cu^{2+} + OH^{\cdot} + OH^- \tag{9}$$

$$Fe^{2+} + H_2O_2 \rightarrow Fe^{3+} + OH^{\cdot} + OH^- \tag{10}$$

H_2O_2 resembles water in its molecular structure and is very diffusible within and between cells. As well as arising by dismutation of $O_2^{\cdot-}$ (Eq. 5), H_2O_2 can be produced by the action of several oxidase enzymes in tissues, including amino acid oxidases and xanthine oxidase. Like $O_2^{\cdot-}$, H_2O_2 can have useful metabolic functions. For example, H_2O_2 is used by the enzyme thyroid peroxidase to help make thyroid hormones (Dupuy et al., 1991). H_2O_2 (or products derived from it), can displace the inhibitory subunit from the cytoplasmic transcription factor NF–κB. The active factor migrates to the nucleus and activates genes by binding to specific DNA sequences in enhancer and promoter elements. Thus, H_2O_2 can induce expression of genes controlled by NF–κB. This is of particular interest at the moment because NF–κB can induce the expression of genes of the provirus HIV-1, the major cause of acquired immunodeficiency syndrome (Schreck et al., 1992).

Thus H_2O_2 is a molecule of limited reactivity, very diffusible and probably performing certain metabolic roles. However, if H_2O_2 comes into contact with transition metal ions, $OH^{\cdot}$ will be generated and cause damage at that site (Halliwell and Gutteridge, 1989).

ANTIOXIDANT DEFENCES

Living organisms have evolved antioxidant defence enzymes to remove excess $O_2^{\cdot-}$ and H_2O_2. Superoxide dismutase enzymes (SODs) remove $O_2^{\cdot-}$ by accelerating its dismutation (Eq. 5) by about four orders of magnitude at pH 7.4. Human cells have a SOD enzyme containing manganese at its active site (MnSOD) in the mitochondria. A SOD with copper and zinc at the active site (CuZnSOD) is also present, but largely in the cytosol (Fridovich, 1983). Catalases convert H_2O_2 to water and O_2, but the most important H_2O_2-removing enzymes in human cells are glutathione peroxidases (GSHPX), the only known human enzymes that require selenium for their action.

GSHPX removes H_2O_2 by using it to oxidize reduced glutathione (GSH) to oxidized glutathione (GSSG). Glutathione reductase, a flavoprotein enzyme, regenerates GSH from GSSG, with NADPH as a source of reducing power (Chance *et al.*, 1979).

Another important antioxidant defence is that iron and copper ions are kept safely protein-bound whenever possible, so that reactions (9) and (10) are largely prevented. This sequestration of transition metal ions into 'non-catalytic' protein-bound forms is particularly important in extracellular fluids, such as blood plasma, because their levels of antioxidant defence enzymes are very low (Halliwell and Gutteridge, 1986, 1990). The same is true of synovial fluid (Blake *et al.*, 1981a). This low extracellular activity of antioxidant defence enzymes may be explained because at least some of the $O_2^{\cdot-}$ and H_2O_2 generated extracellularly, for example by endothelial cells, fibroblasts and phagocytes, could play useful physiological roles, for example in intercellular signalling. However, it is important to sequester metal ions safely to prevent $OH^{\cdot}$ formation (Halliwell and Gutteridge, 1986, 1990). For example, there is three times as much transferrin iron-binding capacity in blood plasma from healthy adult humans as iron needing to be transported, so that there are essentially no iron ions available to stimulate free radical reactions in plasma from healthy adults. Iron ions bound to transferrin cannot convert H_2O_2 into $OH^{\cdot}$ (Aruoma and Halliwell, 1987). The same is true of copper ions bound to the plasma protein ceruloplasmin (Gutteridge and Stocks, 1981). Hence, both iron and copper in forms 'catalytic' for free radical reactions are absent from the plasma of healthy humans (Gutteridge and Halliwell, 1987; Evans *et al.*, 1989).

The value of this sequestration of metal ions is illustrated by an inspection of the severe pathology suffered by patients with iron or copper overload diseases. For example, in patients with idiopathic haemochromatosis, iron ion chelates 'catalytic' for free radical reactions circulate in the blood (Gutteridge *et al.*, 1985; Grootveld *et al.*, 1989), and these patients can suffer liver damage, diabetes, joint inflammation, cardiac malfunction and hepatoma (McLaren *et al.*, 1983).

As well as the primary antioxidant defences (scavenger enzymes and metal-ion sequestration), there are secondary defences. Thus, cell membranes and plasma lipoproteins contain α-tocopherol, which functions as a chain-breaking antioxidant (reviewed by Burton and Traber, 1990). It is a lipid-soluble molecule, located inside biological membranes and lipoprotein particles. Attached to the hydrophobic structure of α-tocopherol is an –OH group whose hydrogen atom is very easy to remove. Thus, when peroxyl radicals are generated as intermediates during lipid peroxidation (Table 1), they abstract hydrogen preferentially from the tocopherol:

$$-CO_2^{\cdot} + TOH \rightarrow -CO_2H + TO^{\cdot} \tag{11}$$

This stops the peroxyl radical from attacking an adjacent fatty acid side-chain or protein and terminates the chain reaction, hence the name chain-breaking antioxidant. It also converts the α-tocopherol into a radical, tocopherol-$O^{\cdot}$. This radical is poorly reactive in that its reaction with adjacent fatty acid side-chains is much slower than that of peroxyl radicals, so that the chain reaction is drastically slowed. It is widely thought, on the basis of experiments *in vitro*, that the tocopherol radical can migrate to the surface of membranes or lipoproteins and be converted back to α-tocopherol by reaction with ascorbic acid (vitamin C). Thus, both vitamin C and α-tocopherol may co-operate to minimize the consequences of lipid peroxidation in membranes and lipoproteins (Burton and Traber, 1990).

The antioxidant defences of the human body are not 100% efficient, and systems that repair oxidative damage are needed. Thus, cells contain systems that can repair DNA after attack by radicals (Breimer, 1991), degrade proteins damaged by radicals (Marcillat *et al.*, 1988) and metabolize lipid hydroperoxides in membranes (Maiorino *et al.*, 1991). It may be that antioxidant defence is not perfect because some free radical formation is useful, as already explained. Like most things, whether free radicals are good or bad is largely a question of amount, time, and location. Indeed, it seems that the antioxidant defence enzymes operate as a balanced, co-ordinated system (Amstad *et al.*, 1994). Thus, too much SOD, in relation to the activities of H_2O_2-destroying enzymes, may be harmful rather than beneficial (Amstad *et al.*, 1994), although it is not clear exactly why. For example, the gene for the copper, zinc-containing SOD is located on chromosome 21 in humans. Trisomy 21 results in a 50% elevation of this enzyme in human tissues, and experiments with transgenic mice are consistent with the view that this increased SOD may contribute to the symptoms of Down's syndrome (Groner *et al.*, 1990). Perhaps, therefore, the use of SOD to treat RA (Flohe, 1988) was not the best choice of antioxidant.

Oxidative stress (a term introduced by Sies, 1991) is said to result when reactive oxygen species are generated in excess in the human body. This can occur if antioxidant levels are too low. For example, malnutrition can cause low body levels of nutritional antioxidants such as α-tocopherol and vitamin C. Oxidative stress can also be caused by increased free radical formation, which can happen by a number of mechanisms. For example, several toxins are metabolized so as to increase free radical formation *in vivo* (reviewed by Halliwell and Gutteridge, 1989).

Cells can tolerate mild oxidative stress, and often respond to it by increased synthesis of antioxidant defence enzymes (Frank 1991; Storz and Tartaglia, 1992). However, severe oxidative stress can lead to cell injury or death. Depending on the cell type used and the means by which oxidative stress is imposed, injury and death can result from damage to DNA, proteins and/or lipids. In mammalian cells, oxidative stress appears to cause increased levels of free intracellular Ca^{2+} (Orrenius *et al.*, 1989) and free intracellular iron (Halliwell, 1987). The latter can lead to OH˙ generation. Some of this OH˙ generation seems to occur within the nucleus (Halliwell and Aruoma, 1991; Dizdaroglu *et al.*, 1991). The hydroxyl radical attacks DNA in a multiplicity of ways. One of the major products of OH˙ attack upon the DNA bases is 8-hydroxyguanine. An excessive rise in intracellular free Ca^{2+} can also activate endonucleases and cause DNA fragmentation (Orrenius *et al.*, 1989).

Thus, several molecular targets must be considered when attempting to measure, or to explain the consequences of, oxidative stress *in vivo* (Halliwell *et al.*, 1992a).

FREE RADICALS AND HUMAN DISEASE: GENERAL PRINCIPLES

What is the exact role played by free radicals in human disease? Limitations in methodology have, until very recently, precluded precise answers to this question although the situation is improving rapidly (reviewed by Halliwell *et al.*, 1992a).

Some human diseases may be caused by oxidative stress. Thus, ionizing generates OH˙ directly by splitting water molecules (von Sonntag, 1987):

$$H_2O \rightarrow H^\cdot + OH^\cdot \qquad (12)$$

Many of the biological consequences of excess radiation exposure may be due to free radical damage to lipids, proteins, and DNA (von Sonntag, 1987). The signs produced by chronic dietary deficiencies of selenium (Keshan disease) or of α-tocopherol (neurological disorders seen in patients with inborn errors in the mechanism of intestinal fat absorption) might also be mediated by oxidative stress (Levander, 1987; Muller and Goss-Sampson, 1990).

SECONDARY PRODUCTION OF RADICALS IN HUMAN DISEASE

For most human diseases, however, the oxidative stress is secondary to the primary disease process (Fig. 1). For example, activated neutrophils produce $O_2^{\cdot-}$, H_2O_2 and

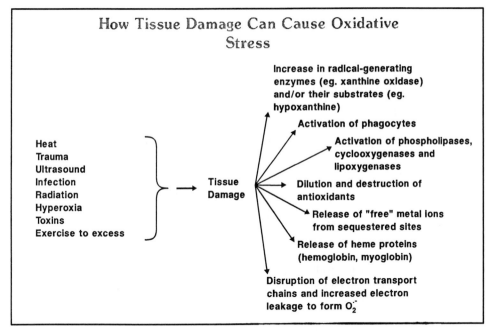

Figure 1. Mechanisms by which tissue injury can cause oxidative stress. Adapted with permission from Halliwell *et al.* (1992a).

HOCl in order to kill bacteria. However, if a large number of phagocytes become activated in a localized area, they can produce tissue damage. Tissue injury can release iron ions, catalytic for free radical reactions, from their normal storage sites within the cell (Halliwell *et al.*, 1988a). It may also lead to disruption of electron transport chains in mitochondria and endoplasmic reticulum, so that more electrons leak to oxygen to form $O_2^{\cdot-}$. Tissue injury frequently causes bleeding, leading to haemoglobin release from erythrocytes. Haemoglobin and myoglobin are potentially dangerous proteins (see Fig. 2; Gutteridge, 1986; Puppo and Halliwell, 1988). Exposure of 'free' haemoglobin to excess H_2O_2 causes haem degradation with release

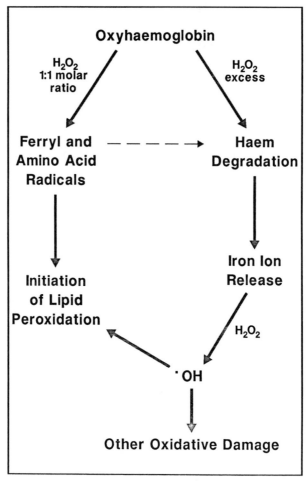

Figure 2. Haemoglobin: a dangerous protein. Haemoglobin is normally transported inside erythrocytes, cells rich in antioxidant defence enzymes. Free haemoglobin is very sensitive to attack by H_2O_2, resulting in an exacerbation of oxidative damage. Haemoglobin is also an avid binder of nitric oxide.

of 'catalytic' iron ions (Gutteridge, 1986). Free haem, another pro-oxidant, might also be released (Prasad *et al.*, 1989). In addition, haemoglobin can react with H_2O_2 to form oxidizing species capable of stimulating lipid peroxidation (Kanner and Harel, 1985) although the chemical nature of this oxidizing species is not yet known with certainty. Reaction of H_2O_2 with the protein probably generates a haeme ferryl species plus an amino acid radical, perhaps on tyrosine (McArthur and Davies, 1993).

THE MAJOR QUESTION

Oxidative stress is an inevitable accompaniment of tissue injury during human disease (Fig. 1). Thus, the main question in RA or in any other human disease is not 'can we demonstrate oxidative stress?' but rather 'does the oxidative stress that occurs make a significant contribution to disease activity?'. The answer to the latter question is as yet uncertain in RA. Let us look at the information available.

OXYGEN-DERIVED SPECIES IN RA

Following the pioneering work of McCord (1974), Halliwell (1978) showed that hyaluronic acid depolymerization by $O_2^{\cdot-}$-generating systems *in vitro* is not caused by $O_2^{\cdot-}$ or H_2O_2 themselves, but by iron-dependent formation of $OH^{\cdot}$. Hydroxyl radical causes fragmentation of hyaluronate in a random fashion to give oligosaccharide species (Grootveld *et al.*, 1991). Both copper and iron ions can catalyse $OH^{\cdot}$ formation from H_2O_2 *in vitro* (Eqs 9 and 10), but 'catalytic' copper has not been detected in synovial fluid freshly aspirated from the knee joints of patients with RA (Winyard *et al.*, 1987). However, the bleomycin assay, an assay that appears to measure iron 'catalytic' for free radical reactions (reviewed by Gutteridge and Halliwell, 1987) detects such iron in about 40% of synovial fluids aspirated from inflamed knee joints of patients with RA (Gutteridge, 1987). Indeed, the iron within such synovial fluid samples has been directly demonstrated to be capable of stimulating lipid peroxidation (Gutteridge *et al.*, 1982). Kaur *et al.* (unpublished observations) found that aspiration of synovial fluid from some RA patients into a solution of phenylalanine produced a pattern of hydroxylation products characteristic of $OH^{\cdot}$ attack upon the phenylalanine aromatic ring (Kaur *et al.*, 1988), suggesting that constituents of synovial fluid can indeed lead to $OH^{\cdot}$ formation in the inflamed rheumatoid joint.

What is the origin of the 'bleomycin-detectable' iron? It could be released from dead cells after lysis (Halliwell *et al.*, 1988a), and by H_2O_2-mediated degradation of haemoglobin released from erythrocytes, liberated as a consequence of traumatic microbleeding in the joint (Blake *et al.*, 1981). Another potential source of iron is synovial fluid ferritin (Biemond *et al.*, 1986). Superoxide can reductively release small amounts of iron from ferritin, although ferritin-bound iron is much safer than an equivalent amount of free iron (Halliwell and Gutteridge, 1986; Bolann and Ulvik, 1990). Indeed, the iron status of patients with RA influences the disease pathology (Blake *et al.*, 1981b; Trenam *et al.*, 1992). A pattern of damage to hyaluronate in synovial fluids from RA patients that is consistent with attack by $OH^{\cdot}$ has been demonstrated by using high-field proton nuclear magnetic resonance spectroscopy (Grootveld *et al.*, 1991), although hyaluronate may additionally be secreted in abnormally low molecular mass forms in rheumatoid disease. The contribution of these two mechanisms has been reviewed (Henderson *et al.*, 1991). The influence of free radicals on connective tissue components is also discussed by Poole and coworkers in Chapter 9, this volume.

The reaction of $O_2^{\cdot-}$ with $NO^{\cdot}$ is another potential source of $OH^{\cdot}$ in the inflamed rheumatoid joint, since the synthesis not only of $O_2^{\cdot-}$ but also of $NO^{\cdot}$ appears to be increased in RA (Farrell *et al.*, 1992). Demonstration of the presence of nitrotyrosines in patients with active RA is consistent with formation of peroxynitrite *in vivo* (Kaur and Halliwell, 1994).

SOURCES OF OXYGEN-DERIVED SPECIES IN RA

Where do $O_2^{\cdot-}$ and H_2O_2 come from in the inflamed rheumatoid joint? One possibility is the activation of the large numbers of neutrophils present (Nurcombe *et al.*,

1991; Robinson *et al.*, 1992; McCarthy *et al.*, 1992). Activated neutrophils liberate $O_2^{\cdot-}$, H_2O_2, elastase, hypochlorous acid, and eicosanoids. Indeed, IgG aggregates in synovial fluid may activate neutrophils (Robinson *et al.*, 1992). Neutrophil production of $O_2^{\cdot-}$ and H_2O_2 may be very much affected by pO_2, and hence might be limited if the joint is hypoxic (Edwards *et al.*, 1984). Activated neutrophils produce little lipid $OH^{\cdot}$ unless transition metal ions are available to convert H_2O_2 into this radical (Britigan *et al.*, 1986; Kaur *et al.*, 1988), but such metal ions do appear to be present in the fluid of at least some patients with RA (Gutteridge, 1987). Hypochlorous acid and $O_2^{\cdot-}$ both react with ascorbate and may contribute to the depletion of this molecule in RA patients (Blake *et al.*, 1981; Halliwell *et al.*, 1987). Hypochlorous acid is a powerful inactivator of α_1-antiproteinase, the major inhibitor of elastase in human body fluids (Weiss, 1989). Indeed, the amount of active α_1-AP appears to be decreased in RA, possibly due to oxidative inactivation (Chidwick *et al.*, 1991).

Hypochlorous acid reacts rapidly with collagen to fragment it (Davies *et al.*, 1993). The pannus overgrowing the cartilage contains many macrophage-like cells, presumably secreting $O_2^{\cdot-}$, H_2O_2, eicosanoids, interleukin-1 and, possibly, $NO^{\cdot}$ (it is not yet clear if macrophages in the rheumatoid joint make $NO^{\cdot}$ but neutrophils and chondrocytes are capable of making $NO^{\cdot}$). These would be another potential source of oxidative damage.

It has also been proposed that the inflamed rheumatoid joint, upon movement and rest, undergoes a hypoxia–reperfusion cycle, which may result in free radical generation by several mechanisms (Merry *et al.*, 1991; Grootveld *et al.*, 1991). It is interesting to reflect that one of these mechanisms may be the enzyme xanthine oxidase, which is present in human synovium (Stevens *et al.*, 1991), in view of the fact that the original work of McCord (1974) used xanthine oxidase to generate $O_2^{\cdot-}$. Xanthine oxidase oxidizes hypoxanthine to xanthine and then to uric acid; O_2 is simultaneously reduced both to $O_2^{\cdot-}$ and to H_2O_2 (Fridovich, 1983).

DRUG-DERIVED RADICALS

A few anti-inflammatory drugs may be able to scavenge reactive oxygen species *in vivo*, but this ability is not widespread (Wasil *et al.*, 1987; Halliwell *et al.*, 1988b). Indeed, the reverse may often be true. Halliwell *et al.* (1992b) have argued that several of the drugs used in the treatment of RA may become converted into damaging free radicals *in vivo*. Thus, several drugs might suppress the symptoms of RA whilst actually aggravating oxidative damage. For example, free radicals derived from penicillamine (Aruoma *et al.*, 1989), the aminosalicylate component of sulphasalazine (Grisham *et al.*, 1992), phenylbutazone (Evans *et al.*, 1992) and some feranic acids (Evans *et al.*, 1994) can be oxidized into products (presumably free radicals) that inactivate α_1-antiproteinase, react with ascorbic acid and may accelerate lipid peroxidation.

CONSEQUENCES OF OXIDATIVE STRESS IN RA

There is no doubt that oxidative stress occurs in RA patients. There is damage to lipids, proteins, DNA and small molecules such as ascorbic acid and uric acid. Table 2 summarizes the available data. Lunec *et al.* (1985) have argued that oxidative damage

Table 2. Evidence consistent with increased oxidative stress in rheumatoid disease

Observation	Reference	Comment
Increased lipid peroxidation products in serum and synovial fluid	Rowley *et al.* (1984)	The methods used were somewhat unspecific and better assays give lower peroxide levels than those found by Rowley *et al.* (unpublished data). However, they are still higher than control values and the decrease in levels of α-tocopherol (per unit lipid) reported in synovial fluid (Fairburn *et al.*, 1992) is suggestive of increased lipid peroxidation *in vivo*, as is the report of increased levels of 4-hydroxy-2-nonenal, a cytotoxic product generated by the decomposition of lipid peroxides (Selley *et al.*, 1992)
Depletion and oxidation of ascorbate in serum and synovial fluid	Blake *et al.* (1981a); Situnayake *et al.* (1991)	Presumably due to consumption of ascorbate during its antioxidant action. Activated neutrophils also take up ascorbate rapidly (Washko *et al.*, 1989)
Increased exhalation of pentane	Humad *et al.* (1988)	A putative end-product of lipid peroxidation although its specificity has been questioned (Phillips *et al.*, 1994)
Increased concentrations of oxidation products of uric acid	Grootveld and Halliwell (1987)	Products measured appear to be end-products of free radical attack upon uric acid (Kaur and Halliwell, 1990)
Formation of 2,3-dihydroxybenzoate (2,3-DHB) from salicylate in increased amounts	Grootveld and Halliwell (1986)	2,3-DHB appears to be a product of attack of OH⁻ upon salicylate in patients taking aspirin (Ingelman-Sundberg *et al.*, 1991)
Degradation of hyaluronic acid by free radical mechanisms	Grootveld *et al.* (1991)	See text
Formation of 'fluorescent' proteins	Lunec *et al.* (1985)	Fluorescence presumably due to oxidative damage to proteins
Increased urinary excretion of 8-hydroxydeoxyguanosine	Lunec *et al.* (1994)	A product of oxidative damage to DNA. DNA damage is increased in RA and SLE (Blount *et al.*, 1991; Lunec *et al.*, 1994)
Increased levels of 'protein carbonyls'	Chapman *et al.* (1989)	Protein carbonyls are an end-product of oxidative damage to proteins (Stadtman, 1990)

to IgG generates IgG aggregates that can activate neutrophils (e.g. see Robinson *et al.*, 1992) and set up a 'vicious cycle' of free radical production. Such damage to IgG could be caused by OH⁻ (Lunec *et al.*, 1985; Griffiths *et al.*, 1988) and by HOCl (Jasin, 1988). There is considerable interest in the role of TNFα in human RA (e.g. Williams *et al.*, 1992; see Chapter 2, this volume) and TNFα is known to cause oxidative stress in cells (Zimmermann *et al.*, 1989; Pogrebniak *et al.*, 1991; Baud *et al.*, 1992; Schulze-Osthoff *et al.*, 1992).

However, what contribution do reactive oxygen species make to the destruction of cartilage and bone in RA? Free radicals such as OH⁻ can degrade isolated proteoglycans (McCord, 1974; Halliwell, 1978) and HOCl degrades collagen (Davies *et al.*,

1993) but their effect on the intact cartilage matrix is probably limited. However, H_2O_2 is a very powerful inhibitor of proteoglycan synthesis (Bates *et al.*, 1985) and interferes with ATP synthesis in cartilage (Baker *et al.*, 1991). Indeed, intra-articular injection of systems generating H_2O_2 produces severe joint damage in animals (Schalkwijk *et al*, 1986). This inhibition of cartilage repair systems could aggravate the effects of proteolytic cartilage degradation and promote cartilage destruction in RA (Halliwell *et al.*, 1988b). Hypochlorous acid can degrade collagen and activate the latent forms of neutrophil collagenases and gelatinase *in vitro* (Weiss, 1989; Weiss and Peppin, 1986), although the extent to which this happens *in vivo* is uncertain (Michaelis *et al.*, 1992). Fibroblasts and chondrocytes can be damaged by H_2O_2 (e.g. Vincent *et al.*, 1991), and it has also been suggested that low levels of H_2O_2 and/or $O_2{}^{.-}$ can accelerate bone reabsorption by osteoclasts (Garrett *et al.*, 1990; Bax *et al.*, 1992), whereas NO' inhibits this process (Alam *et al.*, 1992). In addition, ascorbate is essential for normal cartilage function (Shapiro *et al.*, 1991), and it is not impossible that the very low levels of ascorbate found in synovial fluid of some RA patients could impair cartilage metabolism.

In summary, we do not as yet know the exact contribution made by oxygen-derived species to joint damage in RA. The development of improved assays of oxidative damage that are applicable to humans should help us to address this point (Halliwell *et al*, 1992a) and allow a rational selection of antioxidants (from the many available; see Halliwell, 1991) for possible use in the treatment of RA.

REFERENCES

Alam ASMT, Huang CLH, Blake DR & Zaidi M (1992) A hypothesis for the local control of osteoclast function by Ca^{2+}, nitric oxide and free radicals. *Biosci Rep* **12**: 369–380.

Allen RE, Outhwaite J, Morris CJ & Blake DR (1987) Xanthine oxido-reductase is present in human synovium. *Ann Rheum Dis* **46**: 843–845.

Amstad P, Moret R & Cerutti P (1994) Glutathione peroxidase compensates for the hypersensitivity of Cu, Zn-superoxide dismutase overproducers to oxidant stress. *J Biol Chem* **269**: 1606–1609.

Arroyo CM, Carmichael AJ, Bouscarel B, Liang JH & Weglicki WB (1990) Endothelial cells as a source of oxygen free radicals: an ESR study. *Free Rad Res Comms* **9**: 287–296.

Aruoma OI & Halliwell B (1988) The iron-binding and hydroxyl radical scavenging action of anti-inflammatory drugs. *Xenobiotica* **18**: 459–470.

Aruoma OI, Halliwell B, Butler J & Hoey BM (1989) Apparent inactivation of α_1-antiproteinase by sulphur-containing radicals derived from penicillamine. *Biochem Pharmacol* **38**: 4353–4357.

Babbs CF, Creger MD, Turek JJ & Badylak SF (1991) Endothelial superoxide production in the isolated rat heart during early reperfusion after ischemia. A histochemical study. *Am J Pathol* **139**: 1069–1080.

Baker MS, Bolis S & Lowther DA (1991) Oxidation of articular cartilage glyceraldehyde-3-phosphate dehydrogenase (G3PDH) occurs *in vivo* during carrageenin-induced arthritis. *Agents Actions* **32**: 299–304.

Bates EJ, Johnson CC & Lowther DA (1985) Inhibition of proteoglycan synthesis by hydrogen peroxide in cultured bovine articular cartilage. *Biochim Biophys Acta* **838**: 221–228.

Baud L, Fouqueray B, Philippe C & Affres H (1992) Modulation of tumor necrosis factor by reactive oxygen metabolites. *News Physiol Sci* **7**: 34–37.

Bax BE, Alam ASMT, Banerji B, Bax CMR, Bevis PJR, Stevens CR et al. (1992) Stimulation of osteo-clastic bone resorption by hydrogen peroxide. *Biochem Biophys Res Commun* **183**: 1153–1158.

Beckman JS, Beckman TW, Chen J, Marshall PA & Freeman BA (1991) Apparent hydroxyl radical production by peroxynitrite: implications for endothelial injury from nitric oxide and superoxide. *Proc Natl Acad Sci USA* **87**: 1620–1624.

Beckman JS, Chen J, Ischiropoulos H & Crow JP (1994) Oxidative chemistry of peroxynitrite. *Meth Enzymol* **233**: 229–240.

Biemond P, Swaak AJG, Van Eijk HG & Koster JF (1986) Intraarticular ferritin-bound iron in rheumatoid arthritis. A factor that increases oxygen free radical-induced tissue destruction. *Arthritis Rheum* **29**: 1187–1193.

Blake DR, Hall ND, Treby DA, Halliwell B & Gutteridge JMC (1981a) Protection against superoxide and hydrogen peroxide in synovial fluid from rheumatoid patients. *Clin Sci* **61**: 483–486.

Blake DR, Hall ND, Bacon PA, Dieppe PA, Halliwell B & Gutteridge JMC (1981b) The importance of iron in rheumatoid disease. *Lancet* **2**: 1142–1144.

Blount S, Griffiths HR & Lunec J (1991) Reactive oxygen species damage to DNA and its role in systemic lupus erythematosus. *Mol Aspects Med* **12**: 93–105.

Bolann BJ & Ulvik RJ (1990) On the limited ability of superoxide to release iron from ferritin. *Eur J Biochem* **93**: 899–904.

Breimer LH (1991) Repair of DNA damage induced by reactive oxygen species. *Free Rad Res Comms* **14**: 159–171.

Britigan BE, Rosen GM, Thompson BY, Chai Y & Cohen MS (1986) Stimulated human neutrophils limit iron-catalyzed hydroxyl-radical formation as detected by spin-trapping techniques. *J Biol Chem* **261**: 17026–17032.

Burton GW & Traber MG (1990) Vitamin E: antioxidant activity, biokinetics and bioavailability. *Ann Rev Nutr* **10**: 357–382.

Carreras MC, Pargament GA, Catz SD, Poderoso JJ & Boveris A (1994) Kinetics of nitric oxide and hydrogen peroxide production and formation of peroxynitrite during the respiratory burst of human neutrophils. *FEBS Lett* **341**: 65–68.

Chance B, Sies H & Boveris A (1979) Hydroperoxide metabolism in mammalian organs. *Physiol Rev* **59**: 527–605.

Chapman ML, Rubin BR & Gracy RW (1989) Increased carbonyl content of proteins in synovial fluid from patients with rheumatoid arthritis. *J Rheumatol* **16**: 15–18.

Chidwick K, Winyard PG, Zhang Z, Farrell AJ & Blake DR (1991) Inactivation of the elastase inhibitory capacity of α_1-antitrypsin in fresh samples of synovial fluid from patients with rheumatoid arthritis. *Ann Rheum Dis* **50**: 915–916.

Curnutte JT & Babior BM (1987) Chronic granulomatous disease. *Adv Human Genet* **16**: 229–245.

Davies JMS, Horwitz DA & Davies LJA (1993) Potential roles of hypochlorous acid and N-chloramines in collagen breakdown by phagocytic cells. *Free Rad Biol Med* **15**: 637–643.

Dizdaroglu M, Nackerdien Z, Chao BC et al. (1991) Chemical nature of *in vivo* DNA base damage in hydrogen peroxide-treated mammalian cells. *Arch Biochem Biophys* **285**: 388–390.

Dupuy C, Virion A, Ohayon R et al (1991) Mechanism of hydrogen peroxide formation catalyzed by NADPH oxidase in thyroid plasma membrane. *J Biol Chem* **266**: 3739–3743.

Edwards SW, Hallett MB & Campbell AJ (1984) Oxygen radical production may be limited by oxygen concentration. *Biochem J* **217**: 851–854.

Evans PJ, Bomford A & Halliwell B (1989) Non-caeruloplasmin copper and ferroxidase activity in mammalian serum. *Free Rad Res Comms* **7**: 55–62.

Evans PJ, Cecchini R & Halliwell B (1992) Oxidative damage to lipids and α_1-antiproteinase by phenylbutazone in the presence of haem proteins: protection by ascorbic acid. *Biochem Pharmacol* **44**: 981–984.

Evans PJ, Akarnu D & Halliwell B (1994) Promotion of oxidative damage to arachidonic acid and α_1-antiproteinase by anti-inflammatory drugs in the presence of the haem proteins myoglobin and cytochrome C. *Biochem Pharmacol* in press.

Fairburn K, Grootveld M, Ward RJ, Abiuka C, Kus M, Williams RB et al. (1992) α-Tocopherol, lipids and lipoproteins in knee-joint synovial fluid and serum from patients with inflammatory joint disease. *Clin Sci* **83**: 657–664.

Farrell AJ, Blake DR, Palmer RMJ & Moncada S (1992) Increased concentrations of nitrite in synovial fluid and serum samples suggest increased nitric oxide synthesis in rheumatic diseases. *Ann Rheum Dis* **51**: 1219–1222.

Flohe L (1988) Superoxide dismutase for therapeutic use: clinical experience, dead ends and hopes. *Mol Cell Biochem* **84**: 123–131.

Frank L (1991) Developmental aspects of experimental pulmonary oxygen toxicity. *Free Rad Biol Med* **11**: 463–494.

Fridovich I (1983) Superoxide radical, an endogenous toxicant. *Ann Rev Pharm Tox* **23**: 239–257.

Garrett IR, Boyce BF, Oreffo ROC, Bonewald L, Poser J & Mundy GR (1990) Oxygen-derived free radicals stimulate osteoclastic bone resorption in rodent bone *in vitro* and *in vivo*. *J Clin Invest* **85**: 632–639.

Greenwald RA (1991) Oxygen radicals, inflammation, and arthritis: pathophysiological considerations and implications for treatment. *Semin Arthritis Rheum* **20**: 219–240.

Griffiths HR, Lunec J, Gee CA & Willson RL (1988) Oxygen radical induced alterations in polyclonal IgG. *FEBS Lett* **230**: 155–158.

Grisham MB, Ware K, Marshall S, Yamada T & Sandhu IS (1992) Pro-oxidant properties of 5-aminosalicylic acid. Possible mechanism for its adverse side effects. *Digestive Disease Sci* **37**: 1383–1389.

Groner Y, Elroy-Stein O, Avrahan KB et al. (1990) Down syndrome clinical symptoms are manifested in transfected cells and transgenic mice overexpressing the human Cu/Zn-superoxide dismutase gene. *J Physiol* **84**: 53–77.

Grootveld M & Halliwell B (1986) Aromatic hydroxylation as a potential measure of hydroxyl radical formation *in vivo*. Identification of hydroxylated derivatives of salicylate in human body fluids. *Biochem J* **237**: 499–504.

Grootveld M & Halliwell B (1987) Measurement of allantoin and uric acid in human body fluids. A potential index of free radical reactions *in vivo*. *Biochem J* **243**: 803–808.

Grootveld M, Bell JD, Halliwell B, Aruoma OI, Bomford A & Sadler PJ (1989) Non-transferrin-bound iron in plasma or serum from patients with idiopathic hemochromatosis. Characterization by high performance liquid chromatography and nuclear magnetic resonance spectroscopy. *J Biol Chem* **254**: 4417–4422.

Grootveld M, Henderson EB, Farrell A, Blake DR, Parkes HG & Haycock P (1991) Oxidative damage to hyaluronate and glucose in synovial fluid during exercise of the inflamed rheumatoid joint. *Biochem J* **273**: 459–467.

Gutteridge JMC (1986) Iron promoters of the Fenton reaction and lipid peroxidation can be released from haemoglobin by peroxides. *FEBS Lett* **201**: 291–295.

Gutteridge JMC (1987) Bleomycin-detectable iron in knee-joint synovial fluid from arthritic patients and its relationship to the extracellular antioxidant activities of caeruloplasmin, transferrin and lactoferrin. *Biochem J* **245**: 415–421.

Gutteride JMC & Halliwell B (1987) Radical-promoting loosely bound iron in biological fluids and the bleomycin assay. *Life Chem Rep* **4**: 113–142.

Gutteridge JMC & Stocks J (1981) Ceruloplasmin: physiological and pathological perspectives. *CRC Crit Rev Clin Lab Sci* **14**: 257–329.

Gutteridge JMC, Rowley DA & Halliwell B (1982) Superoxide-dependent formation of hydroxyl radicals and lipid peroxidation in the presence of iron salts. Detection of catalytic iron and anti-oxidant activity in extracellular fluids. *Biochem J* **206**: 605–609.

Gutteridge JMC, Rowley DA, Griffiths E & Halliwell B (1985) Low-molecular-weight iron complexes and oxygen radical reactions in idiopathic haemochromatosis. *Clin Sci* **68**: 463–467.

Halliwell B (1978) Superoxide-induced generation of hydroxyl radicals in the presence of iron salts. Its role in degradation of hyaluronic acid by a superoxide-generating system. *FEBS Lett* **96**: 238–242.

Halliwell B (1987) Oxidants and human disease: some new concepts. *FASEB J* **1**: 358–364.

Halliwell B (1989) Superoxide, iron, vascular endothelium and reperfusion injury. *Free Rad Res Comms* **5**: 315–318.

Halliwell B (1991) Drug antioxidant effects. A basis for drug selection? *Drugs* **42**: 569–605.

Halliwell B & Aruoma OI (1991) DNA damage by oxygen-derived species. Its mechanism and measurement in mammalian systems. *FEBS Lett* **281**: 9–19.

Halliwell B & Gutteridge JMC (1986) Oxygen free radicals and iron in relation to biology and medicine. Some problems and concepts. *Arch Biochem Biophys* **246**: 501–514.

Halliwell B & Gutteridge JMC (1989) *Free Radicals in Biology and Medicine*. Oxford, UK: Clarendon Press.

Halliwell B & Gutteridge JMC (1990) The antioxidants of human extracellular fluids. *Arch Biochem Biophys* **280**: 1–8.

Halliwell B & Gutteridge JMC (1992) Biologically relevant metal ion-dependent hydroxyl radical generation – an update. *FEBS Lett* **307**: 108–112.

Halliwell B, Wasil M & Grootveld M (1987) Biologically-significant scavenging of the myeloperoxidase-derived oxidant hypochlorous acid by ascorbic acid. Implications for antioxidant protection in the inflamed rheumatoid joint. *FEBS Lett* **213**: 15–18.

Halliwell B, Aruoma OI, Mufti G & Bomford A (1988a) Bleomycin-detectable iron in serum from leukaemic patients before and after chemotherapy. *FEBS Lett* **241**: 202–204.

Halliwell B, Hoult JRS & Blake DR (1988b) Oxidants, inflammation and anti-inflammatory drugs. *FASEB J* **2**: 2867–2873.

Halliwell B, Gutteridge JMC & Cross CE (1992a) Free radicals, antioxidants and human disease: where are we now? *J Lab Clin Med* **119**: 598–620.

Halliwell B, Evans PJ, Kaur H & Chirico S (1992b) Drug-derived radicals: mediators of the side effects of anti-inflammatory drugs? *Ann Rheum Dis* **51**: 1261–1263.

Henderson EB, Grootveld M, Farrell A, Smith EC, Thompson PW & Blake DR (1991) A pathological role for damaged hyaluronan in synovitis. *Ann Rheum Dis* **50**: 196–200.

Hogg N, Darley-Usmar VM, Wilson MT & Moncada S (1992) Production of hydroxyl radicals from the simultaneous generation of superoxide and nitric oxide. *Biochem J* **281**: 419–424.

Huie RE & Padmaja S (1993) The reaction of NO with superoxide. *Free Rad Res Comms* **18**: 195–199.

Humad S, Zarling E, Clapper M & Skosey JK (1988) Breath pentane excretion as marker of disease activity in rheumatoid arthritis. *Free Rad Res Comms* **5**: 101–106.

Ingelman-Sundberg M, Kaur H, Terelius Y, Persson JO & Halliwell B (1991) Hydroxylation of salicylate by microsomal fractions and cytochrome P-450. Lack of production of 2,3-dihydroxybenzoate unless hydroxyl radical formation is permitted. *Biochem J* **276**: 753–757.

Jasin HE (1988) Oxidative cross-linking of immune complexes by human polymorphonuclear leukocytes. *J Clin Invest* **81**: 6–15.

Kanner J & Harel S (1985) Initiation of membranal lipid peroxidation by activated metmyoglobin and methaemoglobin. *Arch Biochem Biophys* **237**: 314–321.

Kaur H & Halliwell B (1990) Action of biologically-relevant oxidizing species upon uric acid. Identificaiton of uric acid oxidation products. *Chem Biol Interac* **73**: 235–247.

Kaur H & Halliwell B (1994) Evidence for nitric oxide mediated oxidative damage in chronic inflammation. *FEBS Lett* in press.

Kaur H, Fagerheim I, Grootveld M, Puppo A & Halliwell B (1988) Aromatic hydroxylation of phenylalanine as an assay for hydroxyl radicals. *Anal Biochem* **172**: 360–367.

Laurindo FRM, da Luz PL, Uint L et al. (1991) Evidence for superoxide radical-dependent coronary vasospasm after angioplasty in intact dogs. *Circulation* **83**: 1705–1715.

Levander OA (1987) A global view of human selenium nutrition. *Ann Rev Nutr* **7**: 227–250.

Lunec J, Blake DR, McCleary SJ, Brailsford S & Bacon PA (1985) Self-perpetuating mechanisms of immunoglobulin G aggregation in rheumatoid inflammation. *J Clin Invest* **76**: 2084–2090.

Lunec J, Herbert K, Blount S, Griffiths HR & Emery P (1994) 8 hydroxydeoxyguanosine: a marker of oxidative DNA damage in systemic lupus erythematosus. *FEBS Lett* **348**: 131–138.

Maiorino M, Chu FF, Ursini F et al. (1991) Phospholipid hydroperoxide glutathione peroxidase is the 18 kDa selenoprotein expressed in human tumor cell lines. *J Biol Chem* **266**: 7728–7732.

Marcillat O, Zhang Y, Lin SW & Davies KJA (1988) Mitochondria contain a proteolytic system which can recognize and degrade oxidatively-denatured proteins. *Biochem J* **254**: 677–683.

McArthur KM & Davies MJ (1993) Detection and reactions of the globin radical in haemoglobin. *Biochim Biophys Acta* **1202**: 173–181.

McCarthy DA, Bernhagen J, Taylor MJ, Hamblin AS, James I, Thompson PW et al (1992) Morphological evidence that activated polymorphs circulate in the peripheral blood of patients with rheumatoid arthritis. *Ann Rheum Dis* **51**: 13–18.

McCord JM (1974) Free radicals and inflammation. Protection of synovial fluid by superoxide dismutase. *Science* **185**: 529–531.

McLaren GD, Muir WA & Kellermeyer RW (1983) Iron overload disorders: natural history, pathogenesis, diagnosis and therapy. *CRC Crit Rev Clin Lab Sci* **19**: 205–266.

Meier B, Radeke HH, Selle S, Raspe HH, Sies H, Resch K et al. (1990) Human fibroblasts release reactive oxygen species in response to treatment with synovial fluids from patients suffering from arthritis. *Free Rad Res Comms* **8**: 149–160.

Merry P, Grootveld M, Lunec J & Blake DR (1991) Oxidative damage to lipids within the inflamed human joint provides evidence of radical-mediated hypoxic-reperfusion injury. *Am J Clin Nutr* **56**: 362S–369S.

Michaelis J, Vissers MC & Winterbourn CC (1992) Different effects of hypochlorous acid on human neutrophil metalloproteinases: activation of collagenase and inactivation of collagenase and gelatinase. *Arch Biochem Biophys* **292**: 555–562.

Moncada S (1992) Nitric oxide gas: mediator, modulator, and pathophysiologic entity. *J Lab Clin Med* **120**: 187–191.

Muller DPR & Goss-Sampson MA (1990) Neurochemical, neurophysiological and neuropathological studies in vitamin E deficiency. *Crit Rev Neurobiol* **5**: 239–265.

Nakazano K, Watanabe N, Matsuno K et al. (1991) Does superoxide underly the pathogenesis of hypertension? *Proc Natl Acad Sci USA* **88**: 10045–10048.

Nurcombe HL, Bucknall RC & Edwards SW (1991) Neutrophils isolated from the synovial fluid of patients with rheumatoid arthritis: priming and activation *in vivo*. *Ann Rheum Dis* **50**: 147–153.

Orrenius S, McConkey DJ, Bellomo G & Nicotera P (1989) Role of Ca^{2+} in toxic cell killing. *Trends Pharm Sci* **10**: 281–285.

Palmer RMJ, Hickery MS, Charles IG, Moncada S & Bayliss MT (1993) Induction of nitric oxide synthase in human chondrocytes. *Biochem Biophys Res Commun* **193**: 398–405.

Phillips M, Greenburg J & Sabas M (1994) Alveolar gradient of pentane in normal human breath. *Free Rad Res Comms* **20**: 333–337.

Pogrebniak H, Matthews W, Mitchell J et al. (1991) Spin-trap protection from tumor necrosis factor cytotoxicity. *J Surg Res* **50**: 469–474.

Prasad MR, Engelman RM, Jones RM & Das DK (1989) Effects of oxyradicals on oxymyoglobin. Deoxygenation, haem removal and iron release. *Biochem J* **263**: 731–736.

Puppo A & Halliwell B (1988) Formation of hydroxyl radicals from hydrogen peroxide in the presence of iron. Is haemoglobin a biological Fenton reagent? *Biochem J* **249**: 185–190.

Robinson J, Watson F, Bucknall RC & Edwards SW (1992) Activation of neutrophil reactive-oxidant production by synovial fluid from patients with inflammatory joint disease. *Biochem J* **286**: 345–351.

Rowley DA, Gutteridge JMC, Blake DR, Farr M & Halliwell B (1984) Lipid peroxidation in rheumatoid arthritis: thiobarbituric acid-reactive material and catalytic iron salts in synovial fluid from rheumatoid patients. *Clin Sci* **66**: 691–695.

Saran M, Michel C & Bors W (1990) Reactions of NO with O_2^-. Implications for the action of endothelium-derived relaxing factor. *Free Rad Res Comms* **10**: 221–226.

Schalkwijk J, Van den Berg WB, Van de Putte LBA & Joosten LAB (1986) An experimental model for hydrogen peroxide-induced tissue damage. Effects of a single inflammatory mediator on (peri) articular tissues. *Arthritis Rheum* **29**: 532–538.

Schreck R, Albermann K & Baeuerle PA (1992) Nuclear factor kappa B: an oxidative stress-responsive transcription factor of eukaryotic cells (a review). *Free Rad Res Comms* **17**: 221–237.

Schulze-Osthoff K, Bakker AC, Vanhaesebroeck B et al. (1992) Cytotoxic activity of tumor necrosis factor is mediated by early damage of mitochondrial functions. Evidence for the involvement of mitochondrial radical generation. *J Biol Chem* **267**: 5317–5323.

Selley ML, Bourne DJ, Bartlett MR, Tymms KE, Brook AS, Duffield AM et al. (1992) Occurrence of (E)-4-hydroxy-2-nonenal in plasma and synovial fluid of patients with rheumatoid arthritis and osteoarthritis. *Ann Rheum Dis* **51**: 481–484.

Shapiro IM, Leboy PS, Tokuoka T, Forbes E, DeBolt K, Adams SL et al (1991) Ascorbic acid regulates multiple metabolic activities of cartilage cells. *Am J Clin Nutr* **54**: 1209S–1213S.

Sies H (1991) *Oxidative Stress II*. Oxidants and antioxidants. New York and London: Academic Press.

Situnayake RD, Thurnham DI, Kootathep S, Chirico S, Lunec J, Davis M et al. (1991) Chain-breaking antioxidant status in rheumatoid arthritis. Clinical and laboratory correlates. *Ann Rheum Dis* **50**: 81–86.

Stadtman ER (1990) Metal ion-catalyzed oxidation of proteins: biochemical mechanism and biological consequences. *Free Rad Biol Med* **9**: 315–325.

Stevens CR, Benboubetra M, Harrison R, Sahinoglu T, Smith EC & Blake DR (1991) Localization of xanthine oxidase to synovial endothelium. *Ann Rheum Dis* **50**: 760–762.

Storz G & Tartaglia LA (1992) Oxy R – a regulator of antioxidant genes. *J Nutr* **122**: 627–630.

Trenam CW, Winyard PG, Morris CJ & Blake DR (1992) Iron-promoted oxidative damage in rheumatic diseases. In Lauffer RB (ed) *Iron and Human Disease*, pp 395–417. Boca Raton: CRC Press.

Vincent F, Corral M, Defer N & Adolphe M (1991) Effect of oxygen free radicals on articular chondrocytes in culture: C-*myc* and C-HA-*ras* messenger RNAs and proliferation kinetics. *Exp Cell Res* **192**: 333–339.

Van der Vliet A, O'Neill CA, Halliwell B et al. (1994) Aromatic hydroxylation and nitration of phenyl-alanine and tyrosine by peroxynitrite. *FEBS Lett* **339**: 89–92.

Von Sonntag C (1987) *The Chemical Basis of Radiation Biology*. London: Taylor and Francis.

Washko P, Rotrosen D & Levine M (1989) Ascorbic acid transport and accumulation in human neutrophils. *J Biol Chem* **264**: 18996–19002.

Wasil M, Halliwell B, Moorhouse CP, Hutchison DCS & Baum H (1987) Biologically-significant scavenging of the myeloperoxidase-derived oxidant hypochlorous acid by some anti-inflammatory drugs. *Biochem Pharmacol* **36**: 3847–3850.

Weiss SJ (1989) Tissue destruction by neutrophils. *N Engl J Med* **320**: 365–376.

Weiss SJ & Peppin GL (1986) Collagenolytic enzymes of the human neutrophil. *Biochem Pharmacol* **335**: 3189–3197.

Williams RO, Feldmann M & Maini RN (1992) Anti-tumor necrosis factor ameliorates joint disease in murine collagen-induced arthritis. *Proc Natl Acad Sci USA* **89**: 9784–9788.

Winyard PG, Pall H, Lunec J & Blake DR (1987) Non-caeruloplasmin copper (phenanthroline-copper) is not present in fresh serum or synovial fluid from patients with rheumatoid arthritis. *Biochem J* **247**: 245–247.

Zimmerman RJ, Chan A & Leadon SC (1989) Oxidative damage in murine tumor cells treated *in vitro* by recombinant human tumor necrosis factor. *Cancer Res* **49**: 1644–1648.

16 Neuropeptides and the Synovium

P.I. Mapp and D.R. Blake

INTRODUCTION

In general, body homeostasis is maintained by three systems that interact closely with each other. These are the immune network, the endocrine organs and the nervous system. Whilst the first two of these effector arms have been extensively studied in relation to rheumatoid arthritis (RA), investigations of the role of the nervous system, and the neuropeptides contained within it, have received relatively little attention.

In common with other structures in the body, the nervous system supplies the articular joints. Three major classes of nerves may be identified. Firstly, the large myelinated proprioceptive fibres, which are located primarily in the joint capsule and deliver spatial information to the brain. Whilst this class of nerve fibre is of obvious importance it will not be dealt with in relation to inflammation within the joint. Of much greater interest, in the context of inflammation, are the thinly myelinated and unmyelinated nerve fibres that innervate the synovium. This class of nerve fibre may be subdivided into the sensory fibres and the unmyelinated sympathetic efferent fibres. The sympathetic efferent fibres innervate the synovial blood vessels and exert vasoconstrictor tone, the sensory nerve fibres relay information relating to painful stimuli. A summary of the classification of nerves supplying the joint is given in Table 1. The thinly myelinated and unmyelinated fibres contain within their cytoplasm

Table 1. The diameters of nerve fibres, their classification and location

Afferent fibre diameter (μm)	Conduction velocity (m/s)	Class	Location	Function
Myelinated (10–18)	60–100	I (Aα)	Ligaments	Proprioceptive
Myelinated (5–12)	20–70	II (Aβ)	Capsule	Proprioceptive
Myelinated (1–5)	2.5–20	III (Aδ)	Capsule and synovium	Nociceptive
Unmyelinated (<1)	<1	IV (C)	Capsule and synovium	Nociception

neuropeptides, which are small polypeptides with a wide variety of effects. The nerve fibres may be separated on the basis of the neuropeptides they contain, such that sensory fibres contain substance P and calcitonin gene-related peptide (CGRP), whilst postganglionic sympathetic fibres contain neuropeptide Y (NPY).

This review describes the development and normal innervation of the joints, in particular the synovium, and then show how this changes in the RA joint in the human. Some neuropeptides are described in more detail: substance P, CGRP and NPY. The concepts surrounding neuropeptide release and the role of neuropeptides in inflammatory joint disease are then explored – neurogenic inflammation. The *in*

Mechanisms and Models in Rheumatoid Arthritis
ISBN 0–12–340440–1

317

vitro and *in vivo* effects of some of the peptides are described, mainly those of substance P the most important proinflammatory peptide and about which most is known. The receptors for substance P and the effects of antagonists, peptide and synthetic, for the receptor on inflammatory models are also discussed. Finally the distribution of the enzyme systems in the synovium that break down neuropeptides and how this may lead to functional compartmentalization is described.

DEVELOPMENT OF THE NERVOUS SYSTEM AND APPEARANCE OF THE VARIOUS PEPTIDES

Some information is available about the appearance of nerve fibres and neuropeptides within the embryonic human joint (Hukkanen *et al.*, 1991). The structural elements of nerve fibres have been demonstrated in the knee joint as early as 8 weeks; nerve fibres being present in synovium, periosteum, muscle and adjacent skin. However, there is no immunoreactivity for neuropeptides or catecholamine-synthesizing enzymes at this stage. In periosteum and bone the sensory neuropeptides substance P and CGRP appear at 11 weeks but the sympathetic innervation, as evidenced by neuropeptide Y and tyrosine hydroxylase, is absent until 13 weeks. In bone vascularization and innervation occurred at 13 weeks, neuropeptide Y and tyrosine hydroxylase appearing at 17 weeks.

NORMAL INNERVATION OF THE JOINT

Joints are supplied by both primary and accessory nerves. Primary nerves are branches of peripheral nerves passing near to the joint whilst accessory nerves are branches of intramuscular nerves crossing the joint capsule. Some joints such as the knee and ankle also receive a nerve supply from cutaneous nerves in the overlying skin. The nerves to any one particular joint always arise from more than one level in the spinal cord. About 50% of the axons that comprise articular nerves are less than 5 μm in diameter, those that are less than 2 μm in diameter are unmyelinated. These fibres carry nociceptive information with a slow conduction velocity. The nerve supply to the synovium was, until relatively recently, thought to be sparse. However, it is now known that the synovium contains a good supply of thinly myelinated or unmyelinated nerve fibres (Mapp *et al.*, 1990). These are of two types. The postganglionic sympathetic adrenergic fibres located around the larger blood vessels are responsible for the control of articular blood flow. The unmyelinated C fibres, on the other hand, are responsible for pain transmission. This latter group of fibres is not normally active and is thought only to fire during tissue damage, either mechanical or chemical. They are therefore sometimes referred to as nociceptive fibres. They are not responsive to normal range of movement. During an inflammatory response these fibres may be sensitized by mediators, such as prostaglandin E_2, whereupon even movement in the normal range can cause these fibres to discharge, signalling pain. The typical appearance of the total innervation of the normal human joint is shown in Fig. 1.

INNERVATION OF RHEUMATOID SYNOVIUM

The rheumatoid synovium is a chronically inflamed tissue showing villous hypertrophy of the synovial layer, with an underlying infiltrate of inflammatory cells. Perivascular

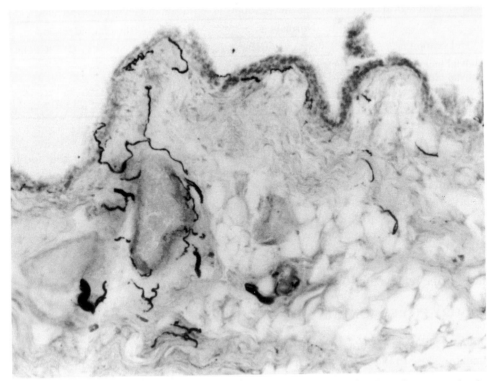

Figure 1. A frozen section through a normal human synovium that has been immunostained to show the total innervation. Note that nerve fibres surround the blood vessels in the subintimal layer and that free fibres extend to the junction between the synovium and the joint space.

cuffs of lymphocytes are seen and the tissue may organize itself to resemble a lymphoid follicle. The innervation of the synovium in RA is markedly different from that of the normal synovium. The initial observations in the human synovium, outlined below, were made by Gronblad *et al.* (1988) and subsequently extended Mapp *et al.* (1990) and confirmed independently by Pereria da Silva and Carmo-Fonseca (1990).

Whilst the deeper vessels in the synovium have a nerve population surrounding them, the superficial vessels are apparently not innervated. Also, the number of free fibres as when compared to normal synovium, is greatly reduced. No immunoreactive fibre are seen in intensely inflamed and 'lymphoid' areas of the synovium. Free sensory fibres are not seen in the intimal layer, nor in the tissue immediately underlying the intima. Staining for specific peptides shows that the free sensory fibres, present in the intimal layer of normal synovium, are absent in the rheumatoid specimens. The perivascular innervation of the deeper blood vessels is predominantly sympathetic efferent fibres. The histological changes to the nerve supply in RA are summarized in Table 2. Similar changes in the innervation of the synovium have been reported in a rat model of adjuvant arthritis (Konttinen *et al.*, 1990).

In summary, it would appear that sensory and sympathetic nerve fibres are absent from the superficial synovium and areas of intense inflammation, whilst the deeper synovium retains its innervation. Staining for specific neuropeptides in the deep syno-

Table 2. Histological evaluation of the nerve supply in normal and rheumatoid synovium

Location	Normal tissue				Rheumatoid tissue			
	PGP	SP	CGRP	CPON	PGP	SP	CGRP	CPON
Synovial membrane	+++	++	++	+	−	−	−	−
Synovial blood vessels	+++	+	+	+++	+	−	−	−
Deep blood vessels	+++	+	+	+++	+++	+	+	++++
Deep free fibres	++	+	+	−	++	+	+	+

+++, abundant; ++, moderate; +, sparse; −, not seen.

vium is weaker and shows a more varicose distribution than in normal controls and it is possible that this reflects an increased release of these peptides, the absence of nerve fibres in the superficial synovium may reflect damage to the peripheral terminals of nerve fibres due to mediators released during the inflammatory response. However, it is possible that the proliferating synovium outstrips the capacity of the nerve supply to innervate it. How these changes in the nerve supply affect the ability of the nervous system to maintain joint homeostasis is a key question and is the subject of much debate and research. The sensory and sympathetic fibres exert some of their influences by the release of neuropeptides and this concept is described below.

SENSORY FIBRES CONTAIN NEUROPEPTIDES

The unmyelinated C fibres arise from cell bodies which are located in the dorsal root ganglion, close to the spinal cord. In addition to its peripheral projection the cell body also has a central projection to the spinal cord. The fine diameter nerve fibres terminate in the superficial layers of the spinal cord, laminae I and II of the dorsal horn, from where they synapse with ascending fibres in the spinal cord. The cell bodies are the site of manufacture of neuropeptides which are transported both centrally and peripherally along the nerve axons. The functions of these peptides are not clearly understood in the central nervous system but some, for instance substance P, are thought to be involved in the modulation of pain transmission. Peripherally where the effects of these peptides are much easier to investigate they are clearly involved in the inflammatory process, both its induction and modulation. They have the capacity individually or in synergism with other neuropeptides or mediators to modulate, mediate or prime for an inflammatory response. In addition, they have an effect on vascular tone.

SENSORY AFFERENT FIBRES CAN HAVE AN EFFERENT FUNCTION

As well as their sensory afferent function the small unmyelinated fibres present in the synovium, and throughout the body, are able to release the neuropeptides they contain when challenged by a nociceptive stimulus. The production of a nociceptive stimulus within a sensory afferent fibre results in an orthodromic electrical signal (in the direction of the spinal cord) and results in a sensation of a dull pain. However, within the extensive peripheral branches of that same fibre an antidromic electrical signal (away from the spinal cord) is propagated and this leads to the peripheral release of neuropeptides. This effect is known as the axon reflex. The peripheral release of neuropeptides stimulates an acute reaction – neurogenic inflammation (Foreman, 1987). The principal peptides known to be involved in the induction of neurogenic inflammation are substance P and CGRP. These peptides have a direct effect on the vasculature, causing vasodilation and oedema, the classical wheal and flare reaction. In addition they may generate indirect effects mediated by stimulation of effector cells, particularly mast cells, with the release of histamine and other inflammatory mediators.

NEUROPEPTIDES SO FAR DEMONSTRATED IN SYNOVIUM

Numerous neuropeptides have been demonstrated in the synovium, the list probably only being limited to those that have actually been looked for. The three major neuropeptides, substance P, CGRP and NPY are described in greater detail below. Those that have also been shown to be present include the opioid peptide met-enkephalin, vasoactive intestinal peptide, somatostatin and galanin. Two other peptides, not derived from neurones but which do interact with them as well as the vasculature are bradykinin and endothelin. These are often mentioned in the same context as neuropeptides.

SUBSTANCE P

In 1931 von Euler and Gaddum extracted from equine brain and intestine a material that was hypotensive and smooth muscle stimulating (von Euler and Gaddum, 1931). They designated this activity preparation P (for powderable) and in later publications referred to it as substance P. It was not until 1971 that the peptide was purified (Chang et al., 1971), sequenced and later synthesized (Tregear et al., 1971).

Substance P is a small polypeptide of 11 amino acids and is one of a family of peptides, the tachykinins, which share four common amino acids at a carboxyl terminal. There appears to be two preprotachykinin (PPT) genes, the SP/NKA PPT I gene and the NKB or PPT II gene. Substance P is encoded by mRNAs from the PPT 1 gene alternative RNA splicing resulting in the production of three (α, β and γ) mRNAs, all of which may produce substance P (Helke et al., 1990). Substance P is distributed widely throughout the central and peripheral nervous system. In the central nervous system substance P is thought to play a role in pain transmission, whilst in the periphery vascular and numerous other effects have been reported (see later: in vitro investigations).

CALCITONIN GENE-RELATED PEPTIDE

CGRP is a 37 amino acid peptide produced by alternative splicing of the primary transcript of the calcitonin gene. It is particularly abundant in the sensory nervous system, being present in approximately 50% of primary sensory neurones. Behavioural and electrophysiological studies have shown that CGRP may play a part in pain perception and reports have indicated that it can potentiate the hyperalgesia caused by intradermal injection of substance P. In addition to its presence in primary sensory nerves, CGRP has also been found in motor end plates and is stored and synthesized in motor neurones (Gibson et al., 1988). This is consistent with reports describing motor-related actions for this peptide, including a role as a muscle trophic factor. In both human and animal studies, CGRP has been shown to be a potent vasodilator, capable of inducing a protracted increase in microvascular blood flow when injected extravascularly. Although relatively inactive on its own, CGRP potentiates oedema induced by other mediators of increased microvascular permeability, including substance P.

The majority of substance-P containing nerve fibres also contain CGRP, and electron immunocytochemical studies have revealed that secretory granules in sensory nerves contain immunoreactivity for both peptides (Merighi et al., 1987). It is interesting to note that co-injection of CGRP with substance P into human skin converts the long-lasting vasodilation induced by CGRP into a transient response. Experiments in animals reveal that this phenomenon is dependent on the action of proteases from mast cells stimulated by substance P (Brain and Williams, 1988). Thus if both CGRP and substance P are released simultaneously from nerve terminals, CGRP will exert a relaxant effect on vascular smooth muscle. The increased blood flow can then be controlled by proteolysis of CGRP by enzymes released from the mast cells in response to substance P. If this inactivation mechanism is overruled by an excess of CGRP, generated locally by depletion of substance P or by loss of mast cell proteases, protracted erythema, as occurs following local infection or injury, could result.

Since CGRP and substance P are colocalized, it might be expected that CGRP has a similar distribution to substance P in articular tissues. However, substance-P immunoreactive nerves are less abundant than CGRP neurones, while CGRP immunoreactivity is found in motor nerves of muscles surrounding the motor nerves and long bones.

NEUROPEPTIDE Y

Neuropeptide Y is a 36 amino acid peptide. Neuropeptide Y is associated with catecholaminergic nerves because of its colocalization with tyrosine hydroxylase and dopamine beta-hydroxylase in sympathetic peripheral ganglion cells. Potent vasoconstrictor effects on the vasculature and presynaptic inhibition of transmitters released from noradrenergic, cholinergic and non-adrenergic, non-cholinergic nerves are among the reported actions (Allen and Bloom, 1986). Neuropeptide-Y containing nerve fibres have been localized (Mapp et al., 1990) almost exclusively to blood vessels in synovial tissues and periosteum, unlike the peptides substance P and CGRP which also occur as free nerve fibres.

IN VITRO INVESTIGATIONS

In vitro the effects of substance P on a wide variety of cell types have been investigated. These data show release of inflammatory mediators from various cell types including the degranulation of mast cells (Mazarek et al., 1981), the simulation of PGE$_2$ and collagenase from synoviocytes (Lotz et al., 1987), secretion of prostaglandins (Hartung et al., 1986), and thromboxane (Hartung and Toyka, 1983) from macrophages and the modulation of immunoglobulin production from lymphoid tissue (Stanitz et al., 1986). Substance P is also reported to induce the release of IL-1 from cultured mouse macrophages (Kimball et al., 1985). Thus tachykinins may contribute to the maintenance of chronic arthritis. These activities of substance P require doses of the peptide in the nanomolar range which is consistent with published figures for the dissociation constant of substance P with its receptor (0.5–2.0 nM). Other cells, such as neutrophils, only appear to be activated directly by much larger concentrations of the peptide ($>10\,\mu$M) suggesting a lack of physiological relevance. However, lower concentrations of substance P, in the nanomolar range, appear to be able to prime neutrophils to respond to other mediators. In particular, neutrophils have been shown to act in a synergistic manner with substance P to other chemotactic peptides such as complement-derived C5a or bacterial fMLP (Perianin et al., 1989). Low doses of substance P have also been shown to modulate the action of other peptides, such as CGRP (Brain and Williams, 1988). Collectively these results suggest that in addition to a direct effect of substance P on several cell types a second modulatory mechanism is also operative. The nervous system may therefore be capable of priming cells to respond to lower doses of certain agents, than might otherwise be the case, leading to an apparent hypersensitivity. This mechanism may be particularly important in allergic responses, such as that seen in asthma.

IN VIVO INVESTIGATIONS

Since neuropeptides are synthesized in the dorsal root ganglion cell bodies an alternative approach to determine the involvement of neuropeptides in arthritis would be to induce an inflammatory response in a single joint and then to monitor changes in neuropeptide levels in the dorsal root ganglia that supply that joint. In the case of the knee joint, nerve tracing studies show that L4 to L6 are the appropriate ganglia to examine. Using this method Smith et al. (1992) found a 70% increase in immunoreactive substance P in the ipsilateral dorsal root ganglia. In a Freunds adjuvant model of hind paw inflammation substance P was found to be raised by 30–40% in the L4 to L6 dorsal root ganglia, 5 days after the induction of the inflammation (Donnerer et al., 1992). In this same study the substance P content of the sciatic nerve supplying the inflamed paw was raised by 60–75%. The increased biosynthesis of substance P in the dorsal root ganglia of the monoarthritic rat is reflected by the finding of increases in the mRNA levels of preprotachykinin A, the precursor of substance P (Donaldson et al., 1992). These data suggest that, in the early stages of the inflammatory response, both the amount of substance P synthesized and transported to the inflammatory site is increased.

The involvement of substance P in arthritis has also been studied directly in animal models. Levine et al. (1984) found that infusion of substance P into rat knees increased the severity of adjuvant induced arthritis. This work was extended to show that the substance P receptor was directly involved in this effect. Further experiments are described in the section on receptors.

EVIDENCE FOR THE RELEASE OF SUBSTANCE P IN HUMAN JOINT INFLAMMATION

One of the most obvious ways to implicate substance P, or any other neuropeptide, in arthritis is to demonstrate that the peptide is present in the inflammatory joint fluid. Many groups have reported the presence of substance P in the synovial fluid, but the agreement between the values obtained is poor. The initial report of the possible presence of substance P in the synovial fluid came from Chapman and Tsao (1980) using high performance liquid chromatography (HPLC). They reported that a rheumatoid patient had a concentration of 0.1 µg/ml in the knee joint synovial fluid. Devillier *et al.* (1986) reported elevated levels of tachykinin-like immunoreactivity in the synovial fluid of patients with rheumatic inflammatory diseases (3.94 ± 1.21 ng/ml compared to 1.91 ± 0.56 ng/ml in the non-inflammatory fluids. By contrast, Larsson *et al.* (1989, 1991) have been unable to detect substance P in arthritic or control groups, despite the fact that they have employed an antiserum specific for substance P rather than the other tachykinins in the same family (neurokinins A and B). Of note in these studies is that neurokinin A was detected. Marshall *et al.* (1990) report levels of 946 ± 82.8 pg/ml, whilst most recently Hernanz *et al.* (1993) give figures of 120 ± 69 pg/ml for rheumatoid synovial fluid. The different methodologies used may go some way to explaining the differences in the results, HPLC being used in the first study. Of more concern is the reliance on antisera prepared from rabbit plasma for the radioimmunoassay. Since each study employed a different antiserum the results are not strictly comparable. Of even greater concern must be the handling of the specimens after withdrawal from the joint; there are numerous enzymes within the joint that are capable of the degradation of substance P (see Degradation of peptides). These enzymes are often unaffected by broad spectrum enzyme inhibitors, such as aprotinin, and may therefore continue to be active *ex vivo*. A further contribution to the confusion surrounding these measurements may be that the substance P is bound to serum albumin (Corbally *et al.*, 1990) in the joint fluid and therefore the extraction procedure for the peptide is critical to the final amount observed.

Taking the limitations of the measurements into account, those studies that have compared the levels of substance P in the synovial fluid with that in the serum have shown higher levels in the synovial fluid. This would indicate that production of substance P is from within the joint. The C fibres are the probable source although there is one report (Loesch and Burnstock, 1988) that a subpopulation of endothelial cells may also contain substance P. Whether these cells acquire substance P by uptake or by synthesis remains to be determined.

RECEPTORS FOR NEUROPEPTIDES

There are currently three pharmacologically distinct receptors for tachykinins, termed NK1, NK2 and NK3. They are usually defined by the rank order of potency of tachykinins in binding studies. Substance P has the greatest affinity for the NK1 receptor (Regoli and Nantel, 1991), although it may interact with NK2 and NK3 receptors at higher concentrations. Substance P has effects on many different cell types from which it may be concluded that each cell type possess a receptor, either constitutive or inducible.

Peptide receptors can be localized and their kinetics studied by quantitative *in vitro* receptor autoradiography with computerized image analysis (Palacois and Dietl 1989). This method, which employs ^{125}I-Bolton-Hunter labelled substance P, has enabled the investigation of receptors for substance P in the synovial membrane. Specific high affinity, low capacity binding sites are present on the endothelial cells of human synovial blood vessel. The ratio of the IC_{50} values for these sites for substance P, neurokinin A and neurokinin B is 1.25:175:>1000 respectively and is characteristic of the NK1 class of tachykinin receptor (Walsh *et al.*, 1992). The interaction of substance P with NK1 receptors on endothelial cells may be important in the regulation of vascular tone. Vasodilation induced by substance P has been shown to be endothelium dependent and is inhibited by N^G monomethyl-L-argenine, indicating a probable mediation by nitric oxide, the endothelium-derived relaxing factor (Rees *et al.*, 1989).

The distinct localization of substance-P receptors on endothelial cells in human synovium suggests that proinflammatory actions of substance P may be predominantly due to direct vascular action.

PEPTIDE ANTAGONISTS

The involvement of substance P and its receptors in inflammation and arthritis has been studied using a number of animal models. Levine *et al.* (1984) found that infusion of substance P into rat knees increased the severity of adjuvant induced arthritis but administration of the substance-P analogue (D-Pro^2, D-Trp^{7,9})-SP, a putative substance-P receptor antagonist (Engberg *et al.*, 1981), only produced moderate soft tissue swelling and osteoporosis. Lam and Ferrell (1989a) showed that the carrageenan model of acute joint inflammation could be virtually abolished by prior administration of the substance-P antagonist d-Pro^4, d-Trp^{7,9,10}-SP (4-11). It has also been shown that injection of capsaicin, the hot component of the chilli pepper, into the synovial cavity of the rat knee inhibited the inflammation seen following substance-P injection. Capsaicin causes the depolarization of afferent C fibres leading to the release of substance P and the degranulation of mast cells, but in this case may have been acting by causing a depletion of substance-P receptors in the target tissue (Lam and Ferrell, 1989b).

NON-PEPTIDE ANTAGONISTS

Until recently antagonists of the NK1 receptor were limited to peptide analogues, such as those described in the previous section. However, the commercial pressure to develop non-metabolizable synthetic antagonists has led to the development of a number of compounds. The first to be described was CP-96,345 by Snider *et al.* (1991) from the Pfizer Company, arising from a high throughput chemical file screening strategy using a ^{3}H substance-P binding assay as the primary screen. This compound is a potent, reversible and competitive antagonist of the NK1 receptor. Their *in vivo* studies show that the compound lacks agonist activity and is highly selective. Since the development of CP-96,345 a number of other NK1 antagonists have become available, the structures of some of these are shown in Fig. 2. Note that the structures are very different when presented in a two-dimensional form, but one assumes that the three-dimensional structures have some similarities. Investigations using such compounds has shown that NK1 receptors display heterogeneity. CP-96,345 has a higher affinity for human and guinea pig NK1 receptors, than for those in the rat (Gitter *et al.*, 1991; Beresford *et al.*, 1991). FK888 has similarly been found to have a higher affinity for guinea pig than rat receptors (Fujii *et al.*, 1992). There is also evidence for differences in NK1 receptor specificities between different tissues of a single species (Petitet *et al.*, 1992), and suggestions that receptor expression and/or affinity may be influenced by inflammation (Scott *et al.*, 1992). Therefore results from studies on

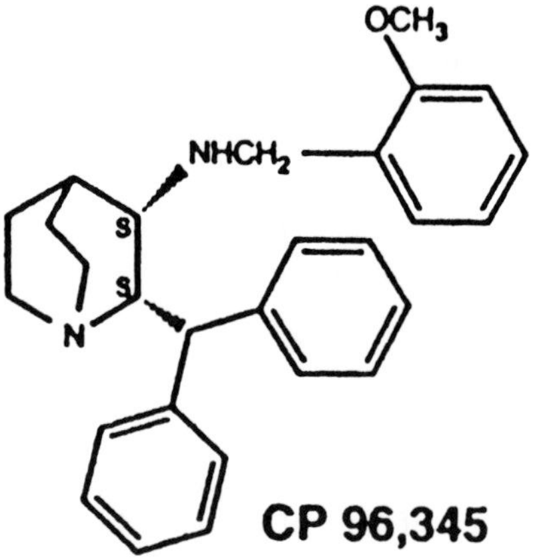

CP 96,345

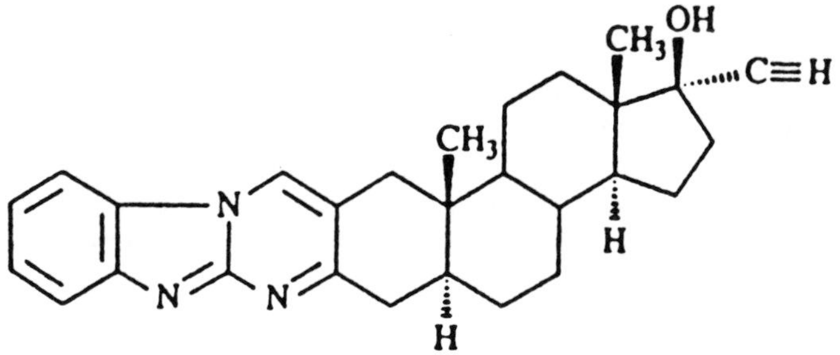

WIN 51,708

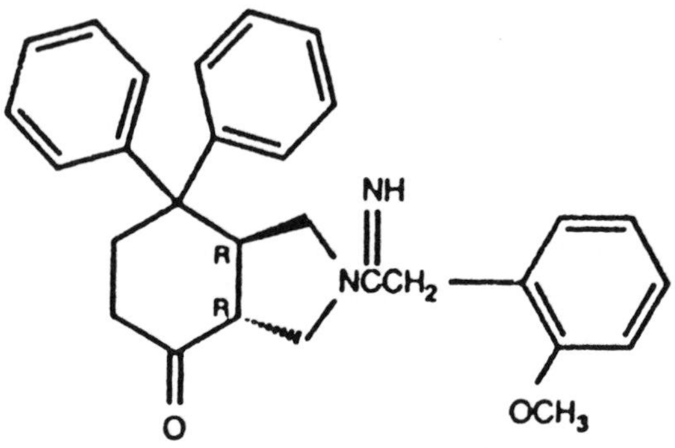

RP 67580

Figure 2. The structures of some of the recently developed antagonists to the substance-P receptor.

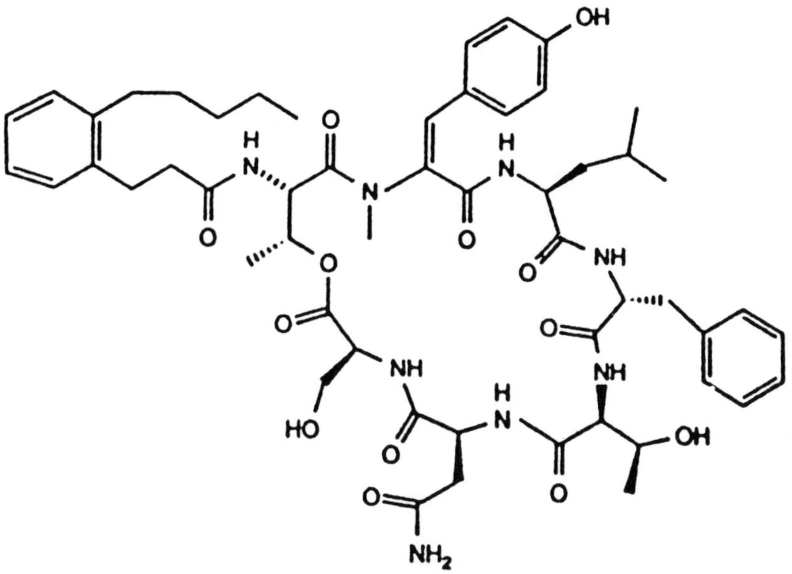

FK 224

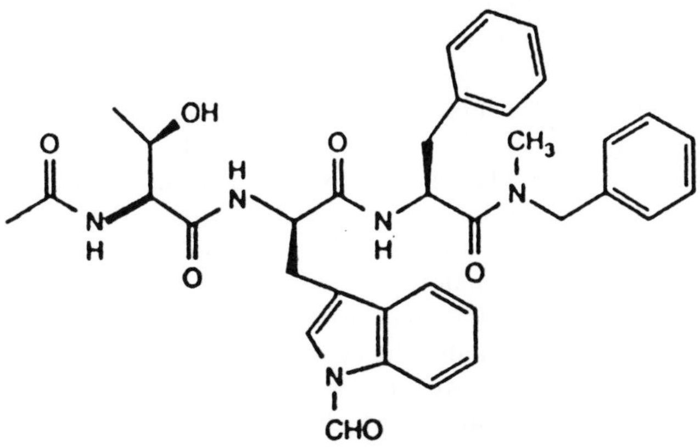

FR 113680

Figure 2. (*cont.*)

different tissues in different species or in different pathological states should be interpreted with caution.

DEGRADATION OF PEPTIDES

The local activities of regulatory peptides depend on a combination of release and clearance from the vicinity of their receptors. Many peptides have short half-lives, rapid clearance being due to membrane-bound peptidases. These enzymes have characteristic regional distributions, and their activities may vary during inflammation. Understanding the local topography of membrane-bound peptidases and their relation to the sites of release and action of those peptides that may act as substrates is therefore essential to understanding peptidergic regulatory systems in the normal and diseased synovium. The first enzyme to be studied in this regard was neutral endopeptidase (NEP).

NEUTRAL ENDOPEPTIDASE

NEP (EC 3.4.24.11) is responsible for the majority of the degradation of substance P in the human synovium. NEP is capable of the hydrolysis of many peptides including substance P (Skid *et al.*, 1984) and CGRP (Katyama *et al.*, 1991). This enzyme has been shown to be indentical to the common acute lymphoblastic leukaemia antigen (CALLA) (Letarte *et al.*, 1988; Shipp *et al.*, 1988) and is the CD10 determinant.

NEP is an integral membrane metalloproteinase with a characteristic zinc-binding motif in the extracellular carboxyterminal domain (Devault *et al.*, 1987). The enzyme hydrolyses peptide bonds at the amino side of hydrophobic amino acids (Kerr and Kenny, 1974), and is thought to inactivate regulatory peptides at the cell surface (Mumford *et al.*, 1981; Fulcher *et al.*, 1982; Gafford *et al.*, 1983; Connelly *et al.*, 1985). NEP has been hypothesized to modulate neurogenic inflammation, for example in the lung (Nadel and Borsin, 1991). Its activity has been shown in the synovium of patients with chronic arthritis (Sreedharan *et al.*, 1990). The activity of NEP was found to be higher in all patients with RA and some patients with degenerative joint disease, when compared to traumatic arthritis controls. Since mature B and T lymphocytes and macrophages which constitute the major inflammatory cell populations in RA contain no detectable NEP activity (Malfroy *et al.*, 1989) it has been speculated that synovial fibroblasts may be the source of this enzyme. Both human fibroblasts (Lorkowski *et al.*, 1987) and rabbit synovial fibroblasts (Werb and Clark, 1989) can be induced to synthesize this enzyme *in vitro*. Our own data show the localization of this enzyme in human synovium, as determined by immunocytochemistry, and support the hypothesis that fibroblasts are its source, a restricted population of cells surrounding blood vessels being responsible for the majority of the activity (Mapp *et al.*, 1992). These may represent a specialist subpopulation of fibroblasts.

Since the function of NEP is probably the degradation of locally released regulatory peptides its presence around the blood vessels makes it ideally located to inactivate vasoactive peptides, such as substance P, which are released from perivascular nerve fibres. There is good evidence from experiments done *in vivo* to support this hypothesis. Substance P in induced oedema in guinea pig skin is potentiated by the NEP inhibitors phosphoramidon and thiorphan (Iwamoto *et al.*, 1989), and attenuated by coadministration of NEP. Furthermore NEP may also limit the activity of endogenously released regulatory peptides. The bronchial contraction induced by capsaicin, which acts by releasing neuropeptides, including substance P, from peripheral nerve endings, is also enhanced by phosphoramidon (Djokic et al., 1989a,b).

In addition to NEP we have also localized several other peptide degrading enzymes to the synovium including angiotensin converting enzyme (ACE), dipeptidyl peptidase IV (DPPIV) and aminopeptidase M (APM).

ANGIOTENSIN CONVERTING ENZYME

ACE acts as a peptidyl peptidase, inactivating bradykinin and activating angiotensin I by removal of C-terminal dipeptides. In addition, ACE can act as an endopeptidase, cleaving substance P to liberate the C terminal di- or tripeptide, and subsequently as a peptidyl peptidase, cleaving successive dipeptide from the unprotected C terminus (Turner et al., 1987). The localization of ACE to the endothelia of all vessels, with the most intense staining on capillaries and arterioles, is similar to that seen in other tissues.

DIPEPTIDYL PEPTIDASE IV

The serine protease DPPIV, is identical to the leukocyte antigen CD26 (Ulmer et al., 1990) and cleaves unprotected N-terminal dipeptides where the penultimate residue is proline. In the case of substance P this may not abolish biological activity, which resides at its C-terminus, but renders it susceptible to further inactivation by successive cleavage of further N-terminal peptides by APM.

AMINOPEPTIDASE M

APM has been identified as the leukocyte antigen CD13 and also participates in the inactivation of enkephalins (Look et al., 1989). In the inflamed synovium APM is found in a similar distribution to NEP; that is, in spindle shaped fibroblast-like cells surrounding the blood vessels and also in similarly shaped cells in a layer underlying the hypertrophic intimal cell layer.

FUNCTIONAL COMPARTMENTALIZATION

The localization of membrane peptidases in the human synovium suggests not only a role limiting the duration of action of regulatory peptides but also in localizing their activities to the vicinity of their release. This functional compartmentalization of vascular and stromal regions in synovium is essential to the local regulatory function of peptides and is likely to influence responses to exogenous peptide administered into non-physiological compartments in experimental investigations. Depletion of neuropeptide-immunoreactive nerves in the chronically inflamed synovium implies a loss of normal neurovascular regulation, and the abundance of membrane peptidases in inflamed synovial tissue would be expected to exacerbate this situation further. Inhibition of specific peptidases may have a therapeutic role in restoring the protective effects of vasoactive regulatory peptides. Inhibitors of aminopeptidases have anti-inflammatory activity *in vivo* and the specific ACE inhibitor, captopril, may have slow antirheumatic activity (Martin *et al.*, 1984).

CONCLUSION

This review has dealt with select aspects of neuropeptides as they relate to inflammation within the joint. However, there is also a wealth of other data on the acute effects of neuropeptides, in such systems as the skin.

Arguments persist as to the relevance of acute effects of neuropeptides as opposed to their contribution to chronic disease, such as RA. Furthermore, it is not clear whether some aspects of their action are protective or deleterious. For instance, there is evidence to suggest that oedema formation in adjuvant arthritis of the rat is protective, since increasing oedema correlates with a decrease in severity of joint disease, as judged by X-ray scores. At the same time it appears that there is also a component, arising from the sympathetic nervous system, that exacerbates joint injury. Our understanding of these chronic aspects of the involvement of the nervous system in joint disease still has some way to go.

REFERENCES

Allen JM & Bloom SR (1986) Neuropeptide Y: a putative neurotransmitter. *Neurochem Int* **8**: 1–8.
Beresford IJM, Birch PJ, Hagan RM & Ireland SJ (1991) Investigation into species variants in tachykinin NK1 receptors by use of the non-peptide antagonist, CP-96,345. *Br J Pharmacol* **104**: 292–293.
Brain SD & Williams TJ (1988) Substance P regulates the vasodilator activity of calcitonin gene-related peptide. *Nature* **335**: 73–75.
Chang MM, Leeman SE & Niall HD (1971) The amino acid sequence of substance P. *Nature New Biology* **232**: 86–87.
Chapman LF & Tsao MU (1980) Possible presence of substance P in the synovial fluid of the knee joint of an arthritic patient. *Fed Proc* **39**: 603.
Connelly JC, Skidgel RA, Schulz WW, Johnson AR & Erdos EG (1985) Neutral endopeptidase 24.11 in human neutrophils: cleavage of chemotactic peptide. *Proc Natl Acad Sci USA* **82**: 8737–8741.
Corbally N, Powell D & Tipton KF (1990) The binding of endogenous and exogenous substance P in human plasma. *Biochem Pharmacol* **39**: 1161–1166.
Devault A, Lazure C, Nault C, Le Moual H, Seidah NG & Chrétien M (1987) Amino acid sequence of rabbit kidney neutral endopeptidase 24.11 (enkephalinase) deduced from complementary DNA. *EMBO J* **6**: 1317–1322.
Devillier P, Weill B, Renoux M, Menkes C & Pradelles P (1986) Elevated levels of tachykinin-like immunoreactivity in joint fluids from patients with rheumatic inflammatory diseases. *N Eng J Med* **314**: 1323.
Djokic TD, Sekizwa K, Borson DB & Nadel JA (1989a) Neutral endopeptidase inhibitors potentiate substance P-induced contraction in gut smooth muscle. *Am J Physiol* **256**: G39–G43.
Djokic TD, Nadel JA, Dusser DJ, Sekizawa K, Graf PD & Borson DB (1989b) Inhibitors of neutral endopeptidase potentiate electrically and capsaicin-induced non-cholinergic contractions in guinea pig bronchi. *J Pharmacol Exp Ther* **248**: 7–11.
Donaldson LF, Harmer AJ, McQueen DS & Seckl JR (1992) Increased expression of preprotachykinin A, calcitonin gene-related peptide, but not vasoactive intestinal peptide, messenger RNA in dorsal root ganglia during the development of adjuvant monoarthritis in the rat. *Mol Brain Res* **16**: 143–149.
Donnerer J, Schuligoi R & Stein C (1992) Increased content and transport of substance P and calcitonin gene-related peptide in sensory nerves innervating inflamed tissue: evidence for a regulatory function of nerve growth factor *in vivo*. *Neuroscience* **49**: 693–698.
Engberg G, Svensson TH, Rosell S & Folkers K (1981) A synthetic peptide as an antagonist of substance P. *Nature* **293**: 222–223.
von Euler US & Gaddum JH (1931) An unidentified depressor substance in certain tissue extracts. *J Physiol (Lond)* **72**: 74.
Foreman JC (1987) Peptides and neurogenic inflammation. *Brit Med Bull* **43**: 386–400.

Fujii T, Murai M, Morimoto H, Maeda Y, Yamaoka M, Hagiwara D et al. (1992) Pharmacological profile of a high affinity NK1 receptor antagonist, FK 888. *Br J Pharmacol* **107**: 785–789.

Fulcher IS, Matasa R, Turner AJ & Kenny AJ (1982) Kidney neutral endopeptidase and the hydrolysis of enkephalin by synaptic membranes show similar sensitivity to inhibitors. *Biochem J* **203**: 519–522.

Gafford J, Skidgel RA, Erdos EG & Hersch LB (1983) Human kidney enkephalinase, a neutral metallo-proteinase that cleaves active peptides. *Biochemistry* **22**: 3265–3271.

Gibson SJ, Polak JM, Giaid A, Hanid QA, Kar S, Jones PM et al. (1988) Calcitonin gene-related peptide messenger RNA is expressed in the sensory neurones of dorsal root ganglia and also in the spinal motorneurones in man and rat. *Neurosci Lett* **91**: 283–288.

Gitter BD, Waters DC, Bruns RF, Mason NR, Nixon JA & Howbert JJ (1991) Species differences in affinities of non-peptide antagonists for substance P receptors. *Eur J Pharmacol* **197**: 237–238.

Gronblad M, Konttinen YT, Korkala O, Liesi P, Hukkanen M & Polak J (1988) Neuropeptides in the synovium of patients with rheumatoid arthritis and osteoarthritis. *J Rheumatol* **15**: 1807–1810.

Hartung H-P & Toyka KV (1983) Activation of the macrophage by substance P: induction of oxidative burst and thromboxane release. *Eur J Pharmacol* **89**: 301–306.

Hartung H-P, Woiters K & Toyka KV (1986) Substance P binding properties and studies on cellular responses in guinea pig macrophages. *J Immunol* **136**: 3856–3861.

Helke CJ, Krause JE, Mantyh PW, Couture R & Bannon MJ (1990) Diversity in mammalian tachykinin peptidergic neurons: multiple peptides, receptors and regulatory mechanisms. *FASEB J* **4**: 1606–1615.

Hernanz A, DeMiguel E, Romera N, Perez-Alaya C, Gijon J & Arnalich F (1993) Calcitonin gene-related peptide, substance P and vasoactive intestinal peptide in plasma and synovial fluid from patients with inflammatory joint disease. *Br J Rheumatol* **32**: 31–35.

Hukkanen M, Mapp PI, Moscoso G, Konttinen YT, Blake DR & Polak JM (1991) Innervation and neuropeptide-containing nerves in the human foetal knee joint. *J Pathol* **163**(2): 181A.

Iwamoto I, Ukei IF, Borson DB & Nadel JA (1989) Neutral endopeptidase activity modulates tachykinin-induced increase in vascular permeability in guinea pig skin. *Int Arch Allergy Appl Immun* **88**: 288–293.

Katyama M, Nadel JA, Bunnet NW, DiMaria GU, Haxhiu M & Borson DB (1991) Catabolism of calcitonin gene-related peptide and substance P by neutral endopeptidase. *Peptides* **12**: 563–567.

Kimball ES, Persico FJ & Vaught JL (1985) Substance P, neurokinin A, and neurokinin B induce generation of IL1-like activity in P388D1 cells: possible relevance to arthritic diseases. *J Immunol* **141**: 3564–3569.

Kerr MA & Kenny AJ (1974) The purification and specificity of a neutral endopeptidase from rabbit kidney brush border. *Biochem J* **137**: 477–488.

Konttinen YT, Rees R, Hukkanen M, Gronblad M, Tolvanen E, Gibson SJ et al. (1990) Nerves in inflammatory synovium: immunohistochemical observations on the adjuvant arthritic rat model. *J Rheumatol* **17**: 1586–1591.

Lam FY & Ferrell WR (1989a) Inhibition of carrageenan induced inflammation in the rat knee joint by substance P antagonist. *Ann Rheum Dis* **48**: 928–932.

Lam FY & Ferrell WR (1989b) Capsaicin suppresses substance P-induced joint inflammation in the rat. *Neurosci Lett* **105**: 155–158.

Larsson J, Ekblom A, Henriksson K, Lundeberg T & Theodorsson E (1989) Immunoreactive tachykinins, calcitonin gene-related peptide and neuropeptide Y in human synovial fluid from inflamed knee joints. *Neurosci Lett* **100**: 326–330.

Larsson J, Ekblom A, Henriksson K, Lundeberg T & Theodorsson E (1991) Concentration of substance P, neurokinin A, calcitonin gene-related peptide, neuropeptide Y and vasoactive intestinal polypeptide in synovial fluid from knee joints in patients suffering from rheumatoid arthritis. *Scand J Rheumatol* **20**: 326–335.

Letarte M, Vera S, Tran R, Addis JBL, Onizuka RJ, Quackenbush E et al. (1988) Common acute lymphocytic leukaemia antigen is identical to neutral endopeptidase. *J Exp Med* **168**: 1247–1253.

Levine JD, Clark R, Devor M, Helms C, Moskowitz MA & Basbaum AI (1984) Intraneuronal substance P contributes to the severity of experimental arthritis. *Science* **226**: 547–549.

Loesch A & Burnstock G (1988) Ultrastructural localisation of serotonin and substance P in vascular endothelial cells of rat femoral and mesenteric arteries. *Anat Embryol* **178**: 137–142.

Look AT, Ashmun RA, Shapiro LH & Peiper SC (1989) Human myeloid plasma membrane glycoprotein CD13 (gp150) is identical to aminopeptidase N. *J Clin Invest* **83**: 1299–1307.

Lorkowski R, Zijderhand-Bleekemolen JE, Erdos EG, Von Figura K & Haslik A (1987) Neutral endopeptidase-24.11 (enkephalinase): synthesis and localisation in human fibroblasts. *Biochem J* **248**: 345–350.

Lotz M, Carson DA & Vaughan JH (1987) Substance P activation of rheumatoid synoviocytes: neural pathways in the pathogenesis of arthritis. *Science* **235**: 893–895.

Malfroy B, Giros B, Llorens-Cortes C & Schwartz J-C (1989) Metabolism of the enkephalins in the central nervous system. In Szekley JI & Rambadran K (eds) *Opioid Peptides*, Vol. 4, p 27. Orlando, FL: CRC Press.

Mapp PI, Kidd BL, Gibson SJ, Terry JM, Revell PA, Ibrahim NBN et al. (1990) Substance P-, calcitonin gene-related peptide- and C flanking peptide of neuropeptide Y-immunoreactive fibres are present in normal synovium but depleted in patients with rheumatoid arthritis. *Neuroscience* **37**: 143–153.

Mapp PI, Walsh DA, Kidd BL, Cruwys SC, Polak JM & Blake DR (1992) Localisation of the enzyme neutral endopeptidase to the human synovium. *J Rheumatol* **19**: 1838–1844.

Marshall KW, Chiu B & Inman RD (1990) Substance P and arthritis: analysis of plasma and synovial fluid levels. *Arthritis Rheum* **33**: 87–90.

Martin MFR, Surrall KE, McKenna F, Dixon JS, Bird HA & Wright VA (1984) Captopril a new treatment for rheumatoid arthritis. *Lancet* **1**: 1325–1328.

Mazarek N, Pecht I, Teichburg VI & Blumberg S (1981) The role of the N-terminal tetrapeptide in the histamine releasing action of substance P. *Neuropharmacology* **20**: 1025–1027.

Merighi A, Polak JM, Gibson SJ, Gulbenkian S, Valentino KL & Peirone SM (1987) Ultrastructural studies on calcitonin gene-related peptide-, tachykinins- and somatostatin-immunoreactive nerves in rat dorsal root ganglia: evidence for the colocalisation of different peptides in single secretory granules. *Cell Tiss Res* **254**: 101–109.

Mumford RA, Pierzchala PA, Strauss AW & Zimmermann M (1981) Purification of a membrane-bound metalloendopeptidase from porcine kidney that degrades peptide hormones. *Biochem Biophys Res Comm* **102**: 59–66.

Nadel JA & Borsin DB (1991) Modulation of neurogenic inflammation by neutral endopeptidase. *Am Rev Resp Dis* **143**: S33–S36.

Palacois JM & Dietl MM (1989) Regulatory peptide receptors: visualisation by autoradiography. In Polak JM (ed) *Regulatory Peptides*, 1st edn. Basle: Birkhauser Verlag.

Perianin A, Snyderman R & Malfoy B (1989) Substance P primes neutrophil activation: a mechanism for neurological regulation of inflammation. *Biochem Biophys Res Comm* **161**: 520–524.

Pereria da Silva A & Carmo-Fonseca M (1990) Peptide containing nerves in human synovium: immunohistochemical evidence for decreased innervation in rheumatoid arthritis. *J Rheumatol* **17**: 1592–1599.

Petitet F, Saffroy M, Torrens Y, Lavielle S, Chassaing G, Loeuillet D et al. (1992) Possible existence of a new tachykinin receptor subtype in the guinea pig ileum. *Peptides* **13**: 383–388.

Rees DD, Palmer RMJ & Moncada S (1989) A specific inhibitor of nitric oxide formation from L-argenine attenuates endothelium-dependant relaxation. *Br J Pharmacol* **96**: 418–424.

Regoli D & Nantel F (1991) Pharmacology of neurokinin receptors. *Biopolymers* **31**: 777–783.

Scott DT, Lam FY & Ferrell WR (1992) Acute inflammation enhances substance P-induced plasma protein extravasation in the rat knee joint. *Regulatory Peptides* **39**: 227–235.

Shipp MA, Vijayaraghavan J, Schmidt EV, Masteller EL, D'Adamio L, Hersch LB et al. (1988) Common acute lymphoblastic leukaemia antigen (CALLA) is active neutral endopeptidase 24.11 ('enkephalinase'): Direct evidence by cDNA transfection analysis. *Proc Natl Acad Sci* **86**: 297–301.

Skid RA, Engelbrecht A, Johnson AR & Erdos EG (1984) Hydrolysis of substance P and neurotensin by converting enzyme and neutral endopeptidase. *Peptides* **5**: 769–776.

Smith GD, Harmer AJ, McQueen DS & Seckl JR (1992) Increase in substance P and CGRP, but not somatostatin content of innervating dorsal root ganglia in adjuvant monoarthritis in the rat. *Neurosci Lett* **137**: 257–260.

Snider RM, Constantine JW, Lowe III JA, Longo KP, Lebel WS, Woody HA et al. (1991) A potent non-peptide antagonist of the substance P (NK1) receptor. *Science* **251**: 435–437.

Sreedharan SP, Goetzl EJ & Malfroy B (1990) Elevated tissue concentration of the acute common lymphoblastic leukaemia antigen (CALLA)-associated neutral endopeptidase (3.4.24.11) in human chronic arthritis. *Immunology* **71**: 142–144.

Stanitz AJ, Befus D & Bienenstock J (1986) Differential effects of vasoactive intestinal peptide, substance P, and somatostatin on immunoglobulin synthesis and proliferation of lymphocytes from Peyers patches, mesenteric lymph nodes and spleen. *J Immunol* **136**: 152–156.

Tregear GW, Niall HD, Potts JT, Leeman SE & Chang MM (1971) Synthesis of substance P. *Nature – New Biology* **232**: 87–89.

Turner AJ, Hooper NM & Kenny AJ (1987) Metabolism of neuropeptides. In Kenny AJ & Turner A (eds) *Mammalian Ectoenzymes*, pp 211–248. Oxford: Elsevier.

Ulmer AJ, Mattern T, Feller AC, Heyman E & Flad HD (1990) CD 26 antigen is a surface dipeptidyl peptidase IV (DPPIV) as characterized by monoclonal antibodies clone T11-19-4-7 and 4EL1C7. *Scand J Immunol* **31**: 429–435.

Walsh DA, Mapp PI, Wharton J, Rutherford RAD, Kidd BL, Revell PA et al. (1992) Localisation and characterisation of substance P binding to human synovial tissue in rheumatoid arthritis. *Ann Rheum Dis* **51**: 313–317.

Werb Z & Clark EJ (1989) Phorbol diesters regulate the expression of the membrane neutral metalloendopeptidase (EC 3.4.24.11) in rabbit synovial fibroblasts and mammary epithelial cells. *J Biol Chem* **264**: 9111–9113.

17 Proteinases and Connective Tissue Breakdown

T.E. Cawston

INTRODUCTION

The breakdown of cartilage and bone in the arthritides prevents the joints from functioning normally. In severe cases a large proportion of the cartilage that lines the articular surface as well as the underlying bone can be destroyed. Cartilage tissue is made up of small numbers of relatively isolated cells placed within an extensive extracellular matrix made up of collagens and proteoglycan (PG). The main collagen in cartilage is type II which forms the fibrillar network with the minor collagens IX and XI. Proteoglycans fill the spaces in this network; by interacting with hyaluronic acid and link proteins they draw water into the tissue to give a swelling pressure that allows cartilage to resist compression. The chondrocytes maintain this matrix and in normal adult cartilage a steady state exists where the turnover of these molecules is in equilibrium. This means that the rate of synthesis equals the rate of degradation. Any change in this steady state situation will rapidly affect the functional integrity of the cartilage. The structure and composition of articular cartilage is reviewed in detail in Chapter 9, this volume.

The primary cause of cartilage and bone destruction in the arthritides involves the elevated levels of active proteinases degrading the collagen and proteoglycan (Fig. 1). The sources of these proteinases will depend on the type of disease. In osteoarthritis (OA) there are often very few inflammatory cells during the initial stages of the disease and so the proteinases produced by chondrocytes are likely to play a major role. In contrast in a highly inflamed rheumatoid joint there are many cell types present and, although proteinases are produced by chondrocytes, other cells such as synovial cells and inflammatory cells produce proteinases and mediators which also play a part in the destruction that is found (Fig. 1). In this chapter the role of proteinases and their inhibitors found in the arthritic joint is reviewed and their participation in the destruction of collagen and proteoglycan from joint tissues is discussed.

CONNECTIVE TISSUE MATRIX

Collagen is the major protein of connective tissue and is the most common protein of the vertebrate body. There are 14 distinct forms of collagen and they all have a unique triple helical structure (Van der Rest and Garrone, 1991). Three coils of polypeptide are wound round each other to produce a long rod-shaped molecule $1.5 \times 300\,\text{nm}$ for types I, II and III collagen. Every third residue in the triple helical part of the molecule is the smallest amino acid glycine and a high proportion of proline and hydroxyproline is found along the polypeptide chain. On leaving the cell the collagen

Mechanisms and Models in Rheumatoid Arthritis
ISBN 0–12–340440–1

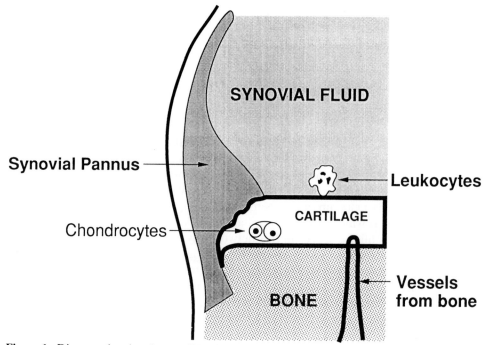

Figure 1. Diagram showing the possible cellular origin of the proteinases involved in joint destruction.

molecules align to produce the characteristic staggered arrangement and crosslinks form between molecules which further stabilize the structure. This aggregate of self-aligned collagen molecules forms the collagen fibres that give connective tissues their strength and rigidity (see Fig 2). Of the 14 collagens so far characterized some have interrupted helices, some form sheets rather than fibres and others have associated carbohydrate or glycosaminoglycan side-chains but all contain the repeating glycine residue and the resulting triple helical structure.

The other major proteins found in connective tissue, particularly as far as cartilage is concerned are the PGs. These large molecules consist of a polypeptide chain containing three globular domains (G1–G3) interspersed by extended linear regions of heavily glycosylated and sulphated polypeptide (Fig. 3) (Hardingham and Fosang, 1992). The first globular domain (G1) is known to associate with hyaluronic acid and link protein and this property enables PG molecules to form highly charged aggregates that are responsible for pulling water into the tissue, creating a swelling pressure thus allowing cartilage to resist compression. Other components of connective tissue are found in bone and cartilage and the possible association of some of these components is shown in Fig. 4.

PROTEOLYTIC PATHWAYS OF CONNECTIVE TISSUE BREAKDOWN

The proteins of the extracellular matrix in connective tissues can be broken down by different proteolytic pathways. Four main classes of proteinase exist and these are

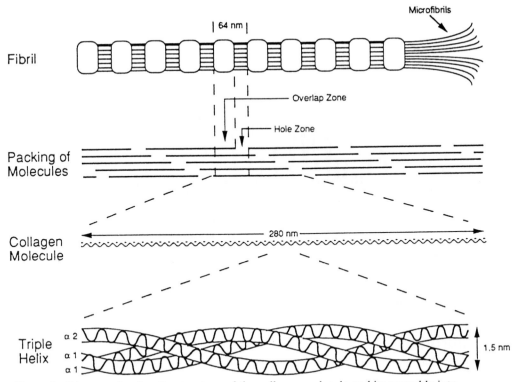

Figure 2. Diagram showing the structure of the collagen molecule and its assembly into collagen fibrils.

classified according to the amino acid or chemical group at the active centre of the enzyme. This chemical group cleaves the peptide bond within the target protein. Specific inhibitors are used to determine which proteinase class an enzyme belongs to: cysteine proteinases are inhibited by iodoacetamide, N-ethyl-maleimide or E64; aspartic proteinases by pepstatin; metalloproteinases by chelating agents such as 1,10-phenanthroline and serine proteinases by diisopropylflourophosphate. All these enzymes are listed in Table 1 and the relevant connective tissue protein cleaved shown for each enzyme. The cysteine and aspartate proteinases cleave protein at acid pH and are thought to be responsible for intracellular proteolytic activity whilst the serine and metalloproteinases act at neutral pH and are thought to be responsible for extracellular digestion. In addition some of these enzymes are stored within neutrophils and can be instantly released in certain situations. Some enzymes may not participate in the cleavage of matrix proteins but are able to activate proenzymes that can then degrade the matrix. An example of this is the ability of mast cell tryptase to activate prostromelysin which, once activated, can activate procollagenase and so lead to collagen loss (Gruber et al., 1989; reviewed by Woolley in Chapter 6, this volume).

Very few serine proteinases are found in cartilage although many have been characterized from mammalian tissues. Those involved in cartilage destruction are thought to enter from outside and elastase and cathepsin G from polymorphonuclear leukocytes have potent PG-degrading activity as well as acting on the telopeptide regions of collagen II.

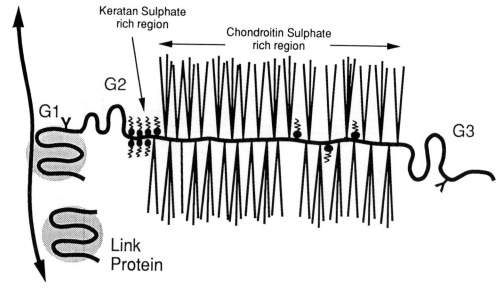

Figure 3. Diagram showing the structure of the major proteoglycan found in cartilage aggrecan.

There is no doubt that all these different pathways play a part in the turnover of the connective tissues and it is likely that the pathway that predominates varies with the different resorptive situations. In some instances one pathway may precede another as in the removal of the osteoid layer by metalloproteinases secreted by the osteoblast prior to the attachment of osteoclasts. These cells adhere to the exposed bone surface and create a tiny pocket under their ruffled border of low pH where the cysteine proteinases are secreted and remove the calcified bone matrix (Vaes *et al.*, 1992; also see Chapter 10, this volume). In septic arthritis there is a massive influx of neutrophils into the joint space. These cells release their granular contents which contain elastase, cathepsin G, neutrophil collagenase and gelatinase. These enzymes far exceed the local concentration of inhibitors and a rapid stripping of the cartilage matrix then occurs (Cawston *et al.*, 1989).

EXTRACELLULAR PROTEOLYSIS

Matrix Metalloproteinases

In the 1950s collagen was regarded as a protein that was totally resistant to proteolytic attack by enzymes from within the body as only bacterial enzymes were known to be able to break down this protein. In 1962, Gross and Lapierre discovered an enzyme that could specifically cleave the collagen in the resorbing tadpole tail. They named this enzyme collagenase and showed that it cleaved collagen at one point through all

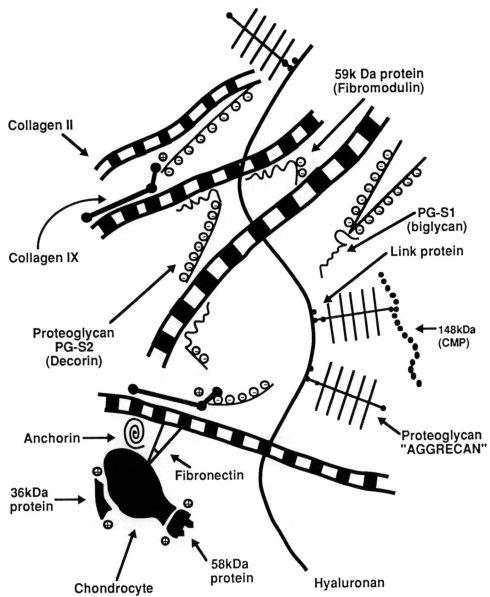

Figure 4. Diagram showing the possible associations between the major and minor proteins found in cartilage.

three alpha chains three quarters of the way from the N-terminal end of the protein. Since this discovery a whole family of enzymes has been discovered that can destroy all the proteins of the extracellular matrix. These enzymes, called the matrix metalloproteinases (MMPs), are made up of common sequences of amino acids as shown in Fig. 5 and fall into three main groups which differ in size: the stromelysins, collagenases and gelatinases (Woessner, 1991). The catalytic mechanism depends on zinc at the active centre and each enzyme is secreted with a propeptide attached which has to

Table 1. Proteinases that degrade connective tissue matrix

Proteinase	Class	Inhibitors	pH range	Core protein	Insoluble helical collagen	Solubilized helical collagen
Cathepsin B	Cys	Cystatins, α_2M		Yes	Yes	Yes
Cathepsin L	Cys	Cystatins, α_2M	3–5.5	Yes	Yes	Yes
Cathepsin H	Cys	Cystatins, α_2M		?	Yes	Yes
Cathepsin D	Asp	α_2M	4–6	Yes	No	No
Plasmin	Ser	α_2M, α_1AC, α_1PI		Yes	No	No
Elastase	Ser	α_2M, α_1AC, α_1PI	6–9	Yes	No	No
Cathepsin G	Ser	α_2M, α_1PI		Yes	No	No
Stromelysin	Metallo	TIMP, TIMP-2, α_2M	4.5–9	Yes	No	No
Collagenase	Metallo	TIMP, TIMP-2, α_2M	7–8	No	Limited	Yes
Gelatinase	Metallo	TIMP, TIMP-2, α_2M	7–8	?	No	No

α_2M, α_2 macroglobulin; α_1PI, α_1 antiproteinase inhibitor; α_1AC, α_1 antichymotrypsin.

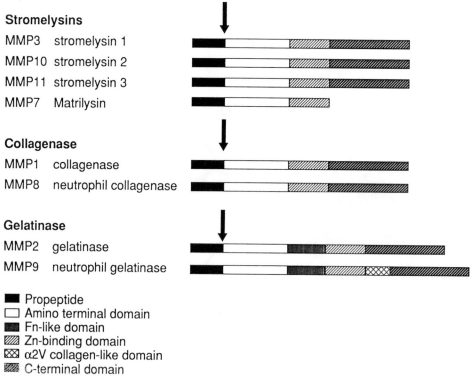

Stromelysins

MMP3   stromelysin 1

MMP10   stromelysin 2

MMP11   stromelysin 3

MMP7   Matrilysin

Collagenase

MMP1   collagenase

MMP8   neutrophil collagenase

Gelatinase

MMP2   gelatinase

MMP9   neutrophil gelatinase

■ Propeptide
☐ Amino terminal domain
▨ Fn-like domain
▨ Zn-binding domain
⊠ α2V collagen-like domain
▨ C-terminal domain

Figure 5. Diagram showing the structure of different members of the MMP family.

be removed proteolytically before the enzyme becomes active and degrades the matrix. This activation possibly involves plasminogen activators acting on plasminogen to generate plasmin which can then activate other metalloproteinases, or may involve membrane-bound proteinases. Two of the metalloproteinases (MMP8 and

MMP9) are found stored within the specific granules of the neutrophil, whilst the others are produced by a variety of cells after stimulation by a number of cytokines (see below).

The first class of MMPs are the stromelysins, so named because of their broad substrate specificity. Two highly homologous enzymes stromelysin 1 (MMP3) and stomelysin-2 (MMP10) and a third, smaller enzyme, now named matrilysin (MMP7) have been described. The natural substrates of these enzymes are probably proteoglycans, fibronectin and laminin. Type IV collagen is cleaved in the globular, but not the helical, domain and there are conflicting data regarding the ability of matrilysin to cleave native type IV collagen. It appears that matrilysin, but not the stromelysins, can cleave elastin efficiently although all these enzymes appear to have some activity against this substrate (Matrisian, 1992). Stromelysin-1 is not normally widely expressed but can be readily induced by growth factors, cytokines such as IL-1 and tumour promotors in cultured mesenchymal cells such as chondrocytes and connective tissue fibroblasts. The expression pattern of these enzymes is often distinct. Stromelysins are expressed in mature macrophages (Welgus *et al.*, 1990) whilst matrilysin is found at the promonocyte stage (Busiek *et al.*, 1992). The differential expression of the different members of this class of MMP may help to explain why there are different enzymes with very similar substrate specificity.

There are two distinct collagenases; interstitial collagenase (MMP1) and neutrophil collagenase (MMP8). Both enzymes cleave fibrillar collagens and have the unique ability to cleave all three α chains of types I, II and III collagens at a single site between residues 775 and 776 producing fragments approximately 3/4 and 1/4 the size of the original molecule (Miller *et al.*, 1976). The two enzymes differ slightly in their specificity for the different fibrillar collagens; neutrophil collagenase has a preference for type I collagen, while the interstitial collagenase preferentially digests type III collagen. Interstitial collagenase is synthesized by connective tissue fibroblasts and macrophages when these cells are stimulated with inflammatory mediators (Welgus *et al.*, 1985; Birkedal-Hansen *et al.*, 1993) and then promptly secreted. Neutrophil collagenase is only synthesized by cells of the neutrophil lineage; it is stored after secretion in the specific granules which are released upon stimulation of the cell (Lazarus *et al.*, 1968). These enzymes can hydrolyse other peptide bonds in other proteins, including proteoglycan, to an extent but the ability to cleave collagen in this specific way is limited to these two enzymes. Once this initial cleavage takes place then the two fragments of collagen are no longer stable at body temperature, the triple helical structure is lost and the polypeptide chains can be further degraded by other proteinases such as the gelatinases.

The third class of MMP, the gelatinases are often thought of as having substrate specificity for denatured collagens as described above and for type IV basement membrane collagen. Type V collagen and elastin are also reported to be degraded by these enzymes. Expression of the 72-kDa gelatinase (MMP2) is the most widespread of all the MMPs and is frequently elevated in malignant tumours as well as being produced by chondrocytes, endothelial cells, keratinocytes, skin fibroblasts, monocytes and osteoblasts (Birkedal-Hansen, 1993). MMP9 (92-kDa) gelatinase is expressed in transformed and tumour-derived cells, neutrophils, corneal epithelial cells, monocytes and alveolar macrophages and keratinocytes (Opdenakker *et al.*, 1991; Matrisian, 1992).

Recently a new member of the MMP family, a metalloelastase, has been identified and cloned (Shapiro *et al.*, 1992). This enzyme may represent a fourth elastin-degrading class of MMP although the stromelysins are also able to degrade elastin. This enzyme also degrades casein, α_1-antiproteinase inhibitor and fibronectin and is found as a 21-kDa protein in macrophages after processing at both the N- and C-terminus from a 53-kDa precursor form.

Another MMP has been found expressed in stromal tissue surrounding breast adenocarcinoma (Basset *et al.*, 1990; Wolf *et al.*, 1993). The cDNA clone was named stromelysin-3 although the protein had not been expressed and consequently its substrate specificity is not yet known. The main substrates of the enzymes are summarized in Table 2.

Table 2. Connective tissue proteins degraded by different MMPs

Enzyme	Matrix substrate
Interstitial collagenase MMP1	Collagen types I, II, III, VII, X Gelatin
Neutrol collagenase MMP8	Collagen types I, II, III
72-kDa gelatinase MMP2	Gelatin types I, II, III elastin Collagen types IV, V, VII, X, fibronectin
92-kDa gelatinase MMP9	Gelatins I, V Collagen types IV, V
Stromelysin-1 MMP3	Proteoglycan, fibronectin, laminin Gelatin types, I, III, IV, V Collagen types III, IV, V, IX Procollagen propeptides, activates procollagenase
Stromelysin-2 MMP10	Gelatin types I, III, IV, V Weak on collagen types III, IV, V Fibronectin, activates procollagenase
Matrilysin MMP7	Gelatin types I, III, IV, V Activates procollagenase, proteoglycan, fibronectin

The involvement of these proteinases in the normal turnover of connective tissue matrix that takes place during growth and development is well established (Case *et al.*, 1989b). A large number of studies indicate that they are also involved in the pathological destruction of joint tissue. Several studies have shown increased collagenase (Harris *et al.*, 1975; Cawston *et al*, 1984; Clark *et al.*, 1992a, 1993) and stromelysin in rheumatoid synovial fluid and in culture media from rheumatoid synovial tissues and cells (Woolley *et al.*, 1978 and Chapter 6, this volume; MacNaul *et al.*, 1990). A number of studies have localized both collagenase and stromelysin at the cartilage–pannus junction and in synovial tissue from rheumatoid joints (Woolley *et al.*, 1977 and Chapter 6, this volume; Okada *et al.*, 1989, 1990; McCachren *et al.*, 1990; Gravellese *et al.*, 1991; McCachren, 1991) and in animal models of arthritis (Case *et al.*, 1989; Hembry *et al.*, 1993). Recent studies have shown by *in situ* hybridization that both mRNA for collagenase and stromelysin can be found in raised amounts within the rheumatoid joint (Brinkerhoff, 1991). In a comparative study Case *et al.* (1989a) found higher levels of stromelysin mRNA and protein in human rheumatoid synovium than in osteoarthritic synovium. Stromelysin was identified in lining cells, in the underlying stromal tissues and in chondrocytes and osteoclasts of rat joints with a model arthritis. Transforming growth factor β (TGFβ) interfered with the development of the disease in these rats presumably by down-regulation of enzyme activity or up-regulation of tissue inhibitors of metalloproteinases (TIMP) (Brandes *et al.*, 1991; Wright *et al.*, 1991a). Dean *et al.*, 1989 were able to extract raised amounts of the MMPs from osteoarthritic cartilage.

Control of the MMPs

Because these enzymes are so potent they are carefully controlled. The synthesis and secretion of the collagenase and stromelysins is stimulated by proinflammatory cytokines such as interleukin-1 (IL-1) and tumour necrosis factor (TNF). However once activated the enzymes can be blocked if sufficient available TIMP is present. TIMP blocks the activity of all the active forms of the enzymes by binding very tightly to form a 1:1 complex (Cawston *et al.*, 1983). Therefore if TIMP levels exceed those of active enzyme then connective tissue turnover is prevented. The main mechanisms that control extracellular proteinase activity are illustrated in Fig. 6. All these events are likely to occur very close to the cell membrane in a tightly controlled environment.

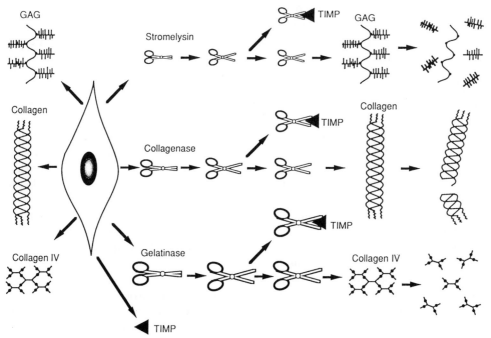

Figure 6. Diagram showing the different mechanisms to control the extracellular activity of the matrix metalloproteinases.

Control of the MMPs – synthesis and secretion

Within arthritic tissues there are areas of cartilage where synthesis of new matrix is occurring and areas where net loss of the extracellular matrix occurs. The chondrocytes are intimately involved in both of these processes and, in addition to the mediators mentioned above, a range of cytokines and growth factors can affect both cartilage matrix synthesis and resorption.

The response of chondrocytes to the polypeptide growth factors has only recently been recognized (see Table 3) and it is apparent that these factors play a major role in

Table 3. The effect of different cytokines and growth factors on chondrocytes

Growth factor	Major function in cartilage
TGFβ	Chondrocyte proliferation, promotes formation of matrix, modulates IL-1 effects, promotes synthesis of proteinase inhibitors
PDGF	Proliferation of chondrocytes
bFGF	Proliferation and differentiation of chondrocytes, proteinase production
IGF-1	Proliferation of chondrocytes, GAG synthesis
IL-1	Induction of proteinases, PGE_2 and other cytokines, inhibition of GAG synthesis
TNFα	Similar catabolic effects as IL-1
IL-6	Proteinase inhibitor production, proliferation of chondrocytes

the regulation of the synthesis of normal matrix and also in the processes that are involved in the destruction of cartilage in disease. It is not yet clear exactly how these agents act on cartilage but many involve the presence of cell surface receptors coupled to intracellular signalling pathways.

The early work of Fell and coworkers (Fell and Jubb, 1977; Dingle *et al.*, 1979) established that a soluble factor produced by porcine synovium could stimulate chondrocytes to degrade their own matrix. At the same time a soluble mediator produced by mononuclear cells was also identified (Dayer *et al.*, 1977) which stimulated collagenase release from rheumatoid synovial fibroblasts. These factors were identified as IL-1. IL-1 and TNF can induce secretion of each other and these cytokines have very similar properties and are produced by the same cell types. They both affect numerous cells to produce proinflammatory and degradative effects. When added to cartilage, IL-1 and TNF both stimulate the degradation of the matrix and the release of proteoglycan fragments within 12–24 h. At the same time the synthesis of matrix components is also down-regulated (Krane *et al.*, 1990). IL-1 is 100–1000 times more potent than TNF although these agents act synergistically if added together. The release of collagen fragments from cartilage in response to these agents occurs much later and does not appear to be as reproducible as the release of PG fragments especially in adult human cartilage. Irreversible damage to cartilage structure does not occur until the collagen framework has been removed. It is not known how PG and collagen turnover is increased after treatment with IL-1 and TNF, but these cytokines are known to stimulate the synthesis and secretion of stromelysin and collagenase.

Various growth factors can affect cartilage turnover (see Table 3), insulin-like growth factor (IGF-1) was found to stimulate DNA and matrix synthesis in growth plate and both immature and adult articular cartilage (McQuillan *et al.*, 1986), particularly the synthesis of aggrecan. TGFβ potentiates the stimulation of DNA synthesis achieved with other growth factors rather than initiating this itself and is locally synthesized by chondrocytes and stimulates PG synthesis (Hiraki *et al.*, 1988). It is also known to stimulate the production and release of TIMP by connective tissue cells (Edwards *et al.*, 1987; Wright *et al.*, 1991b) and other proteinase inhibitors suggesting that it may prevent cartilage destruction by both stimulating synthesis and blocking breakdown pathways through the increased production of inhibitory proteins (Sporn *et al.*, 1987). When TGFβ is added to cartilage in addition to IL-1 it blocks the release of PG fragments in a dose-dependent fashion. This could be accomplished by reversing the effect that IL-1 has on PG synthesis, or it could stimulate the production of TIMP by chondrocytes thus preventing cartilage degradation (Fig. 7).

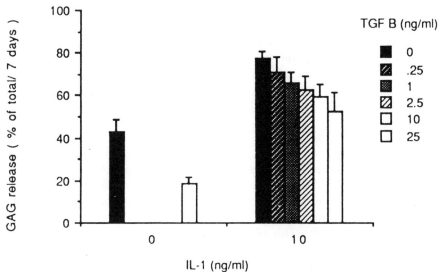

Figure 7. Inhibition of IL-1 stimulated cartilage degradation by TGFβ.

Platelet-derived growth factor (PDGF) has a mitogenic effect on chondrocytes (Howes *et al.*, 1988) and can stimulate collagenase production in some connective tissue fibroblasts (Chua *et al.*, 1986) but regulation of collagenase synthesis in chondrocytes has not been reported (Andrews, 1989a, 1990a). Fibroblast growth factor (bFGF), previously described as cartilage growth factor, stimulates DNA synthesis in adult articular chondrocytes in culture (Osbourne *et al.*, 1989) and plasminogen activators, collagenase and stromelysin as well as plasminogen activator inhibitors and TIMP in fibroblasts and endothelial cells (Edwards *et al.*, 1987; Matrisian and Hogan, 1990). In rabbit chondrocyte cultures bFGF synergizes with IL-1 to enhance the synthesis of collagenase, stromelysin and gelatinase (Phadke, 1987).

The role of interferon-gamma (IFNγ) in the destruction of cartilage in joint diseases is not clear. Although it appears to have differing effects, little attention has been paid to its modulation of the proteinases produced by chondrocytes and synovial cells. IFNγ inhibits cytokine-stimulated bone resorption (Gowen *et al.*, 1986; see Chapter

10, this volume) and inhibits IL-1- or TNF-stimulated collagenase production by chondrocytes as well as reducing IL-1-stimulated PG release from cartilage (Andrews *et al.*, 1989, 1990).

It is likely that these factors are involved in stimulating repair within cartilage. All these growth factors are unlikely to act on their own and many are known to act synergistically in promoting matrix synthesis. Some growth factors, such as TGFB and IGF, can be synthesized within the cartilage by the chondrocytes and these two growth factors are known to antagonize the effects of the proinflammatory cytokines IL-1 and TNF (Tyler, 1989). Further information on the role of growth factors in rheumatoid joint pathology is given in Chapter 12, this volume.

Within the arthritic joint there are large numbers of different cell types (Fig. 1). Specific cytokines and growth factors differ in their action on individual cell types. Agents may suppress the release of one enzyme whilst promoting that of another. For example, 72-kDa gelatinase is down-regulated by TGFβ in fibroblasts (Kerr *et al.*, 1988) but stimulated in keratinocytes (Salo *et al.*, 1991). However, the same cytokine can have different effects on separate cell types. For example IL-1 induces the expression of collagenase and stromelysin in human fibroblasts but not in keratinocytes (Peterson *et al.*, 1987; MacNaul *et al.*, 1990). Effects are seen with some connective tissue fibroblasts and reverse effects seen in others (Andrews *et al.*, 1990). These differences make it sometimes difficult to predict the outcome of blocking the action of individual cytokines to prevent cartilage destruction.

Control of the MMPs – activation of the proenzymes

All the metalloproteinases are produced in a proenzyme form that requires activation before the enzyme is able to degrade its respective substrate. Activation is achieved proteolytically and a 10 000-Da sequence of polypeptide chain is removed in several pieces from the amino terminal of the protein. This process removes a cysteine residue, present in the propeptide sequence, that previously blocked the active site zinc atom (Andrews, 1990b). This allows the enzyme to hydrolyse susceptible peptide bonds in the protein substrates. *In-vitro* activation can be achieved with chemicals that perturb this cysteine–zinc interaction but *in vivo* it is likely that the process involves just proteolysis. It is of interest that stromelysin, once activated, can activate procollagenase suggesting that *in vivo* a carefully controlled cascade activation mechanism occurs that involves different members of the metalloproteinase family (He *et al.*, 1989). Activation of these enzymes is an important control point in connective tissue breakdown. Plasmin can also activate some members of the MMPs and so plasminogen activators are thought to be important (see later section). Many factors, such as IL-1, promote the synthesis and secretion of procollagenase but in many situations little activation of the proenzyme occurs. Measurement of the levels of enzymes whether *in vivo* or *in vitro* needs to distinguish between the levels of total collagenase and that of active collagenase as it is only the active form of the enzyme that can degrade connective tissue. However tissues that have large amounts of proenzyme present obviously have the potential to resorb matrix rapidly.

Control of the MMPs – inhibition of the active enzymes

All the active enzymes are inhibited by TIMPs (Cawston *et al.*, 1981) and all connective tissues contain members of the TIMP family (Cawston, 1986). TIMP is a glycoprotein of Mr 28 000 containing 184 amino acids held together by six disulphide bonds to form two main domains (Fig. 8) (Docherty *et al.*, 1985). The mechanism of inhibition is not yet known but TIMP is very similar to a second inhibitor TIMP-2 which contains 194 amino acids (Stetler-Stevenson *et al.*, 1989; DeClerk *et al.*, 1989). Both proteins are very stable and bind very tightly to the active forms of the MMPs in a 1 : 1 ratio (Cawston *et al.*, 1983). More recent work has shown that the inhibitory portion of the molecule resides in the N-terminal domain (Murphy *et al.*, 1991) and several specific sequences of amino acids are thought to be important in the inhibitory mechanism (O'Shea *et al.*, 1992) as these are conserved between the structures of TIMP and TIMP-2 (Woessner, 1991). A third member of the family has recently been described which has been named TIMP-3. This 21 000-kDa protein is produced by transformed chick fibroblasts and appears to have some similar properties to the other two TIMPs. It appears to be secreted into the connective tissue matrix; it is highly charged and is difficult to study as it is relatively insoluble (Yang and Hawkes, 1992).

TIMPs play an important role in controlling connective tissue breakdown by blocking the action of the activated proenzymes and preventing activation of the proenzymes.

Endogenous Serine Proteinases

There are low levels of endogenous serine proteinases in cartilage compared to the levels of metalloproteinases. It is difficult to decide how much serine proteinase activity found in cartilage originates from outside the tissue as much of the serine proteinase activity found in cartilage is likely to be derived from polymorphonuclear leukocytes. The serine proteinases detected in cartilage include a fibrinolytic enzyme independent of plasminogen (Walton *et al.*, 1981), serine proteinases capable of degrading PG (Martel-Pelletier *et al.*, 1984) and a serine proteinase that breaks down PG and gelatin (Martel-Pelletier *et al.*, 1985). These few activities that have been detected have not always been purified and characterized or been shown to be derived from chondrocytes. Cartilage also contains plasminogen activators and plasmin activity (see below). Some of the other serine proteinases might also activate metalloproteinases although no correlation was observed between the levels of serine proteinase and active MMPs in OA cartilage (Martel-Pelletier *et al.*, 1984). When rabbit cartilage was cultured with IL-1 no reduction of matrix degradation was observed when aprotonin, a serine proteinase inhibitor, was present indicating that serine proteinases were probably not involved in the activation of proMMPs assuming that the aprotonin was able to penetrate the cartilage matrix (Ghosh *et al.*, 1987).

Plasminogen-dependent Pathways

The plasminogen-dependent pathway is implicated in a wide variety of situations where connective tissue matrix is remodelled (Saksela and Rifkin, 1988). Plasminogen is cleaved by specific activating enzymes called plasminogen activators to produce plasmin which is a serine proteinase that can rapidly cleave a broad spectrum of substrates. The concentration of plasminogen in serum, lymph and interstitial fluids is approximately 100–200 µg/ml. Plasminogen-dependent proteolysis is thus initiated by secretion of one or both plasminogen activators at local tissue sites by a wide variety of

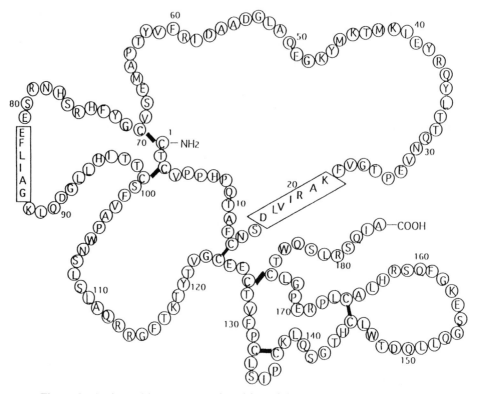

Figure 8. Amino acid sequence and position of the disulphide bonds in TIMP.

cells. The activity of plasminogen and the activating enzymes is maximized by binding to fibrin or the cell surface and so this localizes the degradation that occurs whilst at the same time possibly protecting the proteinases from inhibitors such as α_2-macroglobulin, α_1-antiproteinase inhibitor and α_1-antiplasmin and also specific inhibitors of the plasminogen activators.

It is not known how the matrix metalloproteinases become activated in cartilage breakdown. Many workers have postulated (Werb *et al.*, 1977) that the plasminogen activator plasmin cascade might be involved since it was established that plasmin could activate procollagenase (Vaes and Eeckhout, 1975). As these components are widely distributed in tissues and are found in the extracellular matrix they could well function in this way. Two types of plasminogen activator are recognized: tissue plasminogen activator (tPA) and urokinase (uPA). Both enzymes cleave plasminogen to the active plasmin and the system is regulated by a number of inhibitors as well as by protease nexins that can bind to, and inactivate, the released enzymes (Hart and Fritzler, 1989).

Meats *et al.* (1985) were the first to show that human chondrocytes produced plasminogen activators when stimulated with retinoic acid and IL-1. They showed that often the enzyme was not released from the cell but remained attached to the cell surface, and IL-1 stimulated the production of tPA but not uPA (Bunning *et al.*, 1987). Later work suggested (Campbell *et al.*, 1990) that IL-1 and TNF could stimulate both tPA and uPA although uPA was not released but associated with the cell layer. Retinoic acid caused an increase in uPA (Hamilton et al., 1991) and a major role for this plasminogen activator in matrix degradation was proposed (Campbell et al., 1990). When rabbit cartilage explant cultures are stimulated with IL-1, 30% of the PG is released in the absence of plasminogen but 85% when plasminogen is added (Collier and Ghosh, 1988). A similar loss was found in the presence of activators of metalloproteinases. Experiments with cultured rabbit chondrocytes on collagen films showed that addition of plasminogen led to collagen degradation and this release of collagen could be prevented in the presence of TIMP (Gavrilovic and Murphy, 1989). All these experiments point to a role for the plasminogen–plasmin system in the activation of proMMPs in some situations of matrix turnover.

Neutrophil-dependent Pathways

In many joint diseases a large influx of polymorphonuclear leukocytes are found within the joint. These cells store large quantities of both serine and metalloproteinases. Some evidence is available that discharge of enzyme-containing granules close to, or whilst attached to, the cartilage surface leads to binding of elastase and damage to the cartilage (Sandy et al., 1981; Velvart et al., 1981; Velvart and Fehr, 1987). It is not possible for enzymes released into the synovial fluid to avoid the inhibitors present. Synovial fluid contains large amounts of the plasma proteinase inhibitor α_2-macroglobulin which can inhibit all the classes of proteinases (Barrett and Starkey, 1973). It also contains specific inhibitors such as α_1-antiproteinase inhibitor, TIMP and TIMP-2 (Cawston et al., 1984, 1993; Osthues et al., 1992). Once enzymes are complexed they are often rapidly cleared from the joint (Ekerot et al., 1985). In most synovial fluids an excess of inhibitory activity is found and so it is unlikely that neutrophil proteinases are able to cause damage to the matrix from the fluid phase. Schalwijk et al. (1987) were able to show that neutrophil elastase could cause damage to cartilage and escape inactivation by α_1-antiproteinase inhibitor when discharged at the cartilage surface. In septic arthritis the influx of neutrophils is so great that the normal inhibitory capacity of the synovial fluid is exceeded and these fluids contain active metalloproteinases, derived from the neutrophils, which are active in the fluid phase and can rapidly strip the cartilage from the surface of the joint. Treatment with antibiotics reduces cell numbers, the inhibitory proteins α_2-macroglobulin TIMP reappear and after 1–2 days no active proteinases are detectable (Cawston et al., 1989). Large amounts of TIMP–collagenase complex and α_2-macroglobulin–proteinase complexes are present in these fluids as well as α_1-proteinase inhibitor–elastase complexes (Cawston et al., 1990).

There is considerable evidence that suggests that the neutrophil serine proteinases have a limited role in matrix turnover within the joint. The levels of PG fragments released into rheumatoid synovial fluid do not correlate with markers of neutrophil granule release (Männson et al., 1990) although this could be due to complicated differences in the rate of clearance of these components. Beige mice lack leukocyte elastase and cathepsin G and antigen-induced arthritis in these mice produces severe cartilage loss although these enzymes are absent from the neutrophils in these animals (Schalkwijk et al., 1990; Pettipher et al., 1990). If rabbits are depleted of neutrophils by nitrogen mustard and then made arthritic, the extent of the loss of the matrix is identical to that found when neutrophils are present (Pettipher *et al.*, 1989). A single injection of IL-1 into joints produces rapid matrix loss with no neutrophil involvement (Dingle *et al.*, 1987). Whilst these enzymes are obviously capable of degrading cartilage matrix it is unlikely that they are involved in the turnover of cartilage deep within the matrix. However, where the pannus meets cartilage, where cells adhere to the cartilage surface, or where the inhibitory capacity of body fluids is exceeded, then these enzymes are likely to play a part in the degradation of connective tissues.

Osteoclastic Bone Resorption

In rheumatoid arthritis (RA), in addition to the destruction of cartilage, bone is also destroyed. The mechanisms involved in this process are not well understood. However, recent evidence would suggest that both the MMPs and the lysosomal thiol-proteinases are involved. Osteoblasts can respond to parathyroid hormone and other agents that induce bone resorption, such as IL-1, by increasing the secretion of collagense (Heath *et al.*, 1985; Delaisse *et al.*, 1988) and yet this enzyme has no activity within the low pH regime generated underneath the osteoclast.

Some workers have proposed that the osteoblasts produce collagenase to remove the layer of osteoid on the surface of the bone; the exposure of the mineralized matrix allows the osteoclast precursors to adhere and differentiate. Studies by Hill *et al.* (1993) have shown that both TIMP and TIMP-2 can prevent bone resorption in model systems where mouse bone samples have been induced to resorb with parathyroid hormone and 1,25 dihydroxy vitamin D_3.

Once the osteoid layer is removed then differentiated osteoclasts form a tightly sealed microenvironment beneath their lower surface into which they pump protons to lower the pH and remove mineral and lysosomal proteinases to resorb the exposed decalcified matrix. A single adherent osteoclast was reported to lower the pH in this microenvironment below the plasma membrane from pH 7.0 to pH 3.0 in 6 min (Silver *et al.*, 1988). This low pH is sufficient to remove the mineral and so expose the collagen framework. Cathepsin-B like enzymes extracted from chicken osteoblasts have been isolated (Blair *et al.*, 1986) and would be capable of destroying crosslinked collagen matrix. The studies of Etherington and Birkedal-Hanson (1987) showed that the collagen network of bone is susceptible to cleavage by cathepsins at low pH and in the presence of high concentrations of calcium. The cellular mechanisms resulting in bone loss in RA is reviewed by Skerry and Gowen in Chapter 10, this volume.

INTRACELLULAR PATHWAYS

Lysosomal Proteinases

The involvement of an intracellular route for the breakdown of cartilage was first suggested by the work of Lucy *et al.* (1974) on cultured chick embryo limb buds. Although these studies identified lysosomal enzymes, the individual enzymes responsible were not identified until much later. Cathepsin D, an aspartate proteinase, was shown to be raised in osteoarthritic tissue but this enzyme was unable to degrade PG at physiological pH (Sapolsky *et al.*, 1973). Cathepsin B is raised in osteoarthritic cartilage (Bayliss and Ali, 1978) and cathepsins B, L, and H (all cysteine proteinases) are found in cartilage in antigen-induced rat arthritis (Van Noorden *et al.*, 1988). It is clear that lysosomal proteinases are important in the degradation of cartilage explants incubated below pH 5. Cathepsin D is released from cells in cultured chick limb bone after stimulation with reinol (Poole *et al.*, 1974). The release of PG from human foetal epiphyseal cartilage is inhibited after the addition of antiserum specific for cathepsin D (Morrison *et al.*, 1973). Some workers have proposed that the pH might fall to pH 5.5 at the chondrocyte surface in normal cartilage (Dingle and Knight, 1985). However inhibitors of cathepsin D and cathepsin B have no effect on the release of PG fragments from explants cultured at neutral pH and antiserum to cathepsin D also fails to block this resorption (Hembry *et al.*, 1982). More recent work has suggested that cathepsin B may play a role in cartilage resorption. After incubation of cartilage induced to resorb with IL-1 with specific cathepsin B inhibitors, which are designed to cross cell membranes and so enter the cell, the release of PG fragments was prevented (Buttle *et al.*, 1992).

Lysosomal enzymes probably play a secondary role in connective tissue turnover where fragments of cleaved matrix are engulfed and digested intracellularly. Most of the evidence that indicates that an intracellular pathway exists comes from ultrastructural studies where fragments of material containing the characteristic banding pattern of collagen have been seen within the cell and in some cases associated with lysosomal enzymes (Melcher and Chan, 1981). Inhibition studies suggest that aspartate and cysteine proteinases are involved but not MMPs (Everts *et al.*, 1985, 1989). It is difficult to determine the precise sequence of events that occurs and it could be that the extracellular pathways involving the MMPs are required to fragment collagen partially before it can be internalized and digested within the lysosomal system. Phagocytic collagen degradation is often observed where a rapid turnover of collagen is required, such as the periodontal ligament (Melcher and Chan, 1981) and uterine involution (Parakkel, 1969). This process has also been observed in several different cultured cell lines (Svoboda, 1979).

MODEL SYSTEMS OF CARTILAGE BREAKDOWN

Investigations have shown that much useful information can be obtained using cartilage model systems. Initiaton of breakdown can be induced with either IL-1 or retinoic acid and the release of either proteoglycan fragments or collagen fragments followed in the presence or absence of inhibitors (Caputo *et al.*, 1987; Dodge and Poole, 1989; Marley *et al.*, 1991; Andrews *et al.*, 1992; Buttle *et al.*, 1992). It is likely that the enzyme pathways responsible for cartilage destruction involve the metalloproteinases as the release of PG and collagen from resorbing cartilage in experimental systems can be prevented with highly specific low molecular weight synthetic inhibitors. The effect of adding increasing amounts of such an inhibitor to pig articular cartilage fragments incubated with IL-1 for 3 days is shown in Fig. 9. The release of PG fragments was completely prevented at the highest concentration of inhibitor. It is expected that such inhibitors could be of therapeutic benefit in preventing the destruction of cartilage seen in the arthritides.

Much interest has been shown in the role of stromelysin in the degradation of PGs released into OA synovial fluid and from cartilage in organ culture systems. Stromelysin can readily degrade PGs and IL-1 stimulates its synthesis and secretion and

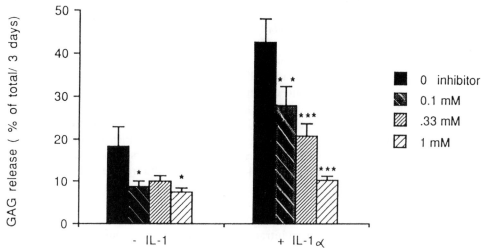

Figure 9. Inhibition of IL-1 stimulated cartilage degradation by low Mr synthetic collagenase inhibitor.

promotes cartilage resorption. In addition stromelysin is found in raised amounts of OA cartilage and it was assumed that stromelysin was responsible for the cleavage of proteoglycan. However, recent data suggest that a further enzyme may be involved. It is known that the cleavage of aggrecan in IL-1 stimulated and osteoarthritic cartilage occurs between the G1 and G2 domains. Although it is known that stromelysin cleaves in this region sequence analysis of PG fragments in synovial fluids (Sandy *et al.*, 1992) and in released fragments from organ culture experiments (Flannery *et al.*, 1992) reveal a different cleavage point from that expected if stromelysin was responsible for cleaving the polypeptide chain. This cleavage is thought to be made by an unidentified enzyme, prematurely named aggrecanase, as it has yet to be purified and characterized.

Inhibitors of cysteine proteinases that are targeted to cross cell membranes (and so enter cells) may also block cartilage resorption (Buttle *et al.*, 1992). Later studies (Buttle *et al.*, 1993) suggest that both metalloproteinase and cysteine proteinase inhibitors can both block the breakdown of proteoglycan release from cartilage but only the metalloproteinase inhibitors are able to block release of PG fragments after treatment of cartilage with retinoic acid. This implies that multiple pathways that depend on other classes of proteinases may be involved and that a mixture of extracellular and intracellular breakdown of cartilage components occurs. In addition, cartilage resorption induced by different agents may proceed by different pathways or include different activation mechanisms.

Much of this recent work has focused on PG breakdown in cartilage resorption to the exclusion of other matrix components. It is known that the turnover of PG is rapid and reversible compared to collagen and so is much more convenient to investigate. Injection of IL-1 into rabbit knee joints causes a rapid loss of PG, which is rapidly replaced by new synthesis (Dingle *et al.*, 1987; Thomas *et al.*, 1991). The gross loss of the collagen fibrillar network from cartilage is thought to be irreversible in the sense that any attempt at repair does not lead to restoration of normal cartilage. In future greater attention should be paid to preventing the loss of collagen from cartilage rather than studying the rapid PG loss which, although important to maintain the resistance to compression of the tissue, does not lead to irreversible damage. In our own recent studies of model cartilage systems using bovine nasal cartilage we have shown that both low molecular weight synthetic inhibitors of collagenase and TIMP-1 and TIMP-2 added to cartilage induced to resorb with IL-1 were able to prevent the release of collagen fragments from the cartilage (Ellis *et al.*, 1994). This is in contrast to the inability of TIMP to prevent the loss of PG fragments from cartilage (Andrews *et al.*, 1992).

Retinoic acid, retinol and lipopolysaccharide can also initiate the release of proteoglycan fragments from cartilage. Interestingly, retinoic acid is known to down-regulate the metalloproteinases and increase the production of TIMP, actions which would be expected to reduce cartilage breakdown (Wright *et al.*, 1991b) and this apparent contradiction in the actions of retinoic acid on cartilage has not, as yet, been adequately explained.

MEASUREMENT OF CARTILAGE BREAKDOWN *IN VIVO*

There is increasing interest in the use of biochemical markers to monitor the progress of joint destruction in individual patients. These have included the measurement of cytokines (involved in the stimulation of cartilage to resorb or synthesize new matrix), released fragments of matrix components, enzymes involved in cartilage destruction, or inhibitors that prevent breakdown. There are obvious difficulties in knowing which marker accurately reflects the processes and there are some conflicting data as to the usefulness of individual components (Poole, 1994). Additionally, although synovial fluid levels reflect the situation in an individual joint, it is difficult to use synovial fluid measurements routinely as joints are aspirated relatively infrequently. Some patients may present with a large effusion which may have been present for a number of months whilst others may have experienced an effusion for a very short period of time. Also the rate of removal of synovial fluid components will vary depending on the size and the degree of inflammation found within each individual joint and treatment with intra-articular steroid will interfere with the production of synovial fluid. Some investigators favour the measurement of marker concentrations whilst others would support the reporting of total amount of marker lost by multiplying the volume of synovial fluid by the marker concentration. There are, of course, profound difficulties in measuring accurately the volume of synovial fluid within a joint as pockets of fluid in some joints are inaccessible with a single aspiration and this leads to inaccuracies (Silverman *et al.*, 1990). These factors need to be taken into consideration when assessing results of synovial fluid studies.

Serum measurements overcome some of these difficulties and these samples are easily available. However, considerable dilution occurs of any individual marker and markers may arise from other sites within the body apart from joints and so an inaccurate assessment may be obtained. Measurement of proteinases and inhibitors in serum samples is difficult as levels are often very low and usually below the level of detection for the assay used (Lohmander, 1993a).

A number of workers have measured the levels of a variety of proteinases and inhibitors in synovial fluid with the view to determining the mechanism of destruction. Collagenase and TIMP are both present in rheumatoid synovial fluid but attempts to quantitate levels were initially difficult as the fluids had to be treated to separate proteinse from inhibitor (Cawston et al., 1984). Subsequently we, with others, have developed immunoassays to measure these enzymes and inhibitors in synovial fluids (Kodama et al., 1990; Cooksley et al., 1990; Clark et al., 1991, 1992a,b). In a study of rheumatoid and osteoarthritic synovial fluids we showed that the levels of both collagenase and TIMP were significantly higher in rheumatoid patients when compared to osteoarthritic patients (Clark et al., 1993). Similar results have also been reported by other workers in this field who have measured TIMP and stromelysin levels in synovial fluids (Lohmander et al., 1993).

However, these studies have investigated single samples from patients. More detailed information will become available when serial samples of individual patients have been completed. In a recent study, Lohmander et al. (1993) showed that the levels of stromelysin and TIMP remained raised for long periods of time after traumatic injuries in knee joints but the significance of these findings is not clear. We have found that a large variation in TIMP levels is found when serial samples of 18 patients with OA were investigated (Cawston et al., unpublished observations). Some patients had high initial levels of TIMP and these tended to remain high throughout the study. Correspondingly patients with low initial levels of TIMP maintained these low levels throughout the 6-month study.

Measurement of proteinases in synovial fluids using immunological methods can lead to results that are easily misinterpreted. In measuring collagenase the assays measure procollagenase as well as active collagenase and complexed enzyme. Whilst the levels of procollagenase may be high in any one sample this will bear no relationship to the amount of damage within the cartilage as the enzyme has never been activated. We have recently developed an ELISA that specifically measures collagenase–TIMP complexes (Clark et al., 1992b). If activation of collagenase occurs within the synovial fluid then collagenase will bind to α_2-macroglobulin, the large proteinase inhibitor found in plasma (Cawston and Mercer, 1986). Collagenase, even in the presence of equimolar TIMP will preferentially bind to α_2-macroglobulin. The measurement of collagenase–TIMP complexes in synovial fluid must mean that the activation of collagenase occurred in a location from which α_2-macroglobulin was excluded, that is, the cartilage matrix or synovium (Fig. 10). We believe that this marker, collagenase–TIMP complex, could be a specific marker for cartilage destruction. In an initial study we have shown that 3/80 osteoarthritic synovial fluids and 16/80 rheumatoid synovial fluids contained measurable complex (Clark et al., 1993). We are currently screening substantial numbers of synovial fluid samples from a variety of rheumatic diseases to determine if patients known to be rapidly destroying cartilage matrix have raised levels of this marker in their synovial fluids.

FUTURE PROSPECTS FOR THE THERAPEUTIC INHIBITON OF PROTEINASES

The future prospects for the prevention of connective tissue breakdown using low molecular weight synthetic proteinase inhibitors look promising at the present time.

Synovial Fluid

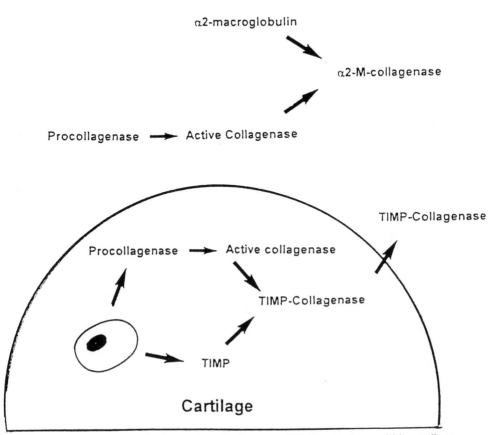

Figure 10 Diagram illustrating the formation of collagense–TIMP complexes within cartilage prior to release into the synovial fluid.

There are differing opinions as to the best enzyme to inhibit but progress to design compounds that target the MMPs are the most advanced to date. There is some discussion as to whether inhibition of stromelysin to prevent MMP activation and possibly some PG degradation is the best way to proceed. Some workers have proposed that as PG synthesis is so rapid and represents a normal response of cartilage then the enzyme to target is collagenase as irreversible cartilage damage appears to occur only after the collagen network is destroyed. Others have proposed that inhibition of these enzymes may lead to an excess deposition of matrix within connective tissues. It is likely that treatment with such agents will shift the balance away from degradation of matrix to prevent the loss of connective tissue matrix without leading to excess synthesis.

Highly specific collagenase inhibitors have been synthesized and patented by a number of different pharmaceutical companies (Henderson *et al.*, 1990; Gordon *et al.*, 1993). One difficulty that has had to be overcome is to ensure that these inhibitors remain biologically active after oral ingestion. As most of these inhibitors mimic the peptide sequence cleaved in substrates digested by collagenase they are often susceptible to peptidases within the gut where they are cleaved and inactivated. However, some inhibitors have been shown to be active in animal models (DiMartino *et al.*, 1991) and initial clinical trials will begin soon. It will be interesting to see if the blocking of one enzyme in the MMP family with some inhibition of the others is sufficient to halt the progressive and chronic destruction of connective tissue seen in the arthritides. If the release of connective tissue fragments drives joint inflammation leading to a greater destruction of connective tissue and so causing a chronic cycle of damage, then these compounds could be effective on their own. It may be necessary to combine proteinase inhibitors, either in sequence or with other agents that hit other specific steps in the pathogenesis, before the chronic cycle of joint destruction found in these diseases can be broken.

Future studies will concentrate on determining the structure of the MMPs (Lloyd *et al.*, 1989) both alone and in combination with the TIMPs in order to determine the precise mechanism of inhibition. This should lead to the synthesis of compounds that are specifically targeted to individual MMPs and that are sufficiently dissimilar from peptides to avoid digestion within the gut.

REFERENCES

Andrews HA, Bunning RAD, Dinarello CA & Russell RGG (1989) Modulation of human chondrocyte metabolism by recombinant human interferon gamma. *Biochim Biophys Acta* **1012**: 128–134.

Andrews HJ, Edwards TA, Cawston TE & Hazleman BL (1989) TGFβ causes partial inhibition of IL-1 stimulated cartilage degradation *in-vitro*. *Biochem Biophys Res Comm* **162**: 144–150.

Andrews HA, Bunning RAD, Plumpton TA, Clark IM, Russell RGG & Cawston TE (1990) Inhibition of IL-1 induced collagenase production in human articular chondrocytes *in vitro* by IFN-gamma. *Arthritis Rheum* **33**: 1733–1738.

Andrews HA, Cawston TE & Hazleman BL (1990) Modulation of plasminogen activator production by IL-1. *Biochim Biophys Acta* **1051**: 84–93.

Andrews HA, Plumpton TA, Harper GP & Cawston TE (1992) A synthetic peptide metalloproteinase inhibitor, but not TIMP, prevents the breakdown of PG within articular cartilage *in vitro*. *Agents Actions* **37**: 147–154.

Barrett AJ & Starkey PM (1973) The interaction of a2-macroglobulin with other proteinases. *Biochem J* **133**: 709–724.

Bassett P, Bellocq JP, Wolf C, Stoll I, Hutin P, Limacher JM et al. (1990) A novel metalloproteinase gene specifically expressed in stromal cells of breast carcinomas. *Nature* **348**: 699–704.

Bayliss MT & Ali SY (1978) Studies on cathepsin B in human articular cartilage. *Biochem J* **171**: 149–154.

Birkedal-Hansen H, Moore WGI, Bodden MK, Windsor LJ, Birkedal Hansen B, De Carlo A et al. (1993) Matrix metalloproteinases: a review. *Crit Rev Oral Biol Med* **4**: 197–250.

Blair HC, Kahn AJ, Crouch EC, Jeffrey JJ & Teitelbaum SL (1986) Isolated osteoclasts resorb the organic and inorganic components of bone. *J Cell Biol* **102**: 1164–1172.

Brandes ME, Allen JB, Ogawa Y & Wahl SM (1991) Transforming growth factor a1 supresses acute and chronic arthritis in experimental animals. *J Clin Invest* **87**: 1108–1113.

Brinkerhoff CE (1991) Joint destruction in arthritis: metalloproteinases in the spotlight. *Arthritis Rheum* **34**: 1073–1075.

Bunning RAD, Crawford A, Richardson HJ, Opedenakker G, Van Damme J & Russell RGG (1987) IL-1 preferentially stimulates the production of tissue type plasminogen activator by human articular chondrocytes. *Biochim Biophys Acta* **924**: 473–484.

Busiek DF, Ross FP, McDonnell S, Murphy G, Matrisian LM & Welgus HG (1992) The matrix metalloproteinase matrilysin (PUMP) is expressed in developing human mononuclear phagocytes. *J Biol Chem* **267**: 9087–9092.

Buttle DJ, Saklatvala J, Tamai M & Barrett AJ (1992) Inhibition of IL-1 stimulated cartilage proteoglycan degradation by a lipophilic inactivator of cysteine endopeptidases. *Biochem J* **281**: 175–177.

Buttle DJ, Handley CJ, Ilic MZ, Saklatvala J, Murata M & Barrett MJ (1993) Inhibiton of cartilage proteoglycan release by a specific activator of cathepsin B and an inhibitor of matrix metalloproteinase:

evidence for two converging pathways of chrondocyte-mediated proteoglycan degradation. *Arthritis Rheum* **36**: 1709–1717.

Campbell IK, Piccoli DS, Roberts MJ, Muirden KD & Hamilton JA (1990) Effects of tumour necrosis factor on resorption of human articular cartilage and production of plasminogen activators by human articular chondrocytes. *Arthritis Rheum* **33**: 542–552.

Caputo CB, Sygowski LA, Wolanin DJ, Patton SP, Caccese RG, Shaw A et al. (1987) Effect of synthetic metalloproteinase inhibitors on cartilage autolysis *in vitro*. *J Pharm Exper Therap* **240**: 460–465.

Case JP, Lafyatis R, Remmers EF, Kumkumian GK & Wilder RL (1989a) Stromelysin expression in rheumatoid synovium. *Am J Pathol* **135**: 1055–1064.

Case JP, Sano H, Lafyatis R, Remmers EF, Kukkumian GK & Wilder RL (1989b) Stromelysin expression in the synovium of rats with experimental erosive arthritis. *J Clin Invest* **84**: 1731–1740.

Cawston TE (1986) Protein inhibitors of metalloproteinases. In Barrett AJ & Salveson G (eds) *Proteinase Inhibitors*, pp 589–606. Amsterdam: Elsevier.

Cawston TE & Mercer E (1986) Preferential binding of collagenase to a2-macroglobulin in the presence of TIMP. *FEBS Letters* **209**: 9–12.

Cawston TE, Galloway WA, Mercer E, Murphy G & Reynolds JJ (1981) Purification of rabbit bone inhibitor of collagenase. *Biochem J* **195**: 159–165.

Cawston TE, Murphy G, Mercer E, Galloway WA, Hazleman BL & Reynolds JJ (1983) The interaction of purified rabbit bone collagenase with purified rabbit bone metalloproteinase inhibitor. *Biochem J* **211**: 313–318.

Cawston TE, Mercer E, De-Silver M & Hazleman BL (1984) Metalloproteinases and collagenase inhibitors in human rheumatoid synovial fluid. *Arthritis Rheum* **27**: 285–290.

Cawston TE, Weaver L, Coughlan RJ, Kyle MV & Hazleman BL (1989) Synovial fluids from infected joints contain active metalloproteinases and no inhibitory activity. *Br J Rhematol* **28**: 386–392.

Cawston TE, McLaughlan P, Coughlan R, Kyle MV & Hazleman BL (1990) Synovial fluids from infected joints contain metalloproteinase-TIMP complexes. *Biochim Biophys Acta* **1033**: 96–102.

Cawston TE, Bigg HF, Clark IM & Hazleman BL (1993) Identification of TIMP-2-progelatinase complex as the third metalloproteinase inhibitor peak in rheumatoid synovial fluid. *Ann Rheum Dis* **52**: 177–181.

Cawston TE & Hazleman BL (1994) The measurement of collagenase and TIMP in serial samples of osteoarthritic synovial fluid. In preparation.

Chua CC, Geiman DE, Keller GH & Ladda RL (1986) Induction of collagenase secretion in human fibroblast cultures by growth promoting factors. *J Biol Chem* **260**: 5213–5216.

Clark IM, Powell LK, Wright JK & Cawston TE (1991) Polyclonal and monoclonal antibodies against human TIMP and the design of an ELISA to measure TIMP. *Matrix* **11**: 76–85.

Clark IM, Powell LK, Wright JK, Cawston TE & Hazleman BL (1992) Monoclonal antibodies against human fibroblast collagenase and the design of an ELISA to measure total collagenase. *Matrix* **12**: 475–480.

Clark IM, Wright JK, Cawston TE & Hazleman BL (1992) Polyclonal antibodies against human fibroblast collagenase and the design of an ELISA to measure TIMP–collagenase complexes. *Matrix* **12**: 108–115.

Clark IM, Powell LK, Hazleman BL & Cawston TE (1993) The measurement of collagenase, TIMP and collagenase–TIMP comples in synovial fluids from patients with osteoarthritis and rheumatoid arthritis. *Arthritis Rheum* **36**: 372–379.

Collier S & Ghosh P (1988) The role of plasminogen in IL-1 mediated cartilage degradation. *J Rheumatol* **15**: 1129–1137.

Cooksley S, Hipkiss JB, Tickle SP, Holmes-Ievers E, Docherty AJP, Murphy G et al. (1990) Immunoassays to detect human collagenase, stromelysin, TIMP and enzyme inhibitor comlexes. *Matrix* **10**: 285–291.

Dayer J-M, Russell RGG & Krane SM (1977) Collagenase production by rheumatoid synovial cells: stimulation by a lymphocyte factor. *Science* **195**: 181–183.

Dean DD & Woessner JF (1984) Extracts of human articular cartilage contain an inhibitor of tissue metalloproteinases. *Biochem J* **218**: 277–280.

Dean DD, Martel-Pellitier J, Pelletier JP, Howell DS & Woessner JF (1989) Evidence for metalloproteinase and metalloproteinase inhibitor imbalance in human osteoarthritic cartilage. *J Clin Invest* **84**: 678–685.

DeClerk YA, Yean TD, Ratskin BJ, Lu HS & Lasngly KE (1989) Purification and charcterisation of two related but distinct metalloproteinase inhibitors secreted by bovine aortic endothelial cells. *J Biol Chem* **264**: 17445–17455.

Delaisse JM, Eeckhout Y & Vaes G (1988) Bone resorbing agents affect the production and distribution of procollagenase as well as the activity of collagenase in bone tissue. *Endocrinology* **123**: 264–276.

DiMartino MJ, Wolff CE, High W, Crimmin MJ & Galloway WA (1991) Antiinflammatory and chondroprotective activities of a potent metalloproteinase inhibitor. *J Cell Biochem* (**supplement E**): 179.

Dingle JT & Knight CG (1985) The role of the chondrocyte microenvironment in the degradation of the cartilage matrix. In Verbruggen G & Veys EM (eds) *Degenerative Joints, 2. Excerpta Med* **2**: 69–77.

Dingle JT, Saklatvala J, Hembry R, Tyler J, Fell HB & Jubb RW (1979) A cartilage catabolic factor from synovium. *Biochem J* **184**: 177–180.

Dingle JTD, Page-Thomas DP, King B & Bard DR (1987) *In vivo* studies of articular tissue damage mediated by catabolin/IL-1. *Ann Rheum Dis* **46**: 527–533.

Docherty AJP, Lyons A, Smith BJ, Wright EM, Stephens PE, Harris TJR et al. (1985) Sequence of human TIMP and its identity to erythroid potentiating activity. *Nature* **318**: 66–69.

Dodge GR & Poole AR (1989) Immunohistochemical detection and immunochemical analysis of type II collagen degradation in human normal, rheumatoid and osteoarthritic articular cartilages and in explants of bovine articular cartilage cultured with IL-1. *J Clin Invest* **83**: 647–661.

Edwards DR, Murphy G, Reynolds JJ, Whitham SE, Docherty AJP, Angel P et al. (1987) TGFB modulates the expression of collagenase and metalloproteinase inhibitor. *EMBO J* **6**: 1899–1904.

Ekerot L, Ohlsson K & Necking L (1985) Elimination of protease inhibitor complexes from the arthritic joint. *Int J Tiss React* **7**: 391–396.

Ellis AJ, Powell LK, Curry VA & Cawston TE (1994) TIMP and TIMP-2 prevent the release of collagen fragments in cartilage stimulated with IL-1. *Biochem Biophys Res Comm* **201**: 94–101.

Etherington DJ & Birkedal-Hansen H (1987) The influence of dissolved calcium salts on the degradation of hard tissue collagens by lysosomal cathepsins. *Coll Rel Res* **7**: 185–199.

Everts V, Beertsen W & Tigchelaar-Gutter W (1985) The digestion of phagocytosed collagen is inhibited by the proteinase inhibitors leupeptin and E-64. *Collagen Rel Res* **5**: 315–336.

Everts V, Hembry RM, Reynolds JJ & Beersten W (1989) Metalloproteinases are not involved in the phagocytosis of collagen fibrils by fibroblasts. *Matrix* **9**: 266–276.

Fell HB & Jubb RW (1977) The effect of synovial tissue on the breakdown of articular cartilage in organ culture. *Arthritis Rheum* **20**: 1359–1371.

Flannery CR, Lark MW & Sandy JD (1992) Identification of a stromelysin cleavage site within the interglobular domain of human aggrecan. *J Biol Chem* **267**: 1008–1014.

Gavrilovic J & Murphy G (1989) The role of plasminogen in cell-mediated collagen degradation. *Cell Biol Int Rep* **13**: 367–375.

Ghosh P, Collier S & Andrews J (1987) Synovial membrane–cartilage interactions: the role of serine proteinase inhibitors in IL-1 mediated degradation of articular damage. *J Rheumatol* **14**: 122–124.

Gordon JL, Drummond AH & Galloway WA (1993) Metalloproteinases as therapeutics. *Clin Exp Rheumatol* **11** (**supplement 8**): S91–S94.

Gowen M, Nedwin GE & Mundy GR (1986) Preferential inhibition of cytokine stimulated bone resorption by IFN-gamma. *J Bone Min Res* **1**: 469–474.

Gravelles EM, Darling JM, Ladd AL, Katz, JN & Glimcher LH (1991) *In situ* hybridization studies of stromelysin and collagenase mRNA expression in rheumatoid synovium. *Arthritis Rheum* **34**: 1076–1084.

Gross J & Lapierre CM (1962) Collagenolytic activity in amphibian tissues; a tissue culture assay. *Proc Natl Acad Sci USA* **54**: 1197–1204.

Gruber BL, Marchese MJ, Suzuki K, Schwartz LB, Okada Y, Nagase H et al. (1989) Synovial procollagenase activation by human mast cell tryptase dependence upon matrix metalloproteinase 3 activation. *J Clin Invest* **84**: 1657–1662.

Hamilton JA, Hart PH, Leizer T, Vitti GF & Campbell IK (1991) Regulation of plasminogen activator activity in arthritic joints. *J Rheumatol* **18** (**supplement 27**): 106–109.

Hardingham TE & Fosang AJ (1992) Proteoglycans: many forms and many functions. *FASEB* **6**: 861–870.

Harris ED, Faulkner CS & Brown FE (1975) Collagenolytic systems in rheumatoid arthritis. *Clin Orthop Rel Res* **110**: 303–316.

Hart DA & Fritzler MJ (1989) Regulaton of plasminogen activators and their inhibitors in rheumatic diseases. *J Rheumatol* **16**: 1184–1191.

He C, Wilhelm SM, Pentland AP, Marmer BL, Grant GA, Eisen AZ et al. (1989) Tissue cooperation in a proteolytic cascade activating human interstitial collagenase. *Proc Natl Acad Sci USA* **86**: 2632–2636.

Heath JK, Saklatvala J, Meikle MC, Atkinson SJ & Reynolds JJ (1985) Pig IL-1 is a potent stimulator of bone resorption *in vitro*. *Calcif Tiss Int* **37**: 95–97.

Hembry RM, Bagga MR, Murphy G, Henderson B & Reynolds JJ (1993) Rabbit models of arthritis; immunolocalization of collagenase and TIMP in synovium and cartilage. *Am J Pathol* **143**: 628–642.

Hembry RM, Knight CG, Dingle JT & Barrett AJ (1982) Evidence that extracellular cathepsin D is not responsible for the resorption of cartilage matrix in culture. *Biochim Biophys Acta* **714**: 307–312.

Henderson B, Docherty AJP & Beeley NRA (1990) Design of inhibitors of articular cartilage destruction. *Drugs of the Future* **15**: 495–507.

Hill PA, Reynolds JJ & Meikle MC (1993) Inhibition of stimulated bone resorption *in vitro* by TIMP-1 and TIMP-2. *Biochim Biophys Acta* **1177**: 71–74.

Hiraki Y, Inoue H, Hirai R, Kato Y & Suzuki F (1988) The effect of TGFB on cell proliferation and glycosaminoglycan synthesis by rabbit growth plate chondrocytes in culture. *Biochem Biophys Acta* **969**: 91–99.

Howes R, Bowness JM, Grotendorst GR, Martin GR & Reddi AH (1988) Platelet derived growth factor enhances demineralized bone matrix induced cartilage and bone formation. *Calcif Tiss Int* **42**: 34–38.

Kerr LD, Olashaw NE & Matrisian LM (1988) TGFB and cAMP inhibit transcription of EGF and oncogene induced transin RNA. *J Biol Chem* **263**: 16999–17005.

Kodama S, Iwata K, Iwata H, Yamashita K & Hayakawa T (1990) Rapid one-step sandwich enzyme immunoassay for TIMP. *J Imm Meth* **127**: 103–108.

Krane SM, Conca W, Stephenson ML, Amento EP & Goldring MP (1990) Mechanisms of matrix degradation in rheumatoid arthritis. *Ann NY Acad Sci* **580**: 340–354.

Lazarus GS, Brown RS, Daniels JR & Fullmer HM (1968) Human granulocyte collagenase. *Science* **159**: 1483–1485.

Lloyd LF, Skarzynski T, Wonacott AJ, Cawston TE, Clark IM, Mannix CJ et al. (1989) Crystallization and preliminary X-ray analysis of porcine synovial collagenase. *J Mol Biol* **210**: 237–238.

Lohmander LS, Hoerrner LA & Lark MW (1993) Metalloproteinases, tissue inhibitor and proteoglycan fragments in knee synovial fluid in human osteoarthritis. *Arthritis Rheum* **36**: 181–189.

Lohmander LS, Hoerrner LA, Dahlberg L, Roos H, Bjoonsson S & Lark MW (1993) Stromelysin TIMP and PG fragments in human knee joint fluid after injury. *J Rheumatol* **20**: 1362–1368.

Lucy JA, Dingle JT & Fell HB (1974) Studies on the mode of action of excess Vitamin A. A possible role of intracellular proteases in the degradation of cartilage matrix. *Biochem J* **79**: 500–508.

MacNaul KL, Chartrain N, Lark M, Tocci J & Hutchinson NI (1990) Discoordinate expression of stromelysin, collagenase and TIMP in human rheumatoid synovial fibroblasts: synergistic effects of IL-1 and TNF on stromelysin expression. *J Biol Chem* **265**: 17238–17245.

Mänsson B, Geborek P, Saxne T & Bjornsson S (1990) Cytidine deaminase activity in synovial fluids of patients with rheumatoid arthritis. *Ann Rheum Dis* **49**: 594–597.

Marley J, Bottomley KMK, Broadhurst J, Brown PA, Johnson WJ, Lawton G et al. (1991) Potent collagenase inhibitors prevent IL-1-induced cartilage degradation *in vitro*. *Int J Tiss React* **13**: 237–243.

Martel-Pelletier J, Pelletier JP, Cloutier JM, Howell DS, Ghandur-Mnaymneh L & Woessner JF (1984) Neutral proteinases capable of proteoglycan digesting activity in osteoarthritic and normal human articular cartilage. *Arthritis Rheum* **27**: 305–312.

Martel-Pelletier J, Cloutier JM, Howell DS & Pelletier JP (1985) Human rheumatoid arthritic cartilage and its neutral proteoglycan degrading proteases. *Arthritis Rheum* **28**: 405–412.

Matrisian LM (1992) The matrix degrading proteinases. *Bioessays* **14**: 455–463.

Matrisian LM & Hogan BL (1990) Growth factor regulated proteases and extracellular matrix remodeling during mammalian development. *Curr Top Dev Biol* **24**: 219–259.

McCachren SS (1991) Expression of metalloproteinases and TIMP in human arthritic synovium. *Arthritis Rheum* **34**: 1085–1093.

McCachren SS, Haynes BF & Niedel JE (1990) Localizaiton of collagenase mRNA in rheumatoid arthritis by *in situ* hybridization histochemistry. *J Clin Immunol* **10**: 19–27.

McQuillan DJ, Handley CJ, Campbell MA, Bolis S, Milway VE & Herington AC (1986) Stimulation of proteoglycan biosynthesis and insulin-like growth factor in cultured bovine articular cartilage explants. *Arch Biochem Biophys* **267**: 416–425.

Meats JE, Elford PR, Bunning RAD & Russell RGG (1985) Retinoids and synovial factor stimulate the production of plasminogen activator by cultured human chondrocyutes. *Biochim Biophys Acta* **838**: 161–169.

Melcher AJ & Chan J (1981) Phagocytosis and degradation of collagen by gingival fibroblasts *in vivo*: a study of serial sections. *J Ultrastruct Res* **77**: 1–36.

Miller EJ, Harris ED, Finch FE, Chung E, McCroskery PA & Butler WT (1976) Cleavage of types II and III collagens with mammalian collagenase. *Biochemistry* **15**: 787–792.

Morrison RIG, Barrett AJ, Dingle JTD & Prior D (1973) Cathepsins D and B; action on human cartilage proteoglycans. *Biochim Biophys Acta* **302**: 411–419.

Murphy G, Houbrechts A, Cockett MI, Williamson RA, O'Shea M & Docherty AJP (1991) The N-terminal domain of TIMP retains metalloproteinase inhibitory activity. *Biochemistry* **30**: 8097–8102.

Okada Y, Takeuchi N, Tomita K, Nakanishi I & Nagase H (1989) Immunolocalisation of stromelysin in rheumatoid synoviocytes. *Ann Rheum Dis* **48**: 645–653.

Okada Y, Gonoji Y, Nakanishi I, Nagase H & Hayakawa T (1990) Immunohistochemical demonstration of collagenase and TIMP in synovial lining cells of rheumatoid synovium. *Virchovs Arch B* **59**: 305–312.

Opdenakker G, Masure S, Grillet B & Van Damme J (1991) Cytokine-mediated control of human leukocyte gelatinases and their role in arthritis. *Lymph Cytok Res* **10**: 317–324.

Osbourne KD, Trippel SB & Mankin HJ (1989) Growth factor stimulation of adult articular cartilage. *J Orthop Res* **7**: 35–42

O'Shea M, Willenbrock F, Williamson RA, Cockett MI, Freedman RB, Reynolds JJ et al (1992) Site directed mutagens that after the inhibitory activity of TIMP. *Biochemistry* **31**: 10146–10152.

Osthues A, Knauper V, Oberhoff R, Reinke H & Tscheche H (1992) Isolation and characterization of TIMP-1 and TIMP-2 from rheumatoid synovial fluid. *FEBS Lett* **296**: 16–20.

Parrakel PF (1969) Role of macrophages in collagen resorption. *J Cell Biol* **41**: 345–354.

Peterson MJ, Woodley DT, Striklin GP & O'Keefe EJ (1987) Production of procollagenase by cultured human keratinocytes. *J Biol Chem* **262**: 835–840.

Pettipher ER, Henderson B, Hardingham TE & Ratcliffe A (1989) Cartilage proteoglycan depletion in acute and chronic antigen induced arthritis. *Arthritis Rheum* **32**: 601–607.

Pettipher ER, Edwards J, Cruwys S, Jessup E, Beesley J & Henderson B (1990) Pathogenesis of antigen-induced arthritis in mice deficient in neutrophil elastase and cathepsin G. *Am J Pathol* **137**: 1077–1082.

Phadke K (1987) FGF enhances the IL-1 mediated chondrocytic protease release. *Biochem Biophys Res Comm* **142**: 448–453.

Poole RA (1994) Immunochemical markers of joint inflammation, skeletal damage and repair: Where are we now. *Ann Rheum Dis*, in press.

Poole RA, Hembry RM & Dingle JT (1974) Cathepsin D in cartilage: the immunohistochemical demonstration of extracellular enzyme in normal and pathological conditions. *J Cell Sci* **14**: 139–161.

Saksela O & Rifkin DB (1988) Cell-associated plasminogen activation. Regulation and physiological functions. *Ann Rev Cell Biol* **4**: 93–126.

Salo T, Lyons JG, Rahemtulla F, Birkedal-Hansen H & Larjava H (1991) TFGB upregulates Type IV collagenase in cultured human keratinocytes. *J Biol Chem* **266**: 11436–11441.

Sandy JD, Sriratana A, Brown HLG & Lowther DA (1981) Evidence for polymorphonuclear leukocyte derived proteinases in arthritic cartilage. *Biochem J* **193**: 193–202.

Sandy JD, Boynton RE & Flannery CR (1991) Analysis of the catabolism of aggrecan in cartilage explants. *J Biol Chem* **266**: 8198–8205.

Sandy JD, Flannery CR, Neame PJ & Lohmander LS (1992) The structure of aggrecan fragments in human synovial fluid: evidence for the involvement in osteoarthritis of a novel proteinase. *J Clin Invest* **89**: 1512–1516.

Sapolsky AJ, Altman RD, Woessner JF & Howell SD (1973) The action of cathepsin D in human articular cartilage on proteoglycans. *J Clin Invest* **52**: 624–633.

Schalkwijk J, Joosten LAB, Van den Berg WB & Van de Putte LBA (1990) Antigen induced arthritis in beige mice. *Ann Rheum Dis* **49**: 607–610.

Schalkwijk J, van den Berg WB, van de Putte LBA & Joosten LAB (1987) Elastase secreted by activated polymorphonuclear leukocytes causes chondrocyte damage and matrix degradation in intact articular cartilage: escape from inactivation by alpha-1 proteinase inhibitor. *Br J Exp Path* **68**: 81–88.

Shapiro SD, Griffin GL, Gilbert DJ, Jenkins NA, Copeland NG, Welgus HG et al. (1992) Molecular cloning and bacterial expression of a novel murine macrophage metalloelastase. *J Biol Chem* **267**: 4664–4671.

Silver IA, Murrils RJ & Etherington DJ (1988) Microelectrode studies on the acid microenvironment beneath adherent osteoclasts. *Exp Cell Res* **175**: 266–276.

Silverman B, Cawston TE, Page-Thomas B, Dingle JTD & Hazleman BL (1990) The sulphated GAG levels in synovial fluid aspirates in patients with acute and chronic joint disease. *Br J Rheumatol* **29**: 340–344.

Sporn MB, Roberts AB, Wakefield LM & Crommrugghe B (1987) Some recent advances in the chemistry and biology of TGFB. *J Cell Biol* **105**: 1039–1045.

Stetler-Stevenson WG, Krutsch HC & Liotta LA (1989) Tissue inhibitor of metalloproteinase (TIMP-2). *J Biol Chem* **264**: 17374–17378.

Svoboda ELA, Melcher AH & Brunette DM (1979) Stereological study of collagen phagocytosis by cultured periodontal ligament fibroblasts. *J Ultrastruct Res* **68**: 195–208.

Thomas DPP, King B, Stephens T & Dingle JTD (1991) *In vivo* studies of cartilage regeneration after damage induced by IL-1. *Ann Rheum Dis* **50**: 75–80.

Tyler JA (1989) IGF-1 can decrease degradation and promote synthesis of proteoglycan in cartilage exposed to cytokines. *Biochem J* **260**: 543–548.

Vaes G & Eechhout Y (1975) Procollagense and its activation. In Burleigh PM & Poole AR (eds) *Dynamics of Connective Tissue Macromolecules*, pp 129–146. Amsterdam: North Holland.

Vaes G, Delaisse JM & Eeckhout Y (1992) Relative roles of collagenase and lysosomal cysteine proteinases in bone resorption. In Birkedal-Hansen H, Werb Z, Welgus HG and van Wart H (eds) *Matrix Metalloproteinases and Inhibitors*, pp 383–388. Stuttgart: Gustav Fischer.

Van der Rest M & Garrone R (1991) Collagen family of proteins. *FASEB* **5**: 2814–2823.

Van Noorden CJF, Smith RE & Rasnick D (1988) Cysteine proteinase activity in arthritic rat knee joints and the effects of a systemic inhibitor. *J Rheumatol* **15**: 1525–1535.

Velvart M & Fehr K (1987) Degradation *in vivo* of articular cartilage in rheumatoid arthritis and juvenile chronic arthritis by cathepsin G and elastase from polymorphonuclear leukocytes. *Rheumatol Int* **7**: 195–202.

Velvart M, Fehr K, Baici A, Sommermeyer G, Knoepfel M, Cancer M et al. (1981) Degradation *in vivo* of articular cartilage in rheumatoid arthritis by leukocyte elastase from polymorphonuclear leukocytes. *Rheumatol Int* **1**: 121–130.

Welgus HG, Campbell EJ, Bar-Shavit Z, Senior RM & Teitelbaum SC (1985) Human alveolar macrophages produce a fibroblast like collagenase and collagenase inhibitor. *J Clin Invest* **76**: 219–224.

Welgus HG, Campbell EJ, Cury JD, Eisen AZ, Senior RM, Wilhelm SM et al. (1990) Neutral metalloproteinases produced by human mononuclear phagocytes. *J Clin Invest* **86**: 1496–1502.

Werb Z, Mainardi CL, Vater CA & Harris ED (1977) Endogenous activation of latent collagenase by rheumatoid synovial cells. *N Engl J Med* **296**: 1017–1023.

Woessner J (1991) Matrix metalloproteinases and their inhibitors in connective tissue remodeling. *FASEB* **5**: 2145–2154.

Wolf C, Rouyer N, Lutz Y, Adida C, Loriot M, Bellocq J et al. (1993) Stromelysin 3 belongs to a subgroup of proteinases expressed in breast carcinoma fibroblastic cells and possibly implicated in tumour progression. *Proc Natl Acad Sci USA* **90**: 1843–1847.

Woolley DE, Crossley MJ & Evanson JM (1977) Collagenase at sites of cartilage erosion in the rheumatoid joint. *Arthritis Rheum* **20**: 1231–1239.

Woolley DE, Harris ED, Mainardi CL & Brinkerhoff CE (1978) Collagenase immunolocalization in cultures of rheumatoid synovial cells. *Science* **200**: 773–775.

Wright JK, Cawston TE & Hazleman BL (1991a) TGFB stimulates the production of TIMP by human synovial and skin fibroblasts. *Biochim Biophys Acta* **1094**: 207–210.

Wright JK, Clark IM, Cawston TE & Hazleman BL (1991b) The secretion of TIMP by human synovial fibroblasts is modulated by all-*trans*-retinoic acid. *Biochim Biophys Acta* **1133**: 25–30.

Yang T & Hawkes SP (1992) Role of the 21-kDa protein TIMP-3 in oncogenic transformation of cultured chick embryo fibroblasts. *Proc Natl Acad Sci USA* **89**: 10676–10680.

Animal Models of
Rheumatoid Arthritis

18 Role of Animal Models in the Study of Rheumatoid Arthritis: an Overview

*Jun Zhang, Barry M. Weichman and
Alan J. Lewis*

INTRODUCTION

The cause and pathogenesis of many chronic diseases including rheumatoid arthritis (RA) remain a mystery. Nevertheless, the identification of an animal model representative of human RA is critical to furthering our understanding of the disease pathophysiology and identifying new strategies for its treatment. As reviewed in subsequent chapters numerous experimentally induced models, ranging from adjuvant arthritis and streptococcal cell wall arthritis in the rat to murine models of collagen-induced arthritis and antigen-induced arthritis, have been characterized with the hope of reproducing clinical RA as a means to study this disease from several different viewpoints. As described in Chapter 25, this volume, arthritis also occurs naturally in a number of species (Weinreich *et al.*, 1993). For example, several mouse strains including the MRL/1pr, Biozzi H, NZB/DN and DBA/1 have some features in common with RA. From the pharmacologist's perspective, an animal model predictive of RA is key to characterizing new therapeutic modalities as well as identifying future drug discovery strategies. From the immunologist's vantage, definition of the inciting antigen and ensuing molecular and cellular events that lead to the arthritic symptomatology is critical to understanding the autoimmune process, which in turn could lead to new biologic approaches for regulating RA. With the advent of gene therapy and transgenic animals (Chapter 27, this volume) new models will be defined that focus on the role of various gene products in eliciting the arthritic symptomatology. Regardless of the viewpoint, the unifying factor in studying animal models of RA is the desire to identify approaches to cure this debilitating disease.

Numerous reviews have been written describing the similarities and differences of the commonly employed animal models of RA, yet it remains clear that none of the models is a perfect replica of the clinical disease (Greenwood, 1988; Chang and Lewis, 1989). Patient to patient variability in disease progression is not understood and would not be desirable in animal models, because it would make interpretation of experiments involving mechanism or drug responses problematic. However, there are compelling reasons why these animal models are used so extensively. Firstly, they enable aspects of the disease to be evaluated under tightly controlled conditions using a significant number of subjects which in turn allows for side-by-side comparisons of multiple variables. Secondly, the ease of tissue sampling enables multiple variables at the molecular, cellular and tissue levels to be evaluated. Thirdly, from a pharmacological perspective, the relationship between drug dose (or preferably drug blood levels) and biological response (both efficacy and toxicity) can be precisely quantitated. This in turn provides a starting point for potential clinical trials (see Chapter 4, this volume). The objective of this chapter is to provide an overview on the use of animal models in the study of RA, including a glimpse of the direction new animal model studies are taking.

COMPARATIVE ANALYSIS OF ANIMAL MODELS WITH RA

RA exhibits a sex predilection of 4:1 for females and usually manifests at an age of 40–55 years. Clinically, the disease is typified by a sustained and symmetrical inflammation of the small joints of the hands and feet, wrists, and knees, resulting in the symptoms of morning stiffness, decreased grip strength, and signs of systemic manifestations such as fatigue, weakness, anaemia, and weight loss (as described in Chapter 1, this volume). Despite the ability to treat some of the symptoms with NSAIDs and DMARDs (disease modifying antirheumatic drugs, a misnomer), RA is a progressive disease that is associated with significant morbidity. The clinical view of the value of DMARDs is discussed in Chapter 4, this volume.

The two animal models of RA that have been studied in greatest detail are the adjuvant-induced arthritis model in rats and the type II collagen-induced arthritis model in mice. Other models, including streptococcal cell-wall- and antigen-induced arthritis, and the more recent transgenic models (e.g. HLA-B27 model in rats) have offered additional insights into RA. A comparison of several of these models with clinical RA is presented in Table 1.

Table 1. Comparison of common animal models with RA

	Adjuvant arthritis	Collagen arthritis	Cell wall arthritis	Rheumatoid arthritis
Species	Rats	Mice, rats, monkeys	Rats, mice	Humans
Genetic linkage	+	+	+	+
Sex predilection	M/F	M/F	F	F
Remitting/relapsing	−	−	+	+
Peripheral joints	+	+	+	+
Axial joints	+	−	−	+
Erosions/pannus	+	+	+	+
Periosteal reaction	+	−	+	−
Antibody dependence	−	+	?	?
T-cell dependence	+	+	+	+
Antigen	*Mycobacterium*	Type II collagen	Group A streptococcal cell wall	Unknown
Pharmacology				
• NSAIDS	+	±	+	+
• Corticosteroids	+	+	+	+
• Methotrexate	+	+	+	+
• Gold salts	±	Worsens	−	+
• Penicillamine	−	+	−	+

'+' refers to presence and '−' to absence of the indicated parameter in the top part of the table. Under the pharmacology heading, a '+' indicates that a drug is effective in the disease; a '±' indicates variable results in tests with the drug; and a '−' indicates that the drug is not effective in the model.

Adjuvant arthritis, induced by an intradermal injection of heat-killed *Mycobacterium butyricum*, *M. phlei*, or *M. tuberculosis* suspended in mineral oil or liquid paraffin, has been commonly employed to evaluate the non-steroidal anti-inflammatory drugs as well as other classes of anti-arthritic drugs (Blackham *et al.*, 1977; Weichman, 1989). The symptoms of this systemic disease are usually manifested by day 10 (swelling, initial histologic changes) and progress to ankylosis and bony deformity during the following 2 months. Histologically, pannus formation with polymorphonuclear and mononuclear cell infiltrates is noted in affected joints. Antibodies to type II collagen are usually absent. The genetic linkage of adjuvant arthritis has not been fully characterized, but is based upon susceptibility of certain rat strains (especially Lewis and Fischer 344 rats). This model is discussed in detail by Billingham in Chapter 20, this volume.

Collagen arthritis has been induced in rats and monkeys, but by far the majority of studies have been performed in mice (Trentham *et al.*, 1977). This disease is elicited by the intradermal injection of native type II collagen in incomplete Freund's adjuvant; other collagens (e.g. type I and III) do not induce disease. The development of antibodies to type II collagen represents one similarity with clinical RA, in which low levels of anti-type II are measured. The genetics of collagen arthritis have been extensively studied, with disease linked to the major histocompatibility complex (MHC) (Wooley, 1991). One advantage of collagen arthritis over adjuvant arthritis is that the former is an autoimmune response to a connective tissue component rather than to a bacterial arthritogen. Further, collagen arthritis can be induced in species other than the rat; most interestingly, in the monkey. Disadvantages include the low incidence of the disease and the time it takes to develop, which is especially noted in mice. However, the disease in mice can be accelerated and the incidence increased by the injection of either LPS or IL-1 on day 21, resulting in a model more amenable for pharmacological evaluations of anti-arthritic agents. A detailed discussion of the immunogenetics of collagen arthritis is presented by Wooley (Chapter 19, this volume) and a general review by Trentham and Dynesius-Trentham (Chapter 23, this volume).

Streptococcal cell-wall arthritis is usually elicited by an intraperitoneal injection of a suspension of group A streptococcal cell-wall fragments (Cromartie *et al.*, 1977). Acute inflammatory changes are symmetrical in the distal joints and subside within several days. However, the chronic arthritic changes are noted by 2–3 weeks and consist of pannus formation, cartilage degradation, bone erosions, and an intense T-cell infiltration (Wilder *et al.*, 1989). The T-cell dependency of this chronic arthritis is evidenced by the observation that athymic rats do not develop the chronic synovitis. Females develop the disease with a higher incidence than males, and interestingly, castration of the males or administration of estradiol results in a higher disease incidence. Antibodies to type II collagen are not found in this model. As with the other models, disease susceptibility is dependent upon the rat strain used, with young female Lewis rats a viable choice. This rat model resembles clinical RA in that the disease involves the peripheral joints and usually spares the axial skeleton, and is typified by synovial pannus formation, synovial fibroblast proliferation, and accumulation of polymorphonuclear and lymphocytic cell infiltrates. Unlike its clinical counterpart, subcutaneous nodules do not occur and hepatic granulomas are sometimes observed.

SCID mice have been employed as unique recipients in disease-adoptive transfer experiments. This enables the study of the immunopathological events in the development of RA *in vivo* by using a defined lymphocyte population or specific molecules. The absence of functional B and T cells in SCID mice (Bosma *et al.*, 1983) prevents interference by host lymphocytes in the disease process and rejection of donor cells due to the histo-incompatibility, and moreover, makes antigen presentation by host to donor-derived T cells improbable. Perhaps one of the most successful examples is the adoptive transfer of collagen-induced arthritis to SCID mice (Williams *et al.*, 1992). Spleen cells (10^7–10^8) from arthritic DBA/1 mice, immunized 4–6 weeks previously with bovine type II collagen in adjuvant, were transferred i.p. into SCID mice. Simultaneously, SCID recipients were injected with native soluble type II collagen. Within 2 weeks, 100% of recipients developed arthritis which was clinically more pronounced than that of the original donors. Histological examination revealed severe synovitis, fibrosis and marginal erosion of cartilage and bone. In addition, significant high level production of specific anti-collagen IgG antibody showed strong association with the development of disease, whereas SCID mice injected with the same donor cells plus denatured collagen or ConA produced undetectable levels of anti-collagen antibody and did not show any clinical or histological evidence of arthritis. Furthermore, it seems that there is an association between development of arthritis and lymphocyte migration away from the site of administration, inasmuch as peritoneal lymphocytes can be only found in non-arthritic recipients with donor cells plus denatured collagen, but not in arthritic mice receiving donor cells and native type II collagen.

Adoptive transfer of arthritis into syngeneic recipients with collagen-immunized lymphocytes, collagen-specific T cell lines activated *in vitro* by antigen or Con A, or anti-collagen-containing serum either alone or in combination, has been difficult to achieve, due to low incidence, transient appearance, and/or mild subclinical symptoms (Ranges *et al.*, 1988; Seki *et al.*, 1988).

The principal features associated with successful transfer of arthritis into SCID mice lead to the hypothesis that after transfer to the SCID peritoneum, splenocytes from bovine type II collagen-immunized mice encounter soluble bovine type II collagen and are stimulated to synthesize lymphokines and anti-collagen antibodies and to up-regulate the expression of cell surface adhesion molecules (Williams *et al.*, 1992). The presence of circulating anti-collagen antibodies which crossreact with murine collagen results in the formation of immune complexes in the joint, that lead to activation of the complement cascade, and then infiltration of inflammatory cells culminating in clinical arthritis.

Selective depletion of the cell population used to transfer disease in SCID mice should allow the identification of cells involved in the induction of arthritis. Thus, the use of blocking antibodies should facilitate the study of the interaction between participating cells. The ability to transfer collagen-induced arthritis adoptively in SCID mice should facilitate the study of this arthropathy.

The successful transfer of human immune response with normal human peripheral blood mononuclear cells (PBMC) (Mosier *et al.*, 1988), and the human autoimmune response with PBMC from primary biliary cirrhosis patients (Krams *et al.*, 1989) to SCID mice led to an *in vivo* study of autoimmune mechanisms of RA in SCID mice. Tighe *et al.* (1990) reported that SCID mice reconstituted with RA synovial lymphocytes (SL) produced human IgM rheumatoid factor (RF) for over 20 weeks in the absence of deliberate immunization. In comparison, reconstitution with RA peripheral blood lymphocytes (PBL) or normal PBL produced minimal levels of IgM RF. The enriched production of RF by RA synovial cells transplanted into SCID mice is consistent with other results (Smiley et al., 1968; Cecere et al., 1982), which suggested that Ig found in synovial membranes is mainly produced locally. In addition to the increased production of IgM RF, other autoantibodies such as anti-DNA and anti-cytoplasmic antibodies were also found in SCID mice after reconstitution with SL from RA patients. However, immunization of RA-SL reconstituted SCID mice with immune complexes containing tetanus toxoid and IgG failed to increase IgM RF levels. The low absolute level and transient appearance of RF in the sera of chimeric SCID mice may explain the lack of detectable inflammatory processes in their joints. IL-6 is essential in the formation of antibody responses to autoantigens and is one of the most abundant cytokines in RA synovial fluid (Firestein and Zvaifler, 1987; Guerne et al., 1989). However, IL-6 cannot be detected in RA-SL-SCID chimeric mice. It will therefore be important to determine if administration of IL-6 and/or other cytokines can maintain a greater immune responsiveness and induce subsequent RA in these animals.

FUTURE CHALLENGES

Clearly, current drug therapy is capable of alleviating some of the symptoms of RA, yet the progressive nature of the disease remains unchecked. Immunosuppressive approaches (e.g. using cyclosporin A) offer promise on the efficacy parameter, but the benefit to risk ratio is limited because of severe side-effects (e.g. renal toxicity with CsA). Thus there is a need for more effective and less toxic therapeutics as discussed by Panayi in Chapter 4, this volume. It is clear that animal models will be invaluable in providing directions for these future strategies. The challenge will be on how to use animal models to define and then evaluate these future strategies.

The ability to introduce genes into the whole animal or into joints may be an important means of creating such models. For example, it should be possible to insert any gene or genes of choice into the synovium using gene transfer techniques. Promoters that determine tissue-specific expression of the transduced genes could also simplify delivery.

Transgenic mice expressing human TNF (hTNF) has been suggested as a predictive genetic model for arthritis (Keffer et al., 1991). The 3'-modified hTNF transgene induces chronic inflammatory polyarthritis in mice, with the disease inherited at a 100% frequency in transgenic progeny. The symptoms include swelling of the ankles occurring at around 3–4 weeks of age, and impairment to complete loss of leg movement at about 9–10 weeks of age. Moreover, progressive weight loss is another common feature in these mice. Histological characteristics are also compatible with human RA, which can be divided into two groups: (a) hyperplasia of the synovial membrane and polymorphonuclear and lymphocytic infiltrates of the synovial space were evident at all stages of disease; and (b) pannus formation, cartilage destruction and fibrosis were observed in the advanced stage of the disease. However, serum RF to mouse IgG was not detectable. Other tissues of the transgenic mice did not reveal further abnormalities. Although weight loss could not be associated with detectable levels of serum TNF, evidence for a causative effect of deregulated hTNF production on the development of arthritis was suggested by the inhibitory effects of a mono-clonal antibody against human TNF on the disease development in these transgenic mice. Animals treated with anti-hTNF i.p. developed normally and showed no signs of arthritis (at both macroscopic or histological levels) or weight loss even past 10 weeks of age.

Since the 3'-untranslated region of TNF mRNA is thought to be critical in the regulation of both mRNA stability and translational efficiency (Caput *et al.*, 1986; Shaw and Kamen, 1986; Kruys *et al.*, 1989; Han *et al.*, 1990), transgenic mice carrying TNF gene constructs with a modified 3'-region would cause deregulated patterns of TNF gene expression, then subsequently abnormal TNF cytokine production. Although the mode of TNF deregulation which leads to the development of arthritis in these transgenic mice remains unclear, it has been suggested that quantitative differences in the expression and/or production of TNF resulting from the 3'-modifi-cation may contribute to the disease pathology, and indeed anti-hTNF treatment can completely block the arthritis development in these animals. TNF has been shown to play an important role in the cascade of processes leading to the irreversible destruc-tion of joints. The most striking evidence is that this cytokine drives the proliferation of synovial cells *in vitro* (Beutler *et al.*, 1989; Gitter *et al.*, 1989) and induces synovial cell collagenase production which then leads to cartilage destruction (Dayer *et al.*, 1985, 1986). The transgenic arthritis model, although not addressing the disease at a primary etiology level, provides a unique opportunity for the design of therapeutic protocols to inhibit specifically TNF action and then block the subsequent cascade of pathological processes during arthritis development. The clinical effects of neutraliz-ing TNFα in rheumatoid patients is described in Chapter 2, this volume.

Other transgenes demonstrate inflammatory arthropathy that resembles RA. For example, transgenic mice carrying the human T-cell leukaemia virus type I (HTLV-1), the etiologic agent of adult T-cell leukaemia, produce arthritis after 2–3 months (Iwakura *et al.*, 1991). This suggests HTLV-1 may be one of the etiologic agents of chronic arthritis in humans. HLA-B27 transgenic rats and mice have also been de-scribed. It appears that HLA-B27 is correlated to the occurrence of reactive arthritis and ankylosing spondylitis and that this molecule is responsible for the association between HLA and disease (Ivanyi, 1992). A spontaneous, inflammatory disease involving several additional organs was described in transgenic LEW and F344 rats with human HLA-B27 and human β_2-microglobulin (Hammer *et al.*, 1990). The HLA-B27 transgenic mouse also manifests joint disease of the ankle and tarsal joints that is almost exclusively restricted to males (Ivanyi *et al.*, 1991). Neither of these models has been used extensively but may provide a means of further studying the important association of HLA-B27 with inflammatory disease. The use of transgenic animals to model RA is discussed in detail in Chapter 28, this volume.

With advances in molecular biology has come the opportunity to evaluate a variety of biologics for their potential benefit in RA. Among the biologics are monoclonal antibodies, cytokines, toxins, soluble cytokine receptors and vaccines as described in Chapter 4, this volume. Significant issues on the utility of animal models are evident. For example, if the human reagent does not interact with its rodent counterpart (e.g. non-crossreacting monoclonal or a human biologic that does not bind to a rodent receptor), little useful information regarding either efficacy or toxicity will be gar-

nered from animal studies. The value of pursuing the rodent counterpart of the human biologic in order to perform animal studies is problematic. Despite the inactivity of the human biologic in an animal system, information on non-specific effects can be gained from animal studies, especially in animals that may have compromised organ systems such as renal or hepatic complications, due to disease. Similarly, pursuing the rodent homologue to the human biologic enables animal studies that could be invaluable to the design and conduct of the clinical trials. When the human biologic cross-reacts with the animal, additional useful information, similar to that obtained with small molecules, is obtainable and includes dose-ranging studies to define the efficacious dose range and the maximum tolerated dose, as well as pharmacokinetic/pharmacodynamic studies to define routes of administration, duration, and correlations between drug levels and effect. Animal studies will also be invaluable in combination studies with the human biologic plus a currently available anti-arthritic by helping to define which combinations are efficacious, which is limited from a toxicity standpoint, and what dose ratios of the two agents are optimal.

On a cautionary note it is possible that a lack of effect of a biologic such as a cytokine or peptide in an animal model may not be predictive of ineffectiveness in man. This may be a consequence of a difference in the handling of the agent by the animal or in the disease model itself. It may therefore be premature to exclude an agent that shows poor efficacy in animals but for which *in vitro* data on human cells suggest it may be useful in man.

The use of animal models to evaluate new concepts for therapy is perhaps best evidenced by the potential of gene therapy. One example is the transfer of the gene for IL-1 receptor antagonist (IL-1ra) into synovial fibroblasts as a means of reducing inflammatory arthritis in the rabbit (Bandara *et al.*, 1992). Initial studies demonstrated that these cells containing the IL-1ra gene and injected into the rabbit synovium were morphologically similar to normal synovial fibroblasts several weeks later. These cells appear capable of releasing IL-1ra locally, and therefore provide a selective drug delivery system. The ability of this gene therapy approach to regulate the inflammatory changes produced by exogenous IL-1 injection or another inciting agent remains to be fully demonstrated. However, if viable, this technology provides a potentially selective approach to controlling RA.

MRL lpr/lpr mice spontaneously develop a systemic autoimmune disease which includes increased autoantibody production, glomerulonephritis, RA and lymphadenopathy (Hang *et al.*, 1982; Cohen and Eisenberg, 1991, reviewed in Chapter 25, this volume). The lpr genetic defect has been identified as a mutation in the fas apoptosis gene which results in low expression of fas mRNA (Watanabe-Fukunaga *et al.*, 1992; Wu *et al.*, 1993). This fas apoptosis gene defect, being a very attractive causal mechanism that may lead to autoimmunity and lymphadenopathy in MRL lpr/lpr mice, is genetically corrected in autoimmune T cells by replacement with the normal murine fas gene under the control of the T-cell specific CD2 promoter and enhancer (Wu *et al.*, 1993). These fas-transgenic MRL lpr/lpr mice resulted in an elimination of (a) the abnormal $CD4^-CD8^-B220^+$ T cells and glomerulonephritis at the age of 4.5 months, and (b) arthritis and lymphadenopathy at age of 1 year (personal communication), and in a decreased production of autoantibodies. In this model, early correction of the lpr defect in T cells is sufficient to eliminate the autoimmune symptoms even in the presence of B cells and other cells which express the mutant lpr gene. These findings directly demonstrate that the T cell abnormality is required for production of abnormal, autoreactive antibody producing B cells in MRL lpr/lpr mice. The search for genetic defects in humans with autoimmune diseases such as SLE and RA has been very actively conducted in the scientific community, and the ability to correct auto-immune disease through gene therapy will certainly be a consideration in the future for some patients with autoimmunity.

In employing animal models to evaluate potential new therapeutics, it is necessary to mimic the clinical setting as closely as possible, not only from a mechanistic vantage, but also from a temporal one. Therapeutic modalities can be evaluated for their ability to prevent the onset of disease or for their ability to alter the course of established disease. It is likely that the latter strategy is the more relevant one to the clinical setting. However, with the cyclical nature of RA, it can be argued that the preventative approach is also relevant in that it may predict activity against the flaring phases. Another aspect from a temporal vantage is the stage of disease. Typically when animal models with established disease are employed, the disease is of low severity with a sufficient window for measuring the drug activity. This may reflect early stage disease. However, the severity, and with it, the underlying molecular mechanisms driving RA may be evolving, which in turn could place significant limitations on the predictability of the animal data. Thus consideration of the potential of RA as a moving target must be made in the testing of any new therapeutic strategy.

SUMMARY

As great strides at the molecular level continue to be made, the ability of animal models to RA to continue to meet the demands of the scientific hypothesis testing and of evaluation of new therapeutic modalities will be severely tested. It is clear that available animal model mimic only certain aspects of RA, and additional modeling of RA, taking into account the evolution of the disease severity as well as the cyclical nature of the disease, will be needed. It is in this light that transgenic animals may find a highly significant application as new animal models, that are hopefully increasingly more reflective of RA. However, the ideal model will await a greater understanding of the pathogenesis of the disease.

REFERENCES

Bandara G, Robbins PD, Georgesu HI, Mueller GM, Glorion J & Evans CH (1992) *DNA and Cell Biol* **11**: 227.
Beutler B & Cerami A (1989) *Ann Rev Immunol* **7**: 625–655.
Blackham A, Burns JW, Farmer JB, Radziwonik H & Westwich J (1977) *Agents Actions* **7**: 145–151.
Bosma GC, Custer RP & Bosma MJ (1983) *Nature* **301**: 527–530.
Caput D, Beutler B, Hartog K, Thayer R, Brown-Shimer S & Cerami A (1986) *Proc Natl Acad Sci USA* **83**: 1670–1674.
Cecere F, Lessard J, McDuffy S & Pope RM (1982) *Arthritis Rheum* **25**: 1307–1315.
Chang JY & Lewis AJ (1989) *Pharmacological Methods in the Control of Inflammation*. New York: Alan R. Liss.
Cohen PH & Eisenberg RA (1991) *Ann Rev Immunol* **9**: 243–269.
Cromartie WJ, Craddock JG, Schwab JH, Anderle S & Yang C (1977) *J Exp Med* **146**: 1585–1602.
Dayer JM, Beutler B & Cerami A (1985) *J Exp Med* **162**: 2163–2168.
Dayer JM, DeRochemonteix B, Burrus B, Demczuk S & Dinarello CA (1986) *J Clin Invest* **77**: 645–648.
Firestein GS & Zvaifler NJ (1987) *Arthritis Rheum* **30(8)**: 857–863.
Gitter BD, Labus JM, Lees SL & Scheetz ME (1989) *Immunology* **66**: 196–200.

Greenwald RA (1988) *Handbook of Animal Models of the Rheumatoid Disease*. Boca Rata: CRC Press.

Guerne PA, Zuraw BL, Vaughan JH, Carson DA & Lotz MJ (1989) *J Clin Invest* **83**: 585–592.

Hammer RE, Marka SD, Richardson JA, Tang JP & Tamog JD (1990) **Cell 63**: 1099–1112.

Han J, Brown T & Beutler B (1990) *J Exp Med* **171**: 465–475.

Hang L, Theophilopoulos AN & Dixon FJ (1982) *J Exp Med* **155**: 1690–1701.

Ivanyi P (1992) *Curr Opin Rheumatol* **4**: 484–493.

Ivanyi P, Euldenirk F, Van Alphen L, Caprova Pla M, Enreich S, Zurcha C (1991) In Lipsky P & Taurog J (eds) *HLA-B27 and Spondylarthropathies*, pp 1171–1184, New York: Elseveir.

Iwakura Y, Tosu M, Yoshida E, Takigueki M, Sato K, Kvajima I et al. (1991) *Science* **253**: 1026.

Keffer J, Probert L, Cazlaris H, Georgopoulos S, Kaslaris E, Kioussis D et al. (1991) *EMBO J* **10**: 4025–4031.

Krams SM, Dorshkind D & Gershwin ME (1989) *J Exp Med* **170**: 1919–1930.

Kruys V, Marinx O, Shaw G, Deschamps J & Huez G (1989) *Science* **245**: 852–855.

Mosier DE, Gulizia RJ, Baird SM & Wilson DB (1988) *Nature* **335**: 256–259.

Ranges GE, Furtin S, Barger MT, Sriram S & Cooper SM (1990) *Int Rev Immunol* **4**: 83–90.

Seki N, Sudo Y, Yoshioka T, Sugihara S, Fujitsu T, Sakuma S et al. (1988) *J Immunol* **140**: 1477–1484.

Shaw G & Kamen R (1986) *Cell* **46**: 659–667.

Smiley JD, Sachs C & Ziff M (1968) *J Clin Invest* **47**: 624–632.

Tighe H, Silverman GJ, Kozin F, Tucker R, Gulizia R, Peebles C et al. (1990) *Eur J Immunol* **20**: 1843–1848.

Trentham DE, Townes AS & Kang AH (1977) *J Exp Med* **146**: 857–868.

Watanabe-Fukanaga R, Brannan CI, Copeland NG, Jenkins NA & Nagata S (1992) *Nature* **356**: 314–317.

Weichman BM (1989) In Chang JY & Lewis AJ (eds) *Pharmacological Methods in the Control of Inflammation*, pp 363–380. New York: Alan R. Liss.

Weirich S, Chopin M, Ivanyi P & Pla M (1993) *Clin Exp Rheumatol* **11** (**supplement 11**): 59–514.

Wilder RL, Lafyatis R, Yocum DE, Case JP, Kumkumian GK & Remmers EF (1989) *Clin Exp Rheumatol* **7/S-3**: 123–127.

Williams RO, Plater-Zyberk C, Williams DG & Maini RN (1992) *Clin Exp Immunol* **88**: 455–460.

Wooley PH (1991) *Curr Opin Rheumatol* **3**: 407–420.

Wu JG, Zhou T, He J & Mountz JD (1993) *J Exp Med* **178**: 461–468.

Wu JG, Zhou T, Zhang JJ, He J & Mountz JD (1993) *Proc Natl Acad Sci USA*, in press.

19 Immunogenetics of Animal Models of Rheumatoid Arthritis

Paul H. Wooley

INTRODUCTION

Rheumatoid arthritis (RA) is a disease of unknown etiology characterized primarily by chronic synovitis and a broad spectrum of immune abnormalities, including the production of autoantibodies and cellular immune dysfunction (Harris, 1990). The development of our immunity in RA has been postulated to be antigen-driven. According to this hypothesis, an infectious agent or an antigenic element may be presented in association with a major histocompatability complex (MHC) class II molecule to a T-cell population sequestered within the joint (Janossy *et al.*, 1981). The reactive T cell is predicted to crossreact with a joint component, causing amplification of the immune reaction and consequent tissue damage. Concomitant recruitment of additional mediators of inflammation may increase the range of the autoimmune response as cartilage-derived antigens are exposed. Evidence to support this hypothesis is provided by the association of RA with HLA-DR4, and the suggestion that the T-cell population infiltrating the joint is oligoclonal in nature (Stamenkovic *et al.*, 1988; Paliard *et al.*, 1991; reviewed in detail in Chapters 2 and 11, this volume). However, studies of the regulatory lymphocyte subsets have failed to identify immune reactivity against an infectious agent or an antigenic element common to the development of RA, nor have they detected a specific defect in the T-cell repertoire of RA patients. It is possible that RA may be a heterogeneous disease, occurring as a consequence of the response to a number of etiological agents. If this is so, it may be difficult to establish a single pathogenic mechanism for this disease. Experimental models are valuable as a means to test hypothetical autoimmune disease mechanisms, and in particular they provide a tool to elucidate the immunogenetic regulation of arthritis.

Experimental arthritis occurs spontaneously, or may be induced, in a variety of species including mice, rats, rabbits, goats, dogs and monkeys (see Chapter 25, this volume). This chapter focuses on murine models where genetic mechanisms have been demonstrated to play a significant role. Mice have been subjected to the most rigorous basic research in immune regulation, and thus can provide us with the most complete information on the regulation of disease susceptibility currently available. However, there are a number of experimental models of arthritis, such as adjuvant arthritis and streptococcal wall-induced arthritis, that have not been induced in mice. These models may provide important clues to the regulation of arthritis. The lack of a known immunogenetic association in a particular model may reflect the limits of our understanding of immune regulation, rather than imply a deficit in that model. Transgenic technology now provides us with a valuble tool to dissect the role of individual

Mechanisms and Models in Rheumatoid Arthritis
ISBN 0–12–340440–1

genes, and we may soon be able to evaluate precisely the contributions and interactions of the different gene systems associated with the development of arthritis. The use of transgenic animals in arthritis research is discussed in Chapter 27, this volume.

IMMUNOGENETIC REGULATION

Although multiple gene systems probably contribute to the regulation of the immune response, recent investigations have focused on the role of the class II MHC genes and on T-cell receptor genes. The cell surface proteins encoded by these polymorphic gene systems act as the primary structures used for antigen presentation and immune recognition. Since a number of autoimmune diseases, including RA, are associated with class II MHC (HLA-DR), it is important to consider the trimolecular complex formed by antigen, class II MHC, and the T cells as central to the immunogenetic regulation of autoimmune disease. Association of antigen with class II MHC results from antigen processing, when antigen-presenting cells internalize and degrade antigens in phagolysosomes. Enzymatically degraded portions of the antigenic molecule (typically short peptide chains) are re-expressed at the cell surface, physically associated with the class II MHC molecule. This combination of self (MHC) and non-self (Ag) is recognized by the T-cell receptor (TCR). Different class II MHC molecules may result in different epitopes of a single antigen being presented to the T cell. Alternatively, the same epitope may be presented, but variations in the three-dimensional structure between different class II MHC molecules (due to polymorphic gene variations) may alter its orientation, and thus modify the specificity of the T-cell response. The TCR has marked similarities to the immunoglobulin molecule, due to its membership in the immunoglobulin supergene family. These properties include an antigen-binding site encoded by variable gene regions that provide the diversity of the immune response. The selection and combination of the variable, the junctional, and the diversity region genes will determine the structure of class II MHC Ag-binding molecule, and thus influence the fine specificity of the T-cell response. Variations in this fine specificity may determine whether an immune response is reactive with self components, which may lead to the development of autoimmunity. Autoimmune disease models provide a valuable tool for the molecular dissection of this process. The clonal nature of inbred mouse strains ensures consistency in the class II antigens and the T-cell repertoire, and thus allows the investigation of inappropriate autoimmune responses to antigenic stimuli, and potential mechanism to divert the auto-immune response towards a non-immunopathogenic reaction to non-self target antigens. The arthritogenicity of the two major components of hyaline cartilage (type II collagen and aggrecan) in animal models suggests that antigen presentation and T-cell responses play a critical role in the development of autoimmune arthritis.

IMMUNOGENETIC REGULATION OF MURINE COLLAGEN-INDUCED ARTHRITIS

Type II collagen-induced arthritis (CIA) in the mouse has provided considerable insights into immunoregulation of experimental arthritis, and has provided the benchmark for other models. This model is reviewed in Chapter 24, this volume. The initial description of murine CIA (Courtenay *et al.*, 1980) indicated strain differences, and investigation of the role of MHC genes in mice congenic to the C57.B10 background showed strict regulation by class II MHC genes (Wooley *et al.*, 1981). Using chick type II collagen, CIA in mice occurred only in H-2^q haplotype animals. When recombinant haplotype mice (also congenic to the C57.B10 background) were tested, susceptibility to CIA was specifically associated with the expression of I-A^q cell surface antigens. This immunogenetic regulation is illustrated in Table 1. The only independent haplo-

Table 1. The regulation of collagen-induced arthritis by H-2 genes

Strain	K	I-A	I-E	D	Arthritis incidence (%)
B10	b	b	b	b	0
B10.K	k	k	k	k	0
B10.D2	d	d	d	d	0
B10.S	s	s	s	s	0
B10.M	f	f	f	f	0
B10.Q	q	q	q	q	80
B10.G	q	q	q	q	60
B10.BYR	q	k	k	b	0
B10.AQR	q	k	k	d	0
B10.T(6R)	q	q	q	d	55
B10.RQB-1	q	q	q	b	75
B10.DA	q	q	q	s	65
B10.RQF-1	q	q	–	f	70
B10.AKM	k	k	k	q	0
B10.MBR	b	k	k	q	0

type mice that develop CIA are B10.Q and B10.G; strains that express H-2^q genes at each of the MHC loci. B10.T(6R), B10.DA, B10.RQB-1 and B10.RQF-1 all express I-A^q, and are all CIA susceptible. Independent and recombinant haplotype mice expressing other genes at the I-A region are resistant. Holmdahl *et al.* (1986) have postulated that the motif regulating CIA susceptibility is restricted to the I-Aβ chain, since B10.P mice express an I-Aα chain identical to the I-A^{q}α, and I-A^{P}β only differs from I-A^{q}β at a restricted number of sites.

It appears that this strict regulation of CIA varies in response to the use of type II collagen from different species. Immunization with either bovine, deer, or porcine collagen induced arthritis in H-2^r mice, as well as H-2^q mice (Table 2). B10.RIII mice

Table 2. Incidence of collagen-induced arthritis using different collagen species

Strain	H-2	CII (%)	BII (%)	DII (%)	PII (%)
B10.Q	q	80	63	55	8
B10.G	q	60	15	18	17
B10.RIII	r	0	80	75	95
LP.RIII	r	0	40	ND	50
RIII	r	0	0	0	0
DBA/1	q	85	75	85	90
BUB	q	77	ND	18	17
SWR	q	0	0	0	0

CII, chick type II collagen; BII, bovine type II collagen; DII, deer type II collagen; PII, porcine type II collagen.

are completely resistant to disease induction with chick type II collagen (CII), but develop a high arthritis incidence when immunized with bovine collagen (BII), deer collagen (DII), or porcine collagen (PII). Insufficient recombinant strains involving H-2^r genes are available to elucidate the influence of I-A^r or I-E^r. However, the inhibition of CIA using antibodies directed against class II MHC antigens provides evidence that these molecules are involved in the arthritogenic response (Wooley *et al.*, 1985). The incidence of CIA in B10.RIII mice was significantly reduced by polyclonal anti-Ia antisera (MI 112). MI 112 reacts with I-A and I-E antigens expressed by H-2^r (Ia. 1,3,7). A marked reduction in disease incidence was seen in mice injected with the monoclonal antibodies H10-93.2, 14-4-4, and 13-4. These antibodies are specific for epitope I of the Ia.7 (I-E) molecule. Monoclonal antibodies reactive with either epitope II or epitope III did not suppress the disease incidence. Interestingly, mice treated with the monoclonal antibody 17–3–3 (anti-Ia.22) developed 100% disease incidence, which suggests that monoclonal antibody therapy may increase immune responsiveness. Genetic regulation of the arthritogenic responses to collagen was examined in other H-2^r (non-B10 congenic) mouse strains. The influence of non-MHC genes is apparent from the data shown in Table 2, since LP.RIII mice are susceptible to CIA induction using BII and PII, but the RIII strain (the progenitor of the H-2^r genes translocated to B10.RIII) is resistant to CIA. Non-MHC genes also influenced H-2^q restriction. DBA/1 mice are highly susceptible to arthritis induced by any immunizing collagen source. BUB mice develop an unusual form of the disease, with a high incidence of ear involvement. This inflammatory reaction in the pinna of the ear may represent a model of relapsing polychondritis (unpublished observations), but a detailed evaluation of this model is not currently available. An atypical H-2^q strain was also identified; the SWR mouse does not develop arthritis when immunized with any of the tested type II collagens. These data demonstrate that CIA is regulated by non-MHC genes, MHC genes (particularly I-A), and antigenic determinants. Since autoimmune phenomenon are involved in the pathogenesis of arthritis, it was predicted that the development of disease would correlate with an immune reaction directed against self (mouse) type II collagen. All CIA susceptible mouse strains develop a vigorous antibody response directed against the immunizing collagen; however, CIA-resistant strains (B10 and B10.D2) also develop high antibody titres. Holmdahl *et al.* (1986) showed that the development of disease was dependent upon the production of autologous reacting antibodies, which are restricted to H-2^q mice immunized with chick collagen.

Type II collagen is a highly conserved molecule composed of a triple helical structure with a primary amino acid chain of repeating *Gly-Pro-X* sequences (see Chapters 9 and 17, this volume). The limited genetic variations observed in the sequences between different species should result in relatively subtle changes in the antigenic epitopes on the collagen molecule. Terato *et al.* (1985) have investigated the type II collagen molecule using cyanogen bromide fragments, which maintain the native conformation of the collagen molecule that appears to be essential for arthritis induction. They found that antibodies directed against autologous (mouse) collagen was restricted to determinants on the CB11 peptide, suggesting that this portion of the collagen molecule contains arthritogenic epitopes. The number of such epitopes remains unclear. The resistance of B10.RIII mice to chick collagen, and the relative insensitivity of B10.Q mice to porcine collagen, suggests that at least two independent collagen epitopes possess the capacity to induce disease. Whether both the epitopes are present of CB11 is unknown. The dissection of the arthritogenic epitope on the type II collagen molecule is complicated by the requirement for the native molecule for the induction of disease, although a low incidence of disease occurred in mice immunized with the CB11 fragment. To date, linear peptide sequences have failed to induce arthritis, but peptide constructs that mimic the CB11 fragment in the regions 245–270 and 122–147 have been used successfully to induce tolerance and inhibit the induction of CIA (Myers et al., 1989; Goldschmidt et al., 1990), suggesting that linear amino acid chains may have the capacity to (a) occupy the class II/TCR cleft and (b) induce a tolerogenic response. Site-directed substitutions of amino acid residues abrogated the capacity of these constructs to induce tolerance and suppress CIA, supporting the concept that this region on the collagen molecule is important in the arthritogenic response (Myers et al., 1992).

TCR genes determine the repertoire of diversity by encoding the receptor for the antigen/MHC ligand. If the responding T cells do not include cells bearing receptors specific for autologous (mouse) collagen, it would be predicted that the mouse should not develop arthritis. Data obtained from two strains support this hypothesis. Although SWR mice are H-2^q and generate a strong antibody response to collagen, this strain is CIA resistant. AUss/J mice are also H-2^q, and resistant to disease induction. Both of these strains have major deletions in the TCR genes, with a loss of approximately half of the genetic information (Behlke et al., 1986; Haqqi et al., 1989b). These deletions appear to be similar in AU and SWR mice, and both strains fail to express Vβ8, Vβ9, Vβ11, Vβ12 and Vβ13. The Vβ8 T-cell subset was implicated in the arthritogenic response to collagen (Banerjee et al., 1988; Haqqi et al., 1989b), since this TCR is present in other H-2^q haplotypes and absent from both AU and SWR mice. In addition, Vβ8 T cells appear to play a role in the pathogenesis of EAE (Zamvil et al., 1988). This hypothesis has been tested by a number of groups, with discordant finding. Banerjee et al. (1988) used F1, F2 and F1 backcross matings between SWR and B10 to analyse the T-cell repertoire. The F1 progeny between the two CIA resistant strains (B10 × SWR) developed a low incidence (17%) of mild arthritis and a normal TCR repertoire. Backcrosses to either parent increased the incidence of disease, although (B10 × SWR)× B10 mice develop a higher CIA incidence (68%) than did (B10 × SWR)× SWR mice (33%). Flow cytometric analysis of the Vβ8 T-cell population suggested that the presence of this T-cell population was correlated with CIA susceptibility; however, two of seven arthritic mice did not exhibit circulating Vβ8 T cells. The molecular analysis of TCR mRNA isolated from the joints of B10.Q mice showed restricted Vβ usage in infiltrating T cells during active CIA. Vβ8 was detected by reverse transcription polymerase chain reaction (RT-PCR) techniques in mRNA extracted from the joints of the majority (6/7) of the arthritic animals (Haqqi et al., 1992).

Involvement of TCR genes was also supported by the findings in H-2^r haplotype mice. B10.RIII (CIA susceptible) mice express a full complement of Vβ TCR genes, while RIII/sJ mice (CIA resistant) were found to have a major (70%) deletion of TCR Vβ genes, with an absence of 13 of the 21 genes examined (Haqqi et al., 1989a). F1, F2 and F1 backcross progeny from B10 (CIA resistant) and RIII (CIA resistant) mice were tested for CIA susceptibility to porcine collagen, and the (B10 × RIII)F1 mice were found to be 100% susceptible to CIA. Arthritis susceptibility segregated with the inheritance of the H-2^r haplotype, either as the homozygous $^{r/r}$ or the heterozygous $^{r/b}$ haplotype, and there was a high association (90%) between the development of CIA and the expression of the complete Vβ profile (David, 1990). However, nearly 10% of mice with arthritis were found to have the Vβ deletion defect of the RIII parent. The involvement of TCR genes in RA is reviewed by Cole and Sawitzke in Chapter 3, this volume.

Other groups have published data that do not support the role of the Vβ8 and Vβ6 TCR-bearing T cells in CIA, and the hypothesis remains controversial. Watson and Townes (1985) noted that SWR mice are complementing (C5) deficient, which may account for their resistance to inflammatory disease. The passive transfer of SWR anti-collagen antibodies to DBA/1 mice resulted in arthritis, suggesting that SWR possess the necessary genetic information to develop an autoimmune response (Reife et al., 1991). However, studies in F1 hybrid mice suggested a high correlation between CIA susceptibility and complement sufficiency, since the cross between two C5 deficient strains (SWR × B10.D2/oSn) was disease resistant, while the cross of SWR to a C5 normal strain (SWR × B10.D2/nSn) generated F1 progeny with a 66% CIA incidence (Reife et al., 1991). Spinella et al. (1991) examined the distribution of C5 and Vβ genes in (DBA/1 × SWR)F2 mice, and found that while C5 sufficiency was required for CIA susceptibility, the Vβ gene distribution did not appear to influence the genetic regulation of arthritis. Interestingly, in a similar study also using (DBA/1 × SWR)F2 mice, Anderson et al. (1991) found CIA susceptibility correlated neither with the inheritance of the Vβ repertoire nor the C5 phenotype. It should be noted that the incidence of CIA in the Andersson study was remarkably higher than the incidence observed by the Spinella group. Griffiths et al. (1993) have examined the role of the Vβ genotypes in progeny generated from intercrosses involving the H-2^r haplotype. When (B10.RIII × RIIIs)F1 mice were backcrossed to both parents, a higher incidence of arthritis was seen in (B10.RIII × RIIIs)× B10.RIII mice compared with (B10.RIII × RIIIs)× RIIIs mice, suggesting a correlation of susceptibility with increased Vβ genes inherited from the B10.RIII parent. The influence of both class II MHC and Vβ gene inheritance on CIA susceptibility was also examined in (B10 × RIIIs) × RIIIs mice, and the results suggests that if class II MHC and sex inheritance are disregarded, Vβ expression does not influence CIA incidence. However, if sex and hybrid class II MHC inheritance are included in the analysis, Vβ expression appears to contribute in a hierarchical manner to the level of CIA susceptibility. Readers should refer to the discussions in Chapters 2 and 3, this volume, concerning Vβ expression in the aetiology of RA.

Cell deletion experiments have not clarified the controversial role of the Vβ8 and Vβ6 T cells in CIA. It is accepted that deletion of CD4$^+$ T cells in mice prevents the induction of collagen arthritis (Ranges et al., 1985), and antibodies to the TCR framework also appear to ameliorate disease susceptibility (Moder et al., 1992a). These experiments suggest that elimination of the 'autoimmune' T-cell subset(s) should also prevent the induction of arthritis. Moder et al. (1993) used monoclonal antibody (Mab) therapy with Mab F23.1 to delete Vβ8 cells in B10.RIII mice at the time of immunization with porcine collagen. The level of circulating Vβ8 cell fell from 23 to 2%, and the arthritic incidence was significantly reduced in this treatment group. Mice treated with Mab to Vβ6 T cells were unaffected, and combined treatment (anti-Vβ8 plus anti-Vβ6) showed no increased reduction of disease incidence compared with the use of anti-Vβ8 alone. A similar approach by Goldschmidt *et al.* (1990), using Mabs to Vβ8 and Vβ6 in DBA/1 mice, did not support these findings. The immuno-therapy successfully reduced the level of circulating Vβ8 and Vβ6 cells below 2%, but despite the use of thymectomy to prevent the regeneration of Vβ TCR, the Mab immunotherapy failed to suppress the incidence of CIA in DBA/1 mice. Compare these findings with the clinical use of T-cell directed immunotherapeutics as described in Chapter 4, this volume.

David (1990) has examined the role of minor lymphocyte stimulating (*Mls*) genes in susceptibility to CIA. The neonatal intrathymic recognition of *Mls-1*[a] antigens in context with I-E appears to represent an 'educational' autoimmune response that results in the deletion of certain Vβ phenotypes, including Vβ8 and Vβ6 T cells. Strains that express the *Mls-1*[b] phenotype did not delete Vβ8 or Vβ6 cells. H-2[q] haplotype mice fail to express a functional I-E molecule at the cell surface, and thus also fail to delete Vβ8.1 and Vβ6 T cells. (B10.Q × BALB/c)F1 mice, which express Vβ8.1 and Vβ6 T-cell subsets, develop a parental-like incidence of arthritis in re-sponse to collagen. In contrast, the F1(B10.Q × BALB/c-*Mls-1*[a] mice, which clonally delete the Vβ6 and Vβ8.1 T cells, develop a significantly lower incidence and severity of disease than the parental strain. These data support the concept that the *Mls* gene locus has a role in the selection of T cells involved in the autoimmune response.

The action of the *Mls* antigen system in T-cell selection is mimicked by the activities of staphylococcal enterotoxins. *In vivo* administration of SEB to neonatal mice causes a complete deletion of mature Vβ8[+] and Vβ3[+] T cells, in contrast to the preservation of cells expressing Vβ6[+], possibly as a consequence of neonatal tolerance of SEB (White *et al.*, 1989). In contrast, enterotoxins are strongly mitogenic *in vitro*, and expand particular Vβ T-cell subsets. The mitogenic profile of SEB indicates that Vβ3, 7, 8 and 17 T cells are clonally expanded, while SEA activates Vβ1, 3, 10, 11 and 17 (Marrack and Kappler, 1990; Takimoto *et al.*, 1990). However, it has been suggested that SEB-induced Vβ8 cells may enter a state of profound anergy (Rellahan *et al.*, 1990), characterized by failure to proliferate in response to either anti-Vβ8, SEB or IL-2 *in vitro*. The hypothesis that superantigenic modification of the T-cell repertoire may alter the activity of self-reactive cells and change susceptibility to autoimmune disease has been tested using CIA (Cingel and Wooley, 1992). Mice injected with SEA or SEB developed more severe arthritis than control animals, although flow cytometric analysis of TCR expression in mice 21 days after CII injection showed decreased expression of Vβ6[+] and Vβ8[+] cells in SEB-treated mice, and decreased expression of Vβ8[+] cells in SEA-treated mice. The data suggest that treatment with bacterial enterotoxins prior to the induction of arthritis does not suppress the im-munological or arthritogenic response to CII in DBA/1 mice, despite the modulation of the Vβ8[+] T-cell subset. However, the treatment of CIA induced in B10.RIII mice using SEB caused disease suppression (Moder *et al.*, 1992b). It is possible that TCR usage in B10.RIII mice immunized with porcine collagen varies markedly from the TCR usage in DBA/1 mice injected with bovine collagen. The interactive role of *Mls* and I-E in CIA regulation is currently being tested through the use of H-2[q] haplotype mice that are transgenic for the I-Eα[k] molecule. Preliminary data suggest that CIA can be driven by different combinations of class II MHC molecules and α/β-TCR-bearing T-cell subsets (M. Griffiths, pers. commun.). Overall, despite the clonal nature of inbred strains, which provides homogeneous class II MHC molecules and

TCR profiles, and limited heterogeneity in the antigen under investigation (type II collagen), it is clear that the regulation of CIA is a complex immunogenetic process. The role of superantigens in the aetiology and pathogenesis of RA and experimental arthritis is discussed in Chapters 3 and 21, this volume.

IMMUNOGENETIC REGULATION OF PRISTANE-INDUCED ARTHRITIS

Pristane-induced arthritis (PIA) is an experimental murine disease model elicited by the intraperitoneal administration of pristane (2,6,10,14 tetramethylpentadecane) (Potter and Wax, 1981). The major clinical feature of this model is an inflammatory joint disease, primarily focused in the ankle and wrist joints. Histopathological changes include synovitis, periostitis, and marginal erosions (Hopkins et al., 1984; Wooley et al., 1989). A broad spectrum of autoantibodies, including RF, anti-collagen antibodies, anti-high density proteoglycan antibodies, and antibodies to heat shock proteins are detected in sera from mice injected with pristane (Wooley et al., 1989; Thompson et al., 1990). There is considerable evidence of T-cell involvement in the pathogenesis of PIA. Athymic BALB/c nu/nu mice do not develop PIA (Wooley et al., 1989), and while irradiation prevents the development of PIA, reconstitution of irradiated mice with normal spleen cells restores susceptibility (Bedwell et al., 1987). Pristane injection has been shown to cause T-cell abnormalities in mice including the suppression of mitogen responsiveness and the induction of mediastinal lymphadeno-pathy in arthritis-susceptible mice (Chapdelaine et al., 1991). Flow cytometric analysis has demonstrated alterations in $CD4^+$ and $CD8^+$ T-lymphocyte subsets (Wooley and Whalen, 1991c). Early mediastinal lymph node changes include an accumulation of surface Ig^+ cells and a $CD8^+$ (Lyt-2) lymphocyte population. The expansion of this $CD8^+$ cell population correlates with an early suppression of mitogen response in pristane-treated mice at 2–4 weeks. Prior to the development of arthritis, there is an augmentation of the mediastinal $CD4^+$ cell population, the CD4:CD8 ratio normal-izes, and mitogen responses are restored. The mechanism by which pristane alters T-lymphocyte phenotype and function is presently unclear, but these cellular effects may be of primary importance in the development of PIA. Recently, it has been shown that treatment with anti-CD4 antisera prevents or delays the onset of PIA (Levitt et al., 1992).

Immunogenetic analysis using independent haplotype strains (Wooley et al., 1989) suggests that susceptibility is associated with the MHC and restricted to the $H-2^q$ (DBA/1, BUB), $H-2^d$ (BALB/c, LG), $H-2^r$ (RIIIs, LP.RIII) and $H-2^f$ (A.CA) haplo-types. However, several $H-2^q$ and $H-2^d$ mice are resistant, indicating non-MHC gene involvement in regulation of the disease. Since DBA/1 mice are susceptible and DBA/2 mice are resistant, the genetic analysis has concentrated on the disparate loci mapped in these two strains. Four of these loci are closely associated with the H-2 complex on chromosome 17 (H-2, Ce-2, Tla and Slp), two loci map on chromosome 4 (Akp-2 and Gpd-1), two loci map on chromosome 3 (Car-2 and If-1), whilst one locus (Hc) maps on chromosome 2. When 27 resistant and susceptible strains are analysed with respect to these nine loci, susceptibility is closely associated with both the Hc locus and the If-1 locus (Table 3). These two loci are associated with C5 haemolytic complement and circulating interferon levels induced by Newcastle Disease Virus, respectively. Bedwell et al. (1987) suggested a gene linked to the heavy chain immuno-

Table 3. The incidence of pristane-induced arthritis in inbred mouse strains

Mouse strain	Gene locus				Arthritis incidence (%)
	H-2	IF-1	Hc	Igh-1	
BALB/c	d	l	l	a	100
LG	d	na	na	na	50
DBA/2	d	h	0	c	0
B10.D2	d	h	l	b	0
DBA/1	q	l	l	c	100
BUB	q	na	l	a	63
SWR	q	na	0	c	0
RIIIs	r	na	l	g	20
LP.RIII	r	na	l	b	63
B10.RIII	r	h	l	b	0
A.CA	f	l	na	e	25
C57.BL/10	b	h	l	b	0
129/J	b	na	l	a	0
CBA	k	l	l	j	0
C3H/HeJ	k	l	l	j	0
P	p	na	l	h	0
BDP	p	na	l	h	0
PL	u	na	l	j	0
SM	v	na	l	b	0

globulin locus, Igh-1, controlled the development of arthritis. However the data shown do not support such a correlation of susceptibility with this gene in the tested strains. The possible linkages to several other loci, including Qa-1, Qa-2, Qa-3, Qa-4, Qa-5, Qed-1, Lyt-1, Lyt-2, Lyt-3 and Thy-1, were also investigated but no correlations were found. DBA/1LacJ and BALB/c J mice are most susceptible to the development of disease, with 100% incidence of arthritis. Arthritis was also observed in BUB, LG, RIIIs, LP.RIII and A.CA mice with an incidence of 20–63%. Analysis of recombinant haplotype strains does not identify precisely an association with H-2 complex locus. Three I-A^q strains (DA, B10.DA, B10.T(6R)) are susceptible, and B10.AKM mice (K^b I^k D^q) are resistant, suggesting an association with I-A^q. However, B10.MBR mice (K^k I^k D^q) are highly susceptible with rapidly progressing nodular arthritis. The incidence of arthritis in susceptible recombinant haplotype strains ranged from 22 to 75%. The inbred strain analysis of PIA susceptibility suggests that both MHC and non-MHC genes influence the development of arthritis, and an intriguing similarity to the genetic regulation of CIA is apparent. Both H-2^q and H-2^r strains are susceptible to both experimental diseases, and SWR mice are resistant to both. Recently, genetic restriction by the minor lymphocyte stimulating (*Mls*) genes has been identified in PIA (Wooley *et al.*, 1991a). The PIA model actually provides more convincing evidence than CIA, since PIA is not confined to H-2^q strains, and does not require the complication of F1 hybrids for Mls analysis that have been used in CIA. PIA susceptibility in BALB/c (H-2^d, *Mls-1^b*) mice and resistance in the BALB/c-*Mls-1^a* strain provides direct evidence that the *Mls-1^a* phenotype confers resistance. The *Mls* regulation also explains the resistance to PIA observed in F1 hybrids between the susceptible parents DBA/1 and BALB/c (Chapdelaine *et al.*, 1991). BALB/cJ, a PIA-susceptible strain, expressed the *Mls^b* phenotype and accordingly fails to delete Vβ8.1 and Vβ6 T-cell subsets. Studies in BALB/c-*Mls^a* mutant mice (where the Vβ8.1

Table 4. The influence of the *Mls* phenotype on pristane-induced arthritis

Strain	H-2	Hc	IF-1	*Mls*-1	Vβ6, 8	Arthritis (%)
DBA/1 LacJ	q/q	l/l	l/l	a/a	+	90
DBA/2	d/d	0/0	h/h	a/a	–	0
BALB/cJ	d/d	l/l	l/l	b/b	+	75
BALB/c-*Mls*[a]	d/d	l/l	l/l	a/a	–	0
(DBA/1 × BALB/c)F1	q/d	l/l	l/l	a/b	±	16
(DBA/1 × DBA/2)F1	q/d	1/0	l/h	a/a	±	16
(DBA/2 × BALB/c)F1	d/d	l/0	l/h	a/b	±	0

and Vβ T-cell subsets are deleted) indicate that this strain is PIA resistant (Table 4). Although DBA/1 mice are *Mls*[a], this strain is unable to delete intrathymically the Vβ8.1 and Vβ6 T-cell subsets due to the absence of functional I-E expression in the H-2^q haplotype. The incidence of disease in (DBA/1 × BALB/c)F1 and (DBA/1 × DBA/2)F1 hybrid mice is significantly lower than in the susceptible parental strains (DBA/1 and BALB/c), and complete resistance to arthritis is observed in (DBA/2 × BALB/c)F1 hybrid mice (Chapdelaine *et al.*, 1991). *Mls* and I-E gene complementation could also explain the resistance of hybrid mice, since the offspring of these susceptible parents are I-$E^{q/d}$ and $Mls^{a/b}$, and this phenotype deletes a high percentage of the Vβ8.1 and Vβ6 T cells.

Flow cytometric analysis of lymph node cells has been used to investigate the role of TCR Vβ genes in the regulation of PIA. Using two colour cytometry, cells were analysed for the co-expression of CD3, and a library of 10 monoclonal antibodies reactive with Vβ determinants. Although the Vβ8 population was increased in PIA lymph nodes, the Vβ6 cells were expanded to a similar extent, and the data suggest that the pristane-induced lymphadenopathy represents a polyclonal T-cell expansion. It remains to be determined whether a restricted number of Vβ TCR-bearing T cells infiltrate the joint in PIA. Cells reactive to the two major connective tissue antigens in the synovial joint (type II collagen and cartilage proteoglycans) have been identified in PIA. It remains to be determined whether the immunogenetic regulation controls the occurrence of cartilage-reactive T cells that infiltrate the joint and cause inflammatory disease. Since the ability to infiltrate the joint may also be mediated by cell adhesion molecules, the genes that regulate this class of cell surface antigens may also influence disease, although the interaction between these diverse genetic systems is not understood at present. The role of leukocyte adhesivity in RA pathology is reviewed in Chapter 11, this volume.

IMMUNOGENETIC REGULATION OF PROTEOGLYCAN-INDUCED ARTHRITIS

The recent development of proteoglycan-induced arthritis (PGIA) provides a powerful tool for autoimmunity studies. The injection of cartilage proteoglycans has been shown to induce an inflammatory arthritis in BALB/c mice (Mikecz *et al.*, 1987; Glant *et al.*, 1987). The histopathological features of this model include the development of symmetrical synovitis, marginal erosions, polarized pannus formation, and synovial infiltrate consisting of lymphocytes, plasma cells and histiocytes represent convincing features resembling RA. Immunological analysis of proteoglycan arthritis indicates marked production of anti-proteoglycan antibodies, and recent findings have demonstrated that autoantibody production to murine high density proteoglycans (HDPG) correlates with disease susceptibility (Wooley *et al.*, 1992). However, a precise role for autoantibody has not been established in the pathogenesis of this experimental arthritis, and a requirement for cellular immunity in the development of the joint lesion appears probable. Mikecz *et al.* (1990) have reported that spleen and lymph node mononuclear cells from BALB/c mice with PGIA adoptively transfer disease to naive recipients. It remains to be determined whether antibodies to the murine CD4 (L3T4) marker, which eliminate T helper cells in mice, do not eliminate the capacity to transfer disease adoptively, since these antibodies clearly abrogate the development of CIA and PIA in susceptible mice (Ranges *et al.*, 1985; Levitt *et al.*, 1992). Genetic analysis of PGIA susceptibility has been hindered by the failure to identify susceptible strains beyond BALB/c (Table 5). However, genetic restriction by the *Mls* genes has

Table 5. Genetic regulation of proteoglycan-induced arthritis in mice

Strain	H-2	*Mls*-1	Vβ6, 8	Arthritis (%)
BALB/cJ	d/d	b/b	+	100
BALB/c-*Mls*ª	d/d	a/a	−	0
DBA/2	d/d	a/a	−	0

been identified in PGIA (Wooley *et al.*, 1991b). BALB/c mice express Vβ8 and Vβ6 TCR-bearing T cells due to the *Mls-1*ᵇ phenotype, which does not permit depletion of this subset during the neonatal thymic selection of the T-cell repertoire. Wild type BALB/c and the mutant BALB/c-*Mls-1*ª strains were immunized with human nHDPG in Freund's complete adjuvant (FCA). All BALB/c developed PGIA by 6 weeks postimmunization (8/8), while all BALB/c-*Mls-1*ª remained disease-free through 15 weeks postimmunization (0/8, p<0.001). Higher levels of antibodies to heterologous (human) and autologous (murine) nHDPG were present in BALB/c sera compared to BALB/c-*Mls-1*ª sera 4 weeks and 6 weeks after immunization. However, the presence of autoantibodies in BALB/c-*Mls-1*ª mice suggests that cellular responses may be critical to the development of PGIA.

IMMUNOGENETIC REGULATION OF ANTIGEN-INDUCED ARTHRITIS

Antigen-induced arthritis (AIA) in mice is an experimental model of a monoarticular, chronic arthritis, produced by the single intra-articular injection of methylated bovine serum albumin (mBSA) into the knee joint of a mouse previously sensitized by immunization with mBSA in FCA. The histological appearance of AIA resembles RA but unlike the clinical picture, the disease remains confined to the injected joint. Immunohistochemical analyses of the joint infiltrate has revealed the presence of T lymphocytes (mostly helper T cells), B lymphocytes, mast cells and macrophages. Brackertz *et al.* (1977a,b,c) conducted a series of experiments that demonstrated immonogenetic regulation of the disease susceptibility. Five independent haplotype inbred mouse strains were tested for AIA susceptibility, and only one strain (CBA)

Table 6. Genetic regulation of antigen-induced arthritis in mice

Strain	H-2	Arthritis (%)
C57BL6	b/b	100
CBA	k/k	0
C3H.SW	b/b	100
C3H/HeJ	k/k	100
B10.BR	k/k	0
(C57BL × CBA)F1	b/k	100
(C57BL × CBA)× CBA	b/k	100
	k/k	50
(C57BL × CBA)F2	b/b	90
	b/k	90
	k/k	62

was identified as resistant. This resistance was not immediately associated with H-2^k, since C3H/HeJ and B.10.K mice developed a high disease incidence (Table 6). However, using F1, F2 and backcross studies, the appearance of definite arthritis (defined by histological evaluation) was associated with the inheritance of the H-2^b haplotype (Table 6). F1 hybrid mice (C57BL × CBA) mice were completely susceptible to AIA, suggesting a recessive gene in CBA mice regulating resistance. Mice that expressed homozygous H-2$^{k/k}$ inheritance, in either F1 backcrosses to the CBA parent or in the F2 cross, developed a significantly lower incidence of AIA when compared to either mice that inherited H-2$^{b/b}$ or H-2$^{k/b}$ from the same intercrosses. These data suggest that susceptibility to AIA is regulated in part by major histocompatibility locus (MHC) genes or a closely linked gene(s). The role of the class II MHC antigen in the regulation of AIA is supported by *in vivo* anti-Ia antibody studies. A modification in the antigen sensitization protocol induces an experimental arthritis characterized by limited disease. This model may be exacerbated by intravenous antigen, which causes a flare reaction (van de Putte *et al.*, 1983). The administration of monoclonal antibody reactive with I-A^b suppressed the flare reaction in C57BL10 (H-2^b) mice, and monoclonal antibody reactive with I-A^k suppressed the flare reaction in C3H/HeJ (H-2^k) mice (van den Broek *et al.*, 1986). The non-haplotype specific control injection of monoclonal antibody did not influence the disease exacerbation. Antibodies directed against T lymphocytes (anti-lymphocyte serum and anti-Thy1) have also proved effective in suppressing the AIA flare reaction (Lens *et al.*, 1984). The mechanism of AIA appears to be dependent upon lymphocytes, which can adoptively transfer both AIA and sensitivity to subsequent mBSA challenge (Brackertz *et al.*, 1977b). It appears that the Ia regulation of AIA occurs at the antigen presentation level, since an antigen-specific (anti-MBSA) T helper cell line has been developed which can induce synovitis on intra-articular injection (Klasen *et al.*, 1989). However, the synovial lining in AIA has been shown to express Ia antigens, and immunotherapy with anti-Ia antibodies could prevent flare-up reactions through a direct action on the abnormal expression of class II antigens in the joint.

   The immunogenetic regulation of AIA at the level of the T cell has been investigated by Winterrowd *et al.* (1993). Using a modification of the classical AIA model

(IL-1 as an intra-articular stimulus in an mBSA immunized animal; Staite *et al.*, 1990), the phenotypes of T cells infiltrating the mouse knee joint were examined by flow cytometric techniques. The findings demonstrated that the ratio of B cells to T cells in the joint was elevated compared with lymph node cells from either AIA or naive mice, suggesting that local antibody production may contribute to the immunopathology. In the population of infiltrating cells, $CD4^+$ T cells were overrepresented and $CD8^+$ T cells were underrepresented. Interestingly, a higher number of γ/δ T cells (14%) were present in the joint, compared with the γ/δ T-cell level seen in lymph nodes (2%). However, the TCR analysis of α/β T cells showed no predominant expression of a particular $V\beta$ TCR-bearing T cell in the arthritic joint. The synovial T cells did exhibit a 'memory' T cell phenotype ($CD44^{hi}$, $CD45RB^-$, L-selectin$^-$) and expressed high levels of CD11a, VLA-4 and ICAM-1. This contrasted with the typical 'naive' phenotype of lymph nodes cells from AIA and normal mice ($CD44^{lo}$, $CD45RB^+$, L-selectin$^+$). A similar distribution of different T-cell phenotypes was also seen in joint infiltrating synovial T cells from the knees of mice with classical AIA (N. Staite, pers. commun.; see also Chapter 11, this volume, on leukocyte adhesion). This acumulation of memory T cells in the inflamed joint suggests that the regulation of adhesion molecules and cell differentiation antigens may contribute to arthritis susceptibility. This model is also discussed by Pettipher and Blake in Chapter 24, this volume.

SUMMARY

The murine models of experimental arthritis described in this chapter highlight the complexity of the immunogenetic regulation of arthritis. In spite of the clonal nature of inbred mouse strains and the use of known antigenic elements, it has been difficult to elucidate the mechanisms that contribute to the immunopathogenesis of inflammatory joint disease, and the relative contributions of autoantibodies, soluble factors, and T cells in arthritis models remain controversial. It may be significant that diverse arthritogenic procedures (immunization with connective tissue antigens and the injection of pristane) affect similar mouse strains (BALB/c and DBA/1), and imply analogous immunogenetic regulation of disease susceptibility. We must proceed with great caution when suggesting these findings are relevant to the pathogenesis of RA. Nevertheless, these models do mimic the human disease, and it appears likely that the observations made in animal models of arthritis may be critical to the discovery of both immunopathological mechanisms and novel therapies in rheumatoid disease.

REFERENCES

Andersson M, Goldschmidt TJ, Michaelsson E, Larsson A & Holmdahl R (1991) T-cell receptor V beta haplotype and complement component C5 play no significant role for the resistance to collagen-induced arthritis in the SWR mouse. *Immunology* **73**: 191–196.

Banerjee S, Haqqi TM, Luthra HS, Stuart JM & David CS (1988) Possible role of V beta T cell receptor genes in susceptibility to collagen-induced arthritis in mice. *J Exp Med* **167**: 832–839.

Bedwell AE, Elson CJ & Hinton CE (1987) Immunological involvement in the pathogenesis of pristane-induced arthritis. *Scand J Immunol* **25**: 393–398.

Behlke MA, Chou HS, Huppi K & Loh DY (1986) Murine T cell receptor mutants with deletions of b-chain variable region genes. *Proc Natl Acad Sci* **83**: 767–775.

Brackertz D, Mitchell GF & Mackay IR (1977a) Antigen-based arthritis in mice. I. Induction of arthritis in various strains of mice. *Arthritis Rheum* **20**: 841–850.

Brackertz D, Mitchell GF, Vadas MA & Mackay IR (1977b) Studies on antigen-induced arthritis in mice. III. Cell and serum transfer experiments. *J Immunol* **118**: 1645–1648.

Brackertz D, Mitchell GF, Vadas MA, Mackay IR & Miller JF (1977c). Studies on antigen-induced arthritis in mice. II. Immunologic correlates of arthritis susceptibility in mice. *J Immunol* **118**: 1639–1644.

Chapdelaine JM, Whalen JD & Wooley PH (1991) Pristane-induced arthritis. II. Genetic regulation in F1 hybrid mice and cellular abnormalities following pristane injection. *Autoimmunity* **8**: 215–220.

Cingel B & Wooley PH (1992) Immunotherapy with bacterial superantigens increases the severity of type II collagen induced arthritis in mice. *Arthritis Rheum* **35**: S140.

Courtenay JS, Dallman MJ, Dayan AD, Martin A & Mosedale B (1980) Immunisation against heterologous type II collagen induces arthritis in mice. *Nature* **283**: 666–668.

David CS (1990) Genes for MHC, TCR and MIs determine susceptibility to collagen induced arthritis. *Acta Pathologica Microbiologica et Immunologica Scandinavica* **XX 98**: 575–584.

Glant TT, Mikecz K, Arzoumanian A & Poole AR (1987) Proteoglycan-induced arthritis in BALB/c mice. Clinical features and histopathology. *Arthritis Rheum* **30**: 201–212.

Goldschmidt TJ, Jansson L & Holmdahl R (1990) *In vivo* elimination of T cells expressing specific T-cell receptor V beta chains in mice susceptible to collagen-induced arthritis. *Immunology* **69**: 508–514.

Griffiths MM, Cole BC, Ito J. et al. (1993) T cell receptors and collagen-induced arthritis in H-2r mice. *Autoimmunity*, in press.

Haqqi TM, Banerjee S, Anderson GD & David CS (1989a) RIII S/J (H-2r) – an inbred mouse strain with a massive deletion of T cell receptor Vβ genes. *J Exp Med* **169**: 1903–1909.

Haqqi TM, Banerjee S, Jones WL et al. (1989b) Identification of T-cell receptor V beta deletion mutant mouse strain AU/ssJ (H-2q) which is resistant to collagen-induced arthritis. *Immunogenetics* **29**: 180–185.

Haqqi TM, Anderson GD, Banerjee S & David CS (1992) Restricted heterogeneity in T-cell antigen receptor V beta gene usage in the lymph nodes and arthritic joints of mice. *Proc Nat Acad Sci USA* **89**: 1253–1255.

Harris ED (1990) Mechanisms of disease: rheumatoid arthritis – pathophysiology and implications for therapy. *N Eng J Med* **322**: 1277–1289.

Holmdahl R, Klareskog L, Andersson M & Hansen C (1986) High antibody response to autologous type II collagen is restricted to H-2q. *Immunogenetics* **24**: 84–89.

Hopkins SJ, Freemont AJ & Jayson MIV (1984) Pristane-induced arthritis in BALB/c mice. I. Clinical and histological features of the arthropathy. *Rheumatol Int* **5**: 21–27.

Janossy G, Panayi GS, Duke O, Bofill M, Poulter LW & Goldstein G (1981) Rheumatoid arthritis: a disease of T-lymphocyte/macrophage immunoregulation. *Lancet* **ii**: 839–841.

Klasen IS, Ladestein RM, van den Berg WB & Benner R (1989) Requirements for flare reactions of joint inflammation induced in mice by cloned MT4$^+$, Lyt-2$^-$ T cells. *Arthritis Rheum* **32**: 330–337.

Lens JW, van den Berg WB, van de Putte LB, Berden JH & Lems SP (1984) Flare-up of antigen-induced arthritis in mice after challenge with intravenous antigen: effects of pre-treatment with cobra venom factor and anti-lymphocyte serum. *Clin Exp Immunol* **57**: 520–528.

Levitt NG, Fernandez-Madrid F & Wooley PH (1992) Pristane induced arthritis in mice. IV. Immunotherapy with monoclonal antibodies directed against lymphocyte subsets. *J Rheumatol* **19**: 1342–1347.

Marrack P & Kappler J (1990) The staphylococcal enterotoxins and their relatives. *Science* **248**: 705–711.

Mikecz K, Glant TT & Poole AR (1987) Immunity to cartilage proteoglycans in BALB/c mice with progressive polyarthritis and ankylosing spondylitis induced by injection of human cartilage proteoglycan. *Arthritis Rheum* **30**: 306–318.

Mikecz K, Glant TT, Buzas E & Poole AR (1990) Proteoglycan-induced polyarthritis and spondylitis adoptively transferred to naive (nonimmunized) BALB/c mice. *Arthritis Rheum* **33**: 866–876.

Moder KG, Luthra HS, Kubo R, Griffiths M & David CS (1992a) Prevention of collagen induced arthritis in mice by treatment with an antibody directed against the T cell receptor alpha beta framework. *Autoimmunity* **11**: 219–224.

Moder KG, Nabozny G, Bull M, Luthra HS & David CS (1992b) Modulation of the T cell receptor Vβ repertoire with superantigens reduces susceptibility to collagen-induced arthritis. *Arthritis Rheum* **35**: S193 (Abstract).

Moder KG, Luthra HS, Griffiths MM & David CS (1993) Prevention of collagen induced arthritis in mice by deletion of T cell receptor Vβ8 bearing T cells with monoclonal antibodies. *Br J Rheumatol* **32**: 26–30.

Myers LK, Stuart JM, Seyer JM & Kang AH (1989) Identification of an immunosuppressive epitope of type II collagen that confers protection against collagen-induced arthritis. *J Exp Med* **170**: 1999–2010.

Myers LK, Terato K, Seyer JM, Stuart JM & Kang AH (1992) Characterization of a tolerogenic T cell epitope of type II collagen and its relevance to collagen-induced arthritis. *J Immunol* **149**: 1439–1443.

Paliard X, West SG, Lafferty JA et al. (1991) Evidence for the effects of a superantigen in rheumatoid arthritis. *Science* **253**: 325–329.

Potter M & Wax JS (1981) Genetics of susceptibility to pristane-induced plasmacytomas in BALB/cAn: reduced susceptibility in BALB/cJ with a brief description of pristane-induced arthritis. *J Immunol* **127**: 1591–1595.

Ranges GE, Sriram S & Cooper SM (1985) Prevention of type II collagen-induced arthritis by *in vivo* treatment with anti-L3T4. *J Exp Med* **162**: 1105–1110.

Reife RA, Loutis N, Watson WC, Hasty KA & Stuart JM (1991). SWR mice are resistant to collagen-induced arthritis but produce potentially arthritogenic antibodies. *Arthritis Rheum* **34**: 776–781.

Rellahan BL, Jones LA, Kruisbeek AM, Fry AM & Matis LA (1990) *In vivo* induction of anergy in peripheral V beta 8[+] T cells by staphylococcal enterotoxin B. *J Exp Med* **172**: 1091–1100.

Spinella DG, Jeffers JR, Reife RA & Stuart JM (1991) The role of *C5* and T-cell receptor *Vb* genes in susceptibility to collagen-induced arthritis. *Immunogenetics* **34**: 23–27.

Staite ND, Richard KA, Aspar DG, Franz KA, Galinet LA & Dunn CJ (1990) Induction of an acute erosive monarticular arthritis in mice by interleukin-1 and methylated bovine serum albumin. *Arthritis Rheum* **33**: 253–260.

Stamenkovic I, Stegagno M & Wright KA (1988) Clonal dominance amongst T-lymphocyte infiltrates in arthritis. *Proc Nat Acad Sci USA* **85**: 1179–1183.

Takimoto H, Yoshikai Y, Kishihara K et al. (1990) Stimulation of all T cells bearing V beta 1, V beta 3, V beta 11 and V beta 12 by staphylococcal enterotoxin A. *Eur J Immunol* **20**: 617–621.

Terato K, Hasty KA, Cremer MA, Stuart JM, Townes AS & Kang AH (1985) Collagen-induced arthritis in mice. Localization of an arthritogenic determinant to a fragment of the type II collagen molecule. *J Exp Med* **162**: 637–646.

Thompson SJ, Rook GA, Brealey RJ, Van der Zee R & Elson CJ (1990) Autoimmune reactions to heat shock proteins in pristane-induced arthritis. *Eur J Immunol* **20**: 2479–2484.

van den Broek MF, van den Berg WB & van de Putte, LB (1986) Monoclonal anti-Ia antibodies suppress the flare up reaction of antigen induced arthritis in mice. *Clin Exp Immunol* **66**: 320–330.

van de Putte LB, Lens JW, van den Berg WB & Kruijsen MW (1983) Exacerbation of antigen-induced arthritis after challenge with intravenous antigen. *Immunology* **49**: 161–167.

Watson WC & Townes AS (1985) Genetic susceptibility to murine collagen II autoimmune arthritis. Proposed relationship to the IgG2 autoantibody subclass response, complement C5, major histocompatibility complex (MHC) and non-MHC loci. *J Exp Med* **162**: 1878–1891.

White J, Herman A, Pullen AM, Kubo R, Kappler JW & Marrack P (1989) The V beta-specific superantigen staphylococcal enterotoxin B: stimulation of mature T cells and clonal deletion in neonatal mice. *Cell* **56**: 27–35.

Winterrowd GE, Chin JE & Staite ND (1993) Phenotype and adhesion molecule expression on synovial tissue from T cells from mice with acute erosive arthritis. *Clin Exp Rheumatol* **11**: s191.

Wooley PH & Whalen JD (1991) Pristane-induced arthritis in mice. III. Lymphocyte phenotypic and functional abnormalities precede the development of pristane-induced arthritis. *Cell Immunol* **138**: 251–259.

Wooley PH, Luthra HS, Stuart JM & David CS (1981) Type II collagen-induced arthritis in mice. I. Major histocompatibility complex (I region) linkage and antibody correlates. *J Exp Med* **154**: 688–700.

Wooley PH, Luthra HS, Lafuse WP, Huse A, Stuart JM & David CS (1985) Type II collagen-induced arthritis in mice. III. Suppression of arthritis by using monoclonal and polyclonal anti-Ia antisera. *J Immunol* **134**: 2366–2374.

Wooley PH, Seibold JR, Whalen JD & Chapdelaine JM (1989) Pristane-induced arthritis. The immunological and genetic features of an experimental murine model of autoimmune disease. *Arthritis Rheum* **32**: 1022–1030.

Wooley PH, Whalen JD & David CS (1991a) The Mls gene locus regulates susceptibility to pristane-induced arthritis. *Arthritis Rheum* **34**: S66.

Wooley PH, Whalen JD, Karvonen RL & David CS (1991b) Mls phenotype influences susceptibility to proteoglycan-induced arthritis in mice. *Arthritis Rheum* **34**: S67.

Wooley PH, Siegner SW, Whalen JD, Karvonen RL & Fernandez-Madrid F (1992) Proteoglycan-induced arthritis in BALB/c mice is dependant upon the development of autoantibodies to high density proteoglycans. *Ann Rheum Dis* **51**: 983–991.

Zamvil SS, Mitchell DJ, Lee NE et al. (1988) Predominant expression of a T cell receptor Vb gene subfamily in autoimmune encephalomyelitis. *J Exp Med* **167**: 1586–1596.

20 Adjuvant Arthritis:
the First Model

M.E.J. Billingham

INTRODUCTION

It is a truism that science generally moves forward by well-conceived hypothesis and experimentation, but also on occasion by mistakes and unexpected observations. The discovery of adjuvant arthritis (AA), some 40 years ago, is an excellent example of the latter; the unintentioned appearance of polyarthritis must have been a real surprise to Stoerk and his colleagues at the time. While studying immune reactivity to homologous tissue in the rat, Stoerk *et al.* (1954) observed that their rats developed red, painful swellings in several joints 2–3 weeks after injection of spleen extracts emulsified in Freund's complete adjuvant. This polyarthritis developed and persisted in the presence of antibiotics, leading the authors to conclude that the polyarthritis was not due to the presence of a pathogen, but may have resulted from sensitization against an 'organ specific antigen'. Carl Pearson (1956) extended these initial observations by showing that tissue extracts were unnecessary and the Freund's adjuvant alone was capable of inducing the polyarthritis. Thus, the first model was born and over the next four decades it has become a major vehicle in the search for anti-arthritic drugs and as a means of gaining insight into inflammatory arthritic diseases of man.

The speculation that AA may be due to sensitization against an 'organ specific antigen' by Stoerk *et al.* (1954) has not been resolved, and investigators are still puzzling over the cause of the polyarthritis in the rat. A plausible hypothesis emerged around the possible involvement of heat shock proteins (HSPs) in the pathogenesis of AA and human rheumatoid arthritis (RA) (van Eden *et al.*, 1988), which will be fully discussed below, but Carl Pearson, who passed away not so long ago, would no doubt smile were he to be aware that modern science remains unable to solve why rats develop polyarthritis when subjected to heat-killed mycobacteria administered in an oil vehicle.

Looking back over the past four decades, since AA entered the literature and this author had reached the grand old age of 11 years, it is salutary to recognize that the original papers, mentioned above, are too old to appear on any of the screens utilizing modern literature searching, which go all the way back to 1964! Also missed by such technology would be the papers describing the initial use of AA, by Newbould (1963), as a means of finding potential drugs for inflammatory arthritis, plus the fact that this polyarthritis could be transferred to naive hosts by passive transfer of primed lymphocytes (Waksman and Wennersten, 1963).

There is a quite understandable tendency nowadays to quote the literature concurring with the tidal wave of recent progress, but this often fails to recognize that others have had similar thoughts over the years. AA exemplifies this well; for example, antibodies to T lymphocytes are very topical for treatment of human disease (Horneff *et al.*, 1991), but Currey and Ziff (1968) were aware of the effectiveness of anti-

Mechanisms and Models in Rheumatoid Arthritis
ISBN 0–12–340440–1

lymphocyte serum against AA over two decades ago. Suppressor cells are now being lauded as targets for therapeutic intervention (Badger and Swift, 1993), but Kayashima and his colleagues (1976, 1978) were advocating their importance in AA in the mid-1970s. Considering the relatively long history of AA, it is not surprising that attention should return to previous ideas and conclusions and even to question some; recently, in fact, some of the cherished dogmas have been challenged. AA has long been considered a phenomenon exclusive to the rat, since the early work of Glenn and Gray (1965) and Graeme *et al.* (1966) who failed to produce AA in a whole range of species, from mice to chickens, pigs and the dog. However, Knight *et al.* (1992) have now shown convincingly that AA can develop in the mouse. Like the very first observation in the rat, the observation of AA in the mouse was a fortuitous accident; Knight *et al.* (1992) were trying to reproduce the experimental lupus syndrome described by Mendlovic *et al.* (1988), only to find a polyarthritis. Even more fundamental, the requirement for the adjuvant itself has been challenged. It has been known for many years that the mycobacterial component of Freund's adjuvant could be replaced by non-antigenic arthritogens such as muramyl dipeptide (Kohashi *et al.*, 1980) or the lipoidal amine CP20961 (Avridene, Pfizer) by Chang *et al.* (1980), but both Kleinau *et al.* (1991) and Cannon *et al.* (1993a) have recently demonstrated that incomplete Freund's adjuvant (IFA), which lacks the mycobacteria, can induce AA in DA strain rats. AA still has some surprises!

This chapter focuses on the way AA has developed over the years, particularly for shedding light, or not, on the pathogenesis of the human conditions. Its use in the discovery of drugs for treatment of human inflammatory arthritis is discussed briefly, but no attempt is made to detail the methodology for producing and measuring AA in the rat, nor to list the numerous agents and drugs that influence this experimental syndrome. These aspects have been reviewed many times in the past and the present author has covered the topic at least three times (most recently in Billingham, 1990).

This review highlights those facets that have stimulated the author's attention over nigh on three decades of involvement.

ADJUVANTS AND THE NATURE OF THE ANTIGEN/S RESPONSIBLE FOR INDUCTION OF POLYARTHRITIS

At the time of their original observations in 1954, Stoerk and his colleagues postulated that the adjuvant properties of the Freund's adjuvant had sensitized their rats to some 'organ specific antigen' which subsequently led to the development of polyarthritis. Following Pearson's (1956) finding that homologous tissue extracts were unnecessary, a view developed that materials in the mycobacteria may crossreact with self components, so a search began to find the arthritogenic substance in mycobacteria. Pearson and Wood (1959) and Waksman *et al.* (1960) showed it to reside in the wax D fraction of mycobacteria and it was subsequently identified as a peptidoglycan (Jolles *et al.*, 1964; Migliore and Jolles, 1968). Coincident with this initial search for the arthritogenic component, it was found that *Mycobacterium tuberculosis* (*M.tb*, the original component in Freund's adjuvant) could be replaced by other mycobacterial strains, provided they were suspended in mineral or vegetable oils; furthermore *Nocardia asteroides* (Flax and Waksman, 1963) and, later on, *Corynebacterium rubrum* (Paronetto, 1970) were also found to be arthritogenic in mineral oil. Azuma *et al.*

(1972) characterized the peptidoglycan further as a mycolic acid–arabinogalactan mucopeptide and found that similar structures could be extracted from corynebacteria and nocardia, thereby explaining why all these species could elicit AA in the rat. The next instalment in this saga was provided by Kohashi and his colleagues (1976, 1977), who were able to extract water-soluble arthritogenic peptidoglycans from arthritogenic and non-arthritogenic bacterial cell walls, including lactobacilli, staphylcoccal, clostridial and streptococcal species. Clearly, a variety of bacteria contain arthritogenic, adjuvant materials and development of arthritis will depend on the availability or extractability, *in vivo*, of the arthritogenic peptidoglycan. Final determination of the arthritogenic component eventually occurred 25 years after Stoerk *et al.*'s original observation, when Kohashi and his colleagues (1980) identified that muramyl dipeptide (MDP), the minimum adjuvant component within mycobacteria and other Gram-positive bacteria, was capable of inducing AA in Lewis rats when emulsified in mineral oil.

In retrospect, the discovery of the ability of MDP to induce AA by Kohashi *et al.* (1980) marked a watershed in the history of this polyarthritis since, in fact, MDP is non-antigenic. Coincidentally, Chang *et al.* (1980) demonstrated that another non-antigenic adjuvant, CP20961, a lipoidal amine from Pfizer, could also induce an AA which was 'essentially identical to classical AA induced by mycobacteria'. These results called into question the earlier thoughts that immunity to mycobacteria, or other arthritogenic bacteria, was necessary for the induction of the polyarthritis, and would also appear to rule out the thesis that these bacteria contain an antigen that crossreacts with self, thereby eliciting arthritis. However, the adjuvant properties of even the non-antigenic arthritogens may well activate reactivity to some component within joints which leads to induction of AA. This, in part, lies at the heart of the thesis of the proponents of the heat shock protein (HSP) driven aetiology of AA and human RA, of which more will be discussed below. Intriguingly, the results of Kleinau *et al.* (1991) and Cannon *et al.* (1993a), demonstrating the ability of IFA to induce AA in the highly susceptible DA strain, add a new twist to the role of adjuvants in the process of arthritis induction. Devoid of mycobacteria, IFA is not a strong adjuvant but can elicit T-lymphocyte responsiveness against a number of antigens, including mycobacterial HSPs (Kingston *et al.*, manuscript submitted). Thus 40 years down the track, we are still not certain if an antigen, either endogenous or exogenous, is responsible for inducing AA when a variety of materials with the ability to boost immune reactivity are administered to the rat in oil vehicles, though scientists with an immunological viewpoint are convinced that an antigen/s exists that initiates and drives this arthritic disease process.

THE HSP SAGA

It is clear from the experiments involving non-antigenic adjuvants as arthritogens, for example MDP and CP20961, that epitopes on the bacterial walls which crossreact with host components are not essential for initiation and development of the polyarthritis. Nevertheless, it seems reasonable to suggest that such powerful immune stimulants could boost reactivity to some component within the joint which subsequently leads on to arthritis. Two potential candidates have arisen during the past 20 years and have been extensively studied for a pathogenic role in AA and human RA, namely type II collagen, the cartilage phenotype (Trentham *et al.*, 1977), and HSPs (van Eden *et al.*, 1988). Collagen-induced arthritis is essentially a separate entity to AA, despite considerable similarities in relation to time of onset after challenge and histopathology, and will not be discussed further in the context of initiating antigens. This model is discussed in detail in Chapters 21 and 23, this volume. HSPs, however, have enjoyed considerable publicity as antigens which could be responsible for initiation and chronicity of inflammatory arthritis.

The story leading to the proposal that HSPs may be pathogenic for arthritis began with the isolation by Irun Cohen's group in Israel of an arthritogenic T-cell line that could initiate AA in Lewis rats (Holoshitz *et al.*, 1983). Essentially, two cell lines were isolated, one which initiated arthritis in irradiated rats, A2b, and another, A2c, which could suppress the developing and established phases of the disease. The group showed a little later that these cloned T-cell lines proliferated in the presence of cartilage extracts (van Eden *et al.*, 1985) and also that T lymphocytes from RA patients showed augmented reactivity to a fraction of mycobacteria crossreactive with with cartilage (Holoshitz *et al.*, 1986). This fraction of mycobacteria, recognized by the T lymphocytes in AA, was eventually cloned by van Eden *et al.* (1988) and shown to be a nonapeptide that shared homology with a peptide on the mammalian cartilage link protein, with four of the amino acids identical. Therefore it appeared at the time, that a breakthrough had occurred in our understanding of the pathogenesis if AA, and perhaps human RA.

In their initial reports on the epitope, and with the recombinant mycobacterial HSP (r65 kDa HSP), van Eden *et al.* (1988) administered the r65 kDa HSP in saline intraperitoneally to rats, but instead of initiating arthritis the rats were rendered tolerant to further attempts to induce arthritis with mycobacteria in oil vehicles. Along similar lines, van den Broek *et al.* (1989) showed that streptococcal cell wall (SCW) induced arthritis could also be prevented by pretreatment with mycobacterial r65 kDa HSP. These initial experiments failed to establish any potential arthritogenic properties of the HSP, but the optimal way for inducing AA is to administer the arthritogen intradermally in the foot pad of at the base of the tail, in an oily vehicle. Billingham and his colleagues (1990a) addressed these remaining issues surrounding the arthritogenic potential of the 65 kDa HSP, though, even at the time, knowledge from histopathological studies that articular cartilage is usually spared from degradative destruction during development of AA, posed a question in the mind of the author as to the validity of this otherwise intriguing hypothesis.

When whole mycobacteria are administered in oil to rats to initiate AA, normally between 100 and 250 μg are given and the 65 kDa HSP would represent just a fraction of this (reviewed in Billingham, 1990). The experiments undertaken by Billingham *et al.* (1990a) involved giving 1–250 μg of mycobacterial r65 kDa HSP emulsified in IFA into the base of the tail; no arthritis was seen at any level, even those way above the amount present in whole mycobacteria. However, the HSP antigen given as whole mycobacteria would have the benefit of the presence of an adjuvant to boost reactivity to the HSP, namely the peptidoglycans containing MDP. To compensate for this, Billingham *et al.* (1990a) emulsified the r65 kDa HSP with a small non-arthritogenic level of the adjuvant CP20961, yet still no arthritis was observed. What was found, however, was that the rats pretreated with the HSP were resistant to further attempts to induce arthritis with mycobacteria or the lipoidal amine adjuvant CP20961, though protection was not as complete as with mycobacterial rechallenge. In the same series of experiments r65 kDa HSP pretreatment reduced the severity of type II collagen-induced arthritis.

Whilst these experiments demonstrated that the 65 kDa HSP was unable to initiate AA, they do not preclude a role in the maintenance of arthritis in those few strains of rat with persistent disease nor in human RA. The fact that T lymphocytes from arthritic rats and RA patients proliferate on contact with the antigen is suggestive of such a role, but many other antigenic epitopes could also provide such a stimulus to chronicity of arthritis. The most interesting aspect of this work is the protection afforded against arthritis development following pretreatment with the HSP, which was specific and total for mycobacterial rechallenge, but which also limited the development of CP20961 and type II collagen arthritis. This will be discussed below when mechanisms of natural remission are described, since this is where AA could provide real insight for the control of human arthritis and novel therapy.

Before leaving HSPs, however, the story has become more complicated by observations by Cannon and his colleagues (1993b) where IFA, when administered alone to DA strain rats, also has the ability to prevent the development of AA in these rats when rechallenged with mycobacteria in oil. We have observed the same effect in Lewis rats using both paraffin oil or IFA pretreatment; these observations call into question the absolute need for the HSP for protection against AA. Our own experience is that IFA and paraffin oil pretreatment increases lymphocyte proliferative activity to antigens such as the 65 kDa HSP and PPD from mycobacteria when the lymphocytes are cultured with these antigens (Hicks *et al.*, manuscript submitted). Additionally, if cyclosporine (CSA) is administered at the same time as the pretreatment with 65 kDa HSP, IFA or paraffin oil, then the protective effect of all these against arthritis development on rechallenge with arthritogens is abrogated, indicating that the phenomenon requires a lymphokine activated phase (Hicks *et al.*, manuscript submitted). Clearly, IFA and paraffin oil with or without the HSP can perturb the immune system, a conclusion also reached by Cannon *et al.* (1993a) who found that IFA could induce a mild transient arthritis in the DA rat. All such treatments may induce a suppressor population of lymphocytes with the ability to protect against arthritis; more on this later.

AETIOLOGY AND PATHOGENESIS

A diverse collection of materials, both antigenic and non-antigenic, leads to the expression of a polyarthritis in the rat which tends to have a broadly similar histopathology, regardless of the initiating arthritogen (Billingham, 1990). Pannus tissue forms within many of the articulating joints of the fore and hind feet leading to destruction of cartilage and bone in a manner similar to that seen in human RA, though over a period of just a few weeks. However, the most prominent reaction is a periostitis outside the joint, which occurs at sites of ligament and muscle insertion, resulting in bone loss and massive new bone and osteoid formation along the areas of periosteal reactivity. There is also profound bone removal and reformation within the tarsals, metatarsals, carpals and metacarpals and other small bones of the wrists and feet. Similar bone remodelling also occurs in the spine, scapulae and skull, again at sites of ligament and muscle insertion.

Despite the fact that we remain unaware of the identity of the antigen/s responsible for the induction of such pathological changes during AA in the rat, we are undoubtedly a little, perhaps much, wiser for undertaking the search. Similarly, our inability to prove or disprove the premise of Stoerk *et al.* in 1954, that AA is due to sensitization to an 'organ specific antigen', does not detract from what we have learnt along the way, namely, a great deal about cellular and molecular mechanisms that are responsible for initiation, maintenance and, finally, natural remission of this experimental arthritis. These are fully described below as they may throw light on aspects of the human inflammatory arthritic disease.

CELLULAR INDUCTION MECHANISMS

There is considerable evidence now that all the arthritogenic adjuvants stimulate a series of cellular events leading to T-lymphocyte activation which in turn initiates the polyarthritis. The first real evidence for this was way back in 1963 when Flax and Waksman demonstrated that 'sensitized' lymphocytes from the thoracic duct of rats stimulated with mycobacteria could transfer arthritis passively to naive syngeneic hosts. The validity of these early experiments was questioned by Quagliata and Phillips-Quagliata (1972) on the grounds that washed thoracic duct cells did not transfer arthritis; they had found it necessary to add small amounts of mycobacteria to the thoracic duct lymphocytes for successful transfer of arthritis. However, such quibbles became irrelevant when Taurog and his colleagues (1983) adoptively transferred arthritis to naive rats with T lymphocytes from *M. tb* stimulated rats which had been expanded and stimulated in culture with the mitogen conconavalin A (con A); the successful development of arthritogenic T-cell lines by Holoshitz *et al.* (1983) also confirmed this primary role for the T lymphocyte in arthritis induction. Prior to this, however, evidence from Currey and Ziff (1968), showing that anti-lymphocyte serum could inhibit AA, and that the disease would not develop in athymic nude mice (Kohashi *et al.*, 1982), clearly pointed to T-lymphocyte involvement. The results of Taurog *et al.* (1983) suggested that the lymphocytes involved in the adoptive transfer of arthritis were of the helper T-lymphocyte subset, since they bound the anti-CD4 mAb W3/25 originally described by White *et al.* (1978); this was finally proven in studies by Billingham *et al.* (1990b) who demonstrated that the anti-CD4 mAbs OX35 and W3/25 were very effective inhibitors of the development of AA induced by both mycobacteria and the non-antigenic adjuvant CP20961 (Billingham, 1994).

The involvement of $CD4^+$ T-helper lymphocytes in the induction of arthritis implies interaction with an antigen-presenting cell, leading to cell-mediated reactivity. Springer (1990) has illustrated the main molecular interactions involved in this process (see Fig. 1) although there are other peripheral interactions which modulate the overall reactivity, for example with cytokines and their receptors such as IL2/IL2r. mAbs have proved invaluable in working out which cells and receptors are essential for the induction of AA, a topic which has been extensively reviewed recently (Billingham, 1994).

It is now clear that mAbs to any of the receptors shown in Fig. 1 can inhibit the development of AA induced by mycobacteria and, where investigated, the disease induced CP20961. Historically, Larsson *et al.* (1985) were the first to use mAbs in AA, demonstrating that anti-pan T was moderately effective against the disease and that anti-CD8 (anti-cytotoxic/suppressor) was ineffective. In terms of Fig. 1, a comprehen-

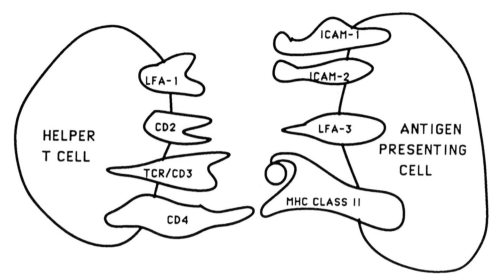

Figure 1. Molecular interactions involved in MHC class II restricted antigen presentation to helper T lymphocytes. After Springer (1990).

sive study was undertaken by Billingham *et al.* (1990b) in AA induced by mycobacteria. Anti-CD4 mAbs were found to be very effective inhibitors of the development of AA, in fact, complete suppression of symptoms could be obtained. This was associated with profound depletion of circulating cells bearing CD4, and when these returned to normal levels, 15–20 days after treatment, arthritis remained suppressed despite the persistence of arthritogenic mycobacteria within the tissues; it appeared that such rats had become resistant/tolerant to the arthritis-inducing properties of the mycobacteria. The inhibitory properties of the anti-CD4 mAb, OX 35, are shown in Fig. 2, where it is clear that the response is dose related; mAbs act like other anti-inflammatory and anti-arthritic drugs in this respect. Anti-Ia mAbs, directed to the MHCII complex on antigen-presenting cells, similarly produced a dose-related effect against arthritis development (Billingham *et al.*, 1990b) and in a series of elegant experiments in Frank Emmrich's laboratory in Erlangen, Yoshino *et al.* (1990a,b) demonstrated that a mAb to the rat αβ T-cell receptor (TCR) R.73, also inhibited development of AA in a dose-related manner. Finally, in relation to Fig. 1, Iigo *et al.* (1991) demonstrated that an antibody to rat ICAM1 inhibited the development of AA induced by mycobacteria. All this evidence is consistent with a mechanism of induction involving MHC class II-restricted antigen presentation to helper T lymphocytes, though we are uncertain of the nature of the antigen. The fact that much of what applies to AA induced by mycobacteria, also applies to AA induced by the non-antigenic arthritogen CP20961 (Billingham, 1994), further implies that the antigen is of host origin. The reader should refer to Chapter 4, this volume, for a review of the use of anti-leukocyte therapy in man.

CELLULAR CHRONOLOGY AT LESION SITES

MAbs to cell surface antigens have proved invaluable for determining which cell types are involved in the induction of AA when used pharmacologically, they can also be

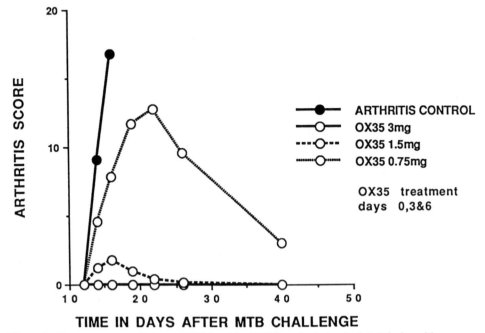

Figure 2. Dose response of the anti/CD4 mAb, OX35 against classical AA induced by mycobacteria in oil. The anti-CD4 mAb produced a dose related inhibition of arthritis development in much the same manner as standard anti-arthritic drugs. The arthritis was scored as described in Billingham *et al.* (1990a). Note the onset of natural remission after day 23 in the low dose OX35 group. This and all the experiments described below were performed in the Lewis rat.

used immunohistochemically to establish the time course of appearance of such cells within arthritic lesion sites. The problem with classical AA, involving mycobacteria, is that this material becomes widely distributed within the tissues of the rat and as it immunogenic in its own right, as well as arthritogenic, sites that develop arthritis may also contain mycobacteria which could attract cells for reasons other than a potential to initiate arthritis. In other words, humoral and cell-mediated immunity to the mycobacteria complicate the unravelling of the cellular events leading to AA, which we now know are due to the adjuvant properties of the non-antigenic muramyl dipeptide component of mycobacteria, as has been discussed above in detail.

To overcome this problem of interpretation, Meacock *et al.* (1994) studied cell traffic to the developing lesion sites of AA induced by the non-antigenic, arthritogenic adjuvant CP20961. This induces an identical arthritis to that seen with mycobacteria in the Lewis rat, but would have largely disappeared from the rat by the time of symptom appearance; visible signs of arthritis occur around 10–12 after injection of this adjuvant (Billingham, 1994; Meacock *et al.*, 1994). These first signs of arthritic swelling were associated with macrophages and polymorphonuclear cells in growing pockets of oedema adjacent to ankle joints and within soft tissue. Rarely, an odd cell bearing a lymphocyte marker was seen in synovial tissue in much the same manner as in control synovial tissue, so it is unlikely that T lymphocytes contributed directly to the initiation of this early phase of inflammation, during days 11–14. From day 18 onwards the predominant invading cells were stained with either macrophage or T lymphocyte markers, often occurring together in joint synovium, at the interface with eroding bone and at tendon and ligament insertion points. Since staining with anti-Ia was also intense at such sites, the opportunity to process and present autoantigen was possible; Meijers *et al.* (1993) demonstrated that local cathepsin activity was also high at such sites of macrophage interaction within eroding pannus in this model of AA (see Chapter 17, this volume, for a discussion of the role of cathepsins in joint damage).

Examination of the lymphoid tissue of these diseased rats revealed an early production of lymphocytes bearing the activation marker IL2r within lymph nodes draining the injection site of CP20961. These may be the cells that initiate AA and transfer the disease to naive hosts, but it is unclear how they might direct the initial wave of macrophages to the sites of disease development. Van de Langerijt *et al.* (1994) have taken this analysis one stage further by labelling the cells that transfer AA with fluorescent dyes to determine where such cells migrate during adoptive transfer of the disease. Interestingly, while blood, lymph nodes, spleen and liver contained many labelled cells up to 14 days after transfer, the authors were unable to detect any fluorescent lymphocytes within putative lesion sites, despite the transfer of 1–500 million labelled lymphocytes of which the majority were IL2r positive. Perhaps a few reactive lymphocytes responsible for arthritis initiation within lesion sites were missed in the experiments of Van de Langerijt *et al.* (1994), but the evidence indicates that while T lymphocytes are responsible for the development of arthritis they appear to do so remotely from outside of the actual lesions. Macrophages are apparently induced to initiate the inflammation and are followed into the lesion by other lymphocytes. Additional evidence for this comes from other studies of Van de Langerijt *et al.* (1994) in which AA was adoptively transferred to nude Lewis rats. Only nude rats reconstituted with naive T lymphocytes were capable of developing AA; by themselves the apparently arthritogenic T lymphocytes were incapable of inducing the disease.

All the available evidence points, therefore, to a CD4$^+$ helper T lymphocyte bearing the $\alpha\beta$ TCR as being responsible for initiating AA. The initial events are very similar to the priming for MHC class II restricted T-cell immunity as illustrated in Fig. 1, though the antigen is unknown. It also remains to be proven whether or not these T lymphocytes initiate the early inflammation; this appears to be the role of the macrophage but the labelling/cell tracking experiments of Van de Langerijt *et al.* (1994) may have missed a very few, very influential T lymphocytes. The lower limit for T cell involvement in RA is discussed by Panayi in Chapter 4, this volume. Later on, T lymphocytes do enter the lesions but these could contain a suppressor population, in addition to effector cells, as will be discussed below. What is interesting is that both macrophages and T lymphocytes are found at tendon and ligament insertion points at such times in AA, the sites which are also associated with the initiation of human RA (Buckland-Wright, 1984).

INDUCTION OF TOLERANCE OF ADJUVANT ARTHRITIS

Part of the folklore amongst those who have worked with AA over several years is the observation that rats who have developed and recovered from AA are resistant to attempts to reactivate the disease by further administration of mycobacteria in oil vehicles. It is also known that pretreatment with small, non-arthritogenic levels of mycobacteria prevents the later development of the disease when full arthritogenic levels are administered (Eugui and Houssay, 1975; Tsukano et al., 1983). Aspects of these early studies may also account for the prevention of AA by pretreatment with mycobacterial HSPs, described above. The studies of Eugui and Houssay (1975), Tsukano et al. (1983) and Larsson et al. (1991) have implicated the induction of suppressor cells which confer the anti-arthritic activity of the various pretreatments.

An interesting observation seen with the prevention of AA using the mAbs directed to the CD4 cluster on helper T lymphocytes, for example W3/25 and OX35, was that these rats were also resistant to further rechallenge with mycobacteria in oil (Billingham et al., 1990b). These rats had received full arthritogenic levels of mycobacteria but disease had been totally inhibited by the mAbs, and remained so even after the depleted T lymphocyte had returned to normal levels; no AA developed after subsequent mycobacterial rechallenge in these animals. It was unclear, however, if this phenomenon involved the emergence of a discreet suppressor T cell population when the CD4$^+$ helper T lymphocytes, which had been totally depleted by anti-CD4 treatment, returned to their normal blood levels (Billingham et al., 1990b), as has been implicated by Eugui and Houssay (1975), Kayashima and colleagues (1976, 1978), Tsukano et al. (1983) and Larsson et al. (1991) for suppression of AA in their low mycobacterial pretreatment studies.

Additional studies (Billingham, 1994) demonstrated that Lewis rats, in which the development of AA induced by the arthritogenic lipoidal amine, CP20961, had been prevented by anti-CD4 treatment, were resistant to rechallenge with CP20961, but even more interestingly, they were resistant to rechallenge with mycobacteria. The converse was also true; rats made tolerant to AA induced by mycobacteria with anti-CD4 mAbs were resistant to rechallenge with CP20961 – this is illustrated in Fig. 3. Van den Broek (1992a) took this story further when they demonstrated that anti-CD4 mAbs could prevent the development of SCW-induced arthritis; interestingly, these Lewis rats were resistant to further attempts to induce SCW arthritis and, more significantly, they were also resistant to classical AA induced by mycobacteria. This phenomenon of induction of resistance to arthritis by anti-CD4 mAbs is analogous to the tolerance to certain soluble antigens induced in mice by anti-CD4 mAb treatment, as described by Benjamin et al. (1988).

The fact that induction of resistance/tolerance to either mycobacterial-, CP20961- or SCW-induced polyarthritis, by anti-CD4 mAbs, confers a cross resistance to the other arthritogens implies that they all induce arthritis by a similar induction pathway, perhaps even via the same antigen/s. Also, the finding that anti-CD4 induced resistance/tolerance to the lipoidal amine CP20961, which is a non-antigenic arthritogen, further implies that the initiating antigen/s is of host origin and, therefore, less likely to be derived from a bacterial source such as mycobacteria or SCW.

In their earlier studies (Billingham et al., 1990b) it was found that type II collagen induced arthritis could also be totally inhibited by anti-CD4 mAb treatment. What was unexpected was that upon rechallenge with type II collagen the rats developed a rapid, florid polyarthritis, demonstrating a surprising lack of tolerance to this arthritogen, though Benjamin et al. (1988) had commented that not all antigens could be tolerized with anti-CD4 treatment. Later experiments (Billingham, 1994) demon-

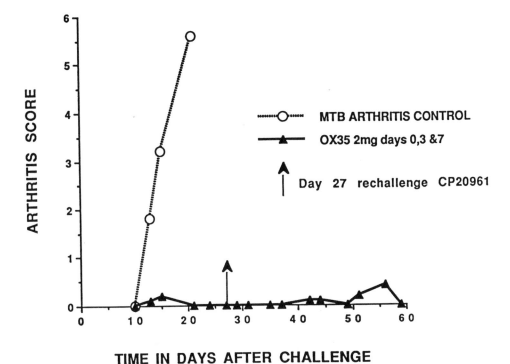

Figure 3. Tolerance to AA induced by mycobacteria, following anti-CD4 treatment, also confers tolerance to AA induced by lipoidal amine CP20961.

strated that the rats in which type II collagen-induced arthritis had been prevented by anti-CD4 mAb treatment remained fully susceptible to CP20961 and mycobacterially induced AA. Further, rats that were tolerant to AA, induced with either mycobacteria or CP20961, were not only susceptible to type II collagen-induced arthritis, but the polyarthritis occurred earlier and was more severe. These experiments added the final touch to the earlier views of Kaibara *et al.* (1984), Cremer *et al.* (1990) and Holmdahl and Kvick (1992) who clearly stated that the adjuvant arthritides and those induced by articular collagens are separate diseases, despite their very similar appearance then viewed histopathologically, as was described above.

SUPPRESSION AND REMISSION MECHANISMS OF ADJUVANT ARTHRITIS

Another facet of AA, familiar to those who use these model diseases, is that they are relatively short lived. Symptoms appear around days 10–12 after giving the arthritogen, but tend to wane visibly shortly afterwards. This can occur as early as day 20–22 after the arthritogen but varies with the strain of rat used (Billingham, 1990, for review). This phenomenon, which is essentially natural remission, can be clearly seen in Figs 2 and 4 where remission occurs early in this strain of Lewis rat (OLAC, Bicester, Oxon, UK). It is clear from what has been said above that a CD4[+] helper T lymphocyte subpopulation is responsible for the initiation of adjuvant AA, but what is responsible (i.e. which cells and molecular mechanisms) for the remission of this

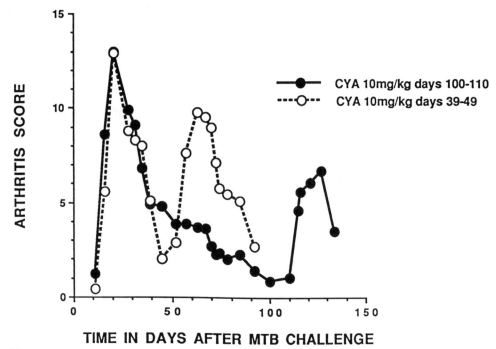

Figure 4. Reactivation of AA by cyclosporin A after natural remission has occurred. A short pulse of therapy can reactivate the disease after a few months of remission. This only occurs, however when the arthritogen persists; it was not seen with the lipoidal amine or after adoptive transfer of arthritis with T lymphocytes.

disease? Furthermore, why are some strains of rat more susceptible than others; are there suppressor mechanisms that limit disease development or intensity; and how is it that pretreatment with small amounts of arthritogens (e.g. mycobacteria or SCW, or bacterial HSPs and even mineral oils or IFA) can limit or prevent the development of these various forms of polyarthritis? Lastly, are these various mechanisms that modulate AA related or are they distinct, and do they have anything in common with the tolerance to arthritis induced by anti-CD4 mAbs, or is this another way of achieving that same end result? These are difficult questions to answer but have been touched upon over the years. They also represent where attention should be focused in future, since, as is the case with many diseases, prevention may well be easier or better than cure.

Eugui and Houssay (1975) were amongst the first to suggest that both the effector and remission phases of AA were controlled by discrete populations of lymphocytes. They investigated the phenomenon of suppression of AA induced by subarthritogenic levels of mycobacterial adjuvant and found that the unresponsiveness so produced could be transferred to naive syngeneic recipients with lymph node cells from the unresponsive donors. Tsukano *et al.* (1983) added to these early results by proving that the suppression induced by low levels of mycobacteria was due to a T-lymphocyte subpopulation, which again could be adoptively transferred to naive recipients. Prior to this Kayashima *et al.* (1976, 1978) concluded that in low responder strains of rat, disease severity was influenced by thymus-derived cells which exerted a modulatory, suppressive influence on disease development. Thymectomy and treatments which abrogated the suppressor population, for example cyclophosphamide or hydrocortisone in appropriate doses, caused a marked enhancement of the severity of AA, leading Kayashima *et al.* (1978) to conclude similarly to Eugui and Houssay (1975), that two subpopulations of T lymphocyte control AA, one initiating the disease and the other modulating the severity. It is clearly possible, therefore that both antigen specific and non-specific regulatory suppressor mechanisms influence disease incidence and severity.

Some interesting experiments with germfree F344 rats (Kohashi *et al.* 1979; van den Broek *et al.* 1992b) shed some light on the origin of the non-specific resistance to AA seen with less susceptible strains of rat. Both groups found that this strain of rat, which is normally resistant to AA and SCW-induced arthritis, was fully susceptible when born and housed under germfree conditions. Kohashi *et al.* (1979) found that specific pathogen free F344 rats had intermediate susceptibility and concluded that presence of a bacterial flora in the gut was not necessary for AA development but could modulate the development of AA through induction of a suppressor population/s. Returning germfree, disease susceptible F344 rats to a conventional environment caused such rats to become resistant to SCW arthritis and to lose their T-lymphocyte responsiveness to SCW (van den Broek *et al.*, 1992b); no doubt these rats would also have been resistant to AA if put to the test.

Whether this is the way in which pretreatment with HSPs or low dose mycobacteria cause a more antigen-specific resistance to AA is unclear, as can also be said for the resistance seen with pretreatment with IFA and mineral oil (Cannon *et al.*, 1993b; Hicks *et al.*, manuscript submitted). T lymphocytes are certainly involved, as the resistance due to HSPs can be transferred to naive recipients (van den Broek *et al.*, 1989); furthermore, resistance to HSPs, and that seen with IFA and mineral oil, can be abrogated by concomitant treatment with CSA, indicating that it is a cytokine-mediated process. Further experiments are required to tie up the loose ends of this aspect, but there are clearly powerful mechanisms available for moderating or preventing the development of AA in different strains of rat, and which may be exploitable in the context of human disease. An additional factor to add to this equation is that the more susceptible strains of rat, for example Lewis, DA, appear to have a deficiency in the hypothalamic–pituitary–adrenal axis resulting in lower levels of corticosterone being secreted for a given stimulus (Sternberg *et al.*, 1989); however, it is unclear how this may influence the suppression and resistance pathways described above.

NATURAL REMISSION

At the beginning of this section, mention was made that AA tends to be short-lived and enters natural remission early after symptoms reach a peak (see Fig. 4). We have investigated this phenomenon to determine if a suppressor T-cell population may be involved in the process. In some early experiments we noticed that treatment of established AA with cyclosporin A was very effective in inhibiting the disease symptoms, but was always associated with a rebound of active arthritis when therapy was stopped; however, this rebound was not seen with an anti-inflammatory drug such as indomethacin. Prud'homme *et al.* (1991) recently reviewed the immunosuppressive properties of cyclosporin A, noting that whilst it is a potent immunosuppressive agent under certain circumstances, it can paradoxically augment some delayed type hypersensitivity reactions, aggravate autoimmune disease and even induce specific forms of autoimmunity. They further commented that cyclosporin A inhibits IL-2 and other cytokine production at the transcriptional level, but does not usually prevent antigen-specific priming of T cells such that these T cells may be poised to respond as soon as the drug is withdrawn. Their conclusions would provide an explanation for the rebound of arthritis described above, and the priming of T cells for AA development, prior to drug withdrawal. If rats are given cyclosporin A for 40 days, and the drug is then withdrawn, arthritis rapidly develops which ultimately goes into remission (Billingham, 1994). This contrasts with the effect of anti-CD4 mAb therapy of adjuvant disease, where tolerance to AA is induced by a short course of treatment, implying that tolerance and remission involve differing mechanisms (see Chapter 4, this volume).

It appears, therefore, that cyclosporin A influences the development and/or function of a suppressor cell population during the evolution of AA whose normal role would be to curtail excessive autoaggressive reactivity. Figure 4 shows that AA can, in fact, be rekindled by cyclosporin A immediately after natural remission and even a few months later, probably by inhibiting production of a suppressor cytokine at the transcriptional level; arthritogenic T-helper cells then gain ascendancy until the suppressor population regains control again. Nanishi and Battisto (1991) have, in fact, described a factor from T-suppressor cells that inhibits the ability of arthritogenic T cells to transfer AA to naive rats.

The identity of the suppressor population responsible for natural remission of AA has not been fully elucidated. Earlier studies (Billingham *et al.*, 1990b) demonstrated that anti-CD4 therapy could reduce established disease activity, but that this rebounded when therapy stopped, as was also described by Yoshino *et al.* (1990a) for their anti-TCR mAb in AA. This rebound was very similar to that seen after cyclosporin A which is suggestive of a T-lymphocyte subset involvement in suppression, possibly $CD4^+$, $\alpha\beta TCR^+$, but $IL-2r^-$, as anti-IL2r mAbs do not affect development of natural remission (Billingham, 1994). We subsequently found that this suppression of arthritis could be adoptively transferred to naive hosts with T lymphocytes obtained from rats in remission from AA. Larsson *et al.* (1989) have provided evidence for a $CD8^+$ T-cell involvement in the resistance to AA produced by pre-immunization with very small amounts of mycobacteria, described above; however, this may be a separate phenomenon to natural remission.

Others have subscribed to T-lymphocyte mediated suppression of arthritis and other models of autoimmunity in rodents. Myers *et al.* (1989) isolated a suppressor population from donors injected with type II collagen and showed they could inhibit development of type II collagen-induced arthritis. Karpus and Swanborg (1989) have described a $CD4^+$ T-suppressor cell that induces the remission of EAE in the rat, suggesting also that it mediates this suppression by differential inhibition of lymphokine production. Later work on the potential mechanism of this suppression by the $CD4^+$ population, suggests that both TGFβ (Karpus and Swanborg, 1991) and IL-4 (Karpus *et al.*, 1992) may be involved; a similar situation may pertain in AA.

It appears, therefore, that separate subsets of T lymphocytes battle for supremacy during the adjuvant models of arthritis described above; a conclusion reached by

Eugui and Houssay some 20 years earlier. Clearly, there are powerful mechanisms existing in animal models of autoimmunity for limiting the destruction that may be induced. However, this aspect has had nowhere near the attention of the effector side of the equation. Encouraging the natural mediation of suppression and down-regulation may be less compromising to host defence mechanisms than the more generally immunosuppressive approaches currently being pursued. The role of CD4 T cells in the pathogenesis of RA is discussed in detail in Chapters 2, 4 and 11, this volume.

USE OF AA FOR DRUG DISCOVERY

Newbould (1963) was the first to use AA as a screening test for potential anti-rheumatic drugs, demonstrating the effectiveness of aspirin, phenylbutazone, corticosteroids and gold, though Pearson and Wood (1959) had shown the model to be drug sensitive a little earlier. Since those pioneering studies, AA has become part of the testing cascade for most of the anti-inflammatory drugs currently in human rheumatology, and a host of 'hopefuls' that failed during development for one reason or other.

With time a major paradox became apparent with use, in AA, of the non-steroidal anti-inflammatory drugs (NSAIDs) which inhibit cyclooxygenase in the arachidonic acid cascade. These were found to inhibit AA and lower biochemical markers such as acute phase proteins (APP), essentially effecting a 'cure' of the model, but they have not been able to achieve this in human RA, exerting mainly symptomatic, anti-inflammatory and analgesic effects. Conversely, many of the drugs which exert the so-called disease modifying effect, associated with a lowering of the APP, and which are of value in the treatment of RA, struggle to demonstrate an effect against AA. This has been reviewed at length relatively recently by Hunneyball et al. (1989) and Billingham (1990). The hope at the height of the search for a 'super-aspirin' was that the troublesome side-effects of gastrointestinal (GI) irritation, associated with the NSAIDs, could be separated from the anti-inflammatory activity and, further, that a more potent agent may demonstrate disease-modifying activity in RA. Despite enormous effort neither objective was fully achieved, the GI side-effects largely remained, though some agents proved less troublesome than others and the goal of achieving disease remission of RA remained stubbornly elusive. Tenidap from Pfizer, however, appears to lower the APP in human RA (Loose et al., 1993) as well as being effective in AA (Otterness et al., 1991), though this is not a typical NSAID, having properties related to modulation of cytokine production, in addition to the inhibition of enzymes in the arachidonic acid cascade (Sipe et al., 1992).

Most commentators point out, in fact, that AA has considerable differences in comparison with human RA, particularly in relation to the histopathology, where AA has very significant periarticular and periosteal components that are never seen in RA. The dramatic osteoporosis seen within the small bones of the wrists and feet and laying down of new bone along the periosteum outside the joint do not occur in RA, but may help to explain the paradox, described earlier, in relation to the efficacy of NSAIDs and disease-modifying drugs in the AA models. Additionally, the lack of real chronicity of AA in most strains of rat could also contribute to this paradox (Billingham, 1990).

Inflammation in all species is associated with peroxidation of lipids and release of inflammatory mediators including reactive oxygen species, prostaglandins, lipoxygenase products and various peroxides including hydrogen peroxide. In the rat, the generation of hydrogen peroxide could be uniquely pertinent to the above paradox, particularly in relation to the excessive osteoporosis and new bone formation that characterize the disease. Hydrogen peroxide is a very potent activator of osteoclastic bone resorption in the rat (Bax *et al.*, 1992) and, from studies on the formation of hydrogen peroxide during lipid peroxidation and administration of peroxisome proliferating drugs (Reddy and Lalwani, 1983), it is known that induction of catalase, which breaks down hydrogen peroxide, is relatively poor in rat liver. Should a similar situation exist during inflammatory episodes within peripheral tissues, such as the periosteum in AA, the potential build up of hydrogen peroxide during the lipid peroxidation (Symans *et al.*, 1988) could result in the excessive osteoporosis seen with this polyarthritis; NSAIDs would be very effective inhibitors of this process through their ability to prevent the generation of peroxide intermediates.

Despite these issues, authors of the many papers describing another series of molecules that affects AA, either prophylactically or therapeutically, always finish on the note that they may be of use for the treatment of human inflammatory arthritis, observing that these models do resemble some aspects of the human disease. The present author (Billingham, 1990) commented that molecules that worked in AA should be taken forward to clinical trial, provided that they had no cyclooxygenase inhibitory properties, since the NSAIDs had not proven to be disease modifying. Tenidap may prove the exception to this rule, but previously only an occasional molecule that was active in AA, without cyclooxygenase activity, demonstrated disease-modifying activity in RA with an attendant fall in the APP and slowing of X-radiographic progression.

One molecule that was truly effective in AA and RA was clobuzarit, or Clozic as it was known during clinical trial. The history of this drug has been reviewed by Billingham and Rushton (1985). This agent emerged from a programme based on hypolipidaemic agents, essentially as a second generation clofibrate, but in early clinical trial was found to have little effect on lipids, though it lowered APP levels in patients with mild diabetes and atherosclerosis. Its profound effects in AA prompted clinical trial in human RA where is was found to induce clinical, biochemical and X-radiographic remission of RA. Development of the drug was abandoned when side-effects occurred, particularly with a new formulation (see Billingham and Rushton, 1985) but it had proven the point that AA could predict activity against human RA.

The most interesting aspect of clobuzarit was that it could lower APP in various chronic, connective tissue diseases, including atherosclerosis, the complications of diabetes and both rheumatoid and psoriatic arthritis, indicating disease modifying activity in all these conditions. Clearly, there are common mechanisms in all the diseases that are susceptible to a drug such as clobuzarit, and the fact that it has thyromimetic properties may suggest an influence via the thyroid receptor, a member of the steroid receptor superfamily. This family of receptors has further modulatory activity in AA via the corticosteroid and retinoid receptors and, of course, the steroids are still used in severe RA. This family of receptors may well provide the next generation of drugs for RA and other connective tissue diseases in the near future.

On the theme of activity in AA and RA, the immunosuppressive agent cyclosporin A is effective in both and so are anti-CD4 mAbs (reviewed by Emmrich *et al.*, 1994).

Antiproliferative agents are effective in both and methotrexate, in particular, is being widely used in RA nowadays (see Chapter 4, this volume).

While it is possible to make certain generalizations about drugs in AA, many scientists will have noticed that the strain of rat can make a difference; clobuzarit was never found by the author to work in Lewis rats and others have found that a particular strain is better for their chosen agent. This should not deter people from their use of AA in a search for anti-rheumatic drugs. Badger and Swift (1993) have found a new class of agent which up-regulates non-specific suppressor T lymphocytes and which is very effective against AA and other autoimmune disease; determination of its effect in the equivalent diseases of man is eagerly awaited.

CONCLUDING COMMENTS

On reflecting upon the last 40 years, it is interesting to speculate where research into inflammatory arthritis would be now if Stoerk and his colleagues had not stumbled upon AA in their attempts to boost immunity in rats with Freund's adjuvant. Perhaps someone else would have been pleasantly surprised whilst using the adjuvant, but it is quite possible that the discovery may never have occurred and we would be much the poorer for it. Research on the human inflammatory arthritides has fed information into studies of the model and vice versa, as exemplified by the HSP story, but it is difficult not to reach the conclusion that AA is a quite different beast from human RA. However, as was stated in the introduction, we have learnt a lot along the way and these polyarthritic models in the rat have provided considerable insight into human disease.

This review has concentrated on the cellular and molecular aspects of the aetiology and pathogenesis of AA rather than drug discovery, mainly because the therapeutic aspects have been covered so many times in the past. The long saga into antigen/s responsible for AA induction has been somewhat like a detective story, and is still unsolved, though we now know that bacterial antigens are unlikely candidates and that even the adjuvant is unnecessary in one highly susceptible DA strain, in which IFA can stimulate reactivity to some endogenous component or other and tip the balance in favour of arthritis. Whether this reactivity includes HSPs remains a speculation at present.

From studies with mAbs which either delete cell types, or inhibit their function, it is clear that this reactivity to endogenous component/s involves mainly, if not exclusively, MHC class II restricted presentation of antigen to induce cell-mediated immunity. However, the intriguing situation exists that these activated T lymphocytes do not appear at the lesion sites to initiate the polyarthritis, at least from adoptive transfer experiments; this role clearly falls to the macrophage from chronological studies of the immunohistopathology during lesion development. It is possible, however, that the comprehensive studies undertaken could have missed a few T lymphocytes! The added value of the mAb studies in AA and other experimental autoimmunities, is that they prompted the human trials which have considerably aided our understanding of the chronicity of RA. Anti-CD4 mAbs have been particularly useful in this respect and, additionally, they have shown by cross-tolerance experiments that the polyarthritis induced bacterial adjuvants, that is mycobacteria and SCW and that induced by the non-antigen lipoidal amine CP20961, probably have the same initiating mechanism; furthermore, this differs from that initiating type II collagen-induced poly-arthritis.

One major issue with AA in comparison with RA is the lack of real chronicity in most strains of rat. The human disease grumbles along for years, slowly destroying cartilage and bone beneath invasive pannus tissue, yet rat polyarthritis can develop and enter remission within a period 10–20 days, with massive destruction and re-modelling of connective tissue structures, This is controlled by different subsets of T lymphocyte in the main, but there is very little of the mesenchymal element described by Fassbender (1994, for review) as typical of RA. Essentially, this involves prolifer-ation and change of fibroblasts to a transformed phenotype, with subsequent erosion of matrix beneath this relatively anoxic pannus tissue. Lack of this mesenchymal element, together with the rapidity of onset and remission of AA, could well contrib-ute to the difficulty generally experienced in demonstrating activity of the well-characterized human disease modifying drugs in the polyarthritis models. Firestein and Zvaifler (1990) have also questioned the importance of T cells in the chronicity of RA, favouring a macrophage-mesenchymal axis; AA models are perhaps overly dominated by T cells.

Rapid remission of the AA models does, however, have its upside, as the aspect of real therapeutic potential that could emerge from AA models in relation to human disease would be an understanding of the molecular mechanisms of natural remission. Drugs that up-regulate the activity of suppressor cells may potentially be less hazard-ous than the general immunosuppressive strategies used at present. This is also the aspect of the HSP saga requiring further study, particularly as cyclosporin A abrogates the protective properties of these materials, and natural remission, in these animal models.

Finally, the credentials for any model of a human disease are established when the model demonstrates activity of drugs that are effective in the human condition. AA fulfils this criterion, despite the fact that not all the disease-modifying anti-rheumatoid drugs work in AA. Clobuzarit and gold salts have demonstrated inhibition of the biochemical parameters of RA activity, that is the APP, in association with a slowing of X-radiographic progression, but the strain of rat was critical to the inhibition of AA. This is likely to be an important consideration in the future, humans are individ-uals and so are strains of rat; as such, the first model will probably remain the one choice for selecting potential drugs to treat inflammatory arthritis in man.

ACKNOWLEDGEMENTS

My thanks are due to Caroline Hicks for her collaboration with the experimental work described herein, to Ann Kingston for her collaboration on the HSP saga and to Eli Lilly and Company for providing an environment which encourages basic studies to assist drug discovery. I would also like to acknowledge that Brian Newbould encour-aged me to elucidate the basis of AA; I have to remind him that it is taking longer than we both anticipated.

REFERENCES

Azuma I, Kanetsuna F, Kada Y, Takashima T & Yamamura Y (1972) Adjuvant polyarthritogenicity of cell walls of mycobacteria, nocardia and corynebacteria. *Jap J Micro Biol* **16**: 333–336.

Badger AM & Swift BA (1993) Therapeutic activity of SK and F 105685, a novel azaspirane with suppressor-cell inducing activity. *Clin Exp Rheumatol* (**supplement 8**): S107–S109.

Bax BE, Alam ASMT, Banerji B, Bax CMR, Bevis PJR, Stevens CR et al. (1992) Stimulation of osteoclastic bone resorption with hydrogen peroxide. *Biochem Biophys Res Comm* **183**: 1153–1158.

Benjamin RJ, Qin XI, Wise WP, Cobbold SP & Waldmann H (1988) Mechanisms of monoclonal antibody-facilitated tolerance induction: a possible role for the CD4 (L3T4) and CD11a (LFA-1) molecules in self-non-self discrimination. *Eur J Immunol* **18**: 1079–1088.

Billingham MEJ (1990) Models of arthritis and the search for anti-arthritic drugs. In Orme M Le (ed) *Int Encycl Pharm Therap*, **133**, *Anti-Rheumatic Drugs*, pp 1–48, New York: Pergamon Press.

Billingham MEJ (1994) Monoclonal antibody therapy of experimental arthritis: comparison with cyclosporin A for elucidating cellular and molecular disease mechanisms. In Davies E & Dingle JT (eds) *Immunopharmacology of Joints and Connective Tissues*, pp 65–86. London: Academic Press.

Billingham MEJ & Rushton A (1985) Clozic In Rainsford KD (ed) *Anti-inflammatory and Anti-rheumatic Drugs*, Vol. III. *Anti-rheumatic Drugs, Experimental Agents, and Clinical Aspects of Drug Use*, pp 31–64. Boca Raton, FL: CRC Press.

Billingham MEJ, Carney SL Butler R & Colston MJ (1990a) A mycobacterial 65kD heat shock protein induces antigen-specific suppression of adjuvant arthritis but is not itself arthritogenic. *J Exp Med* **171**: 339–344.

Billingham MEJ, Hicks CA & Carney SL (1990b) Monoclonal antibodies and arthritis. *Agents Actions* **29**: 77–87.

van den Broek MF, Hogervorst EJM, van Bruggen MCJ, van Eden W, van der Zee R & van den Berg W (1989) Protection against streptococcal cell wall-induced arthritis by pretreatment with the 65-kD mycobacteria heat shock protein. *J Exp Med* **170**: 449–466.

van den Broek MF, van de Langerigt LGM, van Bruggen MCJ, Billingham MEJ & van den Berg WB (1992a) Treatment of rats with monoclonal anti-CD4 induces long-term resistance to streptococcal cell wall-induced arthritis. *Eur J Immunol* **22**: 57–61.

van den Broek MF, van Bruggen MCJ, Koopman JP, Hazenberg MP & van der Berg WB (1992b) Gut flora induces and maintains resistance against streptococcal cell wall-induced arthritis in F344 rats. *Clin Exp Immunol* **88**: 313–317.

Buckland-Wright JC (1984) Microfocal radiographic examination of erosions in the wrist and hand of patients with rheumatoid arthritis. *Ann Rheum Dis* **43**: 160–171.

Canon GW, Woods ML, Clayton F & Griffiths MM (1993a) Induction of arthritis in DA rats with incomplete Freund's adjuvant. *J Rheumatol* **20**: 7–11.

Canon GW, Griffiths MM & Woods ML (1993b) Suppression of adjuvant-induced arthritis in DA rats by incomplete Freund's adjuvant. *Arthritis Rheum* **36**: 126–131.

Chang YH, Pearson CM & Abe C (1980) Adjuvant polyarthritis, IV. Induction by a synthetic adjuvant: immunologic, histopathologic and other studies. *Arthritis Rheum* **23**: 62–71.

Cremer MA, Townes AS & Kang AH (1990) Adjuvant-induced arthritis in rats. Evidence that autoimmunity to homologous collagens types I, II, IX and XI is not involved in the pathogenesis of arthritis. *Clin Exp Immunol* **82**: 307–312.

Currey HLF & Ziff M (1968) Suppression of adjuvant disease in the rat with heterologous anti-lymphocyte serum. *J Exp Med* **127**: 185–203.

van Eden W, Holoshitz J, Nevo A, Frenkel A, Klajman A & Cohen IR (1985) Arthritis induced by an anti-mycobacterial T-cell clone that responds to cartilage proteoglycans. *Proc NY Acad Sci* **82**: 5117–5120.

van Eden W, Thole JER, van der Zee R, Noordzij A, van Embden JDA, Hensen EJ et al. (1988) Cloning of the mycobacterial epitope recognized by T-lymphocytes in adjuvant arthritis. *Nature* **331**: 171–173.

Emmrich F, Schulze-Koops H & Burmester G (1994) Anti-CD4 and other antibodies to cell surface antigens for therapy. In Davies E & Dingle JT (eds) *Immunopharmacology of Joints and Connective Tissues*, pp 87–117. London: Academic Press.

Eugui EM & Houssay RH (1975) Passive transfer of unresponsiveness by lymph node cells. Studies on adjuvant disease. *Immunology* **28**: 703–710.

Fassbender H-G (1994) Inflammatory reactions in arthritis. In Davies E & Dingle JT (eds) *Immunopharmacology of Joints and Connective Tissues*, pp 165–198. London: Academic Press.

Firestein E & Zveifler NJ (1990) How important are T-cells in chronic rheumatoid arthritis. *Arth Rheum* **33**: 768–773.

Flax HM & Wakeman BH (1963) Further immunologic studies of adjuvant disease in the rat. *Int Arch Allergy* **23**: 331–347.

Glenn EM & Gray J (1965) Adjuvant-induced polyarthritis in rats: biological and histologic background. *Am J Vet Res* **26**: 1180–1194.

Graeme ML, Fabry E & Sigg EB (1966) Mycobacterial adjuvant perarthritis in rodents and its modification by anti-inflammatory agents. *J Pharmac Exp Ther* **153**: 373–380.

Holmdahl R & Kvick C (1992) Vaccination and genetic experiments demonstrate that adjuvant-oil-induced arthritis and homologous type II collagen-induced arthritis in the same rat strain are different diseases. *Clin Exp Immunol* **88**: 96–100.

Holoshitz J, Drucker I, Yaretsky A, van Eden W, Klajman A, Lapidot Z et al. (1986) T-lymphocytes from rheumatoid arthritis patients show augmented reactivity to a fraction of mycobacteria cross-reactive with cartilage. *Lancet* **ii**: 305–309.

Holoshitz J, Naparstek Y, Ben-Nun A & Cohen IR (1983) Lines of T-lymphocytes induce or vaccinate against autoimmune arthritis. *Science* (Wash. DC) **217**: 56–58.

Horneff G, Burmester GR, Emmrich F & Kalden JR (1991) Treatment of rheumatoid arthritis with an anti-CD4 monoclonal antibody. *Arthritis Rheum* **34**: 129–140.

Hunneyball IM, Billingham MEJ & Rainsford KD (1989) Animal models of arthritic disease: influence of novel, compared with classical, antirheumatic agents. In Rainsford KD & Velo GP (eds) *New Developments in Antirheumatic Therapy*, pp 93–122. Dordrecht: Kluwer.

Iigo Y, Takashi T, Tamatani T, Miyasaka M, Higashida T, Yagita H et al. (1991) ICAM-1-dependent pathway is critically involved in the pathogenesis of adjuvant arthritis in rats. *J Immunol* **147**: 4167–4171.

Jolles P, Samour-Migliore D, De Wijs H & Lederer E (1964) Correlation of adjuvant activity and chemical structure of mycobacterial wax D fractions. The importance of amino sugars. *Biochem Biophys Acta* **83**: 361–363.

Kaibara N, Hotokebuchi T, Takagishi K, Katsuki I, Morinaga M, Arita C et al. (1984) Pathogenetic difference between collagen arthritis and adjuvant arthritis. *J Exp Med* **59**: 1388–1396.

Karpus WJ & Swanborg RH (1989) CD4$^+$ suppressor cells differentially affect the production of INF-g by effector cells of experimental autoimmune encephalomyelitis. *J Immunol* **143**: 3492–3497.

Karpus WJ & Swanborg RH (1991) CD4$^+$ suppressor cells inhibit the function of effector cells of experimental autoimmune encephalomyelitis through a mechanism involving transforming growth factor-β. *J Immunol* **146**: 1163–1168.

Karpus WJ, Gould KE & Swanborg RH (1992) CD4$^+$ suppressor cells of autoimmune encephalomyelitis respond to T cell receptor-associated determinants on effector cells by interleukin-4 secretion. *Eur J Immunol* **22**: 1757–1763.

Kayashima K, Koga T & Onoue K (1976) Role of T lymphocytes in adjuvant arthritis. I. Evidence for the regulatory function of thymus-derived cells in the induction of the disease. *J Immunol* **117**: 1878–1882.

Kayashima K, Koga T & Onoue K (1978) Role of T lymphocytes in adjuvant arthritis. II. Different subpopulations of T lymphocytes functioning in the development of the disease. *J Immunol* **120**: 1127–1131.

Kleinau S, Erlandsson H, Holmdahl R & Klareskog L (1991) Adjuvant oils induce arthritis in the DA rat. I. Characterisation of the disease and evidence for an immunological involvement. *J Autoimmun* **4**: 871–880.

Knight B, Katz DR, Isenberg DA, Ibrahim MA, Le Page S, Hutchings P et al. (1992) Induction of adjuvant arthritis in mice. *Clin Exp Immunol* **90**: 459–465.

Kohashi O, Pearson CM, Watanabe Y, Kotani S & Koga T (1976) Structural requirements for arthritogenicity of peptidoglycans from *Staphlococcus aureus* and *Lactobacillus plantarum* and analogous synthetic compounds. *J Immunol* **116**: 1635–1639.

Kohashi O, Pearson CM, Watanabe Y & Kotani S (1977) Preparation of arthritogenic hydrosoluble peptidoglycans from both arthritogenic and non-arthritogenic bacterial cell walls. *Infect Immun* **16**: 861–866.

Kohashi O, Kuwata J, Umehara K, Takahashi T & Ozawa A (1979) Susceptibility to adjuvant-induced arthritis among germfree, specific-pathogen-free, and conventional rats. *Infect Immun* **26**: 791–794.

Kohashi O, Tanaka A, Kotani S, Shiba T, Kusumoto S, Yokogawa K et al. (1980) Arthritis inducing ability of a synthetic adjuvant, N-acetyl muramyl dipeptides, and bacterial disaccharide peptides related to different oil vehicles and their composition. *Infect Immun* **29**: 70–75.

Kohashi O, Aihara K, Ozawa A, Kotani S & Azuma I (1982) New model of a synthetic adjuvant, N-acetylmuramyl-L-alanyl-D-isoglutamine-induced arthritis: clinical and histologic studies in athymic nude and euthymic rats. *Lab Invest* **47**: 27–36.

van de Langerijt AGM, Volsen SG, Hicks CA, Craig PJ, Billingham MEJ & van den Berg WB (1994) Cell migration studies in the adoptive transfer of adjuvant arthritis in the Lewis rat. *Immunology* **81**: 414–419.

Larsson P, Holmdahl R, Bencker L & Klareskog L (1985) *In vivo* treatment with W3/13 (anti-pan T) but not OX8 (anti-suppressor/cytotoxic T) monoclonal antibodies impedes the development of adjuvant arthritis. *Immunology* **56**: 383–391.

Larsson P, Holmdahl R & Klareskog L (1989) *In vivo* treatment with anti-CD8 and anti-CD5 monoclonal antibodies alters induced tolerance to adjuvant arthritis. *J Cell Biochem* **40**: 49–56.

Loose LD, Sipe JD, Kirby DS, Kraska AR, Weiner ES, Shanahan WR et al. (1993) Reduction of acute phase proteins with Tenidap sodium, a cytokine-modulating anti-rheumatic drug. *Br J Rheumatol* **33** (**supplement 3**): 19–25.

Meacock SCR, Brandon DR & Billingham MEJ (1994) Arthritis in the Lewis rat induced by the non-immunogenic adjuvant CP20961: and immunohistochemical analysis of the developing disease. *Annals Rheum Dis*, in press.

Meijers MHM, Koopdonk-Kool J, Meacock SCR, van Noorden CJF, Bunning RAD & Billingham MEJ (1993) Cysteine proteinase activity in the development of arthritis in an adjuvant model in the rat. *Agents Actions* **39** (supplement): C219–C221.

Mendlovic S, Brocke S, Shoenfeld Y, Ben-Bassat M, Meshorer A, Bakimer R & Moses E (1988) Induction of a systemic lupus erythematosus-like disease in mice by a common anti-DNA idiotype. *Proc Nat Acad Sci USA* **85**: 2260–2262.

Migliore D & Jolles P (1968) Contribution to the study of adjuvant wax D from mycobacteria, isolation of a peptidoglycan *FEBS Lett* **2**: 7–9.

Myers LK, Stuart JM & Kang AH (1989) A CD4 cell is capable of transferring suppression of collagen-induced arthritis. *J Immunol* **143**: 3976–3980.

Nanishi F & Battisto JR (1991) Down-regulation of adoptive adjuvant-induced arthritis by suppressor factor(s). *Arthritis Rheum* **34**: 180–186.

Newbould BB (1963) Chemotherapy of arthritis induced in rats by injection of mycobacterial adjuvant. *Br J Pharmacol* **21**: 127–136.

Otterness IG, Pazoles PP, Moore PF & Pepys MB (1991) C-reactive protein as an index of disease activity. Comparison of tenidap, cyclophosphamide and dexamethasone in rat adjuvant arthritis. *J Rheumatol* **18**: 505–511.

Paronetto F (1970) Adjuvant arthritis induced by *Corynebacterium rubrum*. *Proc Soc Exp Biol (NY)*. **133**: 296–298.

Pearson CM (1956) Development of arthritis, periarthritis and periostitis in rats given adjuvants. *Proc Soc Exp Biol (NY)* **91**: 95–101.

Pearson CM & Wood FD (1959) Studies of polyarthritis and other lesions induced in rats by injection of mycobacterial adjuvant. I. General clinical and pathologic characteristics and some modifying factors. *Arthritis Rheum* **2**: 440–459.

Prud'homme GJ, Parfrey NA & Vanier LE (1991) Cyclosporin-induced autoimmunity and immune hyper-reactivity. *Autoimmunity* **9**: 345–356.

Quagliata F & Phillips-Quagliata JM (1972) Competence of thoracic duct cells in the transfer of adjuvant disease and delayed hypersensitivity. Evidence that mycobacterial components are required for successful transfer of the disease. *Cell Immunol* **3**: 78–87.

Reddy JK & Lalwani ND (1983) Carcinogenesis by hepatic peroxisome proliferators: evaluation of risk of hypolipidaemic drugs and industrial plasticisers to humans. *Crit Rev Toxicol* **12**: 1–58.

Sipe JD, Bartle LM & Loose LD (1992) Modification of pro-inflammatory cytokine production by the anti-rheumatic agents tenidap and naproxen. A possible correlate with clinical acute phase response. *J Immunol* 1992 **148**: 480–484.

Springer TA (1990) Adhesion receptors of the immune system. *Nature* **346**: 425–434.

Sternberg EM, Hill JM, Chrousos GP, Kamilaris T, Listwak SJ, Gold PW et al. (1989) Inflammatory mediator-induced hypothalamic–pituitary–adrenal axis activation is defective in streptococcal cell wall susceptible Lewis rats. *Proc Natl Acad Sci* **86**: 2374–2378.

Stoerk HC, Bielinski TC & Budzilovich T (1954) Chronic polyarthritis in rats injected with spleen in adjuvants. *Am J Pathol* **30**: 616–621.

Symans AM, Dowling EJ & Parke D (1988) Lipid peroxidation, free radicals and experimentsl inflammation. In Simic MG, Taylor KA & Ward JF (eds) *Oxygen Radicals in Biology and Medicine*, pp 987–990. London: Plenum.

Taurog JD, Sandberg GP & Mahowald ML (1983) The cellular basis of adjuvant arthritis . II. Characterization of the cells mediating passive transfer. *Cell Immunol* **80**: 198–204.

Trentham DE, Townes AS & Kang AH (1977) Autoimmunity to type II collagen: an experimental model of arthritis. *J Exp Med* **146**: 857–868.

Tsukano M, Nawa Y & Kotani M (1983) Characterization of low dose induced suppressor cells in adjuvant arthritis in rats. *Clin Exp Immunol* **53**: 60–66.

Waksman BH & Wennersten C (1963) Passive transfer of adjuvant arthritis in rats with living lymphoid cells of sensitised animals. *Int Arch Allergy* **23**: 129–139.

Waksman BH, Pearson CM & Sharp JT (1960) Studies of polyarthritis and other lesions induced in rats by injection of mycobacterial adjuvant. II. Evidence that the disease is a disseminated immunologic response to exogenous antigen. *J Immunol* **85** 403–417.

White RA, Mason DW, Williams AF, Galfre G & Milstein C (1978) T-lymphocyte heterogeneity in the rat: separation of functional subpopulations using a monoclonal antibody. *J Exp Med* **148**: 664–673.

Yoshino S, Kinne R, Hunig T & Emmrich F (1990a) The suppressive effect of an antibody to the αβ cell receptor in rat adjuvant arthritis: studies on optimal treatment protocols. *Autoimmunity* **7**: 255–266.

Yoshino S, Schlipkoter E, Kinne R, Hunig T & Emmrich F (1990b) Suppression and prevention of adjuvant arthritis in rats by a monoclonal antibody to the αβ T cell receptor. *Eur J Immunol* **20**: 2805–2808.

21 Arthritis Induced by Bacteria and Viruses

Marie M. Griffiths

INTRODUCTION

Rheumatoid arthritis (RA) is an immune mediated disease that is characterized by chronic, erosive inflammation of peripheral joints (Brinkerhoff and Delany, 1991; Morgan and Chow, 1993), autoreactivity to several self-antigens, notably IgG and cartilage components (Sasso, 1992; Sewell and Trentham, 1993), and a clear genetic susceptibility (Gregersen, 1992; Wordsworth, 1992; Nepom, 1993). The etiology of RA is unknown although clues are provided by the association of disease severity with HLA-DR4 molecules (Goronzy and Weyand, 1993). In one scenario, RA is viewed as a self-perpetuating and cytokine-mediated inflammatory process that is neither T-cell nor antigen driven (Firestein, 1992; Koopman and Gay, 1993). An alternative hypothesis is that RA reflects an autoimmune attack on constituents of cartilage or the synovium (Strober and Holoshitz, 1990) that may be genetically predetermined. The pathophysiology and natural history of RA, plus the low concordance of disease among twins, suport a third hypothesis – that RA derives from a transient or chronic exposure to an as yet unidentified, but probably common and widespread, infectious agent (Inman, 1992). Thus, RA may have two stages: (a) an early, acute and antigen-restricted phase that is precipitated by an infectious episode and experienced by a broad segment of the population; and (b) a late, chronic, cytokine-expanded and autoimmune phase that develops only in a subgroup of exposed individuals and that may or may not be accompanied by a persistent infection with the inciting micro-organism. Other views on the aetiology of RA are found in Chapters 2, 3 and 4, this volume.

Genetic susceptibility to RA could reflect an ineffective (or inappropriate) immune response to certain infectious agents (Albani *et al.*, 1992; Winchester *et al.*, 1992). An aberrant immune defence may be compounded by marginal controls over potentially autoreactive lymphocytes, an intrinsically high production of inflammatory cytokines (Jacob, 1992; Duff, 1993) and/or flaws in the neuro-endocrine network (Chapter 16, this volume). A major impediment to deciphering the etiology of RA is identification of the antigen(s) that initiates and promulgates immunoreactivity in the joint (Panayi *et al.*, 1992; Randen *et al.*, 1992). Specifically, is it microbial, self or both? Likewise, the nature and source of infectious agents that might trigger RA are unknown (Rodriguez and Williams, 1989). There are sporadic reports of persisting viral antigens and viral DNA in RA synovia suggesting an occult virus infection (Ford *et al.*, 1992; Murayama *et al.*, 1992). Recent evidence that mycobacteria can persist in tissues in a 'slow-growing' form, not detectable by routine histochemical stains, has reinforced the hypothesis that RA results from anomalous bacterial infections (Wilder and Crofford, 1991; Rook and Stanford, 1992; Hazenberg *et al.*, 1992; McCulloch *et al.*, 1993).

Mechanisms and Models in Rheumatoid Arthritis
ISBN 0–12–340440–1

The hypothesis that RA is caused by an infectious agent has waxed and waned in popularity over the past few decades. This frequent shift in sentiment generally follows a predictable course: First, interest is sparked by the discovery of previously unknown mechanisms of pathological interaction between particular microbes and their hosts or by the development of newer, more sensitive techniques for detecting cryptic infections. Although the initial reports are often promising, subsequent testing of large RA patient and control populations by several different laboratories routinely fails to identify a common etiologic agent. Research efforts then dwindle and other, more provocative, directions of arthritis research are targeted. Current stimuli for investigating the possible infectious etiology of RA are the technological advances of improved serological detection using monoclonal antibodies and signal amplification by fluorescent or enzyme-linked reagents, the exquisitely sensitive polymerase chain reaction (PCR) technique that permits detection and gene identification of DNA and RNA at extremely low levels, and the computerized database and associated software programs that provide very fast and accurate analyses of a tremendous volume of information coalesced from numerous clinical and laboratory-based investigations.

A lack of agreement about the possible infectious etiology of RA is understandable. Myriad problems of data interpretation are encountered when large numbers of patients are screened for evidence of a direct relationship between their existing clinical symptoms and a particular infectious agent (Silman, 1992). Obvious obsfucating factors are differences in age, sex, duration of disease, drug therapy, environmental conditions and individual genetic makeup (Charron, 1992). Other considerations include: RA may be a syndrome that is triggered in genetically susceptible individuals by a variety of different agents (Ford, 1989); the causative infection may be a transient event that initiates autoimmunity; disease causing elements of the infectious agent – DNA, antigen – may remain in the joint but be unrecognizable; the infection may be located in distant, non-articular tissues; opportunist invaders may mask subtle evidence of the etiological agent; one underlying infectious agent may cause several rheumatic syndromes, only a subset of which are classified as RA. One approach to identifying the more promising of these hypothetical mechanisms is to use animal models of experimentally induced arthritis to test their feasibility.

Most models of RA concentrate on the late, chronic and autoreactive stage of arthritis. Thus, autoimmune reactivity to normal joint constituents – type II collagen (Cremer, 1986; Holmdahl et al., 1993), proteoglycans (Glant et al., 1980; Banerjee et al., 1992), heat shock proteins (Wooley et al., 1989; Thompson et al., 1991) – can be induced in an immunologically intact animal and cause a chronic, destructive, peripheral arthritis that histologically mimics RA (Magilavy, 1990). Clear genetic differences among rat and mouse strains in susceptibility to autoimmune disease exist and vary with the target antigen and the induction protocol (Griffiths, 1988; Wooley, 1991; Moder et al., 1992). Such genetic susceptibility is reviewed in Chapter 20, this volume. The antigen-induced arthritis model proved that hyperimmunization to a foreign antigen can cause a monoarticular, granulomatous arthritis when that specific antigen is subsequently deposited in the joint by intra-articular injection. The streptococcal cell wall model of arthritis tests the hypothesis that bacterial antigens, shed from a distant site of infection, can traffic to the joint and there initiate a chronic, undulating arthritis with features of RA. These models, which investigate selected and restricted aspects of arthritis, have helped elucidate the pathogenesis of chronic joint inflammation and continue to identify host genes and traits that protect against – or predispose to – chronic arthritis and autoimmune disease (Brahn, 1991). Importantly, they provide strong circumstantial evidence that RA could have an infectious etiology (Wilder and Crofford, 1991). However, few models investigate the hypothetical first stage of RA – the initial encounter of a susceptible host with a viable, arthritogenic infectious agent.

This chapter describes chronic arthritic conditions caused by infection with viable bacteria or viruses. These are not exact models of RA. However, they emphasize the variety of mechanisms by which infectious agents can both evade and manipulate the human immune–inflammatory system such that destructive arthritis similar to that of RA develops.

MECHANISMS OF ARTHRITIS INDUCTION BY VIABLE INFECTIOUS AGENTS

Three mechanisms are used to explain the historical association of RA with overtones of an infectious etiology: (a) persistence of the infectious agent, part of its genome, or molecular debris, in joint tissues; (b) molecular mimicry and induction of auto-immunity; and (c) immune modulation.

PERSISTENT INFECTION

Chronic infection of joint tissues by viruses or bacteria would provide a constant supply of immunogenic and inflammatory macromolecules capable of provoking local pathologic responses characteristic of RA. Bacterial cell-wall components such as peptidoglycans and lipopolysaccharides can non-specifically activate immune and inflammatory cells. Virus infection of synovial cells or infiltrating mononuclear cells could cause over-expression of a variety of inflammatory molecules. These include potential autoantigens, such as the heat shock proteins, and several cell surface immunoregulatory proteins – Fc-receptors, cytokine receptors, cell adhesion proteins (Span et al., 1991), major histocompatability complex (MHC) antigen presenting molecules. Cartilage degrading proteases and potent inflammatory mediators such as interleukin-1 (IL-1) and tumour necrosis factor alpha (TNFα) would be released into synovial fluid.

Over time, chronic infection with either viruses or bacteria could induce an auto-immune pathology not present during the initital acute phase of infection (Rocken et al., 1992). During maturation of T- and B-cell immune responses to a given antigen, the repertoire of determinants that are recognized gradually expands (Lehmann et al., 1992, 1993). Thus, early primary infections may evoke a very different profile of immune specificities that are under entirely different tolerogenic constraints than that evident during a long-standing infection of the same infectious agent. Studies in mice demonstrated that exposure of damaged host proteins to the immune system during viral infection of a target organ can cause chronic, organ-specific autoimmunity that is not cross-reactive with viral proteins and that persists after the infection clears. Susceptibility to autoimmunity was genetically controlled and unrelated to susceptibility to lethal virus infection (Neumann et al., 1991).

Evidence for persistent infection in RA joints is often questioned because it can usually be explained by alternative mechanisms. For example, synovial lymphocytes from some RA patients exhibit greater *in vitro* proliferative responses to certain viral or bacterial antigens than do autochthonous peripheral blood lymphocytes (Ford *et al.*, 1987). This differential responsivity could indicate local, antigen-driven expansion of these cells within the joint tissues and suggests chronic infection or residual debris from prior infections. This interpretation is tempered by the fact that antigens from distant sites of infection can traffic to the joint as immune complexes or as internally processed antigens within the monocytic precursors of synovial macrophages. Also, heightened immune reactivity to certain foreign antigens could either be due to crossreactivity with joint autoantigens or it could be non-specific and reflect a relatively greater activation state of inflammatory synovial macrophages versus peripheral monocytes (Viner *et al.*, 1993).

'MOLECULAR MIMICRY'

This concept theorizes that infection causes a break in tolerance and initiates an autoimmune response to host or 'self' molecules by presenting to the immune system a structually similar molecule in an immunogenic context. It further predicts that once tolerance to self is broken, autoimmune reactivity can become self-perpetuating (Oldstone and Notkins, 1986; Rocken *et al.*, 1992). For example, murine cytomegalovirus (CMV) infection causes myocarditis and induces the synthesis of anti-CMV antibodies that are cross-reactive with cardiac myosin (Lawson *et al.*, 1992). Similarly, type II collagen (Baboonian *et al.*, 1991), cartilage proteogylcans, heat shock proteins (Res *et al.*, 1991; Cohen, 1991), and HLA-DR4 molecules (Roudier *et al.*, 1989) are possible disease-related autoantigens in RA because of regions of amino acid sequence homology to certain viral and bacterial proteins (Birkenfeld *et al.*, 1990; Vaughan, 1990). Thus, autoreactivity to joint constituents in RA patients could be instigated by an infectious event. Alternatively, these sequence homologies might function as 'tolerogens' and inhibit the development of a vigorous immune response, thereby permitting survival of the infectious agent.

'IMMUNE MODULATION'

This is a more fluid term and refers to the capacity of viral and bacterial products to interact with lymphocytes or macrophages and disrupt the cell to cell communications that are involved in the initiation, amplification and regulation of antigen-specific immune responses. Several pathways exist whereby viruses modify immune reactivity, either in specificity or in degree. Classically, it was assumed that viruses disrupted immune homeostasis by inducing a panel of inflammatory cytokines as part of the normal immune response of the host to foreign antigens (Ramsay *et al.*, 1993). IL-1, IL-2, IL-6 and interferon gamma (INFγ) are of specific interest (Dinarello, 1992; Yoshizaki *et al.*, 1992). These lymphokines are associated with RA and are elevated in animal models of arthritis. More recently, there is recognition of a variety of specialized methods of immune deviation that are inherent to particular viruses. These include molecular mimicry with host immune effector molecules (Stannard and Hardie, 1991), including several cytokines (Moore *et al.*, 1993), and *cis*- and *trans*-activation of host cytokine gene transcription (Boldogh *et al.*, 1990; Iwamoto *et al.*,

1990). Competitive inhibition of the assembly, transport and expression of peptide:class I MHC complexes by CMV class I homologues exemplifies how viral infection might shift the emphasis of developing immune responses (Koszinowski *et al.*, 1992).

T-cell modulation by superantigens predicts novel mechanisms by which infection could induce autoimmune arthritis (Herman *et al.*, 1991). Superantigens are viral and microbial products that form a bridge between MHC class II molecules on antigen processing cells and the beta chain of selected T-cell antigen receptor (TCR) molecules. Formation of this complex causes an antigen-independent but TCR Vβ specific clonal proliferation of T cells. Bacterial superantigens are produced by Gram-positive (streptococci, staphylococci) and Gram-negative (*Pseudomonas*) bacteria (Marrack *et al.*, 1993) and by the murine pathogen, *Mycoplasma arthritidis* (Cole and Atkin, 1991). Superantigen-like activity has also been associated with rabies virus, Epstein-Barr virus, and human immunodeficiency virus (Kotzin *et al.*, 1993). The potential for superantigen-induced proliferation of the small, normally subdued population of potentially autoreactive T cells that escape negative selection in the thymus was quickly recognized (Posnett, 1993). Superantigens might precipitate RA by clonally expanding T-cell subsets bearing TCRs that recognize joint antigens (Drake and Kotzin, 1992). Superantigen activity in RA should therefore be evidenced by a skewing of the TCR repertoire in affected joints (Paliard *et al.*, 1991). Studies investigating this question produced conflicing results. Evidence of both a restricted TCR Vβ usage, indicative of superantigen activity (Friedman *et al.*, 1991), and of an oligoclonal TCR profile, suggesting an antigen-driven expansion, are reported (Richardson, 1992). For discussion of the possible role of superantigens in the aetiology and pathogenesis of RA, see Chapters 3 and 19, this volume.

In summary, viral and/or bacterial infections could potentially initiate a cascade of events that, by a variety of mechanisms, would lead to a chronic, immune-mediated arthritis similar to that of RA. Animal models of chronic arthritis that are induced by viable infectious agents are important for identifying novel, pathologic host–micro-organism interactions that could lead to RA. These models also provide the opportunity to study mechanisms of homing to joint tissues, to identify variances in host response to virulent versus avirulent micro-organisms, and to delineate the host response to an infectious agent that can itself modulate the level and type of immunity that develops during and following the acute infectious episode.

ARTHRITIS INDUCED BY BACTERIA

Until recently, bacteria were not widely considered to be strong candidates for etiologic agents in RA. Evidence supporting this hypothesis, although circumstantial and parenthetical, has accumulated sufficiently to demand re-examination of this question. Candidate bacteria are certain of the mycobacteria (McCulloch *et al.*, 1993), mycoplasmas (Razin, 1992), proteus (Ebringer *et al.*, 1989), and a variety of micro-organisms that produce toxins with superantigen activity and/or express peptidoglycans and lipopolysaccharides in their cell walls. There are several informative models of joint disease that evolve from an experimentally induced bacteraemia and the associated septic arthritis. In concert, these models demonstrate that the presence of viable bacteria in joint tissues can induce a chronic arthritis in a subgroup of exposed individuals and appears to develop from one of three pathways:

(1) Due either to virulence-factors of the micro-organism or to an inadequate host immune response, a few bacteria may persist in the joint tissues as a sparse or slow-growing infection.
(2) The organisms may indeed be eradicated from the joint but inflammation may continue due to persisting bacterial debris in the joints or to an induced autoreactivity to joint constituents.
(3) Viable micro-organisms may persist outside of the joint, perhaps in adjacent bone marrow, peri-articular tissues or in the genito-urinary tract, and continue to produce arthritogenic macromolecules that migrate to joint tissues.

SEPTIC ARTHRITIS

In most cases of septic arthritis, the organisms enter the joint via the haematogenous route (Goldenberg, 1991). Very early rabbit models demonstrated that intravenous injection of virulent pneumococci and streptococci resulted in an acute joint inflammation and demonstrated direct invasion of the joint space by the injected bacteria. Later models were usually based on intra-articular injection of viable or heat-killed organisms and investigated the pathogenesis of septic arthritis caused by *Staphylococcus*, *Haemophilus* and *Mycoplasma*. Irrespective of the invading organism, similar initial events are observed. Bacteria replicate within the joint fluid and synovium. A rapid, massive influx of polymorphonuclear leukocytes occurs in association with vascular congestion, synovial lining cell proliferation, purulent effusions and phagocytosis of bacteria. Evidence of chronic arthritis develops within 1–2 weeks, expressed as marked synovial hypertrophy, mononuclear cell infiltration, and the presence of granulation tissue and areas of necrosis. Eventually, aggressive pannus formation and cartilage erosion are noted. A sterile 'post-infectious' chronic arthritis can occur in response to residual bacterial toxins and debris after eradication of viable infectious agents. This has been attributed to the synergistic action of IL-1 and tumour-necrosis factor α but may also reflect non-biodegradable, immunogenic bacterial debris.

Staphylococcus aureus is the most common cause of non-gonococcal bacterial arthritis in adult humans. In healthy individuals, bacterial arthritis is an infrequent result of bacteraemia and, in the absence of direct trauma to the joint, its occurrence is attributed to 'host factors' including impaired immune responses, genetic predispositions, or underlying chronic arthritis (Mikhail and Alarcon, 1993). Bacterial arthritis is a significant complication for RA patients. Patients with long-standing, chronic and debilitating RA have a higher risk and poorer prognosis than patients of less severe disease (Ho, 1991). Use of the antigen-induced arthritis model in rabbits showed that chronically inflamed joints exhibit more severe changes during experimental *S. aureus* infection than the contralateral control joints. Enhanced bacterial invasion and subchondral bone abscesses developed primarily beneath areas of matrix disruption adjacent to pannus (Mahowald, 1986).

A murine model of bacterial arthritis that evolves into a chronic arthritis resembling RA uses *S. aureus* strain LS-1 isolated from the arthritic joint of an NZB/W mouse during a sponteneous colony outbreak of arthritis and osteitis (Bremell *et al.*, 1992).

Primary symptoms are swelling and ankylosis of rear paws. Secondary symptoms are swelling of the tail, indicating osteitis, and skin sores. When injected into normal mice i.v., LS-1 causes a rapid onset of septic arthritis at 24 h, followed by mononuclear cell infiltration at 72 hr. Pannus formation and other changes typical of chronic destructive arthritis develop over the next several weeks. Serum TNF is increased at 24 h and peaks at 2 weeks. High titres of antigen-specific antibodies reactive with bacterial cell walls and the toxic shock syndrome toxin-1 (TSST-1) occurred. A striking polyclonal B-cell stimulation is evidenced by a 20-fold rise in IgG1 together with rheumatoid factor and anti-DNA antibodies. Because *S. aureus* cell wall constituents, such as protein A and peptidoglycans, primarily stimulate IgM production, the increased IgG response was attributed to the ability of secreted exotoxins to activate T cells and cause the release of cytokines such as IL-6 which are functional in the IgM–IgG switch. This model is noteworthy because of genetic variation in susceptibility to LS-1 induced chronic arthritis among inbred mouse strains. Also, LS-1 binds tightly to bone sialo-protein, suggesting a mechanism of homing to joints and bones. The TSST-1 toxin is a potent superantigen that is not produced by all strains of *S. aureus* and could contribute to the arthritogenicity of LS-1.

Erysipelothrix rhusiopathiae, a Gram-positive bacteria that does not produce lipopolysaccharides, causes spontaneous polyarthritis in swine and rats (Renz *et al.*, 1989). A virulent isolate, T28, is used in experimental models. In pigs, T28 arthritis shows activation of synovial cells and chondrocytes, increased expression of MHC molecules, and depletion of cartilage proteoglycans. In rats, T28 causes an acute septic arthritis with fibrosis, pannus and tendo-vaginitis. Subsequently, bacteria are cleared from the joints, but small numbers are identified in the peri-articular tissue for over a year. A substantial rise in antibody titres, some autoreactive, and a chronic polyarthritis, distinguished by cartilage necrosis and mononuclear cell infiltration, is seen during this time (Ziesenis *et al.*, 1992). There is evidence that the chronic phase of arthritis is caused by products released from viable bacteria residing in sites external to the joint (Meier *et al.*, 1992).

LYME DISEASE

Chronic inflammatory arthritis is one of the many diverse clinical symptoms of Lyme disease which is caused by a tick-borne spirochaete, *Borrelia burgdorferi* (Burgdorfer, 1991). There are three stages of Lyme disease (Steere, 1991). After an initial infection at the site of the tick bite, the spirochaete disseminates and invades multiple organs causing neurologic, dermatologic, rheumatologic and cardiac pathologies. During this intermediate phase of the disease (lasting from months to years), many patients experience intermittent, migratory frank oligoarthritis of the larger peripheral joints. Approximately 10% of Lyme disease patients subsequently develop a chronic arthritis that can be resistant to antibiotic therapy. The immunopathology of chronic Lyme arthritis is very similar to that of RA being characterized by synovial hyperplasia, vascular proliferation, mononuclear cell infiltration and cartilage destruction (Malawista, 1989; Sood *et al.*, 1993).

The pathogenesis of chronic Lyme arthritis is not clearly understood but is postulated to reflect an immune response to either *Borrelia* antigens and/or cross-reactive joint autoantigens. Very few spirochaetes are found in joint tissues and it is difficult to explain the severe arthritis that results from such a sparse infection with this very fastidious micro-organism. Peripheral T cells from patients with chronic Lyme arthritis show strong reactivity to multiple *Borrelia* antigens, a response not characteristic of patients with milder disease. Also, foci of T cells and mature B cells, actively synthezing antibody, are found in the synovium, suggesting an ongoing immune response to local antigens. *Borrelia* DNA is found in joint tissues (Karch and Huppertz, 1993) and a large percentage of chronic Lyme arthritis patients respond to antibiotic therapy, indicating that viable bacteria are a primary cause of the arthritis. However, an overactive host response may amplify this late phase of the disease. US patients with chronic Lyme arthritis have high titres of anti-*Borrelia* antibodies and are often HLA-DR4 or HLA-DR2, two genetic markers associated with severe RA.

Models of Lyme borreliosis exist in mice (Barthold *et al.*, 1992), irradiated hamsters (Schmitz *et al.*, 1988), rats (Moody *et al.*, 1990), and dogs (Appel *et al.*, 1993). These models examine potential host contributions to chronic Lyme arthritis (including genetic predispositions) and question how the spirochaete survives despite a vigorous host immune response. There is no evidence that antigenic variation is used as a means of evasion. One consistent finding is that the duration of chronic arthritis positively correlates with the virulence (and thus survival) of the *Borrelia* inoculum and is inversely correlated with the immunocompetence of the host. Also, there are clear genetic differences in suceptibility to chronic Lyme arthritis that are associated with both MHC (Schaible *et al.*, 1991) and non-MHC genes (Yang *et al.*, 1992). The *B. burgdorferi* cell membrane possesses a potent mitogen that causes polyclonal activation of murine B cells (Schoenfeld *et al.*, 1992). This mitogen differs from superantigens in that it functions independently of accessory cells. The *Borrelia* cell wall components also induce pro-inflammatory cytokines, IL-1β and TNF. Serum antibodies are very important in host resistance to borreliosis. However, both susceptible and resistant mice develop equally high anti-*Borrelia* antibodies suggesting that T cells are more important in the chronic phase. Furthermore, differences in the Th_1 versus Th_2 subset activation may more closely correlate with disease susceptibility (Yang *et al.*, 1992).

REACTIVE ARTHRITIS

Reactive arthritis of humans (ReA) is a sterile, chronic arthritis that develops after gastrointestinal infections with certains strains of shigellae, campylobacters, yersiniae, salmonellae, or genitourinary infection with *Chlamydia trachomatis* or *Ureaplasma* (Maki *et al.*, 1991; Moreland and Koopman, 1992). ReA affects selected joints, primarily the spine and larger peripheral joints, suggesting that arthritis results from immune reactivity to a site-specific autoantigen. However, disease-related autoreactivity is not common to ReA patients. Alternatively, there is substantial evidence that ReA results from a constant, localized immune-inflammatory activity stimulated by bacterial debris lodged in the joint tissues. Bacterial lipopolysaccharide is a prime (but not sole) candidate and other bacterial antigens are identified in ReA joints. During the original infectious episode, arthritogenic bacterial debris may traffic to the joint as immune complexes, as passenger molecules in the mobile population of antigen-processing cells, or be deposited during an acute infection (Gransfors, 1992). Reports of chlamydial DNA and RNA in ReA joints suggest a low-level persistent infection in patients with sexually acquired ReA. Efforts to detect DNA or to culture bacteria from the joints of enteric ReA patients have been negative. ReA occurs predominantly in HLA-B27 positive individuals, suggesting it is caused by an aberrant immune response to the inciting micro-organism. Two theories about the close association of ReA with HLA-B27 are considered (Benjamin and Parham, 1992; Reveille, 1993). Because of its function as an epitope-presenting class I molecule for $CD8^+$ T cells, B27 may be responsible for an ineffective or crossreactive immune response to bacterial antigens. Alternatively, B27 may, in fact, be the target of autoimmune reactivity perhaps complexed with a second joint-specific or bacterial-derived peptide. ReA and its implications for the aetiopathogenesis of RA has been the subject of numerous recent reviews (Hughes and Keat, 1992; Kingsley and Panayi, 1992; Keat, 1992; Kingsley and Sieper, 1993; Koopman and Gay, 1993).

Rodent models of *Yersinia enterocolitica* arthritis (YIA) are used to question the tropism of *Yersinia* for joints, the virulence factors that allow foci of *Yersinia* to persist in non-articular sites, and the host factors, both immune and inflammatory that differentiate between an infection leading to chronic disease and one with no detrimental sequelae (Yong *et al.*, 1988; Toivanen *et al.*, 1988). Experimental factors influencing the development of arthritis include the dose, route and serotype of the challenge *Yersinia*. Host factors are the species, genetic background, specificity of immune response and condition of the gut (Gaede *et al.*, 1992).

In the rat model, live *Y. enterolitica* are injected intravenously and cause a self-limiting, non-suppurative, inflammatory arthritis, at 10–14 days, that histologically mimics ReA. The arthritis is oligoarticular, affecting most frequently the ankles. Achilles tendinitis also occurs. The bacteria are cleared from most organs within 3 months but can persist in inguinal nodes for up to 8 months (Merilahti *et al.*, 1992). In mice, live bacteria are recovered from arthritic joints at 6 months and microcolonies are observed in adjacent bone marrow (de-los-Toyos *et al.*, 1992). Thus, chronic YIA may reflect an inability to eliminate completely the organism from the body.

Pre-exposure of rats to normal rat pathogens inhibits the development of arthritis upon subsequent challenge with *Yersinia* (Gripenberg and Toivanen, 1993). Oral immunization with bacteria expressing 0:3 type lipopolysaccharide also protected mice against the lethal effect of i.v. administered *Yersinia* 0:3 (de-los-Toyos *et al.*, 1991). The microbial flora of the gut modulates other rat models of experimental arthritis as well, including the related models of adjuvant arthritis and bacterial cell wall arthritis. This is attributed to a protective effect generated by pre-exposure of the immune system to crossreactive 65-kDa bacterial heat-shock proteins. Alternatively, it is postulated that differences in the integrity of the intestinal lumen during infectious episodes, caused perhaps by variances in the intensity or type of local immune/ inflammatory responses to certain bacterial components, may dictate arthritic versus non-arthritic outcomes in patients exposed to arthritogenic bacteria. The importance of bacterial infection of a mucosal surface for development of YIA is emphasized by observations that oral challenge caused more severe arthritis than i.v. inoculations in mice.

A promising approach in animal models of arthritis is the development of transgenic mice and rats expressing human disease-related genes. HLA-B27 transgenic mice were used to examine the interaction of this ReA-related, human class I molecule with viable, disease-causing *Yersinia*. When injected intravenously into HLA-B27 transgenic mice, *Y. enterolitica*, did not cause reactive arthritis but B27 positive mice showed a higher incidence of spinal abscesses and higher mortality rates than their B27-negative littermates (Nickerson *et al.*, 1990). In rats, the B27-transgene causes a spontaneous, inflammatory disease affecting the gastrointestinal tract, skin, nails, heart, male genital tract and peripheral and vertebral joints. The B27-rat thus expresses many of the articular and non-articular features of the HLA B27-related human diseases (Hammer *et al.*, 1990). The pathological effects of the B27-transgene in rats require functional T cells. No gut, skin or gastrointestinal–urethral abnormalities developed in athymic nude rats carrying the B27 transgene. Development of a germ-free line of HLA-B27 rats showed that the spontaneous gut inflammation and arthritis do not develop in the absence of a normal gut flora. The dermatological abnormalities and testicular lesions, however, continued to be expressed (Taurog *et al.*, 1993).

CHRONIC ARTHRITIS INDUCED BY VIRUSES

Many of the etiopathogenic mechanisms that have been discussed concerning a bacterial causation of chronic inflammatory arthritis (such as induction of autoimmunity) are also directly applicable to the concept of a virus-induced chronic arthritis. However, there are unique aspects of viruses that must be considered when formulating the hypothesis that RA has a viral etiology.

First, infection of joint tissues with lytic viruses during a viraemic episode can induce a self-limiting acute arthritis. However, because viruses have neither cell walls nor capsular material, the non-immune, inflammatory component of septic arthritis driven by bacterial lipopolysaccharides and peptidoglycans is absent in virus-induced arthropathies. Likewise, a sustained post-viral arthritis is not likely to be caused by non-biodegradable molecular debris.

Secondly, whereas viable bacteria can enter the joint by direct interaction with endothelial cells, virus accumulation in joint tissues is necessarily passive. Filtration of infective virions and immune complexes into joint fluids could occur during acute viraemia. During convalescence, virus-infected mononuclear cells could migrate to joints. Thus, while it is conceivable that lytic infection at a distant site could provide a constant supply of virions, no abnormalities of other organ systems consistently occurs in all RA patients (as for example with the gut in ReA). Indeed, chronic joint inflammation is the one distinguishing, hallmark of rheumatoid disease. Thus, in virus-induced arthropathies, the virus most likely resides either within the joint or peri-articular tissues or it is sequestered in lymphoid tissues from whence it can modulate immune responses to joint antigens.

The third unique aspect of an infectious viral etiology theory for RA derives from the ability of certain viruses to infect lymphocytes, monocytes and synovial cells. These cells are active participants in the chronic arthritis of RA and comprise the pannus that causes cartilage erosion and joint destruction (see Chapter 6, this volume). Non-lytic infection of local synovial cell populations could disrupt their normal metabolism and induce pannus-like bahviour including release of cartilage degrading enzymes. Virus gene products might transactivate host genes encoding inflammatory cytokines or cell surface receptors. Virus encoded molecules that mimic host cytokines could be produced and incite nearby immune-inflammatory cells. Viral proteins with superantigen activity might be released and drive inflammatory synoviocyte–monocyte–lymphocyte interactions. A histologically similar arthritic response could be induced by virus infection of adjacent bone marrow with diffusion of inflammatory molecules or activated lymphoid cells to nearby joint tissues.

Finally, retroviruses possess even more specialized mechanisms of inducing chronic arthritis that could operate in the absence of an overt joint infection (Meltzer *et al.*, 1990). Retrovirus genomes can inegrate into the chromosomes of a host cell and there exist as a silent infection. Virus genes are replicated in tandem with the host genes during cell mitosis. Thus, the influence of virus products constantly expands. Not only are retrovirus proteins synthesized, but retroviral genes, or gene-products, can act to promote or inhibit the transcription of important host genes. Small segments of a retrovirus genome can similarly be incorporated into the host genome and interfere with the normal regulation of particular cell functions. For example, the spontaneous autoimmune disease of MRL/*lpr* mice is attributed to the strategic positioning of a stable, retroviral integrant such that it disrupts the expression of the mouse Fas gene (Mountz and Talal, 1993; see Chapter 25, this volume). Fas is necessary for apoptosis, or programmed cell death, of antigen-stimulated lymphocytes. MRL mice, having a dysregulated Fas gene, develop a mild arthritis and anti-collagen antibodies with age (Wu *et al.*, 1993).

The immunopathology of RA is compatible with the hypothesis of a viral etiology. Several candidate viruses have been proposed including rubella (Ford *et al.*, 1992), Epstein-Barr virus (Vaughan, 1990), cytomegalovirus (Murayama *et al.*, 1992), hepatitis virus C (Sawada *et al.*, 1991), arboviruses (Tai *et al.*, 1993) and the retroviruses (Trabandt *et al.*, 1992; David, 1992). All are ubiquitous viruses that are immunomodulatory and that can potentially establish latent infections in joint or lymphoid tissues. However, as with bacteria, no proof that RA is associated exclusively with any of these viruses has been obtained. Spontaneous arthritis and autoimmune diseases of domestic animals have been more definitively traced to chronic infection with paramyxoviruses and retroviruses. This section chronicles three diseases caused by exogenously acquired viruses that are characterized by arthritis.

ARTHRITIS CAUSED BY PARVOVIRUS

The human parvovirus, B19, is a small, single-stranded DNA virus that replicates in the nucleus. Most adults have been exposed to B19. Symptomatic B19 infection causes a biphasic disease characterized by flu-like symptoms during the first week of viraemia followed by rash, arthralgias, arthritis, and haematologic disorders that are temporally associated with seroconversion and clearance of the virus from the bloodstream. B19 is the etiological agent of hypoplastic crisis in sickle-cell anaemia and erythema infectiosum (fifth disease) of children and is proposed as a triggering agent of fibromyalgia (Thurn, 1988; Rotbart, 1990). In a subset of patients, B19 causes a chronic, episodic arthritis that lasts for months to years. Approximately 50% of patients with chronic B19 arthropathy fulfil the clinical criteria for RA including morning stiffness, a symmetrical polyarthritis of the peripheral joints and transient formation of autoantibodies (rheumatoid factor, anti-DNA antibody), B19 arthritis is distinguished from RA by the absence of rheumatoid nodules, lack of association with DR4 and the presence of significant pain but not erosive disease. PCR analysis identified B19 DNA in bone marrow aspirates, questionably in synovial tissues, but not in the serum of patients with chronic B19 arthritis (Foto *et al.*, 1993). Thus, although synovial cells are non-permissive for parvoviruses (Miki and Chantler, 1992), B19 apparently establishes a persistent infection in the adjacent bone marrow and from there directly effects the health of surrounding tissues. Chronic B19 arthritis develops despite a vigorous host immune response. When overlapping synthetic peptides were used as antigens, serum antibodies from patients with chronic B19 arthritis recognized a more restricted profile of B19 capsid epitopes than serum antibodies from seropositive but non-arthritic controls (Naides, 1993), suggesting that differences in specificity of anti-B19 immune reactivity might allow a persistent virus infection to be established.

Useful models of parvovirus-induced arthritis are not available. Rodent parvoviruses are not arthritogenic. Subclinical infection with Kilham rat virus (KRV) precipitated disease and mildly aggravated the severity of arthritis in rats immunized with type II collagen but did not alter the level of collagen autoimmunity (unpublished observation). Also, infection with canine distemper virus has been associated with 'rheumatoid arthritis' in dogs (Bell *et al.*, 1991).

ARTHRITIS CAUSED BY RETROVIRUSES

An intriguing hypothesis is that RA is caused by infection with a retrovirus (Trabandt *et al.*, 1992; Nakajima *et al.*, 1993). Retroviruses are RNA viruses that replicate by a series of events that includes reverse transcription of the viral RNA genome into DNA, integration of the DNA provirus into the host genome, and subsequent production of viral RNA, viral proteins and daughter virions using host cell machinery. Based on their biological behaviour, the Retroviridae are subdivided into three families: the Lentiviruses, the Oncornaviruses, and the Spumaviruses. The oncornaviruses cause cell transformation *in vitro* and produce leukaemia-lymphomas and solid tumours *in vivo*. The non-oncogenic lentiviruses cause cell fusion and lysis in culture and produce slow, chronic infections in their hosts. Chronic inflammatory arthritis of humans and domestic animals has been traced to exogenously acquired lentiviruses and oncornoviruses.

One of the protean manifestations of infection with the human immunodeficiency virus (HIV), a lentivirus, is a symmetrical, non-suppurative, inflammatory polyarthritis that develops in a subset of patients with acquired immunodeficiency syndrome (AIDS). The arthritic syndromes most commonly associated with AIDS are Reiter's syndrome and psoriatic arthritis (Calabrese, 1993). A group of vaguely defined and heterogeneous arthritic syndromes occurs less frequently (Rynes, 1991). The pathogenesis of these conditions is not well understood. Both HIV DNA and antigenic HIV core protein are detected in synovial tissue of AIDS patients with arthritis. This material may be carried to the joint by macrophages, a major reservoir of HIV (Meltzer and Gendelman, 1992). The possibility that ReA might develop secondary to immune dysfunction at mucosal surfaces is considered but unproven (Espinoza *et al.*, 1992). Relative to rheumatic diseases, it is noteworthy that in HIV-infected individuals chronic arthritis develops in the absence of a normal complement of CD4$^+$ T cells. Also, RA patients that develop AIDS often experience a remission of their arthritis (Furie, 1991), in agreement with other evidence that CD4$^+$ lymphocytes are important host elements in the chronic arthritis of RA. For further reviews of AIDS and RA refer to Chapters 2 and 4, this volume.

A chronic arthritis of goats and sheep is caused by infection with the closely related lentiviruses, caprine arthritis and encephalitis virus (CAEV) and visna maedi virus (VMV) respectively. Lentivirus infections are characterized by prolonged latent periods, thus the original term 'slow growing viruses'. Non-productive, cell-to-cell transfer of infective virions is characteristic and allows the virus to persist in the host for long periods of time despite strong cellular and humoral immune responses. Antigenic variants of CAEV arise frequently during infection but this does not appear to be a primary mechanism of survival (Cheevers et al., 1991). CAEV infects cells of the monocyte-macrophage lineage and there is evidence that CAEV arthritis is driven by the sporadic expression of CAEV antigens on infected synovial macrophages (Narayan et al., 1992). However, as with Lyme disease, this interpretation is difficult to reconcile with the fact that arthritis severity frequently increases at a time when very few virus particles can be identified in the joint. CAEV infects synovial cells (Hullinger et al., 1993), although not exclusively (Zink et al., 1990), and causes multiple anomalies of the host immune system. Most notably, CAEV-infected macrophages are hyperactive, a feature that is detected in vitro as an increased rate of T-cell proliferative response to antigens presented by CAEV-infected versus not-infected macrophages (Banks et al., 1989). The mechanisms by which CAEV amplifies the host immune response is not understood. However, there is some evidence that CAEV elevates surface expression of MHC class II molecules on infected cells. Also, the synthesis of pro-inflammatory cytokines or virokines by CAEV-infected macrophages is possible (Michaels et al., 1991). The visna retrovirus has been less intensively studied. Rheumatoid factor plus autoantibodies to ssDNA and cardiolipin were detected in sheep experimentally infected with visna virus (Harkiss et al., 1993).

HTLV-I, a type C oncovirus, is the etiologic agent of adult human T-cell leukaemia-lymphoma, a malignant proliferation of mature T cells, and is associated with certain progressive neurologic disorders (Hollsberg and Halfer, 1993). HTLV-I contains a gene designated tax that is not found in most retroviruses. The tax protein transactivates transcription of viral RNA and host cell oncogenes, thus intensifying virus replication and promoting cell transformation. The tax gene product also up-regulates host cell synthesis of IL-2, IL-2 receptors and at least two macrophage-activating cytokines. An HTLV-I associated arthropathy develops in humans (Sato et al., 1991) and is characterized by the presence of atypical CD4$^+$ or CD8$^+$ T lymphocytes in an invasive, hyperplastic synovium that exhibits increased expression of HLA-DR antigens (Nishioka et al., 1993). These synovial cell activities could be due to cytokines produced by infiltrating HTLV-I transformed T cells. However, analysis of fresh biopsy material indicated that proviral DNA and HTLV-I gag and env gene products are also present in the non-lymphoid mesenchymal cells. HTLV-I proviral DNA has also been identified in cloned, synovial cells derived from patients with HTLV-I associated arthritis (Kitajima et al., 1991). Thus HTLV-I can directly infect synovial cells, causing a malignant cell activation and proliferation that results in chronic progressive arthritis (Nakajima et al., 1993).

Molecules antigenically related to certain HTLV antigens were reportedly identified in rheumatoid synovial biopsy material (Ziegler et al., 1989). Moreover, rheumatoid synovial cells do have many functional and metabolic characteristics that are reminiscent of a retroviral induced transformation. Thus, it has been proposed that an as yet unknown HTLV-related retrovirus might be etiologically related to RA (Trabandt *et al.*, 1992).

Mice transgenic for the HTLV-I *tax* gene have been developed to study this disorder (Iwakura *et al.*, 1991). *Tax*-transgenic mice develop a spontaneous inflammatory arthritis of the feet at 2–3 months. The involved joints show an invasive, granulomatous lesion in association with mononuclear cell infiltration, pannus and erosion of bone and cartilage. The transgene was expressed most strongly in joints, salivary glands and the central nervous system, tissues that are commonly associated with retrovirus-induced disease. Development of these mice clearly demonstrates the arthritogenic potential of appropriately integrated, retorviral genes.

VIRUS MODULATION OF COLLAGEN-INDUCED ARTHRITIS

No rodent models of chronic arthritis induced by an exogenous virus are available. We therefore used the type II collagen-induced model of autoimmune arthritis (CIA) to test the hypothesis that infection with immunomodulatory viruses could precipitate arthritis in a genetically susceptible host. Rats were subimmunized with type II collagen and simultaneously infected with rat cytomegalovirus (CMV). CMV infection caused significant increases in arthritis severity compared to collagen-immunized but non-infected rats. Antibody titres and skin test reactivity to rat type II collagen were also elevated by CMV infection. CMV alone did not induce arthritis nor autoreactivity to collagen. CMV augmentation of CIA could reflect the release of host defensive cytokines such as interferon and IL-1 which are important pro-inflammatory mediators in the CIA model (Griffiths *et al.*, 1991). However, subsequent analyses have shown that CMV augments arthritis only in rats that are genetically susceptible to CIA, indicating an antigen-specific mechanism, such as molecular mimicry.

In mice, segments of a mouse mammary tumour virus genome have been stably integrated into the murine genome (Marrack *et al.*, 1993). When transcribed, MMTV open reading frame proteins, termed Mls antigens, are expressed on B cells, function as superantigens, and cause thymic, clonal deletion of a subset of T cells that expresses a restricted set of TCRs. In the murine model of CIA, only a subset of T cells is arthritogenic (Haqqi *et al.*, 1992; Moder *et al.*, 1992). Collagen-reactive, arthritogenic T cells utilize TCR Vβ molecules that also bind Mls antigens. Thus, removal of Mls-1 reactive T cells down-regulates arthritis in most mouse strains suggesting that these cells promote arthritis in the CIA model (Anderson *et al.*, 1991). In contrast, preliminary studies suggest that some Mls-reactive T cells may actually be protective. Deletion of Vβ6$^+$ T cells by Mls-1 was associated with selective decreases in IgG1 anti-collagen antibody, suggesting that these cells may have expressed an anti-inflammatory, Th$_2$ phenotype (Griffiths *et al.*, 1993). Thus, retroviral encoded superantigens may possibly be both arthritogenic and protective depending upon the environmental challenge and the host genome.

SUMMARY

Three general conclusions are made. First, joint destruction occurs in RA because of host activity. Because evolution selects for survival, two questions arise: What triggers this self-destructive force? Why is it uncontrolled? Of the current theories about the etiopathogenesis of RA none explains all parameters of the disease. Secondly, if RA is caused by an infectious agent, no single organism has been incriminated. Thirdly, susceptibility to RA is genetically preprogrammed. The term 'syndrome' is frequently used with reference to the etiology of RA to incorporate the concern that the disease may have multiple etiologies. Thus, if RA is in fact precipitated by infectious agents, it is possible that several different microbial infections can result in the same clinical disease expression, given a genetically susceptible host and a viable arthritogenic micro-organism. A testable hypothesis that addresses this possibility can be developed.

Retroviruses are ubiquitous. Retroviral genes can integrate into a host genome and passively determine the T-cell repertoire that develops during thymic 'education' (Herman *et al.*, 1991). Retrovirus-imposed 'holes' in the profile of antigenic determinants recognized by the peripheral T-cell population thus might prevent adequate immune defence mechanisms to be mounted in response to an environmentally imposed secondary viral or bacterial infection. Because multiple retroviral integrants could be scattered throughout the human population, a variety of common organisms might be potential, selective triggers for RA in given individuals dependent upon the specific retroviral genes that are present.

Current animal models are excellent, but they are not a perfect replication of human RA. Until the specific etiology for RA is defined, the relevance of animal models to the pathogenesis of RA will remain a question. However, they continue to be an important asset for the study of rheumatic diseases. First, they provide a medium in which the arthritogenic potential of different microbes and microbial components can be tested. Second, they provide a framework through which genetic susceptibility can be addressed. Finally, they can be manipulated to investigate the variable pathologic responses to known arthritogens. Future theories as to the infectious etiology of RA should be validated using viable micro-organisms in an animal model. This is because there may be subtle aspects of the host–micro-organism interplay that are critical to the development of RA. These may only be detectable in the dynamic relationship that evolves during a triggering event involving a susceptible host and a viable, arthritogenic, infectious agent.

REFERENCES

Albani S, Carson DA & Roudier J (1992) Genetic and environmental factors in the immune pathogenesis of rheumatoid arthritis. *Rheum Dis Clin North Am* **18**: 729–740.

Anderson GD, Banerjee S, Luthra HS & David CD (1991) Role of Mls-1a and clonal deletion of T cells in susceptibility to collagen induced arthritis in mice. *J Immunol* **147**: 1189–1193.

Appel MJ, Allan S, Jacobson RH, Lauderdale TL, Chang YF, Shin SJ et al. (1993) Experimental Lyme disease in dogs produces arthritis and persistent infection. *J Infect Dis* **167**: 651–664.

Baboonian C, Venables PJ, Williams DG, Williams RO & Maini RN (1991) Cross reaction of antibodies to a glycine/alanine repeat sequence of Epstein-Barr virus nuclear antigen-1 with collagen, cytokeratin and actin. *Ann Rheum Dis* **50**: 772–775.

Banerjee S, Webber C & Poole AR (1992) The induction of arthritis in mice by the cartilage proteoglycan aggrecan: roles of CD4$^+$ and CD8$^+$ T cells. *Cellular Immunol* **144**: 347–357.

Banks KL, Jutila MA, Jacobs CA & Michaels FH (1989) Augmentation of lymphocyte and macrophage proliferation by caprine arthritis-encephalitis virus contributes to the development of progressive arthritis. *Rheumatol Int* **9**: 123–128.

Barthold SW, Sidman, CL & Smith AL (1992) Lyme borreliosis in genetically resistant and susceptible mice with severe combined immunodeficiency. *Am J Trop Med Hyg* **47**: 605–613.

Bell SC, Carter SD & Bennett D (1991) Canine distemper viral antigens and antibodies in dogs with rheumatoid arthritis. *Res Vet Sci* **50**: 64–68.

Benjamin R & Parham P (1992) HLA-B27 and disease: a consequence of inadvertent antigen presentation? *Rheum Dis Clin North Am* **18**: 11–21.

Birkenfeld P, Haratz N, Klein G & Sulitzeanu D (1990) Crossreactivity between the EBNA-1 p107 peptide, collagen and keratin: implications for the pathogenesis of rheumatoid arthritis. *Clin Immunol Immunopathol* **54**: 14–25.

Boldogh I, AbuBakar S & Albrecht T (1990) Activation of proto-oncogenes: an immediate early event in human cytomegalovirus infection. *Science* **247**: 561–564.

Brahn E (1991) Animal models of rheumatoid arthritis. Clues to etiology and treatment. *Clin Orthop Rel Res* **265**: 42–53.

Bremell T, Abdelnour A & Tarkowski A (1992) Histopathological and serological progression of experimental *Staphylococcus aureus* arthritis. *Infect Immun* **60**: 2976–2985.

Brinkerhoff CE & Delany AM (1991) Cytokines and growth factors in arthritic diseases: mechanisms of cell proliferation and matrix degradation in rheumatoid arthritis. In Kimball ES (ed) *Cytokines and Inflammation*, pp. 109–145. Boca Raton: CRC Press.

Burgdorfer W (1991) Lyme borreliosis: ten years after discovery of the etiologic agent, *Borrelia burgdorferi*. *Infection* **19**: 257–262.

Calabrese LH (1993) Human immunodeficiency virus (HIV) infection and arthritis. *Rheum Dis North Am* **19**: 477–488.

Charron DJ (1992) New aspects of HLA: perspectives for rheumatoid arthritis. *Clin Exp Rheumatol* **10**: 293–296.

Cheevers WP, Knowles DJ & Norton LK (1991) Neutralization-resistant antigenic variants of caprine arthritis-ecephalitis lentivirus associated with progressive arthritis. *J Infect Dis* **164**: 679–685.

Cohen IR (1991) Autoimmunity to chaperonins in the pathogenesis of arthritis and diabetes. *Annu Rev Immunol* **9**: 567–589.

Cole BC & Atkin CL (1991) The Mycoplasma arthritidis T cell mitogen, MAM: A model superantigen. *Immunol Today* **12**: 271–276.

Cremer M (1986) Type II collagen induced arthritis in rats. In Greenwald RA & Diamond HS (eds) *Handbook of Animal Models for the Rheumatic Diseases*, pp. 17–28. Boca Raton: CRC Press.

Davis P (1992) Viral infections, acquired immunodeficiency syndrome, and rheumatoid diseases. *Curr Opin Rheumatol* **4**: 529–533.

de-los-Toyos JR, Diaz R & Hardisson C (1991) Protection against the lethal effect and arthritogenic capacity of *Yersinia enterocolitica* serotype 0:3 for mice. *Fems Microviol Immunol* **3**: 289–297.

de-los-Toyos JR, Menendez P, Sampedro A & Hardisson C (1992) *Yersinia enterocolitica* serotype 0:3-induced arthritis in mice: microbiological and histopathological information. *Apmis* **100**: 455–464.

Dinarello CA (1992) Interleukin-1 and tumor necrosis factor: effector cytokines in autoimmune diseases. *Semin Immunol* **4**: 133–145.

Drake CG & Kotzin BL (1992) Superantigens: biology, immunology and potential role in disease. *J Clin Immunol* **12**: 149–162.

Duff GW (1993) Cytokines and anti-cytokines. *Br J Rheumatol* **1**: 15–20.

Ebringer A, Khalafpour S & Wilson C (1989) Rheumatoid arthritis and *Proteus*: a possible aetiological association. *Rheumatol Int* **9**: 223–228.

Espinoza LR, Jara LJ, Espinoza CG, Silveira LH, Martinez OP & Seleznick M (1992) There is an association between human immunodeficiency virus infection and spondyloarthropathies. *Rheum Dis Clin North Am* **18**: 257–266.

Firestein GS (1992) Mechanisms of tissue destruction and cellular activation in rheumatoid arthritis. *Curr Opin Rheumatol* **4**: 348–354.

Ford DK (1989) Microbiology will give the real answers to rheumatoid arthritis. *B J Rheumatol* **28**: 436–439.

Ford DK, da Roza DM, Schulzer M, Reid GD & Denegri JF (1987) Persistent synovial lymphocyte responses to cytomegalovirus antigen in some patients with rheumatoid arthritis. *Arthritis Rheum* **30**: 700–704.

Ford DK, Reid GD, Tingle AJ, Mitchell LA & Schulzer M (1992) Sequential follow up observations of a patient with rubella associated persistent arthritis. *Ann Rheum Dis* **51**: 407–410.

Foto F, Saag KG, Scharosch LL, Howard EJ & Naides SJ (1993) Parvovirus B19-specific DNA in bone marrow from B19 arthropathy patients: evidence for B19 virus persistence. *J Infect Dis* **167**: 744–748.

Friedman SM, Posnett DN, Tumang JR, Cole BC & Crow MK (1991) A potential role for microbial superantigens in the pathogenesis of systemic autoimmune disease. *Arthritis Rheum* **34**: 468–480.

Furie RA (1991) Effects of human immunodeficiency virus infection on the expression of rheumatic illness. *Rheum Dis Clin North Am* **17**: 177–188.

Gaede K, Mack D & Heesmann J (1992) Experimental *Yersinia enterocolitica* infection in rats: analysis of the immune response to plasmid-encoded antigens of arthritis-susceptible Lewis rats. *Med Microbiol Immunol Berl* **181**: 165–172.

Glant TT, Csongor J & Scuzs T (1980) Immunopathologic role of proteoglycan antigens in rheumatoid joint disease. *Scand J Immunol* **11**: 247–252.

Goldenberg DL (1991) Septic arthritis and other infections of rheumatologic significance. *Rheum Dis Clin North Am* **17**: 149–156.

Goronzy JJ & Weyand CM (1993) Interplay of T lymphocytes and HLA-DR molecules in rheumatoid arthritis. *Curr Opin Rheumatol* **5**: 169–177.

Granfors K (1992) Do bacterial antigens cause reactive arthritis? *Rheum Dis Clin North Am* **18**: 37–48.

Gregersen PK (1992) T-cell receptor–major histocompatibility complex genetic interactions in rheumatoid arthritis. *Rheum Dis Clin North Am* **18**: 793–807.

Griffiths MM (1988) Immunogenetics of collagen-induced arthritis in rats. *Int Rev Immunol* **4**: 1–15.

Griffiths MM, Smith CB, Wei LS & Ting-Yu SC (1991) Effects of rat cytomegalovirus infection on immune functions in rats with collagen induced arthritis. *J Rheumatol* **18**: 497–504.

Griffiths MM, Nabozny GH, Cannon GW, McCall S, Luthra HS & Davis CS (1994) Colllagen induced arthritis and T cell receptors in SWR and B10.Q mice expressing an Ealpha transgene. *J Immunol* **153**: 2758–2768.

Gripenberg LC & Toivanen P (1993) *Yersinia* associated arthritis in SHR rats: effect of the microbial status of the host. *Ann Rheum Dis* **52**: 223–228.

Hammer RE, Maika SD, Richardson JA, Tang J-P. & Taurog JD (1990) Spontaneous inflammatory disease in transgenic rats expressing HLA-B27 and human beta2m: An animal model of HLA-B27-associated human disorders. *Cell* **63**: 1099–1112.

Haqqi T, Anderson GA, Banerjee S & David DS (1992) Restricted heterogeneity in T cell Vbeta gene usage in the lymph nodes and arthritic joints of mice. *Proc Natl Acad Sci USA* **89**: 1253–1255.

Harkiss GD, Veith D, Dickson L & Watt NJ (1993) Autoimmune reactivity in sheep induced by the visna retrovirus. *J Autoimmun* **6**: 63–75.

Hazenberg MP, Klasen IS, Kool J, Ruseler v EJ & Severijnen AJ (1992) Are intestinal bacteria involved in the etiology of rheumatoid arthritis? Review article. *Apmis* **100**: 1–9.

Herman A, Kappler JW, Marrack P & Pullen AM (1991) Superantigens: mechanism of T-cell stimulation and role in immune responses. *Annu Rev Immunol* **9**: 745–772.

Ho GJ (1991) Bacterial arthritis. *Curr Opin Rheumatol* **3**: 603–609.

Hollsberg P & Hafler DA (1993) Seminars in medicine of the Beth Israel Hospital, Boston. Pathogenesis of diseases induced by human lymphotropic virus type I infection. *N Engl J Med* **328**: 1173–1182.

Holmdahl R, Malmstrom V & Vuorio E (1993) Autoimmune recognition of cartilage collagens. *Ann Med* **25**: 251–264.

Hughes R & Keat A (1992) Reactive arthritis: the role of bacterial antigens in inflammatory arthritis. *Baillieres Clin Rheumatol* **6**: 285–308.

Hullinger GA, Knowles DP, McGuire TC & Cheevers WP (1993) Caprine arthritis-encephalitis lentivirus SU is the ligand for infection of caprine synovial membrane cells. *Virology* **192**: 328–331.

Inman RD (1992) The role of infection in chronic arthritis. *J Rheumatol Suppl* **33**: 98–104.

Iwakura Y, Tosu M, Yoshida E, Takiguchi M, Sato K, Kitajima I, Yamamoto K, Takeda T et al. (1991) Induction of inflammatory arthropathy resembling rheumatoid arthritis in mice transgenic for HTLV-I. *Science* **253**: 1026–1028.

Iwamoto GK, Monick MM & Clark BD (1990) Modulation of interleukin 1 beta gene expression by the immediate early genes of human cytomegalovirus. *J Clin Invest* **85**: 1853–1857.

Jacob CO (1992) Tumor necrosis factor and interferon gamma: relevance for immune regulation and genetic predisposition to autoimmune disease. *Semin Immunol* **4**: 147–154.

Karch H & Huppertz HI (1993) Repeated detection of *Borrelia burgdorferi* DNA in synovial fluid of a child with Lyme arthritis. *Rheumatol Int* **12**: 227–229.

Keat A (1992) Infections and the immunopathogenesis of seronegative spondyloarthropathies. *Curr Opin Rheumatol* **4**: 494–499.

Kingsley G & Panayi G (1992) Antigenic responses in reactive arthritis. *Rheum Dis Clin North Am* **18**: 49–66.

Kingsley G & Sieper J (1993) Current perspectives in reactive arthritis. *Immunol Today* **14**: 387–391.

Kitajima I, Yamamoto K, Sato K, Nakajima Y, Nakajima T, Maruyama I, Osame M & Nishioka K (1991) Detection of human T cell lymphotropic virus type I proviral DNA and its gene expression in synovial cells in chronic inflammatory arthropathy. *J Clin Invest* **88**: 1315–1322.

Koopman WJ & Gay S (1993) Do nonimmunologically mediated pathways play a role in the pathogenesis of rheumatoid arthritis? *Rheum Dis Clin North Am* **19**: 107–122.

Koszinowski UH, Reddehase MJ & Del VM (1992) Principles of cytomegalovirus antigen presentation *in vitro* and *in vivo*. *Semin Immunol* **4**: 71–79.

Kotzin BK, Leung DYM, Kappler J & Marrack P (1993) Superantigens and their potential role in human disease. *Adv Immunol* **54**: 99–166.

Lawson CN, O'Donoghue HL & Reed WD (1992) Mouse cytomegalovirus infection induces antibodies which cross-react with virus and cardiac myosin: a model for the study of molecular mimicry in the pathogenesis of viral myocarditis. *Immunology* **75**: 513–519.

Lehmann PV, Forsthuber T, Miller A & Sercarz EE (1992) Spreading of T-cell autoimmunity to cryptic determinants of an autoantigen. *Nature* **358**: 155–157.

Lehmann, PV, Sercarz EE, Forsthuber T, Dayan CM & Gammon G (1993) Determinant spreading and the dynamics of the autoimmune T-cell repertoire. *Immunol Today* **14**: 203–208.

Magilavy DB (1990) Animal models of chronic inflammatory arthritis. *Clin Orthop* **259**: 38–45.

Mahowald ML (1986) Animal models of infectious arthritis. *Clin Rheum Dis* **12**: 403–421.

Maki IO, Viljanen MK, Tiitinen S, Toivanen P & Granfors K (1991) Antibodies to arthritis-associated microbes in inflammatory joint diseases. *Rheumatol Int* **10**: 231–234.

Malawista SE (1989) Pathogenesis of Lyme disease. *Rheumatol Int* **9**: 233–235.

Marrack P, Winslow GM, Choi Y, Scherer M, Pullen A, White J et al. (1993) The bacterial and mouse mammary tumor virus superantigens; two different families of proteins with the same functions. *Immunol Rev* **131**: 79–92.

McCulloch J, Lydyard PM & Rook GA (1993) Rheumatoid arthritis: how well do the theories fit the evidence? *Clin Exp Immunol* **92**: 1–6.

Meier B, Brunotte CM, Franz B, Warlich B, Petermann M, Ziesenis A et al. (1992) Isolation of a high-molecular mass glycoprotein from culture supernatant of an arthritogenic strain of the bacteria *Erysipelothrix rhusiopathiae* reacting wtih 'inductive' monoclonal antibodies derived from rats with erysipelas polyarthritis. *Biol Chem Hoppe Seyler* **373**: 715–721.

Meltzer MS & Gendelman HE (1992) Mononuclear phagocytes as targets, tissue reservoirs and immuno-regulatory cells in human immunodeficiency virus disease. *Curr Top Microbiol Immunol* **181**: 239–263.

Meltzer MS, Skillman DR, Gomatos PJ, Kalter DC & Gendelman HE (1990) Role of mononuclear phagocytes in the pathogenesis of human immunodeficiency virus infection. *Annual Rev Immunol* **8**: 169–194.

Merilahti PR, Gripenberg LC, Soderstrom KO & Toivanen P (1992) Long term follow up of SHR rats with experimental yersinia associated arthritis. *Ann Rheum Dis* **51**: 91–96.

Michaels FH, Banks KL & Reitz MJ (1991) Lessons from caprine and ovine retorvirus infections. *Rheum Dis Clin North Am* **17**: 5–23.

Mikhail S & Alarcon GS (1993) Nongonoccal bacterial arthritis. *Rheum Dis Clin North Am* **19**: 311–332.

Miki NP & Chantler JK (1992) Non-permissiveness of synovial membrane cells to human parvovirus B19 *in vitro. J Gen Virol* **72**: 1559–1562.

Moder KG, Nabozny GH, Luthra HS & David CS (1992) Immunogenetics of collagen induced arthritis in mice: a model for human polyarthritis. *Reg Immunol* **4**: 305–313.

Moody KD, Barthold SW, Terwilliger GA, Beck DS, Hansen GM & Jacoby RO (1990) Experimental chronic Lyme borreliosis in Lewis rats. *Am J Trop Med Hyg* **42**: 165–174.

Moore KW, O'Garra A, Malefyt RW, Vieira WMR- de P & Mosmann TR (1993) Interleukin-10. *Annu Rev Immunol* **11**: 165–190.

Moreland LW & Koopman WJ (1992) Infection as a cause of reactive arthritis, ankylosing spondylitis and rheumatic fever. *Curr Opin Rheumatol* **4**: 534–42.

Morgan GJ & Chow WS (1993) Clinical features, diagnosis and prognosis in rheumatoid arthritis. *Curr Opin Rheumatol* **5**: 184–190.

Mountz JD & Talal N (1993) Retroviruses, apoptosis and autogenes. *Immunol Today* **14**: 532–536.

Murayama T, Jisaki F, Ayata M, Sakamuro D, Hironaka T, Hirai K, Tsuchiya N, Ito K & Kurukawa T (1992). Cytomegalovirus genomes demonstrated by polymerase chain reaction in synovial fluid from rheumatoid arthritis patients. *Clin Exp Rheumatol* **10**: 161–164.

Naides SJ (1993) Parvovirus B19 infection. *Rheum Dis Clin North Am* **19**: 457–475.

Nakajima T, Aono H, Hasunuma T, Yamamoto K, Maruyama I, Nosaka T. Hatanaka M & Nishioka K (1993) Overgrowth of human synovial cells driven by the human T cell leukemia virus type I tax gene. *J Clin Invest* **92**: 186–193.

Narayan O, Zink MC, Gorrell M, McEntee M, Sharma D & Adams R (1992) Lentivirus induced arthritis in animals. *J Rheumatol Suppl* **32**: 25–32.

Nepom BS (1993) The role of the major histocompatibility complex in autoimmunity. *Clin Immunol Immunopathol* **67**: suppl. 50–55.

Neumann DA, Lane JR, LaFond WA, Allen GS, Wulff SM, Herskowitz A et al. (1991) Heart-specific autoantibodies can be eluted from the hearts of Coxsackievirus B3-infected mice. *Clin Exp Immunol* **86**: 405–412.

Nickerson CL, Luthra HS, Savarirayan S & David CS (1990) Susceptibility of HLA-B27 transgenic mice to *Yersinia enterococolitica* infection. *Hum Immunol* **28**: 382–396.

Nishioka K, Nakajima T, Hasunuma T & Sato K (1993) Rheumatic manifestation of human leukemia virus infection. *Rheum Dis Clin North Am* **19**: 489–503.

Oldstone MBA & Notkins AL (1986) Molecular Mimicry. In Notkins AL & Oldstone MBA (eds) *Concepts of Viral Pathogenesis*, pp. 195–202. New York: Springer-Verlag.

Paliard X, West SG, Lafferty JA, Clements JR, Kappler JW, Marrack P & Kotzin BL (1991) Evidence for the effects of a superantigen in rheumatoid arthritis. *Science* 253: 325–329.

Panayi GS, Lanchbury JS & Kingsley GH (1992) The importance of the T cell in initiating and maintaining the chronic synovitis of rheumatoid arthritis [editorial]. *Arthritis Rheum* 35: 729–735.

Posnett DN (1993) Do superantigens play a role in autoimmunity? *Semin Immunol* 5: 65–72.

Ramsay AJ, Ruby J & Ramshaw IA (1993) A case for cytokines as effector molecules in the resolution of virus infection. *Immunol Today* 14: 155–157.

Randen I, Thompson KM, Pascual V, Victor K, Beale D, Coadwell J, Forre O, Capra JD & Natvig JB (1992) Rheumatoid factor V genes from patients with rheumatoid arthritis are diverse and show evidence of an antigen-driven response. *Immunol Rev* 128: 49–71.

Razin S (1992) Peculiar properties of mycoplasmas: the smallest self-replicating prokaryotes. *Fems Microbiol Lett* 79: 423–431.

Renz H, Gentz U, Schmidt A, Dapper T, Nain M & Gemsa D (1989) Activation of macrophages in an experimental rat model of arthritis induced by *Erysipelothrix rhusiopathiae* infection. *Infect Immun* 57: 3172–3180.

Res P, Thole J & de VR (1991) Heat-shock proteins and autoimmunity in humans. *Springer Semin Immunopathol* 13: 81–98.

Reveille JD (1993) The interplay of nature versus nuture in predisposition to the rheumatic diseases. *Rheum Dis Clin North Am* 19: 15–28.

Richardson BC (1992) T cell receptor usage in rheumatic disease. *Clin Exp Rheumatol* 10: 271–283.

Rocken M, Urban JF & Shevach EM (1992) Infection breaks T-cell tolerance. *Nature* 359: 79–82.

Rodriguez MA & Williams RJ (1989) Infection and rheumatic diseases. *Clin Exp Rheumatol* 7: 91–97.

Rook GA & Stanford JL (1992) Slow bacterial infections or autoimmunity? *Immunol Today* 13: 160–164.

Rotbart HA (1990) Human parvovirus infections. *Annu Rev Med* 41: 25–34.

Roudier J, Petersen J, Rhodes GH, Luka J & Carson DA (1989) Susceptibility to rheumatoid arthritis maps to a T-cell epitope shared by the HLA-Dw4 DR beta-1 chain and the Epstein-Barr virus glycoprotein gp110. *Proc Natl Acad Sci USA* 86: 5104–5108.

Rynes RI (1991) Painful rheumatic syndromes associated with human immunodeficiency virus infection. *Rheum Dis Clin North Am* 17: 79–87.

Sasso EH (1992) Immunoglobulin V genes in rheumatoid arthritis. *Rheum Dis Clin North Am* 18: 809–836.

Sato K, Maruyama I, Maruyama Y, Kitajima I, Nakajima Y, Higaki M, Yamamoto K, Miyasaka N, Osam M & Nishioka K (1991) Arthritis in patients infected with human T lymphotropic virus type I. Clinical and immunopathogenic features. *Arthritis Rheum* 34: 714–721.

Sawada T, Hirohata S, Inoue T & Ito K (1991) Development of rheumatoid arthritis after hepatitis C virus infection. *Arthritis Rheum* 34: 1620–1621.

Schaible UE, Kramer MD, Wallich R, Tran T & Simon MM (1991) Experimental *Borrelia burgdorferi* infection in inbred mouse strains: antibody response and association of H-2 genes with resistance and susceptibility to development of arthritis. *Eur J Immunol* 21: 2397–2405.

Schmitz JL, Schell RF, Hejka A, England DM & Konick L (1988) Induction of lyme arthritis in LSH hamsters. *Infect Immun* 56: 2336–2342.

Schoenfeld R, Araneo B, Ma Y, Yang LM & Weis JJ (1992) Demonstration of a B-lymphocyte mitogen produced by the Lyme disease pathogen, *Borrelia burgdorferi*. *Infect Immun* 60: 455–464.

Sewell KL & Trentham DE (1993) Pathogenesis of rheumatoid arthritis. *Lancet* 341: 283–286.

Silman AJ (1992) The genetic epidemiology of rheumatoid arthritis. *Clin Exp Rheumatol* 10: 309–312.

Sood SK, Rubin LG, Blader ME & Ilowite NT (1993) Positive serology for Lyme borreliosis in patients with juvenile rheumatoid arthritis in a Lyme borreliosis endemic area: analysis by immunoblot. *J Rheumatol* 20: 739–741.

Span AH, Mullers W, Miltenburg AM & Bruggeman CA (1991) Cytomegalovirus induced PMN adherence in relation to an ELAM-1 antigen present on infected endothelial cell monolayers. *Immunology* 72: 355–360.

Stannard LM & Hardie DR (1991) An Fc receptor for human immunoglobulin G is located within the tegument of human cytomegalovirus. *J Virol* 65: 3411–3415.

Steere AC (1991) Clinical definitions and differential diagnosis of Lyme arthritis. *Scand J Infect Dis Suppl* 77: 51–54.

Strober S & Holoshitz J (1990) Mechanisms of immune injury in rheumatoid arthritis: evidence for the involvement of T cells and heat-shock protein. *Immunol Rev* 118: 233–255.

Tai KS, Whelan PI, Patel MS & Currie B (1993) An outbreak of epidemic polyarthritis (Ross River virus disease) in the Northern Territory during the 1990–1991 wet season. *Med J Aust* 158: 522–525.

Taurog JD, Hammer RE, Montanez R, Breban HN, Croft JT & Balish E (1993) Effect of the germfree state on the inflammatory disease of HLA-B27 transgenic rats. A split result. *Arthritis Rheum* **36** (**supplement**): S46.

Thompson SJ, Butcher PD, Patel VK, Rook GA, Stanford J, van-der-Zee R & Elson CJ (1991) Modulation of pristane-induced arthritis by mycobacterial antigens. *Autoimmunity* **11**: 35–43.

Thurn J (1988) Human parvovirus B19: historical and clinical review. *Rev Infect Dis* **10**: 1005–1011.

Toivanen P, Merilahti PR, Gripenberg C, Soderstrom KO & Jaakkola UM (1988) Experimental *Yersinia*-associated arthritis in the spontaneously hypertensive rat. *Br J Rheumatol* **2**: 52–54.

Trabandt A, Gay RE & Gay S (1992) Oncogene activation in rheumatoid synovium. *Apmis* **100**: 861–875.

Vaughan JH (1990) Infection and rheumatic diseases: a review (2). *Bull Rheum Dis* **39**: 1–8.

Viner HJ, Gaston JS & Bacon PA (1993) Synovial fluid antigen-presenting cell function in rheumatoid arthritis. *Clin Exp Immunol* **92**: 251–255.

Wilder RL & Crofford LJ (1991) Do infectious agents cause rheumatoid arthritis? *Clin Orthop* **265**: 36–41.

Winchester R, Dwyer R & Rose S (1992) The genetic basis of rheumatoid arthritis. The shared epitope hypothesis. *Rheum Dis Clin North Am* **18**: 761–783.

Wooley PH (1991) Animal models of rheumatoid arthritis. *Curr Opin Rheumatol* **3**: 407–420.

Wooley PH, Seibold JR, Whalen JD & Chapdelaine JM (1989) Pristane-induced arthritis. The immunologic and genetic features of an experimental murine model of autoimmune disease. *Arthritis Rheum* **32**: 1022–1030.

Wordsworth P (1992) Rheumatoid arthritis. *Curr Opin Immunol* **4**: 766–769.

Wu J, Zhou T, He J & Mountz JD (1993) Autoimmune disease in mice due to integration of an endogenous retrovirus in an apoptosis gene. *J Exp Med* **178**: 461–468.

Yang L, Ma Y, Schoenfeld R, Griffiths M, Eichwald E, Araneo B & Weis JJ (1992) Evidence for B-lymphocyte mitogen activity in *Borrelia burgdorferi*-infected mice. *Infect Immun* **60**: 3033–3041.

Yong Z, Hill JL, Hirofuji T, Mander M & Yu DT (1988) An experimental mouse model of *Yersinia*-induced reactive arthritis. *Microb Pathog* **4**: 305–310.

Yoshizaki K, Kuritani T & Kishimoto T (1992) Interleukin-6 in autoimmune disorders. *Semin Immunol* **4**: 155–166.

Ziegler B, Gay RE, Huang GQ, Fassbender HG & Gay S (1989) Immunohistochemical localization of HTLV-I p19- and p24-related antigens in synovial joints of patients with rheumatoid arthritis. *Am J Pathol* **135**: 1–5.

Ziesenis A, Rollinger B, Franz B, Hart S, Hadam M & Leibold W (1992) Changes in rat leukocyte populations in peripheral blood, spleen, lymph nodes and synovia during *Erysipelas* bacteria-induced polyarthritis. *J Exp Anim Sci* **35**: 2–15.

Zink MC, Yager JA & Myers JD (1990) Pathogenesis of caprine arthritis encephalitis virus. Cellular localization of viral transcripts in tissues of infected goats. *Am J Pathol* **136**: 843–854.

22 Bacterial Cell-wall Induced Arthritis: Models of Chronic Recurrent Polyarthritis and Reactivation of Monoarticular Arthritis

John H. Schwab

INTRODUCTION

Bacterial cell wall structures can induce multisystem acute and chronic inflammatory diseases, including arthritis (Schwab, 1970, 1982; Cromartie *et al.*, 1977). Chronic, remittent inflammation is induced and maintained by the localization in the joint or other tissues of poorly biodegradable, persistent bacterial cell wall fragments derived during *in vivo* degradation of bacterial cells (Ohanian and Schwab, 1967; Cromartie *et al.*, 1977; Schwab, 1979). This hypothesis has evolved from studies on inflammation induced by injection of cell wall fragments, composed of covalently bound polymers of peptidoglycan-polysaccharide (PG-PS) isolated from the cell walls of several bacterial species that colonize humans. Most of our work has utilized PG-PS isolated from the cell walls of group A streptococci (*Streptococcus pyogenes*) for which we use the acronym PG-APS. The tissue involved and the clinical course of disease depend upon host variables such as immunocompetence, the species of animal, genetic background of inbred strains within a species, and route of injection (Schwab, 1982; Wilder *et al.*, 1983). Severity and course of disease are also determined by the molecular size of the PG-PS polymers (Fox *et al.*, 1982) and structural features of both the peptidoglycan and polysaccharide moieties, as reflected in the difference between PG-PS isolated from cell walls of different bacterial species (Stimpson *et al.*, 1986) or by chemical modification of PG-PS (Stimpson *et al.*, 1987b). PG-PS from cell walls of normal intestinal bacteria (Severijnen *et al.* 1988) or from two species prominent in patients with Crohn's disease or rheumatoid arthritis (RA) (Severijnen *et al.*, 1990) are also arthropathogenic. The association of intestinal inflammation and arthritis, and the structure and relevant biological properties of peptidoglycan and polysaccharide moieites, are reviewed elsewhere (Schwab, 1993).

A detailed description of preparation of bacterial cell walls, purification and fractionation of PG-PS; as well as injection of the rats and monitoring of arthritis in the animal models, has been presented (Stimpson and Schwab, 1989).

CHRONIC, EROSIVE SYNOVITIS INDUCED IN RATS BY SYSTEMIC INJECTION OF BACTERIAL CELL WALL FRAGMENTS

Chronic, remittent, erosive polyarthritis is produced in susceptible strains of rats by a single intraperitoneal (i.p.) injection of an aqueous suspension of cell wall fragments,

Mechanisms and Models in Rheumatoid Arthritis
ISBN 0–12–340440–1

of appropriate size, isolated from group A streptococci or certain other bacteria (Cromartie *et al.*, 1977). The disease is characterized by an initial acute inflammation of the ankles, wrists and small joints of the feet which reaches a peak at 3–5 days then recedes. This is followed by a recurrence of inflammation at 2–4 weeks with synovitis, pannus formation and cartilage and bone erosion. In most of the animals repeated cycles of exacerbation and remission occur over the next several months, progressing to fibrosis and ankylosis of the joints (Cromartie *et al.*, 1977; Dalldorf *et al.*, 1980). The arthritis resembles human disease in its clinical course and distribution, and in its radiological and histological features (Clark *et al.*, 1979; Dalldorf *et al.*, 1980). Severity is correlated with the amount of cell wall in the joint (Dalldorf *et al.*, 1980; Eisenberg *et al.*, 1982). Susceptibility is genetically controlled by multiple (more than two) non-MHC genes (Anderle *et al.*, 1979; Wilder *et al.*, 1982, 1983). Outbred Sprague-Dawley and inbred Lewis and some other inbred strains are susceptible, but inbred Buffalo and Fisher-344 (F344) are resistant to development of chronic disease. The precise nature of the genetic regulation continues to be examined. Recent reports indicate that part of the control involves hypothalamus-pituitary-adrenal response, since susceptible Lewis rats have a reduced glucocorticoid production secondary to a defect in corticotropin releasing hormone synthesis and secretion, while resistant F344 rats have a vigorous hormone response (Aksetijevich *et al.*, 1992).

A MODEL OF MONOARTICULAR ARTHRITIS FOR ANALYSING REMISSION AND RECURRENCE

The repeated cycles of remission and exacerbation of arthritis induced in rats by a single i.p. injection of PG-APS is the most remarkable feature of this disease. Since this waxing and waning develops independently and unpredictably in individual rat joints, analysis of regulation and mechanisms is difficult. Therefore, we have developed variations of the model to induce synchronous and predictable recurrence (Esser *et al.*, 1985b). The most useful variation is the model we describe here, in which a monoarticular arthritis is induced by intra-articular (i.a.) injection of PG-APS into the tibiotalar (ankle) joint and a recurrence is induced 1–6 weeks later by i.v. injection of PG-APS (Esser *et al.*, 1985c). The advantages of this model are: (a) it is very sensitive to manipulation by adjustment of dose of PG-APS, or by intervention with inflammatory mediators or inhibitors; (b) it is very consistent and predictable since reactivation occurs in almost all rats, reaching an initial peak at 3–4 days after the i.v. injection; (c) the contralateral joint injected i.a. with saline provides an internal control; and (d) much smaller amounts of PG-APS are needed. The arthritis reactivated in this model is mechanistically related to the spontaneous exacerbations seen in the chronic phase of disease induced by a single i.p. injection of PG-APS. This is shown by: (a) histological evidence of chronic synovitis and erosion; (b) the requirement for T cells, indicated by the greatly reduced severity of reactivation in congenitally athymic rats compared to euthymic littermates and in rats treated with cyclosporin A (Stimpson *et al.*, 1989; Schwab *et al.*, 1993) and (c) reduced reactivation in Buffalo rats, which are resistant to the chronic phase of arthritis induced by i.p. injection of PG-APS (Esser *et al.*, 1985c).

The i.a. injection of 1–5 μg of PG-APS induces an acute, exudative dose-related response which reaches a maximum in 24–48 h and is confined to the injected ankle

(Esser *et al.*, 1986). The swelling resolves by 3 weeks leaving a histologically evident low level of chronic inflammation that is present for at least 8 weeks in most animals. The important difference from the model of polyarthritis induced by i.p. injection of a much larger dose of PG-APS (45 µg/g body wt) is that with the dose injected i.a., the reaction does not progress to joint destruction and episodes of recurrence, although they occur, are moderate (Esser *et al.*, 1985c). We speculate that this may be due to the absence of a reservoir of PG-APS in the liver and spleen, which exists after i.p. injection, and which would provide a source of PG-APS for translocation to the joint, inducing renewed flares. There is some evidence for this from studies on transplantation of livers from donor rats injected i.v. with PG-APS, which induces reactivation of arthritis in the PG-APS-injured ankle joint of recipient rats (Lichtman *et al.*, 1991). Also consistent with this idea is the observation that i.v. injection of ^{125}I-labelled PG-APS showed increased localization in the PG-APS-injured joint, compared to the control joint, accompanying reactivation of arthritis (Esser *et al.*, 1985c).

REACTIVATION BY PG-PS

Arthritis in joints previously injured by PG-APS can be reactivated by i.v. injection of normally subarthropathic doses (300 µg/200 g rat) of PG-APS; or PG isolated from group A streptococci, PG-PS from group D streptococci, or muramyl dipeptide in a much higher dose (30 mg/rat). Group A streptococcal polysaccharide (APS), PG-PS or PG from *Propionibacterium acnes*, and dextran sulphate are inactive (Esser *et al.*, 1985c). Inflammation only develops in the joint previously inflamed by PG-APS. Contralateral saline-injected control joints or joints inflamed initially by lipopolysaccharide (LPS, endotoxin) cannot be activated by PG-APS injected i.v. in this reactivation model. A recurrence can be induced in a PG-APS injected joint that has been clinically normal for as long as 8 weeks. These results indicate that the initial injury of the joint by PG-APS increases the susceptibility of the joint to subsequent insult, perhaps because the milieu of cytokines and other mediators and growth factors creates an environment conducive to inflammatory cell infiltration and activation (this is discussed below in the context of cytokines and T lymphocytes.

REACTIVATION BY LPS

Once the inflammatory reaction is initiated by PG-APS recurrence can be induced by other antigenically related ubiquitous bacterial products, derived from normal flora as well as from infection. Thus, the i.v. injection of LPS 3 weeks after an i.a. injection of PG-APS can also reactivate arthritis (Stimpson *et al.*, 1987a). The lowest effective dose which can induce recurrence in 100% of the test joints is 10 µg/rat. At this dose very little inflammation is induced in contralateral control joints that had been injected i.a. with saline. LPS or Re mutant LPS from *Salmonella typhimurium* or *Escherichia coli*; LPS from *Yersinia enterocolitica* and *Neisseria gonorrhoeae*; and lipid A from *E. coli*, are all active. Reactivation of arthritis is significantly reduced by injecting polymyxin B with LPS. Joints initially inflamed by i.a. injection of LPS cannot be reactivated by i.v. infection of PG-APS, or the same or antigenically different LPS (Stimpson *et al.*, 1987a). LPS injected i.a. or i.v. into naive rats induces only a mild, transient joint swelling that is completely resolved within 2 weeks with no histological evidence of persistent inflammation (Stimpson *et al.*, 1987a). These results indicate that LPS derived from a variety of indigenous or pathogenic bacteria could be involved in chronic erosive arthritis by perpetuating joint injury initiated by peptido-glycan polymers, even though LPS by itself is unable to induce such a disease process.

REACTIVATION BY SUPERANTIGENS

Microbial superantigens are among the most potent activators of T lymphocytes, stimulating as many as 20% of the total T cells, compared to about 0.01% activation by specific antigen binding to the T cell receptor (TCR). They are distinguished from other mitogens on the basis of their requirement for presentation to T cells by class II MHC on antigen-presenting cells (APC) and most importantly, by their selective binding to a limited number of Vβ chains of the TCR. Superantigens differ from classical antigens in that they are not MHC-restricted; and they bind to the outside of the cleft of MHC class II on the APC, and to a limited domain on the outside of the TCR (Kotb, 1992; Richardson, 1992). Paliard *et al.* (1991), in a study of nine RA patients, reported a selective depletion of Vβ14 T cells in the blood and a relative increase of this population in the synovial fluid. Studies of this sort have formed the basis for the hypothesis that superantigens could be involved in RA and other diseases of immune dysfunction (Marrack & Kappler, 1990; Friedman *et al.*, 1991; Paliard *et al.*, 1991; Kotb, 1992). While several other laboratories have confirmed selective Vβ usage in patients with RA, the most prominent Vβ peptide(s) selected varies between different laboratories or subjects (Richardson 1992). Further discussion of superantigens in RA and experimental arthritis is to be found in Chapters 2, 3, 19 and 21, this volume.

We have recently utilized the model of reactivation of monoclonal arthritis to demonstrate that a superantigen can, in fact, induce a recurrence of arthritis (Schwab *et al.*, 1993). Intravenous injection of toxic shock syndrome toxin-1 (TSST-1) produced by *Staphylococcus aureus*, can reactivate arthritis in a rat ankle joint which had been injured previously by i.a. injection of PG-APS. A dose of TSST-1 of 125 μg/kg can induce a recurrence of arthritis characterized as a prolonged, chronic synovitis with pannus formation and some marginal erosion of cartilage and bone. Another superantigen, streptococcal pyrogenic exotoxin (SPE-A) produced by *Streptococcus pyogenes*, induced only a mild acute recurrence and no prolonged chronic synovitis. Intravenous injection of TSST-1 did not induce arthritis in control joints that had been injected previously with saline (Schwab *et al.*, 1993). These studies show that superantigens are incapable of initiating inflammatory arthritis in the rat, but they can contribute to the disease process by sustaining or exacerbating arthritis in appropriately inflamed joints.

Recent studies compare the capacity of other bacterial superantigens to induce recurrence of arthritis in this model (Schwab *et al.*, unpublished data). Staphylococcal enterotoxins A, B, and C1 (SEA, SEB, SEC-1) share some structural and biological properties with TSST-1 and with SPE-A, and all can stimulate Lewis rat T cells *in vitro*. The *in vivo* response to SEA is limited to a moderate acute recurrence with a dose of 125 μg/kg, which is comparable to the *in vivo* effect of SPE-A; but even at a dose of 1.25 mg/kg SEB and SEC-1 display little capacity to induce any flare of arthritis in Lewis rats.

The importance of these observations is the demonstration that bacterial superantigen provides another group of microbial products common in the human environment, in addition to PG-PS and LPS, which could be part of the etiology of RA and other inflammatory diseases. The mechanisms of bacterial arthritis and the role of staphylococcal enterotoxins are reviewed in detail in Chapter 24, this volume.

MECHANISMS OF TISSUE INJURY AND REGULATION OF REMISSION AND RECURRENCE

T CELLS

Evidence that T lymphocytes are required for the chronic relapsing phase of bacterial cell-wall induced arthritis, but not the acute phase, comes from numerous observations. Wilder and co-workers (Allen *et al.*, 1985) using i.p. injection of PG-APS, showed that congenitally athymic nude rats developed a typical acute arthritis, but unlike their euthymic littermates, failed to develop the chronic recurrent phase. Athymic rats also developed much less severe granulomatous hepatitis (Allen *et al.*, 1985). Treatment with cyclosporin A did not effect the acute phase of arthritis, but significantly reduced severity of the chronic phase, even when initial treatment was delayed until 12 days after injection of streptococcal cell wall (Yocum *et al.*, 1986). This group also reported a marked enhancement of expression of MHC class II (Ia) antigen in the synovium, which paralleled severity of arthritis (Wilder *et al.*, 1987). Expression of Ia was thymus dependent in the chronic phase, since it did not occur in athymic rats or rats treated with cyclosporin A. Other laboratories have also found that congenitally athymic rats develop less severe chronic arthritis compared to euthymic littermates after i.p. injection of streptococcal cell wall (Ridge *et al.*, 1985).

Two T-cell lines derived from rats with streptococcal cell-wall induced arthritis could passively transfer a moderate arthritis (DeJoy *et al.*, 1989). In that study the T-cell lines were reactive with both streptococcal cell wall and mycobacterium antigens, but did not proliferate in response to preparations containing the 65-kDa heat-shock protein antigen. Klasen *et al.* (1992) also isolated T-cell lines from the lymph nodes of Lewis rats injected with arthropathogenic PG-PS from *E. aerofaciens*. A T-cell line injected i.v. induced arthritis in Lewis, but not in MHC-compatible F344 rats. The cell lines were stimulated *in vitro* by PG-PS from human intestinal contents. Klasen and co-workers (1992) describe these as autoreactive T cells.

Another approach is to examine the effect of specific suppression or elimination of T cells by antibody. Treatment with monoclonal antibodies specific for rat TCR, beginning at the time of i.p. injection of PG-APS, had no effect on the early acute joint inflammation but significantly reduced development of the chronic phase of polyarthritis and erosion of cartilage and bone (Yoshino *et al.*, 1991). In a very interesting study van den Broek *et al.* (1992b) showed that monoclonal antibody against rat CD4 T cells provided resistance against PG-APS-induced polyarthritis if given before arthritis developed, and reduced disease if treatment was delayed until arthritis was established. Even after CD4 T cells returned to normal levels arthritis did not occur, and reinjection of rats with PG-APS could not induce arthritis, indicating that the rats had developed tolerance to PG-APS antigens. Furthermore, adjuvant arthritis could not be induced in these rats, indicating that 'streptococcal cell walls and

M. tuberculosis may use similar mechanisms of regulation of arthritis' (van den Broek *et al.*, 1992b). This could be related to the long-lasting transplantation tolerance induced by anti-CD4 which was transferable to naive T cells and reportedly maintained by an 'infectious' process (Qin *et al.*, 1993).

Using a model of reactivation of monoarticular arthritis, van den Broek *et al.* (1990) reported that treatment of Lewis rats with a pan T-cell reactive monoclonal antibody prevented reactivation. Recent work from our laboratory shows that cyclosporin A also suppresses reactivation of monoarticular arthritis by PG-APS as well as by TSST-1 (Schwab *et al.*, 1993), again demonstrating the importance of T cells in the chronic recurrent phase of bacterial cell-wall induced arthritis.

However, the function of T lymphocytes in the pathogenesis of bacterial cell-wall induced arthritis is complex. Hunter *et al.* (1980) reported that a delayed-type hypersensitivity (DTH) skin test to peptidoglycan could be elicited in outbred Sprague-Dawley rats 6–14 days after i.p. injection of a subarthropathic dose of PG-APS, but 2–4 weeks later a skin test could not be elicited and these rats could not be sensitized again with peptidoglycan. After an arthropathic dose of PG-APS a DTH skin test could not be elicited at any time. These rats remained hyporesponsive to PG for at least 3 months and lymphocytes from these rats had a severely depressed response to phytothaemagglutinin *in vitro* (Hunter *et al.*, 1980). These observations were extended to show that *in vitro* proliferative depression of T cells was caused by an adherent suppressor cell which had the properties of a macrophage (Regan *et al.*, 1988). Catalase and indomethacin only partially reversed the suppressive activity, indicating that prostaglandin and oxygen metabolites were not the primary molecular mediators of suppression. In addition, lymphocytes from Buffalo rats, which are resistant to induction of arthritis, showed less suppression than Sprague-Dawley or Lewis strains (Regan *et al.*, 1988). Consistent with these findings of suppressed *in vivo* and *in vitro* function T cells is the report of deficiency of IL-2 in rats injected with an arthropathic dose of PG-APS (Ridge *et al.*, 1986). Somewhat different results were reported by van den Broek *et al.* (1988). They found that the *in vitro* T-cell response to streptococcal cell wall antigen was absent in the arthritis-resistant strain of F344 rats, while present in susceptible Lewis rats. They further reported that injection of F344 rats with PG-APS induced a generalized unresponsiveness to the mitogen Con A, and to albumin, if this antigen was injected with PG-APS. Removal of CD8$^+$ T cells with Ox8 monoclonal antibody restored *in vitro* response of F344 T cells to PG-APS and mitogens. From this they suggested that the resistance of F344 rats to chronic arthritis induced by PG-APS is the consequence of a suppressor T-cell population (van den Broek *et al.*, 1988). However, in a subsequent study (van den Broek *et al.*, 1990) depletion of CD8$^+$ T cells from F344 rats did not render these rats susceptible to arthritis.

Studies of Wahl and co-workers (Wahl & Hunt, 1988) show that the suppression of T-cell activity by macrophages, in PG-APS injected rats, involves suppression of cytokine production, as well as growth, and part of this suppression could be accounted for by TGFβ produced by macrophages. Nitric oxide production is also part of the down-regulation by macrophages, since addition of the nitric oxide synthetase inhibitor N^G-monomethyl-L-arginine (N-MMA) to rat spleen cell cultures greatly increases the response to Con A (Mills, 1991) or superantigens (Isobe and Nakashima, 1992). Current work in our laboratory shows that the proliferative response of Lewis rat spleen cells to PG-APS is significantly increased by culturing cells with N-MMA (Brown and Schwab, unpublished), confirming that NO production by rat macrophages stimulated by PG-APS is probably also part of the mechanism of macrophage suppression of T-cell activation, in addition to TGFβ and prostaglandins.

It remains uncertain whether the induced hyporesponsiveness of T lymphocytes, which accompanies the development of PG-APS induced arthritis, is an essential part of the pathogenesis of the disease. As with many features of this experimental model, anergy of T cells is observed in human RA and one report shows an association of clinical improvement with reversal of anergy (Wahl et al., 1983). We hypothesize that a subpopulation of T cells has a protective function, perhaps in determining the trafficking and disposal of bacterial cell wall, and that depressing this function is an essential part of establishment of inflammation. Another T-cell population must have an important role in maintaining the recurrent chronic phase of inflammation, since as summarized above, there is abundant evidence that T cells are required in this phase of experimental arthritis. Thus far, such distinct T-cell populations have not been identified in this model, but protective and arthropathogenic T-cell lines have been obtained from rats with adjuvant arthritis (Holoshitz et al., 1983). These cell lines can be stimulated by a 65-kDa heat-shock protein (HSP) derived from *Mycobacterium tuberculosis*. Therefore, it is significant that van den Broek et al. (1989) have shown that in the bacterial cell-wall induced model, rats can be protected by immunizing with a 65-kDa HSP from *M. tuberculosis*. This protection was accompanied by a suppression of *in vitro* T-cell response, not only to streptococcal cell wall antigens, but also to the 65-kDa HSP and to Con A. There is no obvious explanation why van den Broek et al. (1989) did not observe the suppression of T-cell responses in the rats given systemic arthropathogenic doses of PG-APS, as reported by three other groups (Ridge et al., 1986; Regan et al. 1988; Wahl and Hunt, 1988). It is also uncertain why only spleen cells from rats first immunized with 65-kDa HSP were also anergic to Con A. Although they present strong evidence that the protection stimulated by HSP vaccination against PG-APS induced arthritis is immunologically specific and T-cell mediated, the possibility that this is non-specific immunosuppression must still be considered.

Two observations provide convincing evidence that resistance of F344 rats and susceptibility of Lewis rats to arthritis is dependent upon the capacity of haemopoietic stem cell progeny to recognize the PG-APS antigens. Lethally irradiated Lewis rats, reconstituted with F344 bone marrow, were resistent to PG-APS induced arthritis, and to adjuvant arthritis; whereas, the chimera of F344 strain reconstituted with Lewis bone marrow was susceptible to arthritis in both experimental models (van Bruggen et al., 1991). Thus, they conclude that susceptibility or resistance depends upon the origin of immune cells and not upon the environment provided by the recipient. Furthermore, data presented by this same laboratory show that the resistance of the F344 rats is the result of tolerance to bacterial cell wall antigens, induced by the microbial flora (van den Broek et al., 1992a). This conclusion comes from their demonstration that germ-free F344 rats are susceptible to arthritis and that the T cells from these rats can now respond to PG-APS *in vitro*. Conventionalized F344 rats again become less susceptible to PG-APS induced arthritis (van den Broek et al., 1992a).

CYTOKINES

In a review Wahl (1991a; see Chapter 12, this volume) lists 12 cytokines or growth factors that have been identified as mRNA or protein in human rheumatoid fluid or synovial tissue and describes biological activities which may be relevant in pathogenesis of the disease. The role of cytokines in RA and in animal models is reviewed in Chapters 2, 9, 10, 12, 13 and 26, this volume. Several of these have also been identified, either as mRNA or protein, in joints of rats with bacterial cell-wall induced arthritis; including TGFβ (Wahl and Hunt, 1988; Lafyatis et al., 1989) and IL-1 (Staton et al., 1990).

In another approach, we have examined the capacity of cytokines, injected locally or systemically, to induce or influence reactivation in the monoarticular arthritis model. Inflammation in a PG-APS injured joint can be reactivated by i.v. injection of 1.0 μg of human recombinant IL-1 (Schwab et al., 1991), while i.a. injection of as little as 1.0 ng of human or mouse recombinant IL-1α, or 3 ng of mr IL-1β (Stimpson et al., 1988) also induced an acute, transient, exudative response. Reactivation induced by either i.v. or i.a. injection of IL-1 reached a peak at 6 h and resolved with some residual chronic inflammation which was more severe than observed in control joints that had been injected initially with saline. Repeated i.a. injection of IL-1 induced repeated courses of renewed inflammation. After 5 weekly i.a. injections there was on-going chronic inflammation with marginal cartilage erosion in the PG-APS injured joint that was not observed in the contralateral control ankle (Stimpson et al., 1988). Human recombinant C5a and heated IL-1 were inactive and served as peptide controls (Stimpson et al., 1988). Other cytokines examined by the same assay, which could induce reactivation of joint inflammation, include in decreasing order of activity, TNFα, substance P, IFNγ, and PDGF-BB; while IL-2 and IL-8 were ineffective (Stimpson et al., 1990; Stimpson and Schwab, unpublished). All of the effective mediators had in common the induction of more severe reactions in a PG-APS injured joint compared to a saline-injected joint. However, PDGF was unique in that the peak joint swelling developed much later (48 h after i.a. injection), lasted much longer (5 days) and no pain response was observed (Stimpson et al., 1990).

Remmers et al. (1990) have compared the effects of several cytokines on in vitro growth of synoviocytes from RA patients and from rats with PG-APS induced arthritis. PDGF was the most active stimulator of long-term growth of both human and rat synoviocytes, whereas EGF, TGFβ, IL-1α and IFNγ had little effect. They concluded that PDGF could be important in the pathological proliferation of synoviocytes in arthritis, and this may be down-regulated by TGFβ. This is reviewed in greater detail by Zagorski and Wahl in Chapter 12, this volume.

Another method to establish the importance of a mediator in the pathogenesis of experimental arthritis is to determine the effect of a specific inhibitor. Treatment of rats with a down-regulating cytokine, the human recombinant IL-1 receptor antagonist (IL-1ra), can significantly suppress recurrence of joint swelling and severity of synovitis and erosion induced by reactivation by i.v. injection of PG-APS (Schwab et al., 1991). Polyclonal rabbit anti-murine TNFα is even more effective than IL-1ra in reducing recurrence of inflammation induced by PG-APS (Schwab et al., 1993). It is interesting, however, that neither IL-1ra or anti-TNFα antibody can effectively reduce reactivation of arthritis induced by i.v. injection of LPS or the superantigen TSST-1 (Schwab *et al.*, 1993).

Wahl and co-workers have carefully examined the pro- and anti-inflammatory effects of cytokines in the polyarthritis model induced by i.p. injection of PG-APS. TGFβ injected systemically 1 day before PG-APS suppressed development of both the acute and chronic phases of arthritis; and even when delayed until after the acute phase, further development of arthritis was suppressed (Brandes *et al.*, 1991). In contrast, local i.a. injection of TGFβ greatly increased the severity of ongoing arthritis (Wahl, 1991b; Wahl *et al.*, 1991a), which may be related to the enhanced expression of genes coding for IL-1 and other growth factors (Allen *et al.*, 1990; see Chapter 12, this volume).

Severity of acute and chronic, erosive polyarthritis was also suppressed by systemic injection of IFNγ (Allen *et al.*, 1991; Wahl *et al.*, 1991b). This was associated with a marked reduction in the number of neutrophils and monocytes infiltrating the tissue, which correlated with a decrease in C5a receptors in the inflammatory cells. As with TGFβ, local i.a. injection of IFNγ exacerbated arthritis in that joint (Wahl *et al.*, 1991a). Possibly this enhancement of arthritis reflects the capacity of IFNγ to activate production of pro-inflammatory cytokines such as IL-1 and TNFα by monocytes already recruited into the synovial tissue (Wahl, 1991a).

COMPLEMENT AND ANTIBODY

The chemotactic and vascular permeability effects, and other powerful pro-inflammatory properties of complement components, implicate them as important mediators in the development of joint inflammation. The isolated peptidoglycan moiety of PG-APS is a potent activator of the alternate complement pathway (ACP) (Bokisch, 1975; Greenblatt *et al.*, 1978). The PG-APS complex, however, requires a small amount of antibody to activate the ACP (Eisenberg and Schwab, 1986). The Fab fragment of antibody is effective in activation of the ACP, but only the antibody specific for the *N*-acetyl-D-glucosamine epitope functions in activation of this pathway; and this antibody is present in low but sufficient quantity in normal human serum (Eisenberg and Schwab, 1986).

During the evolving arthritis decreases and elevations of serum haemolytic activity, and of the factor D and C3 components of the ACP, occur *in vivo* after i.p. injection of an arthropathic dose of PG-APS (Lambris *et al.*, 1982). Reduction of serum complement level by treatment with cobra venom factor for 3 days beginning at the time of PG-APS injection significantly suppresses the acute phase of arthritis, but not the chronic course of disease (Schwab *et al.*, 1982). This treatment does not alter the amount of PG-APS in the ankle or wrist joints. Thus, complement does have a role in evolving arthritis, but its effect is not upon the transport of PG-APS into joint tissue (Schwab *et al.*, 1982).

A single i.v. injection of the muralytic enzyme, mutanolysin, prevents the development of chronic arthritis, even if treatment is delayed until severe inflammation has developed (Janusz *et al.*, 1984). The extent of *in vitro* degradation of PG-APS by mutanolysin parallels the loss of complement activation and arthropathogenicity (Janusz *et al.*, 1987). Furthermore, there is also a reduction in the *in vivo* complexing of C3 with PG-APS in the limbs of rats injected i.p. with PG-APS and treated with mutanolysin. This correlation of loss of arthropathic activity and loss of activation of complement supports the hypothesis that complement activation products are an important part of the experimental arthritis (Janusz *et al.*, 1987). Spitznagel *et al.* (1986) also reported that the arthropathic effect of PG-APS is related to capacity to activate the ACP. They found that *in vitro* degradation of cell walls from groups A, B or D streptococci with rat or human lysozyme could increase or decrease complement activation, and this correlated with the extent of exposure of amino-sugar reducing groups.

Using a sensitive radioimmunoassay, serum antibodies specific for peptidoglycan or polysaccharide were measured at intervals following i.p. injection of an arthropathic dose of PG-APS, but no convincing correlation with disease was found (Greenblatt *et al.*, 1980). A detailed analysis of IgG and IgM antibodies against four peptidoglycan epitopes and two polysaccharide epitopes of PG-APS showed that individual rats vary widely in response to the different epitopes and in isotype of antibody specific for each determinant (Esser *et al.*, 1985a). An apparent protective effect of IgM anti-peptidoglycan antibodies in the development of chronic arthritis was the only suggestion of a function of serum antibody in this model.

PROTEASES, KININS, AND OXYGEN RADICALS

Products of the activated coagulation and kallikrein–kinin systems are powerful mediators of increased vascular permeability, vasodilation, and neutrophil chemotaxis. Recent studies (DeLa Cadena *et al.*, 1991) demonstrate an early and persistent decrease in prekallikrein levels, and in high molecular weight kininogen levels in the acute phase, after i.p. injection of rats with an arthropathogenic dose of PG-APS. These changes reflect activation of the kallikrein–kinin system and correlate with severity of arthritis. *In vivo* activation of the contact system releases enzymatically active factor XIIa, a protease that can cleave C1 and thus can be an initiator of the complement cascade. The elevated sedimentation rate, increased leukocyte count, and decreased haematocrit in the arthritic rats also could reflect activation of the contact coagulation system (DeLa Cadena *et al.*, 1991). Further evidence that trypsin-like proteases have an important role in this model of arthritis come from the experiments showing the suppression of arthritis by treatment with synthetic protease inhibitors (Geratz *et al.*, 1990, 1991), although there is no evidence that these inhibitors are functioning *in vivo* through an effect on the clotting or complement systems. The role of proteases in arthritic joint destruction is reviewed by Poole *et al.* in Chapter 9 and Cawston in Chapter 17, this volume.

Oxygen metabolites (superoxide anion, hydrogen peroxide, and hydroxyl radicals) produced by phagocytic cells can be an important part of tissue damage in inflammation (Chapter 15, this volume). We have shown that PG-APS, with bound complement (C3), can activate human polymorphonuclear neutrophil (PMN) metabolism and increase secretion of superoxide anion (Leong *et al.*, 1984). Since PMN and macrophages containing PG-APS are prominent in bacterial cell-wall induced arthritis, especially during recurrences of flares (Dalldorf *et al.*, 1980), the results of Leong *et al.* suggest that oxygen radicals could be contributing to the pathology. Others have shown that monocytes from susceptible Lewis rats produce more oxygen metabolites when stimulated *in vitro* with PG-APS than cells from F344 rats, which are resistant to arthritis (Skaleric *et al.*, 1991). More direct evidence that reactive oxygen is involved is provided by the demonstration that i.a. injection of superoxide dismutase or catalase can reduce PG-APS induced arthritis (Skaleric *et al.*, 1991). See Chapter 15, this volume, for a detailed discussion of the role of free radicals in rheumatoid joint inflammation.

CONCLUSIONS

The bacterial cell wall models of chronic inflammation not only provide experimental approaches for analysing mechanisms of tissue injury, and sensitive assays to test anti-inflammatory agents; but in addition, the data summarized here support the hypothesis that PG-PS polymers from bacterial cell walls are part of the etiology of human arthritides and related chronic inflammatory diseases. Consistent with this concept are several studies showing significantly higher levels of anti-peptidoglycan antibodies in patients with RA and other rheumatic diseases (Pope *et al.*, 1982; Johnson *et al.*, 1984; Burgos-Vargas *et al.*, 1986; Moore *et al.*, 1989; Nesher *et al.*, 1991; Todome *et al.*, 1992). Other studies show that agalactosyl IgG found in patients with RA crossreacts with PG-APS (Rook *et al.*, 1988); and that anti-PG-PS and rheumatoid factor may share idiotypic specificity (Johnson and Smalley, 1988).

Considerable insight into mechanisms of the disease process has been gained by preventing or intervening in evolving arthritis with agents that have specific and well-established modes of action. These have been discussed above and are summarized in Table 1.

Table 1. Prevention or treatment of arthritis induced by PG-PS from bacterial cell walls

Agent	References
Muramidase (peptidoglycan degradation)	Janusz *et al.* (1986, 1987)
BABIM and analogues (protease inhibitors)	Geratz *et al.* (1990, 1991)
Cytokines	
IL-1	Schwab *et al.* (1991)
TGFβ	Brandes *et al.* (1991)
IFNγ	Allen *et al.* (1991)
Cytokine blockers	
IL-1 receptor antagonist	Schwab *et al.* (1991)
Anti-TNFα antibody	Schwab *et al.* (1993)
Cyclosporin A	Schwab *et al.* (1993); Yocum *et al.* (1986)
Anti T-cell antibody	
Anti-pan T cell	van den Broek *et al.* (1990)
Anti-CD4	van den Broek *et al.* (1992b)
Anti-TCR	Yoshino *et al.* (1991)
Superoxide dismutase and catalase	Skaleric *et al.* (1991)

A number of research groups have intensively studied the bacterial cell wall model of arthritis in order to dissect the cellular and molecular components that regulate pathogenesis. Not surprisingly, in a complex reaction progressing over a long period and producing such severe injury, all immune and inflammatory systems examined have been incriminated, and all of these cellular and soluble mediators have also been described in RA. A major problem being addressed is the uncertainty of the sequence in which these components act, and their involvement in circuits which amplify or down-regulate inflammation. Adding to the problem is the fact that many, if not all, of the cells and mediators can be demonstrated to have both pro- and anti-inflammatory activities. Nevertheless, several proposals, with emphasis on different components of inflammation, have been presented to explain the natural history of disease induced by bacterial cell wall debris; often with parallel observations on similar features in human disease (Schwab *et al.*, 1988; Sternberg *et al.*, 1989; van den Broek, 1989; Wahl *et al.*, 1991a; Wilder *et al.*, 1991; Hazenberg *et al.*, 1992).

REFERENCES

Aksetijevich S, Whitfield HJ Jr, Young WS, Wilder RL, Chrousos GP, Gold PW et al. (1992) Arthritis-susceptible Lewis rats fail to emerge from the stress hyporesponsive period. *Development Brain Res* **65**: 115–118.

Allen JB, Malone DG, Wahl SM, Calandra GB & Wilder RL (1985) Role of the thymus in streptococcal cell wall-induced arthritis and hepatic granuloma formation. *J Clin Invest* **76**: 1042–1056.

Allen JB, Manthey CL, Hand AR, Ohura K, Ellingsworth L & Wahl SM (1990) Rapid onset synovial inflammation and hyperplasia induced by TGF-β. *J Exp Med* **171**: 231–247.

Allen JB, Bansal GP, Feldman GM, Hand AO, Wahl LM & Wahl SM (1991) Suppression of bacterial cell wall-induced polyarthritis by recombinant gamma interferon. *Cytokine* **3**: 98–106.

Anderle SK, Greenblatt JJ, Cromartie WJ, Clark RL & Schwab JH (1979) Modulation of the susceptibility of inbred and outbred rats to arthritis induced by cell walls of group A streptococci. *Infect Immun* **25**: 484–490.

Bokisch VA (1975) Interactions of peptidoglycans with anti-IgGs and with complement. *Z Immunitaets-forsch Exp Klin Immunol* **149**: 320–330.

Brandes ME, Allen JB, Ogawa Y & Wahl SM (1991) Transforming growth factor beta 1 suppresses acute and chronic arthritis in experimental animals. *J Clin Invest* **87**: 1108–1113.

Burgos-Vargas R, Howard A & Ansell BM (1986) Antibodies to peptidoglycan in juvenile onset ankylosing spondylitis and pauciarticular-onset juvenile arthritis associated with chronic iridocyclitis. *J Rheumatol* **13**: 760–762.

Clark RL, Cuttino JT, Anderle SK, Cromartie WJ & Schwab JH (1979) Radiologic analysis of arthritis in rats after systemic injection of streptococcal cell walls. *Arthritis Rheum* **22**: 25–35.

Cromartie WJ, Craddock JG, Schwab JH, Anderle SK & Yang C (1977). Arthritis in rats after systemic injection of streptococcal cells or cell walls. *J Exp Med* **146**: 1585–1602.

Dalldorf FG, Cromartie WJ, Anderle SK, Clark RL & Schwab JH (1980) Relation of experimental arthritis to the distribution of streptococcal cell wall fragments. *Am J Pathol* **100**: 383–402.

DeJoy SQ, Ferguson KM, Sapp TM, Zabriskie JB, Oronsky AL & Kerwar SS (1989) Streptococcal cell wall arthritis: Passive transfer of disease with a T cell line and cross-reactivity of streptococcal cell wall antigens with *Mycobacterium tuberculosis*. *J Exp Med* **170**: 369–382.

DeLa Cadena RA, Laskin K, Pixley RA, Sartor RB, Schwab JH, Back N et al. (1991) Role of kallikrein-kinin system in pathogenesis of bacterial cell wall-induced inflammation. *Am J Physiol* **260**: G213–G219.

Eisenberg RA & Schwab JH (1986) Arthropathic group A streptococcal cell walls require specific antibody for activation of human complement by both the classical and alternative pathways. *Infect Immun* **53**: 324–330.

Eisenberg RA, Fox A, Greenblatt JJ, Anderle SK, Cromartie WJ & Schwab JH (1982) Measurement of bacterial cell wall in tissues by solid-state radioimmunoassay: correlation of distribution and persistence with experimental arthritis in rats. *Infect Immun* **38**: 127–135.

Esser RE, Schwab JH & Eisenberg RA (1985a). Immunology of peptidoglycan–polysaccharide polymers from cell walls of group A streptococci. In Stewart-Tull DES & Davis M (eds) *Immunology of the Bacterial Cell Envelope*, pp 91–118. New York: Wiley.

Esser RE, Stimpson SA, Anderle SK, Eisenberg RA, Brown RR, Cromartie WJ et al. (1985b) Mechanisms of recurrence in bacterial cell wall-induced arthritis. In Kimura Y, Kotani S & Shiokawa Y (eds) *Recent Avances in Streptococci and Streptococcal Diseases*, pp 351–352. Bracknell, UK: Reedbooks.

Esser RE, Stimpson SA, Cromartie WJ & Schwab JH (1985c) Reactivation of streptococcal cell wall-induced arthritis by homologous and heterologous cell wall polymers. *Arthritis Rheum* **28**: 1402–1411.

Esser RE, Anderle SK, Chetty C, Stimpson SA, Cromartie WJ & Schwab JH (1986) Comparison of inflammatory reactions induced by intraarticular injection of bacterial cell wall polymers. *Am J Pathol* **122**: 323–334.

Fox A, Brown RR, Anderle SK, Chetty C, Cromartie WJ, Gooder H & Schwab JH (1982) Arthropathic properties related to molecular weight of peptidoglycan–polysaccharide polymers of streptococcal cell wall. *Infect Immun* **35**: 1003–1010.

Friedman SM, Posnett DN & Tumang JR (1991) A potential role for microbial superantigens in the pathogenesis of systemic autoimmune disease. *Arthritis Rheum* **34**: 468–480.

Geratz JD, Tidwell RR, Schwab JH, Anderle SK & Pryzwansky KB (1990) Sequential events in the pathogenesis of streptococcal cell wall-induced arthritis and their modulation by Bis(5-amidino-2-benzimidazolyl) methane (BABIM). *Am J Pathol* **136**: 909–921.

Geratz JD, Tidwell RR, Lombardy RJ, Schwab JH, Anderle SK & Pryzwansky KB (1991). Streptococcal cell wall-induced systemic disease. Beneficial effects of *trans*-Bis(5-amidino-2-benzimidazolyl)ethene, a novel, macrophage-directed anti-inflammatory agent. *Am J Pathol* **139**: 921–931.

Greenblatt JJ, Boackle RJ & Schwab JH (1978) Activation of the alternate complement pathway by peptidoglycan from streptococcal cell wall. *Infect Immun* **19**: 296–303.

Greenblatt JJ, Hunter N & Schwab JH (1980) Antibody response to streptococcal cell wall antigens associated with experimental arthritis in rats. *Clin Exp Immunol* **42**: 450–457.

Hazenberg MP, Lalaen IS, Kool J & Ruseler-van Embden JG (1992) Are intestinal bacteria involved in the etiology of rheumatoid arthritis? *APMIS* **100**: 1–9.

Holoshitz J, Naparster Y, Ben-Nun A & Cohen IR (1983). Lines of T lymphocytes induce or vaccinate against autoimmune arthritis. *Science* **219**: 56–58.

Hunter N, Anderle SK, Brown RR, Dalldorf FG, Clark RL, Cromartie WJ & Schwab JH (1980) Cell-mediated immune response during experimental arthritis induced rats with streptococcal cell walls. *Clin Exp Immunol* **42**: 441–449.

Isobe K-I & Nakashima I (1992) Feedback suppression of staphylococcal enterotoxin-stimulated T lymphocyte proliferation by macrophages through inductive nitric oxide synthesis. *Infect Immun* **60**: 4832–4837.

Janusz MJ, Chetty C, Eisenberg RA, Cromartie WJ & Schwab JH (1984) Treatment of experimental erosive arthritis in rats by injection of the muralytic enzyme mutanolysin. *J Exp Med* **160**: 1360–1374.

Janusz MJ, Esser RE & Schwab JH (1986) *In vivo* degradation of bacterial cell wall by the muralytic enzyme mutalolysin. *Infect Immun* **52**: 459–467.

Janusz MJ, Eisenberg RA & Schwab JH (1987) Effect of muralytic enzyme degradation of streptococcal cell wall in complement activation *in vivo* and *in vitro*. *Inflammation* **11**: 73–85.

Johnson PM & Smalley HB (1988) Idiotypic interactions between rheumatoid factors and other antibodies. *Scand J Rheumatol Suppl* **75**: 93–96.

Johnson PM, Phua KK, Perkins HR, Hart CA & Bucknell RC (1984). Antibodies to streptococcal cell wall peptidoglycan-polysaccharide polymers in seropositive and seronegative rheumatic disease. *Clin Exp Immunol* **55**: 115–124.

Klasen IS, Kool J, Melief MJ, Loeve I, van den Berg WB, Severijnen AJ & Hazenberg MP (1992) Arthritis by autoreactive T cell lines obtained from rats after injection of intestinal bacterial cell wall fragments. *Cell Immunol* **139**: 455–467.

Kotb, M (1992) Role of superantigens in the pathogenesis of infectious diseases and their sequelae. *Curr Opinion Infect Dis 1992* **5**: 364–374.

Lafyatis R, Thompson NJ, Remmers EF, Flanders KC, Roberts AB & Wilder RL (1989) Transforming growth factor-β production by synovial tissues from rheumatoid patients and streptococcal cell wall arthritic rats. *J Immunol* **143**: 1142–1148.

Lambris JD, Allen JB & Schwab JH (1982) *In vivo* changes in complement induced with peptidoglycan–polysaccharide polymers from streptococcal cell walls. *Infect Immun* **35**: 377–380.

Leong PA, Schwab JH & Cohen MS (1984) Interaction of group A streptococcal peptidoglycan–polysaccharide with human polymorphonuclear leukocytes: implications for pathogenesis of chronic inflammation. *Infect Immun* **45**: 160–165.

Lichtman SN, Bachmann S, Bender DE, Holt LC, Schwab JH, Sartor RB & Lemasters JJ (1991) Transplantation of livers from PG-APS treated rats causes reactivation of arthritis. *Gastroenterology* **100**: A766 (Abs).

Marrack P & Kappler J (1990) The staphylococcal enterotoxins and their relatives. *Science* **248**: 705–711.

Mills CD (1991) Molecular basis of suppressor macrophages. Arginine metabolism via the nitric oxide synthetase pathway. *J Immunol* **146**: 2719–2723.

Moore TL, El-Najdawi E & Dorner RW (1989) Antibody to streptococcal cell wall peptidoglycan-polysaccharide polymers in sera of patients with juvenile rheumatoid arthritis but absent in isolated immune complexes. *J Rheumatol* **16**: 1069–1073.

Nesher G, Moore TL, Grisanti MW, El-Najdawi E & Osborn TG (1991) Correlation of antiperinuclear factor with antibodies to streptococcal cell-wall peptidoglycan-polysaccharide polymers and rheumatoid factor. *Clin Exp Rheumatol* **9**: 611–615.

Ohanian SH & Schwab JH (1967) Persistence of group A streptococcal cell walls related to chronic inflammation of rabbit dermal connective tissue. *J Exp Med* **125**

Paliard X, West SG, Lafferty JA, Clements JR, Kappler JW, Marrack P & Kotzin BL (1991) Evidence for the effects of a superantigen in rheumatoid arthritis. *Science* **253**: 325–329.

Pope RM, Rutstein JE & Straus DC (1982) Detection of antibodies to streptococcal mucopeptide in patients with rheumatic disorders and normal controls. *Int Arch Allergy Appl Immunol* **67**: 267–274.

Qin S, Cobbold SP, Pope H, Elliott J, Kioussis D, Davies J & Waldmann H (1993) 'Infectious' transplantation tolerance. *Science* **259**: 974–976.

Regan DR, Cohen PL, Cromartie WJ & Schwab JH (1988) Immunosuppressive macrophages by arthropathic peptidoglycan-polysaccharide polymers from bacterial cell walls. *Clin Exp Immunol* **74**: 365–370.

Remmers EF, Lafyatis R, Kumkumian GK, Case JP, Roberts AB, Sporn MB & Wilder RL (1990) Cytokines and growth regulation of synoviocytes from patients with rheumatoid arthritis and rats with streptococcal cell wall arthritis. *Growth Factors* **2**: 179–188.

Richardson BC (1992) T cell receptor usage in rheumatic disease. *Clin Exp Rheumatol* **10**: 271–283.

Ridge SC, Zabriskie JB, Oronsky AL & Kerwar SS (1985) Streptococcal cell wall arthritis: studies with nude (athymic) inbred Lewis rats. *Cellular Immunol* **96**: 231–234.

Ridge SC, Zabriskie JB, Osawa H, Diamantstein T, Oronsky AL & Kerwar SS (1986) Administration of group A streptococcal cell walls to rats induces an interleukin 2 deficiency. *J Exp Med* **164**: 327–334.

Rook GA, Steele J & Rademacher T (1988) A monoclonal antibody raised by immunising mice with group A streptococci binds to agalactosyl IgG from rheumatoid arthritis. *Ann Rheum Dis* **47**: 247–250.

Schwab JH (1970) Significance of bacterial components in the pathogenesis of connective tissue disease. In Floursheim G (ed) *Proc IV Int Cong Pharmacol*, pp 226–232. Basel: Schwabe.

Schwab JH (1979) Acute and chronic inflammation induced by bacterial cell wall structures. In Schlessinger D (ed) *'Microbiology 1979'*, pp 209–214. Washington DC: Am Soc Microbiology.

Schwab JH (1982) Immune dysfunction associated with arthritis induced by peptidoglycan–polysaccharide polymers from streptococcal cell walls. In Yamamura Y & Kotani S (eds) *Immunumodulation by Microbial Products and Related Synthetic Compounds*, pp 84–93. Amsterdam: Excerpta Medica.

Schwab JH (1993) Phlogistic properties of peptidoglycan–polysaccharide polymers from cell walls of pathogenic and normal flora bacteria which colonize humans. *Infect Immun* **61**: 4535–4539.

Schwab JH, Allen JB, Anderle SK, Dalldorf F, Eisenberg R & Cromartie WJ (1982) Relationship of complement to experimental arthritis induced in rats with streptococcal cell walls. *Immunology* **46**: 83–88.

Schwab JH, Stimpson SA & Bristol LA (1988) Pathogenesis inflammatory arthritis induced by bacterial peptidoglycan–polysacccharide polymers and lipolysaccharide. In Schrinner E, Richmond MH, Seibert G & Schwarz O (eds) *Surface Structures of Microorganisms and their Interactions with the Mammalian Host*, pp 99–112. Weinheim: VCH Verlagsgesellschaft.

Schwab JH, Anderle SK, Brown RR, Dalldorf FG & Thompson RC (1991). Pro- and anti-inflammatory roles of interleukin-1 in recurrence of bacterial cell wall-induced arthritis in rats. *Infect Immun* **59**: 4436–4442.

Schwab JH, Brown RR, Anderle SK & Schlievert PM (1993). Superantigen can reactivate bacterial cell wall-induced arthritis. *J Immunol* **150**: 4151–4159.

Severijnen AJ, Hazenberg MP & van de Merwe JP (1988) Induction of chronic arthritis in rats by cell wall fragments of anaerobic coccoid rods isolated from the faecal flora of patients with Crohn's disease. *Digestion* **39**: 118–125.

Severijnen AJ, Kool J, Swaak AJG & Hazenberg MP (1990) Intestinal flora of patients with rheumatoid arthritis. Induction of chronic arthritis in rats by cell wall fragments from isolated *Eubacterium aerofaciens* strains. *Br J Rheumatol* **29**: 433–439.

Skaleric U, Allen JB, Smith PD, Mergenhagen SE & Wahl SM (1991) Inhibitors of reactive oxygen intermediates suppress bacterial cell wall-induced arthritis. *J Immunol* **147**: 2559–2564.

Spitznagel JK, Goodrum KJ, Warejcka DJ, Weaver JL, Miller HL & Babcock L (1986) Modulation of complement fixation and the phlogistic capacity of group A, B, and D streptococci by human iysozyme acting on their cell walls. *Infect Immun* **52**: 803–811.

Staton LS, Schwab JH & Stimpson SA (1990) Chronic local expression of interleukin-1β mRNA in peptidoglycan-polysaccharide induced arthritis in rats. *Arthritis Rheum* **33**: S76 (Abs).

Sternberg EM, Hill JM, Chrousos GP, Kamilaris T, Listwak SJ, Gold PW & Wilder RL (1989) Inflammatory mediator-induced hypothalamic–pituitary–adrenal axis activation is defective in streptococcal cell wall arthritis-susceptible Lewis rats. *Proc Natl Acad Sci USA* **86**: 2374–2378.

Stimpson SA & Schwab JH (1989) Chronic remittent erosive arthritis induced by bacterial peptidoglycan-polysaccharide structures. In Chang JY & Lewis AJ (eds) *Pharmacological Methods in the Control of Inflammation*, pp 381–394. New York: Alan R. Liss.

Stimpson SA, Brown RR, Anderle SK, Klapper DG, Clark RL, Cromartie WJ & Schwab JH (1986) Athropathic properties of cell wall polymers from normal flora bacteria. *Infect Immun* **51**: 240–249.

Stimpson SA, Esser RE, Carter PB, Sartor RB, Cromartie WJ & Schwab JH (1987a). Lipopolysaccharide induces recurrences of arthritis in rat joints previously injured by peptidoglycan-polysaccharide. *J Exp Med* **165**: 1688–1702.

Stimpson SA, Lerch RA, Cleland DR, Yarnall DP, Clark RL, Cromartie WJ & Schwab JH (1987b) Effect of acetylation on arthropathic activity group A streptococcal peptidoglycan-polysaccharide fragments. *Infect Immun* **55**: 16–23.

Stimpson SA, Dalldorf FG, Otterness IG & Schwab JH (1988) Exacerbation of arthritis by IL-1 in rat joints previously injured by peptidoglycan-polysaccharide. *J Immunol* **140**: 2964–2969.

Stimpson SA, Anderle SK, Noel LS & Schwab JH (1989) Role of T lymphocyte in exacerbation of monoarticular arthritis induced in rats by intravenous peptidoglycan-polysaccharide. *J Leucocyte Biology* **46**: 338 (Abs).

Stimpson SA, Patterson DL, Eastin C & Noel LS (1990) Inflammation induced in rats by intraarticular injection of platelet-derived growth factor. In Dinarello CA (ed) *The Physiological and Pathological Effects of Cytokines*, pp 93–98. New York: Wiley-Liss.

Todome Y, Ohkuni H, Mizuse M, Furuta M, Fujikawa S, Tanaka S, Watanabe N & Zabriskie JB (1992) Detection of antibodies against streptococcal peptidoglycan and the peptide subunit (synthetic tetra-D-alanyl-bovine serum albumin complex) in rheumatic diseases. *Int Arch Allergy Appl Immunol* **97**: 301–307.

van Bruggen MCJ, van den Broek MF & van den Berg WB (1991) Streptococcal cell wall-induced arthritis and adjuvant arthritis in F344 to Lewis and in Lewis to F344 bone marrow chimeras. *Cellular Immunol* **136**: 278–290.

van den Broek MF (1989) Streptococcal cell wall-induced polyarthritis in the rat. Mechanisms for chronicity and regulation of susceptibility. *APMIS* **97**: 861–878.

van den Broek MF, van Bruggen MJC, van de Putte LBA & van den Berg WB (1988) T cell responses to streptococcal antigens in rats: Relations to susceptibility to streptococcal cell wall induced arthritis. *Cellular Immunol* **116**: 216–222.

van den Broek MF, Hogervorst EJM, van Bruggen MCJ & van den Berg WB (1989) Protection against streptococcal cell wall-induced arthritis by pretreatment with the 65-kD mycobacterial heat shock protein. *J Exp Med* **170**: 449–466.

van den Broek MF, van Bruggen MCJ, Stimpson SA & Severijnen AJ (1990) Flare-up reaction of streptococcal cell wall induced arthritis in Lewis and F344 rats: the role of T lymphocytes. *Clin Exp Immunol* **70**: 297–306.

van den Broek MF, van Bruggen MC, Koopman JP, Hazenberg MP & van den Berg WB (1992a) Gut flora induces and maintains resistance against streptococcal cell wall-induced arthritis in F344 rats. *Clin Exp Immunol* **88**: 313–317.

van den Broek MF, van den Langerijt LG, van Bruggen MC, Billingham ME & van den Berg WB (1992b) Treatment of rats with monoclonal anti-CD4 induces long-term resistance to streptococcal cell wall-induced arthritis. *Eur J Immunol* **22**: 57–61.

Wahl SM (1991a) Cellular and molecular interactions in the induction of inflammation in rheumatic diseases. In Kresina TF (ed) *Monoclonal Antibodies, Cytokines, and Arthritis*, pp 101–132. New York: Marcel Dekker.

Wahl SM (1991b) The role of transforming growth factor-β in inflammatory processes. *Immunologic Res* **10**: 249–254.

Wahl SM & Hunt DA (1988) Bacterial cell wall-induced immunosuppression. Role of transforming growth factor-β. *J Exp Med* **168**: 1403–1417.

Wahl SM, Katona IM, Wahl LM, Allen JB, Dedker JL, Scher I & Wilder RL (1983) Leukaperesis in rheumatoid arthritis. Association of clinical improvement with reversal of anergy. *Arthritis Rheum* **20**: 1076.

Wahl SM, Allen JB & Brandes ME (1991a) Cytokine modulation of bacterial cell wall induced arthritis *Agents Actions* **35** (**supplement**): 29–34.

Wahl SM, Allen JB, Ohura K, Chenoweth DE & Hand AR (1991b) IFN-gamma inhibits inflammatory cell recruitment and the evolution of bacterial cell wall-induced arthritis. *J Immunol* **146**: 95–100.

Wilder RL, Allen JB & Hansen C (1987) Thymus-dependent and -independent regulation of Ia antigen expression *in situ* by cells in the synovium of rats with streptococcal cell wall-induced arthritis. *J Clin Invest* **79**: 1160–1171.

Wilder RL, Calandra GB, Garvin AJ, Wright KD & Hansen CT (1982) Strain and sex variation in the susceptibility to streptococcal cell wall-induced polyarthritis in rats. *Arthritis Rheum* **25**: 1064–1072.

Wilder RL, Allen JB, Wahl LM, Calandra GB & Wahl SM (1983) The pathogenesis of group A streptococcal cell wall induced polyarthritis in the rat: comparative studies in arthritis resistant and susceptible rat strains. *Arthritis Rheum* **26**: 1442–1451.

Wilder RL, Case JP, Crofford LJ, Kumkumian GK, Lafyatis R, Remmers EF, Sano H, Sternberg EM & Yocum DE (1991) Endothelial cells and the pathogenesis of rheumatoid arthritis in humans and streptococcal cell wall arthritis in Lewis rats. *J Cell Biochem* **45**: 162–166.

Yocum DE, Allen JB, Wahl SM, Calandra GB & Wilder RL (1986) Inhibition by cyclosprin A of streptococcal cell wall-induced arthritis and hepatic granulomas in rats. *Arthritis Rheum* **29**: 262–273.

Yoshino S, Cleland LG, Mayerhofer G, Brown RR & Schwab JH (1991) Prevention of chronic erosive streptococcal cell wall-induced arthritis in rats by treatment with monoclonal antibody against the T cell antigen receptor α,β. *J Immunol* **146**: 1487–1489.

23 Collagen-induced Arthritis

*David E. Trentham and Roselynn
Dynesius-Trentham*

INTRODUCTION

The intent of this chapter is to update and evaluate important new knowledge derived in the past 5 years using collagen model of arthritis and to reappraise the potential relevance of this animal counterpart for rheumatoid arthritis (RA). Initially described around the time that streptococcal cell wall arthritis was recognized, characterization of the collagen model (Trentham *et al.*, 1977) resulted from an immunologic survey of then recently described and purified human type I, II and III collagen preparations. The experiments involved immunizing rats to raise reference antisera; pure serendipity interceded, in that native type II collagen was found to be an arthritogenic host protein. Subsequent work has shown that collagen arthritis is an autoimmune disease in which T- and B-cell processes probably cocontribute. This conclusion is based on both sensitized cells or collagen antibody mixtures being capable of passively transferring disease; in like manner, when combined they appear to act synergistically to produce the characteristic clinical features and anatomic lesion found in the primary disease. Five years later, in 1982, a review of the evidence, pros and cons, for the value of collagen arthritis as a working representation of RA was published (Trentham, 1982). Now it is again timely that further explorations of this topic occur but first a review of current thinking regarding the pathogenesis of both RA and collagen arthritis is warranted.

PATHOGENESIS OF RHEUMATOID ARTHRITIS

Recently a review of the pathogenesis of RA was published (Sewell and Trentham, 1993). This chronic polysynovitis of unknown etiology is a common disorder. It continues to be deemed a prototype for autoimmune disease, although an infectious agent cannot be dismissed. Potential candidates usually cited are: (a) a bacterium, possibly unidentified; (b) a mycoplasma; or (c) a virus, especially Epstein-Barr virus (EBV). Two fundamental processes are operative in the expression of RA. First, a remarkable immunogenetic predisposition with strong MHC class II linkage has been clearly defined in the last decade. Second, activated, and presumably auto-aberrant, $CD4^+$ T cells provide the cornerstone for the inflammatory process and its perpetration in RA. Other pathways appear to be ancillary and under the governance of these hallmark features. Indeed, the entirety of this disease state might be brought under control or into complete resolution if effective gene alterations protocols or relevant T-cell ablation modalities could be identified. This view is reviewed by Panayi in Chapter 4, this volume.

T-cells appear to be reacting to antigen both in the early and late stages of RA. In active disease, synovial capillaries are characterized by enhanced permeability as well

Mechanisms and Models in Rheumatoid Arthritis
ISBN 0–12–340440–1

as increased expression of intercellular adhesion molecule (ICAM-1), a ligand that promotes adhesion to capillary walls by circulating mononuclear cells. As the pannus thickens, more abundant amounts of ICAM-1 are found concurrently. In established rheumatoid synovitis, the dominant T cell resident in the synovium of the joint has a distinct phenotype. that is CD4$^+$, CD45RO$^+$, CD 29 'bright', connoting a memory population of helper T cells that is undergoing activation *in situ* after being pro-grammed in the thymus (Sewell and Trentham, 1993). The role of leukocyte traffick-ing in RA is reviewed in Chapter 11, this volume. Other unique markers include HLA-DR/DQ and very late antigen (VLA-1), suggesting that the unknown antigen resides within the joint. The major structural protein of cartilage, type II collagen, is one of several possible autoantigens that could perpetuate the disease. The structure of the connective tissue macromolecules of articular cartilage is described in Chapters 9 and 17, this volume.

The synovial fluid within the rheumatoid joint is an abnormal and complex mixture of deleterious cytokines, largely of monocyte/macrophage origin, as well as immuno-globulins of various classes. Memory T cells characteristically respond weakly to antigen and release only low levels of cytokine; however, their promotion of mono-kine generation and stimulation of immunoglobulin synthesis is quite efficient. Hence much of the distinctive biochemical milieu of the rheumatoid joint can be easily understood by a memory T cell influence. A large proportion of the immunoglobulin repertoire consists of antibodies to type II and the minor cartilage collagens (types V, VI, IX), a finding also consistent with the collagen hypothesis for RA. It has also evoked a change in thinking because previously it had been assumed that much of the antibody present in the joint and synovial tissue was predominantly rheumatoid factor.

A restricted set of genetically determined MHC class II molecules, composed of glutamine/lysine residues occupying position #70/71 of the HLA-DR β_2 chain, is a uniquely predictable marker for predisposition for RA. A striking parallel also exists in the collagen model of arthritis, in both mice and rats. Finally, evidence for T-cell oligoclonality in RA, based on T-cell receptor (TCR) Vβ profiling and analysed as an aggregate, is not as convincing as originally anticipated (see Chapters 2, 4 and 19, this volume). This too favours a role for a complex, multi-epitopic autoantigen that could stimulate more of a polyclonal T-cell response in RA, such as type II collagen. In summary, since the earlier equivocal conclusions made in 1982 regarding the rel-evance of collagen and other animal models for RA (Trentham, 1982), the ensuing years have furnished more extensive and persuasive evidence from many quarters that support a role for collagen immunity in the pathogenesis of rheumatoid arthritis. It is predicted that within the next 5 years the possible linkage will be further addressed and supported (or refuted) more directly. For detailed discussions of the aetiology and immunopathogenesis of RA refer to Chapters 1–4, this volume.

PATHOGENESIS OF COLLAGEN ARTHRITIS: BACKGROUND

Clearly collagen arthritis is an autoimmune disease, in that immunologic sensitization to a normal host constituent induces, in an explosive manner, a highly inflammatory joint disorder. Shortly after the clinical description of the model, the co-existence of autoantibodies and cell-mediated immunity to native type II collagen was identified.

Most importantly, there was a close temporal association between the development of both B- and T-cell processes and the onset of macroscopically evident polysynovitis. Even more persuasive for an autoimmune origin was the subsequent demonstration of successful cell transfer of collagen arthritis. Viable and type II collagen specific lymphoid cells were required; control experiments excluded the possibility that antigen (collagen) carryover accounted for transfer of the disease. Later, more elegant isolation procedures and studies in both rat and mouse systems demonstrated that the effector population for the cell transfer phenomenon was a CD4$^+$ T-lymphocyte subset.

Disease transfer by serum fractions enriched for antibodies to native type II collagen was shown to be also capable of passively transferring synovial inflammation in the collagen system. Much debate ensued over the morphology of the antibody-mediated lesion. In contrast to the extensive amount of pannus formation that was generated by cell transfer, or that exists in the primary model, the condition incited by antibody appeared to be a more acute and evanescent process. Rather than a mononuclear infiltrate, the synovium was replete with polymorphonuclear leukocytes and unaccompanied by appreciable degrees of synovial hyperplasia. In further contrast were the large quantities of immunoglobulin that were required to consistently achieve serum transfer. Use of murine monoclonal antibodies raised against type II collagen was even less efficient. Together these observations raised questions of possible covert contamination contributing, at least in part, to 'antibody' transfer. Potential biologically active contaminants would include copurified cytokine material or even serum iron. Intravenous injection of ferric citrate can experimentally trigger changes in the synovium of immunologically naive rats that resemble states of activation. Other studies, using cobra venom factor (CVF), also implicated complement components in the pathogenesis of collagen arthritis. The polyspecificities of CVF make interpretation of the data somewhat difficult. Further studies in rodents with complement deficiencies definitively created with ablative or 'knock-out' techniques have not been performed.

Later work has largely implicated immunogenetics and T-cell mechanisms in the initiation of collagen arthritis (reviewed in Chapter 19, this volume). Virtually all antibody preparations, polyclonal and monoclonal, with varying degrees of T and CD4 specificities have been quite palliative in this model of arthritis (in this context refer to Chapter 4, this volume, for a discussion of novel therapies for RA). Serial histologic assessment of the synovium after immunization has defined the cellular kinetics of collagen arthritis, at least in the rat. Around day 3 postimmunization the first infiltrating cell population egresses from the capillaries into the perivascular spaces of the synovium; it is universally CD4$^+$. The infiltrate expands and remains, phenotypically, solely a helper cell population until day 7 or 8. At this time CD8$^+$ cells also begin to appear and their numbers increase progressively during the next 7–10 days. Clinically apparent disease emerges around day 10 as does serological evidence of collagen autoantibody production around day 9–11. These studies suggest that a delayed-type hypersensitivity (DTH) response is occurring *in situ* in the model during this interval when arthritis is detectable. However, whether antibodies, generated in extrasynovial locations and homing to the joint, further stimulate the arthritogenic response has not been carefully examined. Collagen antibody localization within the joint, at least in the established stage of the disease, seems to be primarily on the surface of the cartilage. A serious shortcoming in our longitudinal studies has been a failure to analyse cartilaginous regions for the inceptual deposition of antibodies.

Another potentially relevant effector pathway in the collagen model is arthritogenic factor (AF). This protein has an apparent molecular weight of 65 kDa and was isolated by its binding to type II collagen affinity columns. This binding property is somewhat similar to members of the collagenase family of enzymes. AF, on the other hand, does not display such degradative reactivities and its origin appears to be exclusively form $CD4^+$ cell populations that expand rapidly after collagen immunization. AF can induce sustained synovial proliferation and inflammation after intra-articular injection. Experiments using systemic injection have been unsuccessful and, due to extremely limited quantitites of the protein, only a modest level of biochemical characterization has been achieved. Recent NH_2-terminal microsequencing results have shown some homology with the supergene family of serpins or α-1 antitrypsins. Further work is presently underway.

In summary, the pathogenesis of collagen arthritis appears to be a T-cell dependent autoimmune process in which both cytokines and antibodies play substantive roles. Their relative contributions need further clarification. Studies from adjuvant arthritis using collagen antibodies and T-cells suggest that synergy can be created through autoantibody pathways and T-cell derived cytokines. Whether this represents the case in RA is unknown, but the existence of autoimmune responses to collagen in the human disease would suggest that it is within the realm of reasonable possibilities.

MORE RECENT INSIGHTS INTO THE PATHOGENESIS OF COLLAGEN ARTHRITIS

DRUG-INFERRED DATA FAVOURING T-CELL MEDIATION

The most potent and T-cell specific pharmacological compound identified to date appears to be FK-506, an extracted metabolite of a yeast with properties analogous to cyclosporin. Paralleling earlier findings with cyclosporin, it is noteworthy that the murine model of collagen arthritis is markedly susceptible to down-regulation with FK-506 (Takagishi et al., 1989). Administration of this compound during the induction stage of disease profoundly ($P < 0.01$) suppressed the development of collagen arthritis and did not merely retard its onset. It also significantly decreased both collagen antibody production, a T-cell dependent process, and DTH to collagen. All of these parameters were altered in a dose-dependent fashion by FK-506. As is generally the case, delivery of FK-506 during established disease had no observable clinical or immunological effect. Investigators working with the collagen model should become more aware and appreciative of the fact that the explosive onset and sheer flagrancy of collagen arthritis, coupled with the vigorous nature of the afferent and efferent autoimmune response that drives the disease, causes a state that is refractory to potentially interventional compounds during the established stage.

VIRAL EFFECTS ON COLLAGEN ARTHRITIS

Viruses continue to be plausible and attractive candidates for the etiology of RA. At the theoretical level, their mode of action could be any one of several: they could directly damage tissue that, in turn, would incite a host response to 'altered self' constituents; viruses might share epitopes with host tissue and, in the process of mounting an appropriate immune response, autoimmunity could emerge and persist; finally viruses might alter the normal immune network, allowing aberrant reactivities to develop, expand and remain unrestrained.

Cytomegalovirus (CMV) infection is known to change immune functions in animals and man. CMV has also been found (Griffiths *et al.*, 1991) to enhance markedly susceptibility to collagen arthritis in rats. Early experiments appeared to exclude the possibility that direct viral infection of joint tissue was involved. Of distinct interest, subsequent work has identified a systemic adjuvant effect for CMV in this model. This work is described in more detail in Chapter 21, this volume.

Infection with CMV promoted serum IgG anti-rat type II collagen antibody titres, augmented DTH responses to collagen, and by day 8 significantly expanded a CD8$^+$ population of cells functioning as natural killer cells and thereby possibly producing an added injurious effect. It also was suggested that CMV infection interfered with tolerance to an autoantigen, collagen, more than with other antigens. It is not entirely clear whether these immunological changes account for the up-regulated expression of collagen arthritis by CMV but these data clearly demonstrate that a viral:auto-immunity interplay can operate in collagen arthritis. Analogous codeterminates could exist in RA as well, as discussed in Chapter 2, this volume.

SPONTANEOUS ARTHRITIS IN RODENTS

A major argument against the relevance of animal models for RA is their dependence on use of exogenous antigens for disease induction, in contrast to the seemingly spontaneous nature of the human disease. However, on rare occasion in older animals, we have noted the appearance of a collagen-like arthritis in non-immunized rats (Trentham *et al.*, 1984). The infrequency of the phenomenon and the lack of success in breeding attempts has stalled progress in this area until a recent report appeared (Bouvet *et al.*, 1990) describing spontaneous arthritis in mice. This is a potentially pivotal paper in the field of arthritis research using animal models and further expanded use of these animals is anticipated. The interested reader is referred to Chapter 25, this volume, for discussion of spontaneously-induced animal models of RA.

Biozzi's selection $I(H_I)$ is a strain of mice that is quite susceptible to collagen arthritis and is known to be a brisk antibody responder to certain antigens. By age 13 months, without prior immunization, 28% of male mice of this strain had developed macroscopically evident arthritis that closely resembled both collagen arthritis and RA. Like the collagen-induced model, male mice were preferentially susceptible to the disorder, in contradistinction to the collagen model, rheumatoid factor, as well as high titres of antibodies to type II collagen, were frequently found in the affected mice and also in their normally appearing littermates. There was no apparent permissive or obligatory role for antibodies in the induction of this arthritis but unfortunately another potential correlate was not evaluated – whether cellular immunity to collagen was associated with subsequent development of an arthritic state. Although the significance of these observations is unclear, the fact that inducible models of disease have spontaneous parallels in nature lends some credence to the prospect that a similar situation may extend to human disease.

IMMUNOGENETICS OF COLLAGEN ARTHRITIS

Differing terminology across species makes perusal of immunogenetic literature difficult at best – but sometimes it is worth the effort! In the mouse, collagen arthritis is unequivocally a classic autoimmune disease, dependent on both appropriate MHC-encoded class II molecules and non-MHC-TCR genes (Banerjee *et al.*, 1988; reviewed in detail by Wooley in Chapter 19, this volume). Similar analyses have now been conducted elegantly in the rat (Griffiths *et al.*, 1992). MHC congenic strains along with different heterologous collagen antigens were used. This study demonstrated an analogous dualistic role (as in the mouse) for both MHC (termed RT 1 in the rat) – and non-MHC-encoded gene products. Still unexplained were the differences in arthritogenic responses to immunizing collagens that were encountered in this study. This is a somewhat unexpected outcome given the high degree of conserved homology that exists for type II collagen between various species.

What is the significance of this complex work? In addition to providing more parallels between experimental arthritis in an animal system and RA, the findings point to the profound influence of heredity in these diseases. TCR molecules function independently of the MHC in governing susceptibility to autoimmune arthritis. Because the MHC class II molecular and TCR structures appear to be exquisitely specific, at least within given strains, strategically targeted modalities such as the use of peptides, may be developed and used as vaccines in model protocols. Unfortunately in humans, individual differences within the rheumatoid patient population could pose a major impediment to any patient-to-patient extended use.

How many epitopes on type II collagen are involved in arthritis? In the rat, sophisticated studies have recently shown (Cremer *et al.*, 1992) that type II collagen, functioning as an arthritogen, is a complex multivalent stimulus. Using purified and renatured cyanogen bromide (CB) fragments of type II collagen, these investigators found a diverse spectrum of antibodies to epitopes situated throughout the molecule. The genetic background of the rat and species source of collagen were again demonstrated to be critical. These data imply that it is unlikely that a single specific arthritogenic epitope will be isolated from type II collagen; this contrasts markedly with the situation in experimental allergic encephalomyelitis (EAE), where finite regions of the inducing antigen, myelin basic protein, are fundamental to the disease process. The observations also predict that if peptide therapy will work for RA, large complex regions of the collagen molecule will have to be delivered rather than small discrete peptides.

SUPPRESSION OF COLLAGEN ARTHRITIS BY ANTIBODY DIRECTED AGAINST THE TCR αβ FRAMEWORK

Although investigations with antibodies directed against fairly widely shared T-cell epitopes might appear arcane, a recent paper (Moder *et al.*, 1992) is of importance. Use of a monoclonal antibody against TCR αβ framework efficiently suppressed the induction of collagen arthritis in mice. This observation argues strongly against the recently popularized notion that cells of the T γδ population are instrumental in the production of inflammatory arthritis, since this subset is left intact after anti-αβ administration. Also, by inference, because T γδ cells react avidly to mycobacterial constituents and heat-shock proteins, these candidates become less attractive as an explanation for inflammatory arthritis in general. This study also provides the ground-work to predict that if there is a bias in TCR Vβ usage that can be defined, mono-clonal antibodies specific for the involved Vβ gene products will be ameliorative for autoimmune disease, because antibody targeted to the entire framework is obviously successful.

DO OTHER DISEASE RELEVANT T-CELL EPITOPES EXIST?

Immunology is usually constrained by the currently available reagents and tech-nology. Such is not the case for an innovative report (Peacock *et al.*, 1992) which provides evidence that unidentified cell-surface markers may exist on T-cell popu-lations that are germane for inflammatory arthritis. First, a type II collagen specific T-cell line was generated from lymphoid tissue harvested from collagen immunized rats; from this line were derived three distinct clones as determined by Southern blot analysis. Next, polyclonal rabbit antibodies, apparently specific for the line, were raised. Using this reagent, it was shown that induction of arthritis in rats could be blocked effectively. However, T-cell phenotyping by flow cytometry showed that the rabbit antibody removed, at most, only a small percentage of T cells suggesting that they represented a minute subfraction. Finally, further experiments suggested that the anti-line cell antibodies might co-recognize TCR Vβ₄ positive cells.

Overall, these outcomes indicate that extremely finite populations of T cells provide the initiating effector force for collagen arthritis and that, possibly, T-cell oligoclona-lity can be identified by Vβ antisera. Regardless of these still somewhat speculative conclusions, the data further show that exquisitely specific anti-T-cell reagents can profoundly palliate experimental arthritis.

WHAT ABOUT GENUINE AUTOIMMUNITY IN COLLAGEN ARTHRITIS?

Unfortunately, because of difficulty in acquiring sufficient quantities of collagen for experimentation, 95% or greater of the literature regarding collagen arthritis reports results using heterologous collagen preparations. From the outset it was demonstrated that homologous collagen could induce this disease (Trentham *et al.*, 1977) but only recently has substantial additional progress added to our understanding (Griffiths *et al.*, 1993). Earlier reports (Banerjee *et al.*, 1988; Griffiths *et al.*, 1992) have clearly shown that both MHC- and non-MHC-gene products influence collagen arthritis but the data gathered had been almost exclusively based on heterologous collagen usage. In the rat, arthritogenic autoimmune reactivity to homologous native type II collagen was found to be under rigorously tight genetic control (Griffiths *et al.*, 1993). Rats with an appropriately susceptible MHC makeup developed severe arthritis and brisk antibody responses after immunization with the homologous preparation. Perhaps what was more revealing was the action of non-MHC gene elements. These latter products acted exclusively to down-regulate the clinical expression of the MHC-related genetic susceptibility! Thus, a permissive and counterbalancing/co-operative influence on collagen arthritis has been recognized. When considered in a broad context, the data in this latter paper support the thesis that an individual's HLA genotype contributes to the total potential for developing autoimmunity to type II collagen – a situation reminiscent of the genetic complexities and mechanisms encountered in RA.

WHAT REALLY IS THE CASE FOR TCR Vβ RESTRICTION IN COLLAGEN ARTHRITIS?

Searches for a restricted TCR in human disease may continue to be unfruitful because of difficulties in sampling tissue from the inceptual or earliest phase of disease. In animal models, TCR restriction has been definitively detected in EAE, where the relevant segments appear to be $V\beta_{8.2}$ and $V\beta_{13.}$ Such is not the case in the spontaneous non-obese diabetic (NOD) mouse model of type I diabetes mellitus, where usage is quite extensive. What actually is the case in collagen arthritis? Recently, 13 clonally distinct T-cell hybridomas were established from mice immunized with bovine type II collagen (Osman *et al.*, 1993). Although usage was somewhat heterogenous, over-representation of $V\beta_{8.2}$ appeared to exist. Limited skewing in Vβ usage has also been observed by C. Lorenzo and coworkers in our laboratory (unpublished data). Although probably not the final answer, the TCR Vβ story continues to point to finite, if not oligoclonal, numbers of autoaggressive cells being the major effector mechanism for inflammatory arthritis, at least in model systems. The current understanding of Vβ gene usage in RA discussed in Chapters 2, 4, 19 and 21, this volume.

HOW RELEVANT IS THE COLLAGEN MODEL FOR RHEUMATOID ARTHRITIS?

Traditionally, immunologists equivocate when working with model systems and conclude, publicly at least, that their pursuits relate only to the acquisition of fundamental knowledge; extrapolation to human disease is another matter entirely. How intellectually dishonest this conclusion really is! Certainly, if true, it would not justify the cruel necessity of rendering animals arthritic solely to satisfy one's own curiosity. Perhaps the problem, in the main, has been an inability to conduct experiments that might 'bridge-the-gap'. Animal models have been rather successful in predicting outcomes for new anti-rheumatic modalities (see Table 1). For example, drugs traditionally considered to have slow-acting properties for RA such as gold and penicillamine, are ineffective overall in collagen arthritis. Curiously, methotrexate has not been subjected to extensive evaluation in this model. Newer compounds currently showing promise in clinical trials, such as minocycline and an interleukin-2:diphtheria toxin conjugate termed $DAB_{486}IL-2$, were first shown to possess anti-arthritic effects in animal models, discoveries that were stimulatory for further developmental scrutiny. This record suggests that pathogenically similar processes exist in animal models and human disease. Recently, however, another therapeutic protocol has emerged whereby the fidelity of animal models for human disease has been tested more directly.

   Oral tolerance is an idea from immunologic antiquity purported to form the basis of immunologic inertness for foodstuff. Whether correct or not, it is certainly a simple

Table 1. Predictive role of animal models for anti-rheumatic therapy

Treatment	Outcome
Gold and penicillamine	→
Total lymphoid irradiation	↓
Cyclosporin and FK-506	↓
Methotrexate	?
Fish oil	↑
Amiprilose hydrochloride	→
Minocycline	↓
Antithymocyte globulin	↓
Pan T-cell monoclonal antibody	↓
DAB$_{486}$ IL-2	↓
T-cell vaccination	↓
Oral tolerance (type II collagen)	↓

and satisfying explanation of why ingestion of a wide variety of foreign substances does not readily lead to hypersensitivity. Recently studies in experimentally induced autoimmune disease, including EAE and experimentally inducible uveitis, have shown that antigen-relevant feeding, myelin basic protein (MBP) and retinal antigen-S for the above models, respectively, can abort the development of the experimental process. What is happening mechanistically is presently under great debate. In different models and in different laboratories, evidence that oral tolerance involves: (a) T-suppressor cell generation: (b) clonal anergy: or (c) a diversion of cytokine profiles from activating and/or proinflammatory species such as interleukin-2 to more palliative products such as transforming growth factor β and interleukin-4.

Because EAE is morphologically equivalent to multiple sclerosis, a report has just appeared describing the results of a study in the human disease in which patients were fed MBP for 1 year (Weiner *et al.*, 1993). The results are inconclusive regarding whether the treatment was effective but the study certainly showed that the approach was safe and did not exacerbate the disease. An extension of this work into RA has become attractive. We are currently evaluating oral type II collagen in a fairly sizable, double-blind placebo-controlled trial; optimal doses in animal models have clearly demonstrated that the protocol efficiently suppresses collagen (Nagler-Anderson *et al.*, 1986; Thompson and Staines, 1986) and adjuvant arthritis (Zhang *et al.*, 1990). A negative result will be uninterpretable but a positive outcome will confirm that the collagen model has been telling us something about RA for some time; it just took 17 years to appreciate it fully.

REFERENCES

Banerjee S, Haqqi TM, Luthra HS, Stuart JM & David CS (1988) Possible role of Vβ T-cell receptor genes in susceptibility to collagen-induced arthritis in mice. *J Exp Med* **167**: 832–839.

Bouvet J-P, Couderc J, Bouthillier Y, Franc B, Ducailar A & Mouton D (1990) Spontaneous rheumatoid-like arthritis in a line of mice sensitive to collagen-induced arthritis. *Arthritis Rheum* **33**: 1716–1722.

Cremer MA, Terato K, Watson WC, Griffiths MM, Townes AS & Kang AH (1992) Collagen-induced arthritis in rats. Examination of the epitope specificities of circulating and cartilage-bound antibodies produced from heterologous and homologous type II collagens. *J Immunol* **149**: 1045–1053.

Griffiths MM, Smith CB, Wei LS & Ting-Yu SC (1991) Effects of rat cytomegalovirus infection on immune functions in rats with collagen induced arthritis. *J Rheumatol* **18**: 497–504.

Griffiths MM, Cremer MA, Harper DS, MacCall S & Cannon GW (1992) Immunogenetics of collagen-induced arthritis in rats. Both MHC and non-MHC gene products determine the epitope specificity of immune response to bovine and chick type II collagens. *J Immunol* **149**: 309–316.

Griffiths MM, Cannon GW, Leonard PA & Reese VR (1993) Induction of autoimmune arthritis in rats by immunization with homologous rat type II collagen is restricted to the RA 1^{avl} haplotype. *Arthritis Rheum* **367**: 254–258.

Moder KG, Luthra LS, Kubo R, Griffiths MM & David CS (1992) Prevention of collagen induced arthritis in mice by treatment with an antibody directed against the T-cell receptor α–β framework. *Autoimmunity* **11**: 219–224.

Nagler-Anderson C, Bober LA, Robinson ME, Siskind GW & Thorbecke GJ (1986) Suppression of type II collagen-induced arthritis by intragastric administration of soluble type II collagen. *Proc Natl Acad Sci USA* **83**: 7443–7448.

Osman GE, Toda M, Kanagawa O & Hood L (1993) Characterization of the T-cell receptor repertoire causing collagen arthritis in mice. *J Exp Med* **177**: 387–395.

Peacock DJ, Ku G, Banquerigo ML & Brahn E (1992) Suppression of collagen arthritis with antibodies to an arthritogenic, oligoclonal T-cell line. *Cell Immunol* **140**: 444–452.

Sewell KL & Trentham DE (1993) Pathogenesis of rheumatoid arthritis. *Lancet* **341**: 283–286.

Takagishi K, Yamamoto M, Nishimura A, Yamasaki G, Kanasawa N, Hotokebuchi T et al. (1989) Effects of FK-506 on collagen arthritis in mice. *Transplant Proc* **21**: 1053–1055.

Thompson HSG & Staines NA (1986) Gastric administration of type II collagen delays the onset and severity of collagen-induced arthritis in rats. *Clin Exp Immunol* **64**: 581–586.

Trentham DE (1982) Collagen arthritis as a relevant model for rheumatoid arthritis. Evidence pro and con. *Arthritis Rheum* **25**: 911–916.

Trentham DE, Townes AS & Kang AH (1977) Autoimmunity to type II collagen: an experimental model of arthritis. *J Exp Med* **146**: 857–868.

Trentham DE, Brahn E, Williams W, McCune WJ & Belli JA (1984) Connective tissue disease can develop in rats either spontaneously or after total lymphoid irradiation. *J Rheumatol* **11**: 410–412.

Weiner HL, Mackin GA, Matsui M, Orav EJ, Khoury SJ, Dawson DM et al. (1993) Double-blind pilot trial of oral tolerization with myelin antigens in multiple sclerosis. *Science* **259**: 1321–1323.

Zhang JZ, Lee CSY, Lider O & Weiner HL (1990) Suppression of adjuvant arthritis in Lewis rats by oral administration of type II collagen. *J Immunol* **145**: 2489–2493.

24 Antigen-induced Arthritis

E.R. Pettipher and S. Blake

INTRODUCTION

Antigen-induced arthritis was first described by Dumonde and Glynn (1962) as an animal model for the study of rheumatoid arthritis (RA). Chronic synovitis was induced by the intra-articular injection of fibrin in rabbits previously sensitized to this protein. Subsequently, it was realized that other protein antigens, such as ovalbumin, could substitute for fibrin and that antigen-induced arthritis can be induced in other species such as the mouse (Brackertz *et al.*, 1977a), guinea pig (Cashin *et al.*, 1980; Yamashita *et al.*, 1991) and rat (Griffiths, 1992), although the guinea pig and rodent species differ from the rabbit in antigenic requirements, histopathology and response to drug therapy.

Antigen-induced arthritis in the rabbit is very similar to human RA in regard to histopathology – the formation of lymphoid follicles and synovial hypertrophy are prominent features and, like RA, the synovitis is persistent, lasting many months to years (Glynn, 1968). Furthermore, the response of antigen-induced arthritis in the rabbit to drug therapy is similar to that in RA and unlike commonly used rodent models of arthritis where NSAIDs display disease-modifying activity (see Hunneyball, 1984).

In this chapter we discuss what has been learned about the processes and mediators involved in antigen-induced arthritis and what implications this has for understanding the pathogenesis of RA. This review focuses on the rabbit model of antigen-induced arthritis, although comparisons to antigen-induced arthritis in other species are made when appropriate.

THE IMMUNOPATHOLOGY OF ANTIGEN-INDUCED ARTHRITIS

In order to induce chronic synovitis in rabbits the animals must be appropriately immunized with antigen. Ovalbumin and bovine serum albumin can both be used as antigens, though a more persistent synovitis is often induced with ovalbumin. In either case, rabbits must display both humoral and cell-mediated immunity to the antigen in order to develop a chronic arthritis. This is achieved by sensitizing animals to antigen in Freund's complete adjuvant (containing heat-killed mycobacteria) to boost cell-mediated immunity. Rabbits immunized in Freund's incomplete adjuvant (mineral oil alone) develop equivalent antibody titres to the immunizing antigen but have very weak cell-mediated immune responses as measured by delayed type hypersensitivity (DTH) reactions. While these animals develop acute synovitis, they fail to develop chronic arthritis (Fox & Glynn, 1975; Pettipher & Henderson, 1988). Thus, acute synovitis, characterized by early swelling and leukocyte infiltration, is presumably a

Mechanisms and Models in Rheumatoid Arthritis
ISBN 0–12–340440–1

consequence of the formation of antigen–antibody complexes. Indeed, deposition of immune complexes in menisci and articular cartilage from joints of rabbits with antigen-induced arthritis has been shown directly (Consden *et al.*, 1971; Cooke *et al.*, 1972) and transfer of immune serum has been shown to induce a transient arthritis subsequent to antigen challenge (Brackertz *et al.*, 1977c; Yoshino & Yoshino, 1992). Although the duration of antigen retention in these collagenous structures is very long (Hollister and Mannik, 1974), the elegant work of Fox and Glynn (1975) have shown that there is equivalent retention of immune complexes in the joints of rabbits immunized to antigen in either Freund's incomplete or complete adjuvant. Furthermore, reimmunization of rabbits in which arthritis had waned did not lead to reappearance of arthritis indicating that the sequestered immune complexes were unable to stimulate chronic synovitis (Fox and Glynn, 1977). Consequently, although immune complex deposition is important in the acute phase of rheumatoid arthritis, it is postulated that T-cell mediated immunity is responsible for the chronic aspects of disease in this model.

This view is supported by the findings that chronic arthritis cannot be induced in athymic mice and that in mice and rats chronic arthritis can be transferred by primary lymphoid cells (Brackertz *et al.*, 1977b; Griffiths *et al.*, 1992) and T-cell clones (Klasen *et al.*, 1989). The ability of cells to transfer disease can be abolished by anti-Thy 1 antibody treatment (Brackertz *et al.*, 1977b). Furthermore, a recent study in the rat demonstrated that antibodies directed against the αβ T-cell receptor block chronic, but not acute, antigen-induced arthritis and that immune serum can transfer only transient arthritis subsequent to antigen challenge (Yoshino and Yoshino, 1992). In the rabbit, FK 506 and cyclosporin suppress chronic, but not acute, synovitis supporting the view that T cells mediate the chronic stages of antigen-induced arthritis in this species (Blackham and Griffiths, 1991).

In mice, guinea pigs and rats, chronic synovitis cannot be induced with ovalbumin or bovine serum albumin. However, if the albumin is methylated or amidated then induction of a more chronic form of arthritis is possible. The ability of methylated or amidated proteins to induce arthritis has been attributed to their cationic charge, thus aiding antigen retention by binding to the negatively charged cartilage. However, high T-cell reactivity to the antigen is also required (van Lent *et al.*, 1987). Therefore, antigen retention during the early stages of disease may be necessary for development of chronic arthritis. The more stringent requirement for antigen retention in rodents may reflect higher antigen clearance rates compared to the rabbit. The greater mobility of rodents compared to rabbits may enhance clearance rates. This may explain why the severity of arthritis can be enhanced when mice are immobilized (van Lent *et al.*, 1990) or reduced in rabbits by continuous passive motion (Kim *et al.*, 1993).

MEDIATORS INVOLVED IN ANTIGEN-INDUCED ARTHRITIS

LIPID MEDIATORS

Cell membranes contain fatty acids esterified into phospholipids which can be metabolized to products with diverse biological activities. The best known group of inflammatory lipids are the eicosanoids (prostaglandins and leukotrienes) which are derived from arachidonic acid and have a well-characterized role in inflammation (Pettipher *et al.*, 1992; see Chapter 14, this volume). Arachidonic acid is liberated from membrane phospholipids, such as phosphatidylcholine by the action of phospholipase A_2. When this arachidonyl moiety is released from a phosphatide with an ether link in the 1 position the precursor for the synthesis of platelet activating factor (PAF) is released at the same time. The important roles of the eicosanoids and PAF in antigen-induced arthritis are discussed below.

Prostaglandins

Prostaglandins of the E series were first detected in the inflamed joints of rabbits with antigen-induced arthritis using a bioassay method (Blackham *et al.*, 1974). In this study, PGE-like activity peaked in the acute phase of arthritis (around 20 ng per knee joint) and was maintained at lower levels during the chronic phase of disease (1–2 ng per joint). These levels have been confirmed using radioimmunoassay (Henderson *et al.*, 1985; Henderson and Higgs, 1987; Pettipher *et al.*, 1989). Prostacyclin is also modestly induced in synovial tissues in antigen-induced arthritis as indicated by the production of its stable breakdown product, 6-keto PGF1α in explant cultures *ex vivo* (Henderson and Higgs, 1987), although PGE_2 is the major cyclooxygenase product generated in inflamed joints in antigen-induced arthritis. Based on their ability to synthesize large amounts of PGE_2 *in vitro* and *ex vivo*, resident synovial cells are likely to be the main cellular source of PGE_2 within the inflamed joint. However, the stimulus for the increased prostaglandin synthesis comes from the invading neutrophils, even though they have only a limited capacity to produce prostaglandins themselves (Pettipher *et al.*, 1988). This phenomenon extends to other systems such as infarcted myocardial tissue where it has been shown that neutrophils infiltrate resident tissue and initiate prostaglandin synthesis (Freed *et al.*, 1989). It is not well understood how neutrophils trigger prostaglandin synthesis by resident tissue but mechanisms involving the release of lysosomal phospholipase A_2 or reactive oxygen species may be involved (see Chapters 14 and 15, this volume).

Prostaglandin E_2 is produced in sufficiently high amounts to increase blood flow to the inflamed joint and consequently, potentiate oedema formation. This explains why cyclooxygenase inhibitors, when administered at doses sufficient to block cyclooxygenase activity completely, can reduce joint swelling in both arthritic rabbits (Pettipher *et al.*, 1989) and rats (Griffiths, 1992). Interestingly, cyclooxygenase inhibitors only inhibit joint swelling in the chronic phase of arthritis and do not affect peak swelling at days 1–3 after antigen when PGE_2 production is maximal (Pettipher *et al.*, 1989). This anomaly cannot be satisfactorily explained but it is likely that the acute response to antigen is so severe that blood flow to the synovial microvasculature is maximal even in the absence of prostaglandins. It should be remembered that although acute joint swelling is almost entirely due to oedema, increased tissue mass and fibrin deposition make a large contribution to increased joint diameter in chronic arthritis. Thus, in antigen-induced arthritis, vascular permeability is much greater in the first few days after antigen challenge compared to the later stages of arthritis, despite equivalent joint swelling (Berry *et al.*, 1973; Pettipher *et al.*, 1990). Furthermore, even in the chronic stages of arthritis, joint swelling is only inhibited by up to 50% by indomethacin in the rabbit, implicating additional mediators and processes in arthritis. In the rat the situation is quite different: although indomethacin does not affect acute swelling it can *completely* suppress joint swelling in chronic arthritis. This is in accord with the effect of indomethacin on synovial histopathology which is completely inhibited by this drug in the rat but is reported to be unaffected (Blackham *et al.*, 1974) or even worsened by indomethacin in the rabbit (Pettipher *et al.*, 1989). The differences in the effects of indomethacin on cartilage proteoglycan loss in rabbits and rats with antigen-induced arthritis are also quite striking. Indomethacin is an effective inhibitor of cartilage proteoglycan loss in the rat model while in rabbits indomethacin exacerbates cartilage damage (Pettipher *et al.*, 1989). The guinea pig model of antigen-induced arthritis responds to cyclooxygenase inhibitors in a manner similar to the rat (Pettipher, unpublished observations). These data illustrate the more profound role to prostaglandins in the manifestation of the immune response in rodents compared to other species. In rodents, cyclooxygenase inhibitors display efficacy comparable to immunosuppressants in models of arthritis – if dosed to inhibit cyclooxygenase activity in tissues *effectively*, NSAIDs will completely suppress the symptoms of collagen arthritis in mice and reduce anti-collagen antibody titres (Griffiths and Pettipher, unpublished observations). In the rabbit model of arthritis, prostaglandins play more of a modulatory role by damping down the immune response and, consequently, their removal by NSAID-treatment may lead to exacerbation of chronic inflammatory processes – see Pettipher and Whittle (1992) for a more detailed account of the role of prostaglandins in the immune response.

Leukotrienes

The 5-lipoxygenase product of arachidonic acid metabolism, LTB_4, has been the focus of much research since it was first discovered to be chemotactic for neutrophils *in vitro* and *in vivo* (Ford-Hutchinson *et al.*, 1980; Bray *et al.*, 1981) and to mediate increased vascular permeability by a neutrophil-dependent mechanism (Wedmore and Williams, 1981a; Bjork *et al.*, 1982). Leukotriene B_4 is produced predominantly from neutrophils and has been detected in neutrophil-rich exudates including the joint fluids from rabbits with acute antigen-induced arthritis (Henderson *et al.*, 1985; Henderson and Higgs, 1987). As acute joint swelling is almost completely inhibited by neutrophil depletion (Pettipher *et al.*, 1988), LTB_4 is a candidate for the substance which mediates the intense neutrophil infiltration and concomitant oedema occurring rapidly in response to antigen in this model. However, complete inhibition of LTB_4 by selective 5-lipoxygenase inhibitors fails to inhibit neutrophil influx or joint swelling in acute antigen-induced arthritis (Higgs *et al.*, 1989). Although the effects of 5-lipoxygenase inhibitors are disappointing in this model when administered alone, more dramatic effects are observed if the drugs are combined with indomethacin. There is a potentiation of the anti-inflammatory action of indomethacin in the chronic stages of disease (as measured by joint swelling and leukocyte numbers in the joint fluid) and the detrimental effects of indomethacin on cartilage integrity are prevented or reversed (Higgs *et al.*, 1989). Similar synergistic effects between cyclooxygenase inhibitors and lipoxygenase inhibitors have been observed in other models of inflammation (Foster and Potts, 1992) which highlight the potential of 5-lipoxygenase inhibitors as adjunctive therapy to NSAIDs in RA. This subject of the synergy between NSAIDs and lipoxygenase inhibitors and its therapeutic implications is discussed more fully in Chapter 14, this volume.

PLATELET-ACTIVATING FACTOR

Platelet-activating factor (PAF) is an ether-linked lipid produced from membrane phospholipids by the sequential action of phospholipase A_2 and an acetyl transferase. PAF has potent proinflammatory activities and is synthesized and released by a large number of cell types relevant to inflammation, including neutrophils, macrophages and endothelial cells. PAF stimulates neutrophil chemotaxis *in vitro* and neutrophil recruitment to sites of inflammation *in vivo*, although it is a much weaker chemotactic factor than LTB_4, C5a or IL-8 *in vivo* (Pettipher, unpublished observations). Probably the most important role for PAF is to increase vascular permeability, which it does by a direct action on the endothelium for which activation of circulating neutrophils is not required (Wedmore and Williams, 1981b; Doebber *et al.*, 1984). As chemotactic factors such as LTB_4 only increase vascular permeability in the presence of circulating neutrophils (Wedmore and Williams, 1981a) and PAF can be released from neutrophils in response to chemotactic factors (Camussi *et al.*, 1981), this led to the proposal that PAF derived from neutrophils may mediate oedema in response to chemotactic factors (Wedmore and Williams, 1981b). Indeed PAF antagonists reduce oedema associated with some neutrophil-dependent inflammatory responses such as the immune-complex mediated Arthus response (Hellewell and Williams, 1986; Issekutz and Szpejda, 1986) but do not decrease vascular permeability in response to exogenous chemotactic factors (Hellewell and Williams, 1986). Thus it seems that PAF is not the ubiquitous mediator or vascular permeability in all neutrophil-dependent reactions. Other mediators such as elastase released from azurophilic granules may play this role (see later).

As PAF appears to play an important role in Arthus-like responses it is not surprising that PAF can be detected in the joint fluids in the acute stages of antigen-induced arthritis (Pettipher *et al.*, 1987). Levels of around 100 pg/ml were detected by specific bioassay and this has since been confirmed by Zarco *et al.* (1992). The presence of an acetyl hydrolase in both plasma and synovial fluid (Hilliquin *et al.*, 1992) may explain the high levels of lysoPAF detected in both the acute and moderately chronic stages of antigen-induced arthritis (Pettipher *et al.*, 1987). However, it should be remembered that lysoPAF is also the precursor PAF synthesis and hence the balance of acetyl transferase and hydrolase activity is critical for the formation of PAF. PAF has since been detected in synovial fluids from patients with inflammatory joint disease (Hilliquin *et al.*, 1992), indicating the predictive value of the rabbit model in studying the mediators involved in arthritis.

One study has examined the effects of two PAF antagonists (BN 50726 and alprazolam) on the progression of antigen induced arthritis in the rabbit (Zarco *et al.*, 1992). Both compounds had profound inhibitory effects on intra-articular oedema and leukocyte infiltration and it was also noted that although PAF alone displayed only modest proinflammatory activity after intra-articular injection, synergistic responses could be achieved when combined with tumour necrosis factor (TNFα). In addition to its proinflammatory effects, PAF may also have detrimental effects on cartilage (Howat *et al.*, 1990) and bone (Zheng *et al.*, 1993). Clinical trials in RA with newly developed PAF antagonists are awaited with interest.

CYTOKINES

Cytokines are potent multi-functional proteins that are produced by a variety of cell types. Much work over the past two decades has shown cytokines to possess important pathophysiological actions in many diseases ranging from RA to AIDS. This research has highlighted two cytokines, interleukin-1 (IL-1) and TNFα as being key mediators in the cartilage and bone loss that is characteristic of inflammatory joint diseases such as RA (Arend and Dayer, 1990). Although it is likely that multiple cytokines are involved in various aspects of the pathogenesis of immune arthritis, this review focuses on studies investigating the role of IL-1 and TNFα since antagonists of, or neutralizing antibodies to, these cytokines are available and have been tested in antigen-induced arthritis. The role of cytokines in the pathology of RA is discussed in Chapters 2, 9, 10, 11, 12, 13, 26 and 27, this volume.

Interleukin-1

IL-1 is produced in two forms (α and β) which are 26% homologous. Both forms are active in inducing neutrophil and monocyte infiltration into synovial joints and in stimulating cartilage degradation (Henderson and Pettipher, 1988). However, IL-1β is the major form of IL-1 that is released from cells, while IL-1α tends to remain cell associated. A natural inhibitor that prevents the binding of IL-1α and β to their cell surface receptors is also produced by leukocytes, especially neutrophils (McColl *et al.*, 1992). This protein, termed IL-1 receptor antagonist (IL-1ra), has been cloned and expressed (Eisenberg *et al.*, 1990) and has efficacy in a variety of animal models including endotoxic shock in several species (Ohlsson *et al.*, 1990; Alexander *et al.*, 1991), colitis in rabbits (Cominelli *et al.*, 1990) and streptococcal cell-wall induced arthritis (Schwab *et al.*, 1991).

IL-1 has been detected by specific bioassay in the joint fluids in the early stages of antigen-induced arthritis in the rabbit (Henderson *et al.*, 1988). Although IL-1 could not be detected to joint fluid in the chronic stages of disease, IL-1-like activity was produced by the synovial tissue *ex vivo* at these times. The failures to detect IL-1 by bioassay is likely due to the presence of IL-1ra, which is detectable in RA synovial fluid at 10–20 ng/ml measured by ELISA (Malyak *et al.*, 1993). This contrasts with IL-1α or β which are present at low picogram levels per millilitre of synovial fluid. Any IL-1 present in synovial fluid is likely to be swamped by IL-1ra and suggests that IL-1 must act locally in the inflamed synovial tissue and at the cartilage–pannus junction.

The contribution of IL-1 to the pathogenesis of antigen-induced arthritis has been investigated using recombinant IL-1ra in the rabbit and by using blocking antibodies in the mouse. Although IL-1ra has shown efficacy in a number of animal models of inflammatory disease including streptococcal cell-wall arthritis (Schwab *et al.*, 1991, see Chapter 22, this volume), it did not supress synovial inflammation or cartilage damage in antigen-induced arthritis in the rabbit using a dosing regimen that inhibited the effects of exogeneous IL-1 (Lewthwaite *et al.*, 1993). However, IL-1ra did reduce the synovial fibrosis in the chronic stages of disease.

The contribution of IL-1α and β to the pathogenesis of antigen-induced arthritis in mice has been examined in some detail using blocking polyclonal antibodies directed against murine IL-1α and IL-1β (van de Loo *et al.*, 1992; see Chapter 26, this volume). The use of neutralizing antibodies that are specific for either form of IL-1 can determine the relative role of IL-1α versus IL-1β, unlike IL-1ra which inhibits both IL-1α and β. Another advantage of using antibodies for experimental studies is that a single injection can block the action of IL-1 for up to a week, while the effects of IL-1ra are transient. In antigen-induced arthritis in the mouse, anti-IL-1 therapy reduced intra-articular oedema at day 4, but not day 1, and also prevented the inhibition of cartilage proteoglycan synthesis seen in this model (van de Loo *et al.*, 1992). Interestingly anti-IL-1α and anti-IL-1β had to be given in combination to achieve these effects, either antibody given alone was without effect (van de Loo *et al.*, 1991), suggesting important roles for both IL-1α and IL-1β in the pathogenesis of immune synovitis.

Tumour Necrosis Factor α

TNFα shares many of the proinflammatory activities of IL-1 and may therefore also promote synovitis and stimulate cartilage and bone breakdown (Arend and Dayer, 1990). TNFα may also be an essential stimulus for the production of other cytokines such as IL-1 in the rheumatoid joint since neutralizing antibodies directed against TNFα reduce the spontaneous production of IL-1 from synovial mononuclear cells derived from the joints of RA patients (Brennan *et al.*, 1989). Furthermore, once synthesized and released from cells in the rheumatoid joint the inflammatory effects of IL-1 and TNFα are synergistic (Henderson and Pettipher, 1989).

As in RA (Di Giovine *et al.*, 1988), TNFα can be detected in high concentrations in the synovial fluid of rabbits with acute antigen-induced arthritis (Lewthwaite, Blake, Morgan and Henderson, unpublished observations). TNFα has also been immuno-localized in macrophage-like cells in the inflamed synovial lining and in the chondro-cytes in the deep zone of articular cartilage (Henderson *et al.*, 1993). Neutralizing monoclonal antibodies against TNFα reduce joint swelling and synovial leukocytosis in rabbits with antigen-induced arthritis but do not protect against cartilage degra-dation in this model (Blake, Lewthwaite, Henderson and Hardingham, unpublished observations). In antigen-induced arthritis in the mouse, anti-TNFα did not suppress synovitis or cartilage degradation (van de Loo *et al.*, 1991).

Conclusions

Taken together the evidence would suggest pathogenic roles for the cytokines IL-1 and TNFα in some aspects of antigen-induced arthritis, although IL-1 appears more important in the mouse model while in the rabbit TNFα is dominant. As anti-TNFα therapy is reported to be effective in patients with severe RA (Elliott *et al.*, 1993), this suggests that the rabbit model of antigen-induced arthritis is reflective of human disease, while the negative results with anti-TNFα in the murine model of antigen-induced arthritis casts doubt on the value of this model.

PROTEASES

Neutrophil Proteases

Neutrophils infiltrate the joints of animals with antigen-induced arthritis in large numbers and, as these cells contain proteases such as elastase and cathepsin G which can degrade the connective tissue components of both basement membrane and articular cartilage (Oronsky and Perper, 1975; Pipoly and Crouch, 1987), it is possible such neutrophil-derived proteases are responsible for mediating both the intra-articular oedema and cartilage destruction that occur in this model.

Although joint swelling in response to antigen is neutrophil-dependent (Pettipher *et al.*, 1988), it appears independent of the enzymatic activity of elastase or cathepsin G, since the formation of intra-articular oedema is unimpeded in beige mice which lack catalytically active elastase and cathepsin G (Pettipher *et al.*, 1990). However, it is now appreciated that the defect in neutrophils from beige mice is not due to the lack of the elastase or cathepsin G proteins but due to the presence of inhibitors of these proteases in the cells (Takeuchi and Swank, 1989). This has important implications for the interpretation of data derived from experiments involving these neutrophils because it is now known that elastase and cathepsin G increase vascular permeability by a mechanism that is related to their cationic charge but independent of their catalytic activity (Peterson, 1989; Rosengren and Arfors, 1991). Thus, elastase-induced vascular leakage is not inhibited by elastase inhibitors and consequently, neutrophil-dependent oedema such as occurs in antigen-induced arthritis may be mediated by non-catalytic properties of elastase or cathepsin G, even in beige mice.

Serine proteases derived from neutrophils have been also implicated in the cartilage proteoglycan loss that occurs rapidly over the first few days after antigen challenge. Sandy *et al.* (1981) extracted a serine protease with elastase-like properties from the articular cartilage from rabbits with antigen-induced arthritis. The method employed measured free enzyme dissociated from enzyme-inhibitor complexes and consequently it is not clear how much free elastase is available to degrade the cartilage. In fact, several studies have highlighted the vast excess of protease inhibitors present at the synovial fluid–cartilage interface and questioned the importance of neutrophil-derived proteases in mediating cartilage damage (Hadler *et al.*, 1979). In contrast to joint swelling, cartilage proteoglycan loss is not reduced in neutropenic animals (Pettipher *et al.*, 1988), suggesting that neutrophil-derived proteases do not contribute to this aspect of joint pathology. Furthermore, cartilage proteoglycan loss, measured histochemically, was found to be similar in beige mice and mice with normal levels of catalytically active neutrophil neutral proteases (Pettipher *et al.*, 1990).

There is some evidence that neutrophils have protective properties that impede cartilage degradation – cartilage damage is accelerated in rabbits if the neutropenia is extended for 4 days (Pettipher *et al.*, 1988). The mechanism of neutrophil-mediated protection of cartilage may be related to the presence of protease inhibitors in inflammatory exudate (Moore *et al.*, 1990) or could be due to the ability of neutrophils to bind IL-1 or produce the IL-1ra (McColl *et al.*, 1992; Malyak *et al.*, 1993). This interpretation of the role of neutrophils in cartilage degradation is attractive because it appears to fit with the clinical picture in RA where the levels of neutrophil-derived proteases in synovial fluid are inversely related to the degree of radiographic progression (Hadler *et al.*, 1979). The importance of neutrophils in RA joint pathology is also considered by Poole *et al.* (Chapter 9) and Cawston (Chapter 17) this volume.

Proteases Derived from Resident Connective Tissue Cells

Blackham *et al.* (1974) suggested that lysosomal enzymes were important in mediating the histopathology of antigen-induced arthritis based on their observations that indomethacin, while reducing prostaglandin levels and joint swelling, did not affect the levels of free acid phosphatase or the extent of tissue damage. It is not clear from this study whether the acid phosphatase was derived from the infiltrating leukocytes or the resident tissue. In a later study the extracellular levels of β-glucuronidase and *N*-acetyl-β-glucosaminidase were measured in the joint fluids of rabbits with antigen-induced arthritis and it was found that the large increase in β-glucuronidase could be significantly reduced by neutrophil depletion while the levels of *N*-acetyl-β-glucosaminidase remained elevated (Pettipher *et al.*, 1988). The fact that the cartilage proteoglycan loss was not inhibited by neutrophil depletion suggests that lysosomal enzymes derived from resident tissue may contribute to joint damage.

Some lysosomal enzymes, such as cathepsins B and L, are capable of cleaving cartilage collagen and proteogylcan. Cathespin L is elevated in the inflamed synovial tissues of rabbits with antigen-induced arthritis (Etherington *et al.*, 1988). Synovial lining cells and infiltrating macrophages play an important role in cartilage degradation and these cells stain heavily for cathepsin L in antigen-induced arthritis in the rabbit (Etherington *et al.*, 1988). In the rat model of antigen-induced arthritis, van Noorden *et al.* (1988) showed that cathepsin B was elevated to a much greater extent than cathepsin L in both the synovial tissue and articular cartilage and treatment with the cysteine proteinase inhibitor, Z-Phe-Ala-CH$_2$F, reduced both synovial inflammation and cartilage damage. This compound inhibits both cathepsin B and L and so it would be of interest to test selective inhibitors of B or L in this model.

Collagenase, stromelysin and the gelatinases belong to a family of metalloproteinases that are induced in connective tissue cells by the action of cytokines such as IL-1 or TNFα. The combined actions of these proteases can lead to the degradation of all components of the extracellular matrix at around neutral pH. The degradation of collagen by synovial cells to chondrocytes is mediated by collagenase (Gavrilovic *et al.*, 1987; Reynolds *et al.*, 1988; Cruwys *et al.*, 1990), although it is less certain whether cartilage proteoglycan degradation is metalloproteinase-dependent as the cleavage sites in aggrecan induced by IL-1 in cultured cartilage differ from those of stromelysin (Sandy *et al.*, 1992). *In vivo*, it has proved difficult to detect any of the metalloproteinases in an active form although synovial tissues from rabbits with antigen-induced arthritis produce elevated amounts of latent collagenase in culture (Henderson *et al.*, 1990). Interestingly, articular cartilage from these rabbits did not produce significant amounts of collagenase. This contrasts with the polycation-induced arthritis model where collagenase was produced by both the synovial tissue and articular cartilage *ex vivo*. The lack of metalloproteinase production in cartilage from rabbits with antigen-induced arthritis may be related to the degree of chondrocyte death that is known to occur in this model and has been seen by some as a limitation of its usefulness as a model for RA (Howson *et al.*, 1986). However, it does suggest that articular chondrocytes play little role in cartilage degradation and that the hypertrophic synovial tissue is the main source of degradative enzymes.

Metal-dependent gelatinase activity has been detected in the synovial homogenates from guinea pigs with antigen-induced arthritis (Yamashita *et al.*, 1991). Based on their findings that the molecular weight was 92 kDa, the authors concluded that the gelatinase was derived from infiltrating neutrophils. This may be true but it is now known that rheumatoid synovial fibroblasts constitutively express the 92-kDa gelatinase (type V collagenase) and normal synovial fibroblasts can be induced to express the 92-kDa gelatinase by the addition of cytokines (Unemori *et al.*, 1991). Consequently, it is likely that the resident synovial cells may contribute to the appearance of gelatinase in this model. It would be of interest to study the effects of leukocyte depletion to determine the cellular source of the gelatinase activity.

GENERAL CONCLUSIONS

Antigen-induced arthritis has served as a useful model for the study of mechanisms and mediators involved in the pathogenesis of RA. Similarities of antigen-induced arthritis in the rabbit to RA include the synovial histopathology, the chronicity of disease, antibody and T-cell responsiveness to cartilage components and the levels of inflammatory mediators in diseased joints. In particular, studies investigating the role of infiltrating leukocytes have given us insights into mechanisms involved in both the acute and chronic aspects of disease and allow us to make some general conclusions regarding the pathogenesis of antigen-induced arthritis. Thus, it seems that the disease activity is orchestrated by activated T-cells which in collaboration with macrophages send signals to recruit neutrophils to the joint. Activated neutrophils directly increase vascular permeability leading to joint swelling (as may occur during a flare). Cytokines produced during T-cell/macrophage interactions also activate the resident cells in the synovial lining to proliferate, grow over the articular cartilage and release proteases to destroy the cartilage matrix. Based on present evidence chondrocyte activation seems only to play a minor role in antigen-induced arthritis.

While the above scheme seems to fit with the clinical picture it does not necessarily mean that this model (like any other) will predict therapeutic efficacy of new classes of compound (see Chapter 28, this volume, for a discussion of the use of animal models in drug development). Ultimately, only careful clinical trials with drugs with well-defined biochemical mechanisms will predict which classes of compound will be successful in the treatment of RA in the future.

REFERENCES

Alexander HR, Doherty GM, Buresh CM, Venzon DJ & Norton JA (1991) A recombinant human receptor antagonist to interleukin 1 improves survival after lethal endotoxemia in mice. *J Exp Med* **173**: 1029–1032.

Arend WP & Dayer J-M, (1990) Cytokines and cytokine inhibitors or antagonists in rheumatoid arthritis. *Arthitis Rheum* **33**: 305–315.

Berry H, Browett JP, Huskisson EC, Bacon P & Willoughby DA (1973) Measurement of inflammation. Application of technetium clearance to rheumatoid arthritis and animal models. *Ann Rheum Dis* **32**: 95–98.

Bjork J, Hedqvist P & Arfors K-E (1982) Increase in vascular permeability induced by leukotriene B₄ and the role of polymorphonuclear leukocytes. *Inflammation* **6**: 189–200.

Blackham A & Griffiths RJ (1991) The effect of FK 506 and cyclosporin A on antigen-induced arthritis. *Clin Exp Immunol* **86**: 224–228.

Blackham A, Farmer JB, Radziwonik H & Westwick J (1974) The role of prostaglandins in rabbit mono-articular arthritis. *Br J Pharmacol* **51**: 35–44.

Brackertz D, Mitchell GF & MacKay IR (1977a) Antigen-induced arthritis in mice. Induction of arthritis in various strains of mice. *Arthritis Rheum* **20**: 841–850.

Brackertz D, Mitchell GF, Vadas MA, MacKay IR & Miller JFAP (1977b) Studies on antigen-induced arthritis in mice. Immunologic correlates of arthritis susceptibility in mice. *J Immunol* **118**: 1639–1644.

Brackertz D, Mitchell GF, Vadas MA & MacKay IR (1977c) Studies on antigen-induced arthritis in mice. Cell and serum transfer experiments. *J Immunol* **118**: 1645–1648.

Bray MA, Ford-Hutchinson AW & Smith MJH (1981) Leukotriene B_4: an inflammatory mediator *in vivo*. *Prostaglandins* **22**: 213–222.

Brennan FM, Chantry D, Jackson A, Maini R & Feldmann M (1989). Inhibitory effect of TNFα antibodies on synovial cell interleukin 1 production in rheumatoid arthritis. *Lancet* **2**: 244–247.

Camussi G, Tetta C, Bussolino F, Caligaris Cappio F, Coda R, Masera C et al. (1981) Mediators of immune-complex-induced aggregation of polymorphonuclear neutrophils. II. Platelet-activating factor as the effector substance of immune-induced aggregation. *Int Arch Allergy Appl Imunol* **64**: 25–41.

Cashin CH, Doherty NS, Jeffries BL & Buckland-Wright JC (1980) An investigation of the effect of anti-inflammatory and anti-rheumatoid drugs in cell-mediated immune arthritis in guinea pigs by microfocal radiography. *Br J Exp Pathol* **61**: 296–302.

Cominelli P, Nast CC, Clark BD, Schindler R, Lierena R, Eysselein VE, Thompson RC & Dinarello CA (1990) Interleukin 1 (IL-1) gene expression, synthesis, and effect of specific IL-1 receptor blockade in rabbit immune complex coloitis. *J Clin Invest* **86**: 972–980.

Consden R, Doble A, Glynn LE & Nind AP (1971) Production of a chronic arthritis with ovalbumin. Its retention in the rabbit knee. *Ann Rheum Dis* **30**: 307–315.

Cooke TD, Hurd ER, Ziff M & Jasin HE (1972) The pathogenesis of chronic inflammation in experimental antigen-induced arthritis. Preferential localization of antigen-induced complexes to collagenous tissues. *J Exp Med* **135**: 323–338.

Cruwys SC, Davies DE & Pettipher ER (1990) Co-operation between interleukin 1 and the fibrinolytic system in the degradation of collagen by articular chondrocytes. *Br J Pharmacol* **100**: 631–635.

Di Giovine FS, Nuki G & Duff GW (1988) Tumour necrosis factor in synovial exudates. *Ann Rheum Dis* **47**: 768–772.

Doebber TW, Wu MS & Shen TY (1984) Platelet activating factor intravenous infusion in rats stimulates vascular lysosomal hydrolase secretion independent of blood neutrophils. *Biochem Biophys Res Comm* **125**: 980–987.

Dumonde DC & Glynn LE (1962) The production of arthritis in rabbits by an immunological reaction to fibrin. *Br J Exp Pathol* **43**: 373–383.

Eisenberg ST, Evans RJ, Verderber E, Brewer MT, Hannun CH & Thompson RC (1990) Primary structure and functional expression from complementary DNA of a human interleukin 1 antag-onist. *Nature* **343**: 341–346.

Elliott MJ, Maini RN, Feldmann M, Long-Fox A, Charles P & Brennan FM (1993) Treatment of rheuma-toid arthritis with chimeric monoclonal antibodies to TNFα. Safety, clinical efficacy and regulation of the acute phase response. *Br J Rheumatol* **32**: 209.

Etherington DJ, Taylor MAJ & Henderson B (1988) Elevation of cathepsin L levels in the synovial lining of rabbits with antigen-induced arthritis. *Br J Exp Pathol* **69**: 281–289.

Ford-Hutchinson AW, Bray MA, Doig MV, Shipley ME & Smith MJH (1980) Leukotriene B: a potent chemokinetic and aggregating substance released from polymorphonuclear leukocytes. *Nature* **286**: 264–265.

Foster SJ & Potts HC (1992) Arachidonic acid-induced mouse ear oedema: synergistic inhibition by combined treatment with ICI D2138, a selective 5-lipoxygenase inhibitor, and non-steroidal anti-inflammatory agents. *Sixth International Conference of the Inflammation Research Association* (Abstr).

Fox A & Glynn LE (1975) Persistence of antigen in nonarthritic joints. *Ann Rheum Dis* **34**: 431–437.

Fox A & Glynn LE (1977) Is persisting antigen responsible for the chronicity of experimental allergic arthritis. *Ann Rheum Dis* **36**: 34–38.

Freed MS, Needleman P, Dukel CG, Saffitz JE & Evers AS (1989) Role of invading leukocytes in enhanced atrial eicosanoid production following rabbit left ventricular myocardial infarction. *J Clin Invest* **83**: 205–212.

Gavrilovic J, Hembry RM, Reynolds JJ & Murphy G (1987) Tissue inhibitor of metalloproteinases (TIMP) regulates extracellular type 1 collagen degradation by chondrocytes and endothelial cells. *J Cell Science* **87**: 357–362.

Glynn LE (1968) The chronicity of inflammation and its significance in rheumatoid arthritis. *Ann Rheum Dis* **27**: 105–121.

Griffiths RJ (1992) Characterisation and pharmacological sensitivity of antigen arthritis induced by methylated bovine serum albumin in the rat. *Agents Actions* **35**: 88–95.

Griffiths RJ, Li SW & Mather ME (1992) Chracterisation of passively transferred antigen arthritis induced by methylated bovine serum albumin in the rat: Effect of FK 506 on arthritis development. *Agents Actions* **36**: 146–151.

Hadler NM, Spitznagel JK & Quinet RJ (1979) Lysosomal enzymes in inflammatory synovial effusions. *J Immunol* **123**: 572–577.

Hellewell PG & Williams TJ (1986) A specific antagonist of platelet activating factor suppresses oedema formation in an Arthus reaction but not oedema induced by leukocyte chemoattractants in rabbit skin. *J Immunol* **137**: 302–307.

Henderson B & Higgs GA (1987) Synthesis of arachidonate oxidation products by synovial joint tissues during the development of chronic erosive arthritis. *Arthritis Rheum* **30**: 1149–1156.

Henderson B & Pettipher ER (1988) Comparison of the inflammatory activities after intraarticular injection of natural and recombinant IL-1α and IL-1β in the rabbit. *Biochem Pharmacol* **37**: 4171–4176.

Henderson B & Pettipher ER (1989) Arthritogenic actions of recombinant IL-1 and tumour necrosis factor α in the rabbit: evidence for synergistic interactions between cytokines *in vivo*. *Clin Exp Immunol* **75**: 306–310.

Henderson B, Higgs GA, Moncada S & Salmon JA (1985) Synthesis of eicosanoids by tissues of the synovial joint during the development of chronic erosive synovitis. *Agents Actions* **17**: 360–362.

Henderson B, Rowe FM, Bird CR & Gearing AJH (1988) Production of interleukin 1 in the joint during the development of antigen-induced arthritis in the rabbit. *Clin Exp Immunol* **71**: 371–376.

Henderson B, Pettipher ER & Murphy G (1990) Metalloproteinases and cartilage proteoglcan depletion in chronic arthritis. *Arthritis Rheum* **33**: 241–246.

Henderson B, Hardingham T, Blake S & Lewthwaite J (1993) Experimental arthritis models in the study of mechanisms of articular cartilage loss in rheumatoid arthritis. *Agents Actions Suppl* **39**: 15–26.

Higgs GA, Pettipher ER & Henderson B (1989) The effect of a novel selective lipoxygenase inhibitor in anaphylactic and inflammatory responses. *Proceedings of the Third Interscience World Conference on Inflammation* (Abstr.).

Hilliquin P, Menkes CJ, Laoussadi S, Benveniste J & Arnoux B (1992) Presence of paf-acether in rheumatic diseases. *Ann Rheum Dis* **51**: 29–31.

Hollister JR & Mannik M (1974) Antigen retention in joint tissue in antigen-induced synovitia. *Clin Exp Immunol* **16**: 615–627.

Howat D, Desa F, Chander C, Moore A & Willoughby D (1990) The synergism between platelet-activating factor and interleukin 1 on cartilage breakdown. *J Lipid Mediators* **2**: 143–149.

Howson P, Shepard N & Mitchell N (1986) The antigen-induced arthritis model: The relevance of the method of induction to its use as a model of human disease. *J Rheumatol* **13**: 379–390.

Hunneyball IM (1984) Use of experimental arthritis in the rabbit for the development of antiarthritic drugs. In Otterness I, Capetola R & Wong S (eds), **Vol. 7**: 249–262. New York: Raven Press.

Issekutz AC & Szpejda M (1986) Evidence that platelet activating factor may mediate some acute inflammatory responses. Studies with the platelet activating factor antagonist, CV 3988. *Lab Invest* **54**: 275–281.

Kim HKW, Kerr RG, Cruz TF & Salter RB (1993) The effect of continuous passive motion on antigen-induced arthritis in rabbits. *Transactions of the 39th Annual Meeting of the Orthopaedic Society February 15–18* (Abstr.).

Klasen IS, Ladestein RMT, Van den Berg WB & Benner R (1989) Requirements for flare reactions of joint inflammation induced in mice by cloned MT4+, LYT-2 T-cells. *Arthritis Rheum* **32**: 330–337.

Lewthwaite JC, Blake SM, Hardingham TE & Henderson B (1993). The effect of interleukin 1 receptor antagonist on the progression of antigen-induced arthritis in the rabbit. *Transactions of the 39th Annual Meeting of the Orthopaedic Research Society February 15–18* (Abstr.).

Malyak M, Swaney RE & Arend WP (1993) Levels of synovial fluid interleukin 1 receptor antagonist in rheumatoid arthritis and other arthropathies. *Arthritis Rheum* **36**: 781–789.

McColl SR, Paquin R, Menard C & Beaulieu AD (1992) Human neutrophils produce high levels of the interleukin 1 receptor antagonist in response to granulocyte/macrophage colony-stimulating factor and tumor necrosis factor. *J Exp Med* **176**: 593–598.

Moore AR, Desa FM, Hanahoe TH, Colville-Nash PR, Chander CL, Howat DW & Willoughby DA (1990) The protective effects of cell-free fluid exudate on cartilage degradation *in vitro*. *Int J Tissue Reactions* **12**: 33–37.

Ohlsson KO, Bjork P, Bergenfeldt M, Hageman R & Thompson RC (1990) Interleukin 1 receptor antagonist reduces mortality from endotoxin shock. *Nature* **348**: 550–552.

Oronsky AL & Perper RJ (1975) Connective tissue-degrading enzymes of human leukocytes. *Ann NY Acad Sci* **256**: 233–253.

Peterson MW (1989) Neutrophil cathepsin G increases transendothelial albumin flux. *J Lab Clin Med* **113**: 297–308.

Pettipher ER & Henderson B (1988) The relationship between cell-mediated immunity and cartilage degradation in antigen-induced arthritis in the rabbit. *Br J Exp Pathol* **69**: 113–122.

Pettipher ER & Whittle BJR (1992) Prostaglandins. In Roitt IM & Delves PJ (eds) *Encyclopaedia of Immunology*, pp 1279–1282. London: Academic Press.

Pettipher ER, Higgs GA & Henderson B (1987) PAF-acether in chronic arthritis. *Agents Actions* **21**: 98–103.

Pettipher ER, Henderson B, Moncada S & Higgs GA (1988) Leucocyte infiltration and cartilage proteoglycan loss in immune arthritis in the rabbit. *Br J Pharmacol* **95**: 169–176.

Pettipher ER, Henderson B, Edwards JCW & Higgs GA (1989) Effect of indomethacin in swelling, lymphocyte influx and cartilage proteoglycan depletion in experimental arthritis. *Ann Rheum Dis* **48**: 623–627.

Pettipher ER, Edwards J, Cruwys S, Jessup E, Beesley J & Henderson B (1990) Pathogenesis of antigen-induced arthritis in mice deficient in neutrophil elastase and cathepsin G. *Am J Pathol* **137**: 1077–1082.

Pettipher ER, Higgs GA & Salmon JA (1992) Eicosanoids (prostaglandins and leukotrienes). In Whicher JT & Evans SW (eds) *Biochemistry of Inflammation*, pp 91–108. Dordrecht: Kluwer.

Pipoly DJ & Crouch EC (1987) Degradation of native type IV procollagen by human neutrophil elastase. Implications for leukocyte-mediated degradation of basement membranes. *Biochemistry* **26**: 5748–5754.

Reynolds JJ, Lawrence CE & Gavrilovic J (1988) Model systems for studying the destruction of the extracellular matrix and their usefulness in testing inhibitors. In Glauert A (ed) *The Control of Tissue Damage*, pp 281–296. Amsterdam: Elsevier.

Rosengren S & Arfors K-E (1991) Polycations induce microvascular leakage of macromolecules in hamster cheek pouch. *Inflammation* **15**: 159–172.

Sandy JD, Sriratana A, Brown HLG & Lowther DA (1981) Evidence for polymorphonuclear leucocyte-derived proteinases in arthritic cartilage. *Biochem J* **193**: 193–202.

Sandy JD, Flannery CR, Neame PJ & Lohmander LS (1992; The structure of aggrecan fragments in human synovial fluid. Evidence for the involvement in osteoarthritis of a novel proteinase which cleaves the Glu 373-Ala 374 bond of the interglobular domain. *J Clin Invest* **89**: 1512–1516.

Schwab JH, Anderle SK, Brown RR, Dalldorg FG & Thompson RD (1991) Pro- and anti-inflammatory roles of interleukin 1 in recurrence of bacterial cell wall-induced arthritis in rats. *Infect Immunol* **59** 4436–4442.

Takeuchi KH & Swank RT (1989) Inhibitors of elastase and cathepsin G in Chediak–Higashi (Beige) neutrophils. *J Biol Chem* **264**: 7431–7436.

Unemori EN, Hibbs MS & Amento EP (1991) Constitutive expression of a 92 kD gelatinase (type V collagenase) by rheumatoid synovial fibroblasts and its induction in normal human fibroblasts by inflammatory cytokines. *J Clin Invest* **88**: 1656–1662.

van de Loo, FAJ, Arntz OJ, Otterness IG, Beuscher HU & van den Berg WB (1991) Specific role for IL-1 in experimental arthritis. *Cytokine* **3**: 406.

van de Loo FAJ, Arntz OJ, Otterness IG & van den Berg WB (1992) Protection against cartilage proteoglycan synthesis inhibition by antiinterleukin 1 antibodies in expermiental arthritis. *J Rheumatol* **19**: 348–356.

van Lent PLEM, van den Berg WB, Schalkwijk J, van de Putte LBA & van den Bersselaar L (1987) Allergic arthritis induced by cationic antigens: relationship of chronicity with antigen retention and T-cell reactivity. *Immunology* **62**: 265–272.

van Lent PLEM, van den Bersselaar L, van de Putte LBA & van den Berg WB (1990) Immobilisation aggravates cartilage damage during antigen-induced arthritis in mice. Attachment of polymorphonuclear leukocytes to articular cartilage. *Am J Pathol* **136**: 1407–1416.

van Noorden CJF, Smith RE & Rasnick D (1988) Cysteine proteinase activity in arthritic rat knee joints and the effects of a selective systemic inhibitor, Z-Phe-AlaCH$_2$F. *J Rheumatol* **15**: 1525–1535.

Wedmore CV & Williams TJ (1981a) Control of vascular permeability by polymorphonuclear leukocytes in inflammation. *Nature* **289**: 646–650.

Wedmore CV & Williams TJ (1981b) Platelet-activating factor, a secretory product of polymorphonuclear leucocytes, increases vascular permeability in rabbit skin. *Br J Pharmacol* **74**: 916P.

Yamashita N, Nakanishi I & Okada Y (1991) Arthritis induced immunologically with cationic amidated bovine serum albumin in the guinea pig. A morphological and biochemical study on the destruction of articular cartilage. *Virchows Archiv B Cell Pathol* **60**: 57–66.

Yoshino S & Yoshino J (1992) Suppression of chronic antigen-induced arthritis in rats by a monoclonal antibody against the T-cell receptor αβ. *Cell Immunol* **144**: 382–391.

Zarco P, Maestre C, Herrero-Beaumont G, Gonzalez E, Garcia-Hoyo R, Navarro FJ et al. (1992) Involvement of platelet-activating factor and tumour necrosis factor in pathogenesis of joint inflammation in rabbits. *Clin Exp Immunol* **88**: 318–323.

Zheng ZG, Wood DA, Sims SM & Dixon SJ (1993) Platelet-activating factor stimulates resorption by rabbit osteoclasts *in vitro*. *Am J Physiol* **264**: E74–E81.

25 Spontaneous Arthritis Models

Frank X. O'Sullivan, Renate E. Gay and Steffen Gay

INTRODUCTION

Although joint diseases due to inherited dysplasias or to degenerative and infectious causes occur frequently in wild and domesticated animals, spontaneous inflammatory arthritides resembling rheumatoid arthritis (RA) are rare. Until recently only the MRL/lpr mouse and the occasional domestic dog were known to develop non-infectious, seropositive, erosive polyarthritis without the administration of an exogenous agent. However in the last 3 years several new murine models have been recognized, and are included in this dicsussion. Ironically, the suitability of any single animal disease entity as a model for RA depends on the definition of the prototypic disease. Since the etiologic agent(s) and pathogenetic mechanisms causing RA have not been fully delineated, it is difficult to judge accurately the true validity of a given spontaneous animal model of this disease. Current views on these subjects are presented in Chapters 1–3, this volume.

The purpose of this chapter is to present the clinical and immunopathologic characteristics of spontaneously occurring animal arthritides resembling RA for comparison with the pathogenetic mechanisms described in previous chapters. Although few in number, these models represent a broad spectrum of etiologies and pathogenetic mechanisms. For instance the polyarthropathy in NZB/KN mice appears to arise from multiple genetic factors, while that of the *ank/ank* mouse appears to be due primarily to the influence of a single gene mutation. In the middle of this pathogenetic spectrum is the MRL/lpr strain in which the expression of joint disease represents a complex interaction between a single gene mutation and the genetic background. These are reviewed in detail as are the arthropathies that occur in normal DBA/1 mice, in the high antibody responding Biozzi (H_I) mouse strain and in canine RA.

MRL/Mp-*lpr/lpr* (MRL/lpr) MOUSE

The MRL/lpr mouse is the most extensively scrutinized model of spontaneous arthritis described in this chapter. The MRL substrains arose in 1976 during the course of a breeding programme originally designed to transfer an achondroplasia mutation, carried by AKR/J mice with a high incidence of leukaemia, on to a genetic background which was free of early onset haematologic malignancies. After a series of crosses involving C57Bl/6, C3H/Di and LG/J mouse strains followed by additional rigid inbreeding, an autosomal recessive mutation occurred which caused massive lymphoproliferation (*lpr*). Selective mating of affected individuals established the homozygous MRL/lpr substrain described below (Murphy and Roths, 1978).

Mechanisms and Models in Rheumatoid Arthritis
ISBN 0–12–340440–1

MRL/lpr mice develop a severe systemic lupus erythematosus (SLE)-like disease characterized by immune-complex mediated glomerulonephritis, dermatitis, production of autoantibodies and rheumatoid factors, systemic vasculitis, hypergamma-globulinaemia, sialoadenitis, inflammatory central nervous system lesions and erosive arthritis (Andrews *et al.*, 1978; Theofilopoulos and Dixon, 1981, 1985; Hang *et al.*, 1982; Alexander *et al.*, 1983; Hoffman *et al.*, 1984; O'Sullivan *et al.*, 1985; Vogelweid *et al.*, 1991). The *lpr* mutation causes massive enlargement of the spleen and lymph nodes due to the accumulation of an unusual T-lymphocyte subset with the phenotype Thy-1$^+$CD4$^-$CD8$^-$B220$^+$ (Morse *et al.*, 1982), and markedly accelerates the mild, late age-associated autoimmune phenomena that occur in congenic MRL/Mp-+/+ (MRL/n) mice (Theofilopoulos and Dixon, 1985). The co-occurrence of spontaneous destructive polyarthritis and high levels of circulating rheumatoid factors (RFs) in these mice has prompted studies in the MRL/lpr strain directed toward the delineation of factors involved in the etiology and pathogenesis of RA.

CLINICOPATHOLOGIC CHARACTERISTICS OF JOINT DISEASE

MRL/lpr mice rarely manifest clinical evidence of articular disease. A few reports have included descriptions of hindpaw swelling without erythema (Andrews *et al.*, 1978; Boissier *et al.*, 1989). However, Edwards and colleagues (1986) attributed the swelling to subcutaneous inflammatory infiltrates rather than to underlying tenosynovitis. Gait and postural abnormalities have not been observed in most reports (Hang *et al.*, 1982; O'Sullivan *et al.*, 1985; Pataki and Rordorf-Adam, 1985; Gilkeson *et al.*, 1989), although one group of investigators detected decreased cage-climbing activity in MRL/lpr compared to control animals (Edwards *et al.*, 1986).

Histopathological abnormalities appear in the joints of affected MRL/lpr mice after 2 months of age. The arthropathy is progressive, such that more than half develop synovial pathology by 3–4 months of age, and 80–100% are affected after the age of 5 months. Males and females are apparently affected equally, and the distribution of the articular disease is symmetric. Hind- and forepaw joints are most frequently affected, followed by the knee and hip. Costovertebral joint abnormalities have also been observed (Hang *et al.*, 1982; O'Sullivan *et al.*, 1985; Pataki and Rordorf-Adam, 1985; Boissier *et al.*, 1989; Gilkeson *et al.*, 1989).

The microscopic appearance of the synovitis in MRL/lpr mice is quite variable between and within individual breeding colonies, regardless of environmental conditions. For example, Hang and coworkers (1982) demonstrated proliferating synovial cells, extensive mononuclear cell infiltration of the subsynovial tissue, and pannus formation associated with destruction of bone and cartilage in joints from mice 3–4 months of age and older. Lymphocytes, plasma cells and macrophages comprised the majority of the infiltrating cells. By transmission electron microscopy (TEM) some of the lymphocytes had ultrastructural characteristics of T-cells, and macrophages were observed interdigitating with adjacent plasma cells and lymphocytes. In contrast, histopathologic analysis of articular tissue from comparably aged MRL/lpr mice by O'Sullivan and colleagues (1985) revealed an initial phase consisting of synovial cell proliferation and subsequent erosion of adjacent cartilage and bone in the absence of significant inflammatory cell infiltration (Fig. 1). In older mice with later stages of joint disease, inflammatory cells were detected in significant numbers in synovial

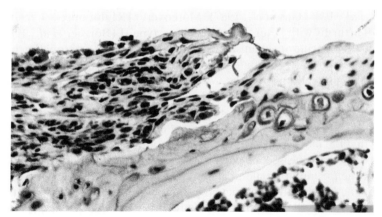

Figure 1. Histopathology of 13-week old MRL/lpr mouse knee joint: proliferating synovial cells at site of cartilage and bone erosion in the initial phase of joint destruction.

tissues. TEM studies of proliferating synovial layers from MRL/lpr mice by the same workers revealed that the majority were type B synovial cells (Tanaka *et al.*, 1988) and strongly resembled those observed in the synovial tissues from patients with early RA (Fassbender, 1983). Variations on these two histopathological themes appear to a greater or lesser degree in studies by other workers. For example, an immunohisto-chemical analysis by Tarkowski *et al.* (1987) found primarily Mac-1^+ proliferating synovial cells in the joints of MRL/lpr mice without infiltrating T or B cells. Gilkeson and coworkers (1989) found both non-inflammatory and inflammatory proliferative synovitis in aged male MRL/lpr mice from the same colony, all of which had been housed under the same conditions.

ASSOCIATED IMMUNOPATHOLOGIC FINDINGS

IgM and IgG RFs are elaborated in significant quantities by MRL/lpr mice. The serum levels of both RF isotypes increase in an age-related manner through 5–6 months of age (Andrews *et al.*, 1978; Hang *et al.*, 1982; Gilkeson *et al.*, 1989). However it is not clear whether there is a relationship between RF levels and the incidence or severity of joint disease. Han *et al.* (1982) found a positive correlation between the presence of IgM RF and arthritis in animals 3–6 months of age. In contrast, Gilkeson and col-leagues (1989) found both IgM RF and histologic evidence of arthropathy in all seven-month-old male mice examined, yet were unable to demonstrate a relationship between the RF titre and severity of arthritis. These data suggest that both RF production and articular pathology are common in MRL/lpr mice, but only loosely associated from a mechanistic standpoint. Interestingly, other studies reviewed by Koopman and Gay (1988) show that MRL/lpr RF share characteristics with those produced in patients with RA including variable subclass binding specificity as well as crossreactivity with heterologous IgG and with antigens other than IgG.

Autoantibodies to collagen type II are readily detectable in the sera of MRL/lpr mice. However, it is doubtful that these antibodies play a role in the induction of the arthritic process since they appear after the onset of joint disease and in low titres compared to those detected in mice with collagen arthritis (Phadke *et al.*, 1984;

Tarkowski *et al.*, 1986; Gay *et al.*, 1987). Moreover, MRL/lpr mice are resistant to the induction of arthritis with heterologous collagen type II (Boissier *et al.*, 1989).

Although the specific mechanisms causing the variable arthropathy in MRL/lpr mice have not been fully elucidated, significant new insights relating to the *lpr* mutation and its interaction with the MRL genetic background are emerging. For example, recent molecular studies have localized this mutation to the Fas gene which encodes a surface protein that mediates apoptosis (Watanabe-Fukunaga *et al.*, 1992). More recently, Wu *et al.* (1993) and Chu and coworkers (1993) have independently discovered that the molecular basis of the *lpr* mutation is the insertion of the retroviral transposon *ETn* into the second intron of the Fas gene. On another level, it is of interest that the *lpr* mutation alone is not arthritogenic in other genetic backgrounds (Gilkeson *et al.*, 1989), and that articular pathology is rare in MRL/n mice (O'Sullivan *et al.*, 1992). Thus, either the MRL background is permissive for the induction of arthritis by the lpr gene, or the *lpr* gene accelerates a weak predisposition for joint disease carried in the MRL genome.

It is also important to discuss the potential role of T cells in the expression of arthritis in MRL/lpr mice. Gay and colleagues found that anti-CD4 immunotherapy reduced the severity of arthritis significantly, but failed to prevent synovial hyperplasia in MRL/lpr mice, suggesting that expression of this pathological phenomenon is not exclusively T-cell dependent (Gay, Reiter and Riethmüller, unpublished observation) and that two cellular mechanisms may explain joint destruction (Gay *et al.*, 1993). In related studies O'Sullivan and colleagues observed abrogation of arthritis in this strain with anti-CD4 treatment (O'Sullivan, Vogelweid, Besch-Wiliford and Walker, unpublished observation) as did Mountz *et al.* (1987) with the use of cyclosporin A. These latter observations may seem unexpected in light of the dearth of T-cell infiltrates in the joints of MRL/lpr mice with proliferative synovitis. Alternative explanations are that only a small number of resident synovial T cells are required to provide the necessary help to drive the proliferative response, or that the influence of T-cells on joint disease is due to soluble mediators elaborated at a distance from target synovial cells.

Recently, our laboratory has been involved in studies designed to investigate the cellular basis of cartilage and bone destruction in these mice. We previously showed by ultrastructural studies that the hyperplastic synovium consisted of both macrophage-like (type A) and fibroblast-like (type B) synoviocytes (Tanaka *et al.*, 1988), and that cartilage destruction appeared to be mediated by the outgrowth of proliferating synovial fibroblast-like cells (O'Sullivan *et al.*, 1992). Since typical erosions of articular structures occurred in areas with these proliferative cells, we examined the role of the proliferation-associated oncogenes *ras* and *myc* as well as the expression of collagenolytic and cysteine proteinases in synovial cells of MRL/lpr mice. Significant levels of the cysteine proteinase cathepsin L, which is the major *ras*-induced protein in *ras*-transformed NIH 3T3 cells, were detected in the proliferating synovial lining cells indicating that this collagen-degrading proteinase contributes to the destruction of cartilage (Trabandt *et al.*, 1990). Related studies also revealed that elevated levels of the *c-fos* gene could be detected in collagenase-expressing cells (Trabandt *et al.*, 1992). It is of interest that collagenase was detected not only at the site of synovial attachment to cartilage and expressed in the proliferating synovial cells, but also in chondrocytes at the initial sites of cartilage erosion in affected MRL/lpr joints.

Although certain cytopathological features common to the articular pathology in MRL/lpr mice and rheumatoid synovium have led to more extensive investigations of the molecular and cellular mechanisms involved in the pathogenesis of RA (Gay and Gay, 1989), it has been widely observed that the severity of the arthropathy in MRL/lpr has been diminished over time. Based on the possibility that unintentional breeding influences are responsible, efforts have been undertaken using selective mating programmes to ensure that this model remains intact for future studies.

NZB/KN MOUSE

Inbred NZB mice were originally derived from an unknown background in the 1950s. These mice manifest autoimmune abnormalities such as haemolytic anaemia and mild glomerulonephritis, but do not develop significant joint disease. This strain is perhaps most well known for the florid SLE-like diathesis that develops in females of the F1 generation resulting from an (NZB × NZW) mating (Theofilopoulos and Dixon, 1981, 1985). In 1991, Nakamura et al., described the high incidence of a spontaneous, progressive polyarthropathy in an NZB substrain designated NZB/KN.

CLINICOPATHOLOGICAL CHARACTERISTICS OF JOINT DISEASE

NZB/KN males developed clinically evident hindlimb swelling and gait disturbance by 4 months of age (Nakamura et al., 1991). However radiographic changes were evident from the age of 2 months and were progressive. The earliest abnormalities included bone resorption and joint space narrowing in the distal portions of the fore- and hindpaws. The lesions increased in number and severity over time, with bony ankylosis appearing by 6 months of age. Caudal vertebrae exhibited arthritic changes by 6 months of age. Female NZB/KN and males of the parent NZB strain were not affected (Nakamura et al., 1991).

Histopathological changes also first appeared at 2 months of age. The lesion was characterized by synovial cell hypertrophy and proliferation, subsynovial infiltration by lymphocytes, monocytes and plasma cells, and erosion of articular cartilage and bone. Tendinitis and proliferation of chondrocytes in a periarticular distribution were also noted. (Nakamura et al., 1991; Nakagawa et al., 1993). Joint pathology became more severe with time, progressing to pannus formation and bony ankylosis by the age of 6 months; and to osteonecrosis, new bone formation and periarticular soft tissue ossification by 14 months (Nakamura et al., 1991).

ASSOCIATED IMMUNOPATHOLOGIC FINDINGS

RFs were readily detected in the sera of male NZB/KN mice, but did not appear to be associated with the arthritic lesions since they were also present in non-arthritic female NZB/KN and aged BALB/c mice. Anti-collagen type II antibodies were also judged not to be useful as a marker for joint disease since significant titres were found in roughly half of arthritic male NZB/KN, as well as in female NZB/KN and males from the parental NZB strain (Nakamura et al., 1991).

The etiology of spontaneous male-associated NZB/KN arthritis is not clear. However joint disease was successfully induced in female NZB/KN mice injected with spleen cells from 4- to 6-month-old males (Nakamura *et al.*, 1991), indicating that male hormonal influences are not necessary to sustain the pathological process once it has been established. Arthritis could also be transferred to male H-2-identical BALB/c mice with unpurified spleen cells but not with T-cell depleted spleen cells (Nakamura *et al.*, 1991). Joint disease could be prevented in male NZB/KN mice the lethal irradiation followed by allogeneic bone marrow transplantation (Nakagawa *et al.*, 1993). These observations suggest that T cells play a pivotal role in the pathogenesis of the articular in this substrain.

DBA/1 MOUSE

Like NZB mice, the DBA/1 inbred strain was derived more than 30 years ago. These mice are known to develop erythrocytosis and are highly susceptible to collagen- and pristane-induced arthritis, but significant immunological abnormalities have not been observed (Altman and Katz, 1979). Nordling and colleagues (1992) recently described the occurrence of spontaneous polyarthritis in aged, male DBA/1 mice.

CLINICOPATHOLOGICAL CHARACTERISTICS OF JOINT DISEASE

Visible swelling and erythema occurred in the hindlimbs of 60–80% of male DBA/1 mice beginning at 4–5 months of age. Proximal interphalangeal, distal interphalangeal and metetarsophalangeal joints were most frequently affected, although ankles and tarsal joint involvement was also seen. The arthritis was intermittent and migratory, developing in an asymmetric fashion. Progression usually ceased 2–3 months after the onset of clinical arthritis (Nordling *et al.*, 1992; Holmdahl *et al.*, 1992).

Early histopathological features of the arthritis were infiltration of the synovium with macrophages and neutrophils, synovial cell proliferation, and adherence of proliferating synovium to articular cartilage. A chronic mononuclear infiltrate persisted in later stages, with formation of pannus, and marked bone and cartilage erosion. Interestingly, the mononuclear infiltrate was devoid of T cells and exhibited very low levels of Ia expression (Nordling *et al.*, 1992; Holmdahl *et al.*, 1992). Compare this with the c-fos transgenic mouse described by Harris in Chapter 27, this volume.

ASSOCIATED IMMUNOPATHOLOGICAL FINDINGS

Given the absence of systemic immunological abnormalities in DBA/1 mice and the noticeable lack of local immune activation in the joint tissue of arthritic joints, it is not surprising tha anti-collagen type II antibodies were not present in the sera of arthritic DBA/1 mice (Holmdahl *et al.*, 1992). However, disease expression is clearly sex-associated. Castration of 11–14 week-old male DBA/1 mice completely prevented the development of arthritis, while testosterone replacement in castrated animals restored the high incidence of joint disease (Holmdahl *et al.*, 1992). Other hormonal and behavioural factors are apparently involved in disease expression, since mice must be housed at a density of three male mice per cage or greater for the arthritis to appear. By introducing systemic autoimmunity via a cross with male or female BXSB mice, the incidence and severity of joint disease in the F1 generation was markedly increased (Holmdahl *et al.*, 1992).

Nordling *et al.* (1992) also demonstrated that the joint disease in their mice was not due to a spontaneous mutation in their breeding colony. New colonies were established with breeding stock obtained from two separate suppliers. Male DBA/1 mice in the newly established colonies developed arthritis at approximately the same rate and age as observed in the original colony.

BIOZZI (H₁) MOUSE

Another example of a spontaneous male-associated arthropathy in inbred mice is that which occurs in the high antibody responder line of Biozzi's selection I (Biozzi (H₁). This strain is the result of a selective breeding programme in Swiss mice for high or low antibody responses to heterologous erythrocytes and a variety of other unrelated antigens (Biozzi *et al.*, 1979). A detailed description of late-occurring arthritis in male Biozzi (H₁) mice has recently been published (Bouvet *et al.*, 1990).

CLINICOPATHOLOGICAL CHARACTERISTICS OF JOINT DISEASE

Twenty eight per cent of 1-year-old male Biozzi (H₁) mice exhibited discrete swelling of one or more digits of the fore- and hindpaws. The joint involvement was symmetric and became progressively more severe over a period of months. Gait was not affected. Radiographs revealed rare instances of bone erosion, joint space narrowing and ossification of periarticular soft tissues (Bouvet *et al.*, 1990).

The histopathological characteristics of the arthritic lesion were that of a mixed inflammatory infiltrate. Synovial proliferation was noted, along with infiltrates containing neutrophils and lymphocytes. Tenosynovitis and pannus associated with erosive changes were also observed (Bouvet *et al.*, 1990).

ASSOCIATED IMMUNOPATHOLOGICAL FINDINGS

Although Biozzi (H₁) mice are susceptible to collagen-induced arthritis, no correlation between autoantibody levels and the presence or severity of arthritis was noted. Anti-type II collagen antibody and RF titres were low, and antinuclear and anti-DNA antibodies were detected in only a few animals (Bouvet *et al.*, 1990).

PROGRESSIVE ANKYLOSIS (*ank/ank*) MOUSE

Sweet and Green (1981) first described the *ank* mutation in mice from a mixed C3HeB/FeJ and C57B1/6J-Aʷ-J background. It caused severe functional deficits that were assumed to be due to rapidly progressive non-inflammatory ankylosis of peripheral and axial joints. However, subsequent detailed histological studies have shown that these animals suffer from a far more remarkable disease process than was first appreciated, and one that bears considerable resemblance to human spondyloarthropathies (SNA).

CLINICOPATHOLOGICAL CHARACTERISTICS OF JOINT DISEASE

Murine progressive ankylosis (MPA) is caused by the autosomal recessive *ank* mutation. The incidence of the condition is 100% in homozygous individuals, while heterozygotes are unaffected. Males and females are affected equally (Sweet and Green, 1981; Hakim *et al.*, 1984). Peripheral joint involvement becomes apparent at an early age and is rapidly progressive. The arthritis reliably follows a distal-to-proximal pattern of progression beginning with the interphalangeal joints, and is symmetrical. The forepaws are first affected at 2–3 weeks of age, the hindlimbs by 4–7 weeks. Swelling and erythema of affected joints may occur, but are not prominent clinical features.

Functional impairment is rapidly progressive. Mice first exhibit difficulty grasping with the forepaws at 3–4 weeks of age. Complete rigidity of the forelimbs and hindlimbs occurs by 8–12 weeks of age, causing a markedly abnormal gait. Elbows, shoulders and axial spine are also severely affected; the hips are generally spared (Hakim *et al.*, 1984; Mahowald *et al.*, 1988).

The histopathological progression of the arthritis parallels the clinical course of the disease. The earliest lesions develop in the interphalangeal and metacarpophalangeal joints of the forepaws by the age of 3 weeks (Hakim *et al.*, 1984; Mahowald *et al.*, 1989). Synovial cells proliferate and form confluent layers attached to the surface of articular cartilage. Within 2–3 days, an inflammatory infiltrate consisting of mononuclear cells and a few neutrophils develops and erosions of cartilage and bone appear. During the following 7–10 days the synovitis intensifies and a remarkable form of chondroid metaplasia develops in which cartilaginous projections arise from the periosteum subjacent to the junction of articular cartilage and subchondral bone on either side of the joint. Opposing cartilaginous projections eventually coalesce and undergo enchondral ossification, resulting in the formation of large bridging osteophytes. Over the ensuing 6–8 weeks the destructive lesion subsides and is replaced by a reparative phase that leads to the development of fibrous and bony ankylosis of opposing articular surfaces. A similar sequence of events occurs in the hindpaws and more proximal joints of upper and lower extremities over the next few weeks. Tenosynovitis and enthesitis with similar inflammatory and proliferative microscopic characteristics are commonly observed (Hakim *et al.*, 1984; Mahowald *et al.*, 1989).

Abnormalities are observed in the axial skeleton by the age of 3 months. The sacroiliac joints contain proliferative inflammatory tissue and are eroded and fibrosed. The intervetebral discs are replaced by chondroid metaplasia with enchondral ossification and synchondroses, and bony syndesmophytes are present. The costovertebral joints are similarly affected (Mahowald *et al.*, 1989). Crystalline hydroxyapatite (basic calcium phosphate) deposits are frequently found in synovial fluid and periarticular soft tissue of ank/ank mice (Hakim *et al.*, 1984). However, detailed light and electron microscopic studies of the early lesions of MPA show that proliferative synovitis is well established prior to the appearance of hydroxyapatite crystals (Mahowald *et al.*, 1989).

MPA is associated with singular radiographic abnormalities. Symmetric erosions, joint space narrowing and joint capsule calcification affect the peripheral joints from 4 weeks of age in a proximal-to-distal progression. By the age of 3–4 months bony ankylosis becomes a prominent feature. Squaring of vertebral bodies is apparent by 2 months of age. After 3 months apophyseal joints fuse and syndesmophyte formation produces a typical 'bamboo spine' appearance. The costosternal joints are also affected by syndesmophyte formation and the sacroiliac joints appear eroded and exhibit pseudowidening by six months of age (Mahowald *et al.*, 1988).

ASSOCIATED IMMUNOPATHOLOGICAL FINDINGS

Extra-articular manifestations are scarce. Balanitis and priapism are noted in males over the age of 10 weeks, and scaling skin lesions on the plantar aspect of the feet occur in mice of both sexes (Mahowald *et al.*, 1988). Mice with MPA appear to be intact immunologically, although the responsiveness of their spleen cells to T-cell mitogens is diminished in comparison to non-arthritic littermates. RFs are not detected in the sera of MPA mice (Krug *et al.*. 1989).

Although the peripheral arthritis in MPA resembles the more severe manifestations of psoriatic arthritis and Reiter's disease, and the axial disease is reminiscent of ankylosing spondylitis, there are important differences from human SNA. The etiology of MPA is strictly genetic, unlike the SNA in which environmental influences play an important role. Moreover, MPA lacks many of the extra-articular manifestations of SNA such as uveitis, pulmonary or endocardial fibrosis, aortic incompetence or amyloidosis (Mahowald *et al.*, 1989). This model may be relevant to the late stages of RA, when bony fibrous ankylosis become prominent components of the articular pathology (Fassbender, 1975).

OTHER ANIMAL MODELS

The most common etiologies of polyarthritis in dogs are systemic lupus erythematosus, infection and degenerative joint disease. However, some of these animals clearly meet strict criteria for the diagnosis of human RA (Liu *et al.*, 1969; Newton *et al.*, 1976; Pederson *et al.*, 1976). The clinical characteristics of canine RA include lameness, pyrexia, anorexia, joint swelling and depression. Joint involvement tends to be bilateral and symmetric. Radiographic abnormalities, including subchondral erosions, closely resemble those seen in the human form of the disease. Early diagnosis is difficult, and the clinical course progressive. No age, sex or breed predilections have been noted (Newton *et al.*, 1976). The macro- and microscopic abnormalities observed in synovial biopsies from patients with RA (Zvaifler, 1973) are generally recapitulated in affected dogs, the main differences being more prominent polymorphonuclear neutrophil infiltration and fewer subsynovial lymphocytic follicles in the latter (Newton *et al.*, 1976; Schumacher *et al.*, 1980). RFs are readily demonstrated in sera and synovial fluids from dogs with RA when canine IgG is used as the target for detection of antiglobulin activity (Newton *et al.*, 1976; Schumacher *et al.*, 1980; Carter *et al.*, 1989), but rheumatoid nodules have not been demonstrated clinically or microscopically (Newton *et al.*, 1976). Interestingly, electron microscopic studies of canine rheumatoid synovium reveal the presence of tubuloreticular structures reminiscent of those seen in tissues of SLE patients and crystalline tubular arrays resembling those seen in viral illnesses (Schumacher *et al.*, 1980).

Spontaneous, seropositive, symmetrical hindlimb arthritis affecting one-third of inbred female and 10% of male 'Old English' laboratory rabbits was reported by Hanglow and colleagues in 1986. Microscopic examination of affected joints revealed a proliferative synovitis associated with a lymphoplasmacytic infiltrate. Significant titres of serum antibodies to *Pasturella multocida*, an organism known to cause respiratory infections in rabbits, were found to correlate with the severity of synovitis in females but not in affected males (Hanglow *et al.*, 1986). These observations suggest that microbial infection and hormonal influences may be involved in the pathogenesis of spontaneous arthritis in this breed of rabbits.

Inbred C57BL/6J mice carrying the autosomal recessive motheaten (*me/me*) and viable motheaten (*me^v/me^v*) mutations of the haematopoietic cell protein–tyrosine phosphatase gene (Schultz *et al.*, 1993) exhibit profound immune dysregulation with features of severe immunodeficiency and autoimmunity (Green and Schultz, 1975; Schultz *et al.*, 1984; Schultz, 1988). Occasional allusions to the presence of arthritis in these short-lived mice have appeared in the literature. However detailed histomorphological studies do not support the existence of this pathological entity (Green and Schultz, 1975; Schultz *et al.*, 1984). The confusion has arisen from the fact that motheaten and viable motheaten mice develop soft tissue inflammation and necrosis of their distal extremities which involves adjacent joints by direct extension (L. Schultz, pers. commun.).

SUMMARY AND CONCLUSIONS

The search for, and use of, animal models of RA has been carried on for several decades. Although much valuable information has been obtained from these models, each has its limitations. Even canine RA, which appears to be closely related to human disease is unsatisfactory because it is extremely difficult to diagnose in its early stages and is too rare to be economical as a laboratory tool. Perhaps the most realistic approach to the use of spontaneous models is to acknowledge their limitations, glean the relevant data from each model and integrate them into the larger scheme of immune injury and tissue repair.

The NZB/KN appears to have potential as a model because, like RA, the arthropathy appears on a background of systemic autoimmunity and is easily detected both clinically and radiographically. Its obvious limitation is its strong association with the male sex, unlike RA, which affects females slightly more frequently than males.

Conversely, the study of the arthropathy of the DBA/1 mice may be limited by the very late age of onset, and the fact that it differs from RA in the total lack of any apparent systemic immune abnormalities. MPA appears to be better suited as a model for SNA, but may have relevance to mechanisms involved in the response of bone and cartilage to immune injury that occurs in the late stages of RA. The experience with the Biozzi strain is too limited for substantial criticism at this point.

Even though a variable spectrum of articular pathology is manifested in the MRL/lpr model, important insights have been derived from histological and immunopathological investigations. Several studies in these mice support the concept that synovial lining cells may proliferate and cause the degradation of articular bone and cartilage without the participation of large numbers of inflammatory cells. Morphological similarities between the transformed-appearing synovial cells associated with cartilage and bone destruction in RA and those observed in arthritic MRL/lpr mice led us to initiate studies of tissue and joint fluid from patients and mice which reveal potential associations between proto-oncogene expression, cell proliferation, induction of matrix-

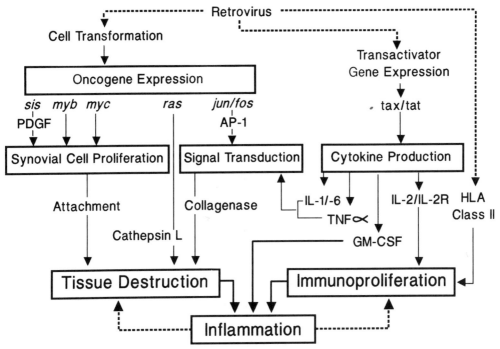

Figure 2. Hypothesis for the aetiopathogenesis of RA. Reproduced with permission from Gay *et al.* (1993).

degrading enzymes and identification of retrovirus-like particles. Based on these findings, we are pursuing the hypothesis that a hitherto unknown HTLV-related retrovirus is involved in the pathogenesis of RA (Fig. 2) (Gay and Gay, 1989; Gay *et al.*, 1993).

In conclusion, the contributions of spontaneous animal arthritis studies toward the elucidation of the etiology and pathogenesis of RA are substantial in spite of the limitations inherent to the use of models having incomplete identity with the prototypic disease. The recent success in deciphering the molecular basis of the *lpr* mutation, the growing body of data on retroviruses, and the discovery of several new models bode well for the continued utility of these tools in the future.

REFERENCES

Alexander EL, Murphy ED, Roths JB & Alexander GE (1983) Congenic autoimmune murine models of central nervous system disease in connective tissue disorders. *Ann Neurol* **14**: 242–248.

Altman PL & Katz DD (1979). In *Inbred and Genetically Defined Strains of Laboratory Animals*, pp. 16–29. Bethesda: Federation of American Societies for Experimental Biology.

Andrews BS, Eisenberg RA, Argyrios N, Theofilopoulos SI, Wilson CB, McConahey PJ et al. (1978) Spontaneous murine lupus-like syndromes: Clinical and immunopathological manifestations in several strains. *J Exp Med*: 1198–1215.

Biozzi G, Muton D, Sant'Anna OA, Passos HC, Gennari M, Reis MH et al. (1979) Genetics of immuno-responsiveness to natural antigens in the mouse. *Curr Top Microbiol Immunol* **85**: 31–98.

Boissier M-C, Texier B, Carlioz A & Fournier C (1989) Polyarthritis in MRL/lpr mice: mouse type II collagen is antigenic but not arthritogenic. *Autoimmunity* **4**: 31–41.

Bouvet J-P, Couderc J, Bouthillier Y, Franc B, Ducailar A & Mouton D (1990) Spontaneous rheumatoid-like arthritis in a line of mice sensitive to collagen-induced arthritis. *Arthritis Rheum* **33**: 1716–1722.

Carter SD, Bell SC, Bari ASM, & Bennett D (1989) Immune complexes and rheumatoid factors in canine arthritides. *Ann Rheum Dis* **48**: 986–1991.

Chu J-L, Drappa J, Parnassa A & Elkon KB (1993) The defect in Fas mRNA expression in MRL/lpr mice is associated with insertion of the retrotransposon. *J Exp Med* **178**: 723–730.

Edwards JCW, Cooke A, Moore AR, Collins C, Hay F & Willoughby DA (1986) Connective tissue abnormalities in MRL/1 mice. *Ann Rheum Dis* **45**: 512–518.

Fassbender HG (1975) In *Pathology of Rheumatic Diseases*, pp. 79–210. Berlin: Springer-Verlag.

Fassbender HG (1983) Histomorphologic basis of articular cartilage destruction in rheumatoid arthritis. *Collagen Rel Res* **3**: 141–155.

Gay S & Gay RE (1989) Cellular basis and oncogene expression of rheumatoid joint destruction. *Rheumatol Int* **9**: 105–113.

Gay S, O'Sullivan FX, Gay RE & Koopman WJ (1987) Humoral sensitivity to native collagen types I–VI in the arthritis of MRL-1 mice. *Clin Immunol Immunopathol* **45**: 63–69.

Gay S, Gay RE & Koopman WJ (1993) Molecular and cellular mechanisms of joint destruction in rheumatoid arthritis: two cellular mechanisms explain joint destruction. *Ann Rheum Dis* **52** (**supplement**): 39–47.

Gilkeson GS, Ruiz P, Grudier JP, Kurlander RJ & Pisetsky DS (1989) Genetic control of inflammatory arthritis in congenic 1pr mice. *Clin Immunol Immunopathol* **53**: 460–474.

Green MC & Shultz LD (1975) Motheaten, or immunodeficient mutant of the mouse: I. Genetics and pathology. *J Hered* **66**: 250–258.

Hakim FT, Cranley R, Brown KS, Eanes ED, Harne L & Oppenheim JJ (1984) Hereditary joint disorder in progressive ankylosis (ank/ank) mice. *Arthritis Rheum* **27**: 1411–1420.

Hang L, Theofilopoulous AN & Dixon FJ (1982) A spontaneous rheumatoid arthritis-like disease in MRL/1 mice. *J Exp Med* **155**: 1690–1701.

Hanglow AC, Welsh CJR, Conn P, Thomas DS & Coombs RRA (1986) Synovitis associated with serum IgM rheumatoid factor arising spontaneously in 'Old English' rabbits. *Ann Rheum Dis* **45**: 331–338.

Hoffman RW, Alspaugh MA, Waggie KS, Durham JB & Walker SE (1984) Sjögren's syndrome in MLR/1 and MRL/n mice. *Arthritis Rheum* **27**: 157–165.

Holmdahl R, Jansson L, Anderson N & Jonsson R (1992) Genetic, hormonal and behavioral influence on spontaneously developing arthritis in normal mice *Clin Exp Immunol* **88**: 467–472.

Koopman WJ & Gay S (1988) The MRL/lpr mouse. A model for the study of rheumatoid arthritis. *Scand J Rheum Suppl* **75**: 284–289.

Krug HE, Mahowald ML & Clark C (1989) Progressive ankylosis (ank/ank) in mice: an animal model of spondyloarthropathy. I. Clinical and radiographic findings. *Clin Exp Immunol* **78**: 97–101.

Lewis RM & Hathaway JE (1967) Canine systemic lupus erythematosus: presenting with symmetrical polyarthritis. *J Small Anim Pract* **8**: 273–284.

Lewis RM & Schwartz RS (1971) Canine systemic lupus erythematosus. *J Exp Med* **134**: 417–438.

Liu S, Suter PR, Fischer CA & Dorfman HD (1969) Rheumatoid arthritis in a dog. *J Am Vet Med Assoc.* **154**: 495–502.

Mahowald ML, Krug H & Taurog J (1988) Progressive ankylosis in mice: an animal model of spondyloarthropathy. *Arthritis Rheum* **31**: 1390–1399.

Mahowald ML, Krug H & Halverson P (1989) Progressive ankylosis (ank/ank) in mice: an animal model of spondyloarthropathy. II. Light and electron microscopic findings. *J Rheumatol* **16**: 60–66.

Morse HC, Davidson WF, Yetter RA, Murphy ED, Roths JB & Coffman RL (1982) Abnormalities induced by the mutant gene lpr: expression of a unique lymphocyte subset. *J Immunol* **129**: 2612–2615.

Mountz JD, Smith HR, Wilder RL, Reeves JP & Steinberg AD (1987) CS-A therapy in MRL-lpr mice: amelioration of immunopathology despite autoantibody production. *J Immunol* **138**: 157–163.

Murphy ED & Roths JB (1978) Autoimmunity and lymphoproliferation: induction by mutant gene lpr, and acceleration by a male associated factor in strain BXSB mice. In Rose NR, Bigazzi PE & Warner NL (eds) *Genetic Control of Autoimmune Disease*, pp 207–219. New York: Elsevier/North Holland.

Nakamura K, Kashiwazaki S, Takagishi K, Tsukamoto Y, Morohoshi Y, Nakano T et al. (1991) Spontaneous degenerative polyarthritis in male New Zealand Black/KN mice. *Arthritis Rheum* **34**: 171–179.

Nakagawa, T, Nagata, N, Hosaka N, Ogawa R, Nakamura K & Ikehara S (1993) Prevention of autoimmune inflammatory polyarthritis in male New Zealand Black/KN mice by transplantation of bone marrow cells plus bone (stromal cells). *Arthritis Rheum* **36**: 263–268.

Newton CD, Lipowitz AJ, Halliwell RE, Allen HL, Biery DN & Schumacher HR (1976) Rheumatoid arthritis in dogs. *J Am Vet Med Assoc* **168**: 113–121.

Nordling C, Karlsson-Parra A, Jansson J, Holmdahl R & Klareskog L (1992) Characterization of a spontaneously occurring arthritis in male DBA/1 mice. *Arthritis Rheum* **35**: 717–722.

Nordling C, Kleinau S & Klareskog L (1992) Down-regulation of a spontaneous arthritis in male DBA/1 mice after administration of monoclonal anti-idiotypic antibodies to a cross-reactive idiotype on anti-collagen antibodies. *Immunology* **77**: 144–146.

O'Sullivan FX, Fassbender H-G, Gay S & Koopman WJ (1985) Etiopathogenesis of the rheumatoid arthritis-like disease in MRL/1 mice. I. Histomorphologic basis of joint destruction. *Arthritis Rheum* **28**: 529–536.

O'Sullivan FX, Koopman WJ & Gay S (1992) Scanning electron microscopic evaluation of the arthritis in MRL/lpr mice, *Rheumatol Int* **12**: 115–120.

Pataki A & Rordorf-Adam C (1985) Polyarthritis in MRL1pr/1pr mice. *Rheumatol Int* **5**: 113–120.

Pederson NC, Pool RC, Castles JJ, Weisner K (1976) Non-infectious canine arthritis: rheumatoid arthritis. *J Am Vet Med Assoc* **169**: 295–303.

Phadke K, Fouts R, Parrish J & Baker RS (1984) Autoreactivity to collagen in a murine lupus model. *Arthritis Rheum* **27**: 313–319.

Schumacher R, Newton C & Halliwell REW (1980) Synovial pathologic changes in spontaneous canine rheumatoid-like arthritis. *Arthritis Rheum* **4**: 412–423.

Schultz LD (1988) Pleiotropic effects of deleterious alleles at the 'Motheaten' locus. *Curr Top Microbiol Immunol* **137**: 216–222.

Schultz LD, Coman DR, Bailey CL, Beamer WG & Sidman CL (1984) 'Viable motheaten', a new allele at the motheaten locus. *Am J Pathol* **116**: 179–192.

Schultz LD, Schweitzer PA, Rajan TV, Yi T, Ihle JN, Matthews RJ et al. (1993) Mutations at the murine motheaten locus are within the haematopoietic cell protein-tyrosine phosphatase (Hcph) gene. *Cell* **73**: 1445–1454.

Sweet HO & Green MC (1981) Progressive ankylosis, a new skeletal mutation in the mouse. *J Hered* **72**: 87–93.

Tanaka A, O'Sullivan FX, Koopman WJ & Gay S (1988) Etiopathogenesis of rheumatoid arthritis-like disease in MRL/1 mice: II. Ultrastructural basis of joint desruction. *J Rheumatol* **15**: 10–16.

Tarkowski A, Holmdahl R, Rubin K, Klareskog L, Nilsson LA & Gunnarsson K (1986) Patterns of autoreactivity to collagen type II in autoimmune MRL/1 mice. *Clin Exp Immunol* **63**: 441–449.

Tarkowski A, Jonsson R, Holmdahl R & Klareskog L (1987) Immunohistochemical characterization of synovial cells in arthritic MRL-lpr/lpr mice. *Arthritis Rheum* **30**: 75–82.

Theofilopoulos AN & Dixon FJ (1981) Etiopathogenesis of murine SLE. *Immunol Rev* **55**: 179–216.

Theofilopoulos AN & Dixon FJ (1985) Murine models of systemic lupus erythematosus. *Adv Immunol* **37**: 269–390.

Trabandt A, Aicher WK, Gay RE, Sukhatme VP, Nilson-Hamilton M & Hamilton RT (1990) Expression of the collagenolytic and ras-induced cysteine proteinase cathepsin L and proliferation-associated onco-genes in synovial cells of MRL/1 mice and patients with rheumatoid arthritis. *Matrix* **10**: 349–361.

Trabandt A, Gay RE, Birkedal-Hansen H & Gay S (1992) Expression of collagenase and potential transcriptional factors in the MRL/1 mouse arthropathy. *S. Arthritis Rheum* **21**: 246–251.

Vogelweid CM, Johnson GC, Besch-Wiliford CL, Basler J & Walker SE (1991) Inflammatory central nervous system disease in lupus-prone MRL/lpr mice: comparative histologic amd immunohistochemical findings. *J Neuroimmunol* **35**: 89–99.

Watanabe-Fukunaga R, Brannan CI, Copeland NG, Jenkins NA & Nagata S (1992) Lymphoproliferation disorder in mice explained by defects in Fas antigen that mediates apoptosis. *Nature (London)* **356**: 314–317.

Wu J, Zhou T, He J & Mountz JD (1993) Autoimmune disease in mice due to integration of an endogenous retrovirus in an apoptosis gene. *J Exp Med* **178**: 461–468.

Zvaifler NL (1973) The immunopathology of joint inflammation in rheumatoid arthritis. *Adv Immunol* **13**: 265–337.

26 Cytokines in Models of Arthritis

Ivan G. Otterness, Fons A.J. van de Loo and Marcia L. Bliven

INTRODUCTION

The possibility that a cytokine may play an important role in arthritis requires the fulfilment of several criteria: first, to demonstrate that the cytokine can cause or contribute to the type of pathology observed in arthritis; second, to demonstrate that there is sufficient cytokine present to cause the postulated effects; and third, to demonstrate that agents which selectively block the action of the cytokine can inhibit arthritis in man.

Pettipher *et al.* (1986) first injected IL-1 into the rabbit knee joint and demonstrated proteoglycan loss and infiltration of inflammatory cells. Others have obtained similar results in the rabbit (Dingle *et al.*, 1987; Arner *et al.*, 1989, 1994; Feige *et al.*, 1990; O'Byrne *et al.*, 1990; McDonnell *et al.*, 1992), mouse (van de Loo and van den Berg, 1990), rat (Gilman *et al.*, 1986; Chandrasekhar *et al.*, 1990, 1992) and hamster (Otterness *et al.*, 1994a). It is the ability of cytokines IL-1, TNF and IL-8 to induce an arthritis or to potentiate an arthritis in predisposed animals that is the focus of this discussion.

GENERAL COMMENTS ON CYTOKINE USE *IN VIVO*

Many investigators have sought to induce an arthritis in animals with IL-1, TNF or IL-8. Most studies have been carried out using human cytokines. Thus when the human cytokine is not fully active in all species, the effects of the cytokine will be underestimated in animal studies. Yet even with IL-1 where activities appear to cross between species, it is clear that the effect of the cytokine depends not only on the amount given, but on the route and timing of its administration, and the state of activation of the animal. Thus IL-1 administered into the joint may induce an arthritis (Pettipher *et al.*, 1986) whereas even much larger amounts of IL-1 given systemically will not cause arthritis in normal animals (Otterness *et al.*, 1988). Intra-articular injections of IL-1 may also diminish a subsequent antigen-induced arthritis (Jacobs *et al.*, 1988) or potentiate it (Stimpson *et al.*, 1988a) depending on the antigen, route and timing. IL-1 given systemically during disease induction (Hom *et al.*, 1988) may potentiate an arthritis and given after disease induction may cause a flare-up of disease (van de Loo *et al.*, 1992). Thus as with many biological processes, individual responses to a cytokine are best rationalized only after they have been examined in their depth and variety. Moreover, cytokines normally do not act in isolation. Thus a description of the effect of a cytokine administered alone may fail to demonstrate the potential richness of actions that can occur when the cytokine acts in concert with other mediators.

Mechanisms and Models in Rheumatoid Arthritis
ISBN 0–12–340440–1

Although this review focuses primarily on intra-articular (i.a.) IL-1, TNF and IL-8, it is important to note that many other biologically active materials have been administered i.a., for example, transforming growth factor β (TGFβ) (Elford *et al.*, 1992), C5a (Stimpson *et al.*, 1988b), and platelet derived growth factor (PDGF) (Stimpson *et al.*, 1990). Some mediators such as TGFβ can induce an arthritis. Others such as C5a induce only a transient influx of polymorphonuclear leukocytes PMNs.

DISTRIBUTION AND CLEARANCE OF CYTOKINES

The effects of chronic administration of cytokine is best underpinned by an understanding of the actual cytokine exposure and distribution. The clearance rate or half-life of a protein usually depends on its physicochemical properties (molecular size, glycosylation, isoelectric point, and hydrophobic/hydrophylic properties), but other effects such as receptor binding may dramatically affect clearance. Lisi *et al.* (1987) injected 100 μg of human (hu) IL-1β intraperitoneally in the mouse and obtained peak plasma levels of *c.* 200 ng/ml 35 min later. A terminal half-life of 24 min can be estimated from their data. Extrapolating back to time zero, it appears that less than 0.5% of the injected IL-1 reached the circulation.

Detailed pharmacokinetic studies have been carried out after i.v. administration. In most studies, clearance of IL-1, radiolabelled according to the method of Bolton and Hunter, was investigated. Although receptor-binding capacity remains unchanged after labelling, Dower *et al.* (1985) found that only 5% of the starting IL-1 was biologically active. Typically, two clearance rates are found: the first, a distribution phase, is *c.* 3 min in rats (Klapproth *et al.*, 1989; Reimers *et al.*, 1991) and 2–10 min in mice (Newton *et al.*, 1988; Banks *et al.*, 1992), and the second rate, an elimination phase, is 14 min (Kudo *et al.*, 1990), 40 min (Reimers *et al.*, 1991), or 240 min (Klapproth *et al.*, 1989), as determined by three different groups using huIL-1β in the rat, and 30–50 min for murine (mu) IL-1α and IL-1β given to the mouse (Banks *et al.*, 1992). Reimers *et al.* (1991) examined the fraction of the circulating iodinated huIL-1β in the plasma that still retained native size (17 kDa). One minute after injection approximately 76% of the IL-1 was of the correct molecular weight. At 2 h, only 10% of the dose originally administered was of correct molecular weight; the majority of radiolabel was in low molecular weight fractions indicating that the IL-1 had been fragmented. The volume of distribution calculated for the IL-1 distribution phase was found to be *c.* 100 ml/kg, typical for substances that distribute in the plasma volume. An apparent concentration of 3.3 ng/ml of IL-1 can be calculated from their data as being available for clearance after the distribution phase. This compares to the extrapolated time 0 concentration of 38 ng/ml; that is, more than 90% of the IL-1 is removed from the circulation during the distribution phase. One possible explanation is that until the concentration falls below the Kd of the receptor, that is 3×10^{-10} M, nearly all the IL-1 is rapidly receptor-bound and removed from the circulation. Organ distribution revealed localization of IL-1 to the liver and kidney, possibly related to hepatic metabolism and excretion of the iodine radiolabel. The nature of the unbound IL-1 can only be speculated on. The IL-1 could be a biologically inactive isomorph that cannot bind to the IL-1 receptor, or it is possible that IL-1 receptors are saturated with IL-1 so the second phase of clearance measures clearance of excess unbound IL-1.

In either case, a half-life of 30–40 min would be expected for a moderate-sized unbound protein during the clearance phase.

Dingle *et al.* (1987) measured clearance of ^{131}I-labelled porcine IL-1α (catabolin) from rabbit knees after i.a. injection. A $t_{\frac{1}{2}}$ of 0.4 h was determined compared to a $t_{\frac{1}{2}} =$ 2.4 h for albumin. The lower molecular weight would be sufficient to account for the rapid clearance of IL-1 from the joint space. Although IL-1α and IL-1β differ considerably in isoelectric point (pI 5 and 7, respectively), neither form has a pI above 8.5 nor a partition coefficient of less than 0.2 indicating that IL-1 does not accumulate in the negatively charged cartilage as do cationic proteins.

Thus, after administration, IL-1 will bind to its receptors, and only that IL-1 in excess of receptor binding capacity or in an inactive form will be available for recirculation. That excess will have a half-life of 20–40 min whether injected into the joint or into the circulation.

Radiolabelled muTNF has also been administered to mice and detailed pharmacokinetics carried out. Naturally occurring TNF isoforms are all glycosylated proteins (Sherry *et al.*, 1990), and this could change their pharmacokinetics compared to the non-glycosylated recombinant TNF used in these studies. In contrast to earlier findings with IL-1, TNF shows non-linear pharmacokinetics. The mean half-life of lymphotoxin (TNFβ) and TNFα increases with increasing dose (Kawatsu *et al.*, 1990). Non-glycosylated TNFβ disappears much faster than TNF with N-type glycosylation. (Mature IL-1 is secreted in a non-glycosylated form although both IL-1 types possess potential glycosylation sites.) Beutler *et al.* (1985) found a half-life of 6 min for clearance of muTNF in mice. Although they detected radiolabel in the blood at later times, none of the radiolabel was associated with intact TNF. They examined the tissue distribution of the radiolabel in various organs both with and without large amounts of unlabeled TNF. Failure to compete labelled TNF with unlabelled TNF was taken as an indication of non-specific radiolabel uptake. The radiolabel in skin and lung were not competed away by unlabelled TNF, and could be decreased by pre-administration of iodine. Liver, kidney and spleen were the major sites of specific TNF localization. Ferraiolo *et al.* (1988) recorded a similar distribution with huTNF. The kidney and liver have both been shown to be major sites of accumulation and catabolism of huTNF, γ-interferon, and insulin suggesting this is a catabolic rather than a functional localization. Beutler *et al.* (1985) note that localization should not be equated with target organ activity. For example, adipose tissue fails to accumulate TNF efficiently, but is a major target of TNF activity.

So far, no pharmacokinetic studies have been carried out with IL-8, In spite of the doubtful utility for defining sites of action, a preliminary nuclear imaging study (Hay *et al.*, 1993) found that systemically administered radioactive IL-8 accumulates in sites of inflammation.

PATHOLOGY

PROTEOGLYCAN LOSS FROM ARTICULAR CARTILAGE

Compromise of articular cartilage is one of the hallmarks of arthritis. After i.a. IL-1, proteoglycan loss from articular cartilage is the most frequently reported result. With proteoglycan loss, articular cartilage loses its resiliency and resistance to compression.

This failure to dampen loading forces in the cartilage leads to increased collagen failure, chondrocyte death, and subchondral sclerosis. In patients with arthritis, articular cartilage loss is read by X-ray as joint space narrowing. Proteoglycan loss can be determined as increased proteoglycan fragments in synovial fluid, and this loss can be followed over time. In animal studies, the loss of proteoglycan can also be measured in the synovial fluid and, in addition, by direct analysis of the cartilage. Further coverage of cartilage breakdown in rheumatoid arthritis (RA) is found in Chapters 9 and 17, this volume.

Pettipher et al. (1986) administered 10 units of human recombinant huIL-1 intra-articularly to rabbits and measured loss of cartilage proteoglycan after 4, 24, and 72 h. (Retrospectively, it is difficult to determine how much IL-1 was present in 10 units. Roughly 100–300 pg would seem likely, but this is much less than most investigators have used and may explain the more transient duration of proteoglycan loss.) They found peak depletion of proteoglycan at 24 h and restoration of the loss by 72 h. Several controls were used to show that the effects were specific for IL-1. IL-2 did not cause depletion of proteoglycan, phenylglyoxal (which destroys the biological activity of IL-1) prevented the proteoglycan loss, and finally, polymyxin B, which inactivates LPS, had no effect on the activity. Dingle et al. (1979) injected a much larger amount of IL-1 protein when they examined the loss of proteoglycan by a partially purified preparation of catabolin (IL-1) and heat-inactivated catabolin at 7 days. Between 5 and 20 ng were required for greater than 60% loss of proteoglycan 2 days after i.a. injection. The femur was more easily depleted than the tibia. Arner et al. (1989) found maximum loss after 10 μg of huIL-1β/knee whereas at least 100 ng were required for significant loss of proteoglycans 3 days after IL-1β injection.

In the mouse, because of the small amounts of cartilage, van den Berg et al. (1982) have used another approach to determine proteoglycan loss. They prelabelled the proteoglycan with ^{35}S-SO$_4$ and then determined rates of loss. With this method, they have shown that muIL-1α and muIL-1β accelerate the loss of proteoglycan in a dose responsive manner both in vitro (van den Berg et al., 1988) and in vivo (van de Loo and van den Berg, 1990). Since the loss of prelabelled proteoglycan is measured, new proteoglycan synthesis does not enter into the loss rate, and a true half-life of proteoglycan can be calculated. IL-1 accelerates the rate of proteoglycan turnover from a half-life of 6.4 days for normal mouse articular cartilage to a half-life of 2.8 days.

McDonnell et al. (1992) measured the protoglycans in synovial fluid from the rabbit rather than directly measuring decreased proteoglycan in articular cartilage at sacrifice. They found normal proteoglycan amounts to be less than 20 μg in joint lavage. It was still unmeasurable after 1 and 2.5 ng/knee of huIL-1β. Peak release of proteoglycan into the synovial fluid (c. 200 μg) was found between 12 and 16 h after 200 ng IL-1β/knee, but release of proteoglycans was found at 12 h with as little as 5 ng. Pettipher et al. (1988, 1989) also examined release of protoglycans into the synovial fluid. After 25 ng of huIL-1α, they found peak concentrations of 160 μg of proteoglycan in synovial fluid at 8 h and 80–90 μg at 24 h. Keratan sulphate release was also measured and rose from c. 3 to 25 μg at 24 h.

Human TNF has also been shown in vitro to cause loss of proteoglycans from intact cartilage (Pratta et al., 1989; Campbell et al., 1990a). In vivo, Henderson and Pettipher (1989) failed to find proteoglycan loss from rabbit articular cartilage after i.a. huTNF. O'Byrne et al. (1990) failed to report whether TNF induced cartilage loss from rabbit articular cartilage using huTNF, Schnyder and Dinarello (1987) have found huTNF to be inactive on rabbit chondrocytes, but huTNF has been shown to be active on human chondrocytes (Bunning and Russell, 1989). These results suggest that failure to use homologous TNF may give an inaccurate picture of TNF activity because not all of TNFs activities cross between species. For example, it has been shown in the mouse that huTNF retains activities dependent on binding to the p55 TNF receptor, but not activities dependent on binding to the p75 TNF receptor (Tartaglia *et al.*, 1991). A similar problem may exist in the rabbit.

In mice i.a. injections of homologous murine recombinant TNFα up to 100 ng resulted in a moderate suppression (<30%) of the chondrocyte proteoglycan synthesis compared to the 50–60% suppression with muIL-1α. TNF did not induce joint swelling, as measured by uptake of ^{99m}Technetium pertechnetate, nor did it enhance proteoglycan breakdown (van den Berg *et al.*, manuscript in preparation).

Human IL-8 has been administered intra-articularly to rabbits. Endo *et al.* (1991) found that IL-8 (5 μg) did not cause loss of proteoglycan 24 h later as measured by analysis of the articular cartilage. By contrast, Forrest *et al.* (1992) found IL-8 (8 μg) increased proteoglycan levels in synovial fluid from 30 (saline control) to 160 μg/ml. They presented data strongly suggesting that the results could not be caused by contaminating endotoxin. The reasons for the difference in results between the two studies is not known. One can speculate that the elevation of proteoglycan in synovial fluid might be a more sensitive method of detection of changes in proteoglycan content. Elford and Cooper (1991) demonstrated that addition of IL-8 to cocultures of neutrophils with bovine nasal cartilage caused rapid neutrophil-mediated proteoglycan degradation.

CHANGES IN THE CHONDROCYTE

Intra-articular IL-1 leads directly to decreased proteoglycan synthesis. Van den Berg *et al.* (1988) and van de Loo and van den Berg (1990) showed in mouse articular cartilage *in vitro* and *in vivo* that muIL-1α caused a marked suppression of proteoglycan synthesis. Chandrasekhar *et al.* (1992) found similar results with huIL-1β in the rat. Arner *et al.* (1989) measured proteoglycan synthesis in the rabbit and found 100 ng of huIL-1β/knee were required for significant suppression. By two independent methods, Otterness *et al.* (unpublished observations) have calculated a synthetic rate of *c.* 0.11 μg/h/mg for proteoglycan synthesis in normal mouse articular cartilage. Administration of muIL-1α causes that rate to fall to about 40% of normal.

Topographical variations in chondrocyte responses towards *in vivo* IL-1 challenge were described (van Osch *et al.*, 1993). The inhibition of proteoglycan synthesis at the periphery of patellar cartilage was considerably smaller than the central part of the patella, femur and tibial plateau. After repeated IL-1 injections, prolonged suppression of chondrocyte proteoglycan synthesis in both the central part of the patella and the medial side of the femur was demonstrated by autoradiography (van Beuningen *et al.*, 1991). They hypothesized that there was an environmental influence (e.g. distance to the synovium) and loading conditions that predisposed certain areas in the joint. As circumstantial evidence, short-term immobilization of the knee joint in extension after IL-1 injection prevented IL-1 induced proteoglycan synthesis inhibition (van Lent *et al.*, 1991). Gender differences are also reported in the responses of cartilage to IL-1 exposure. Femoral head cartilage of the female rat was more sensitive to IL-1 induced proteoglycan synthesis suppression, but male cartilage was more vulnerable to IL-1 induced degradation. The net IL-1 effect on proteoglycan content was the same in both sexes (Da Silva *et al.*, 1992).

If there was no further exposure to IL-1, the rate of synthesis was suppressed for 2–3 days after IL-1 in young mice, whereas the synthetic defect was further prolonged in older animals (van Beuningen *et al.*, 1991; Page-Thomas *et al.*, 1991). Thereafter, enhanced synthesis of proteoglycans of normal hydrodynamic volume occurs. This lasts for several days. Breakdown of these newly synthesized proteoglycans during the recovery phase was decreased compared to normal cartilage (van de Loo *et al.*, 1994). In old mice, it took longer to return to normal synthetic level after the recovery phase. Page-Thomas *et al.* (1991) reported topographical differences in the proteoglycan synthetic recovery rate; that is, slower in patellar than in tibial cartilage of rabbits. Chandrasekhar *et al.* (1992) found impaired recovery of proteoglycan synthesis in tibial cartilage of rats after multiple injections of extremely high IL-1 doses.

CELL INFILTRATION

IL-1 and TNF both induce leukocyte infiltration into the synovial lining and the synovial fluid. This infiltration is due to induction of secondary chemotactic mediators as *in vitro* neither cytokine is directly chemotactic. Pettipher *et al.* (1986) lavaged the rabbit synovial cavity with 1 ml saline and measured leukocyte counts before and after administration of i.a. huIL-1β. At 24 h there was a dose response increase in the number of leukocytes in the lavage with increasing IL-1; however, peak cell numbers were found at 4 h. Interestingly lipopolysaccharide (LPS), at a concentration which resulted in similar leukocyte numbers at 24 h, failed to cause cartilage proteoglycan loss. If the same amount of inflammation was caused by zymosan, there was also no inhibition of proteoglycan synthesis (van de Loo *et al.*, 1991). Further, cartilage proteoglycan depletion by IL-1 was found to be normal in rabbits made neutropenic by nitrogen mustard (Pettipher *et al.*, 1989). These observations suggest that PMN do not contribute to IL-1 induced proteoglycan loss or synthesis inhibition.

Human TNF administered i.a. to rabbits also caused cell infiltration (Henderson and Pettipher, 1989; O'Byrne *et al.*, 1990). Whereas huIL-1α and β caused infiltration of approximately equal numbers of PMNs and monocytes, huTNF preferentially stimulated the infiltration of monocytes (Henderson and Pettipher, 1989). The combination of huIL-1β and huTNF showed a synergistic enhancement of both monocyte and PMN infiltration into the synovial fluid. Neither cytokine affected lymphocyte infiltration.

Human IL-8 administered into rabbit joints causes peak PMN infiltration (10^6 cells/joint) at 4 h and then a decrease until PMNs have largely disappeared by 24 h (Endo *et al.*, 1991). However, when examined at 8, 24 and 72 h, monocytes were present in significant numbers (10^4–10^5 cells/joint). IL-8 is not considered a chemotactic factor for monocytes (Yoshimura *et al.*, 1987) suggesting that other factors secondary to IL-8 are induced which lead to monocyte infiltration. As with other PMN chemotactic factors, intravenous injection of natural endothelium-derived IL-8 caused decreased PMN accumulation at the intradermal injection sites of chemoattractants and cytokines (Hechtman *et al.*, 1991). Cellular infiltration into rheumatoid joints is the subject of Chapter 11, this volume.

JOINT SWELLING

Studies in the rabbit failed to note joint swelling in spite of heavy infiltration of leukocytes (Pettipher *et al.*, 1986). Van de Loo and van den Berg (1990) found no swelling in the murine knee joint up to 10 ng IL-1α/knee (measured as uptake of ^{99m}Technetium). Stimpson *et al.* (1988a) measured ankle joint swelling to muIL-1α in the rat and found a measurable response at around 5 ng i.a. The swelling peaked around 6 h after IL-1 and had waned by 24 h. Chandrasekhar *et al.* (1990) compared the ankle and knee and found a good swelling response from 1 to 10 ng huIL-1β i.a. into the ankle whereas 5 to 10 μg were required for a similar swelling response in the knee. They summarized additional data suggesting that the ankle is more sensitive to swelling changes than the knee.

SECONDARY PRODUCTION OF OTHER MEDIATORS

IL-1 and TNF also lead to the synthesis of other cytokines such as GM-CSF (Fibbe *et al.*, 1986), IL-6 (McIntosh *et al.*, 1989; Libert *et al.*, 1990), and IL-8 (DeMaro and Kunkel, 1991). IL-6 levels in serum and bone marrow aspirates correlated with disease activity of collagen-type-II induced arthritis in mice and rats (Takai *et al.*, 1989; Hayashida *et al.*, 1992). Although their presence has been detected in human rheumatoid synovial fluid, measurements of these secondary mediators have not been reported after i.a. IL-1 and TNF administration in animals. Thus the induction of an array of secondary cytokines after i.a. IL-1 or TNF is suspected but not demonstrated. Recently, we have detected high levels of IL-6 in wash-outs of joint capsules 6 h after i.a. injections of murine recombinant IL-1α and TNFα in mice (van de Loo *et al.*, unpublished). On the other hand, IL-8 does not induce either IL-1 or IL-6 after i.a. administration in the rabbit (Endo *et al.*, 1991).

ENZYMES

MMP

The addition of IL-1 to synovial cells of cultured chondrocytes leads directly to the synthesis of collagenase (Mizel *et al.*, 1981; Lefebvre *et al.*, 1990), stromelysin (Hasty *et al.*, 1990), and gelatinase (Lefebvre *et al.*, 1991), enzymes believed to be directly involved in cartilage degradation (Woessner, 1991). McDonnell *et al.* (1992) injected huIL-1β into rabbit knee joints and examined the synovial fluid for the metalloproteinases stromelysin and collagenase. Synovial fluid stomelysin was increased with as little as 2.5 ng/knee of huIL-1β and stromelysin continued to increase up to the highest IL-1 dose (400 ng). Proteoglycans were elevated in parallel with stromelysin and the correlation was $r = 0.93$ between proteoglycan elevation and stromolysin elevation.

Van de Loo *et al.* (1994) examined the appearance of metalloproteinases in the mouse knee after i.a. muIL-1α. Both the 59-kDa (interstitial type I collagenase or proMMP3 (stromelysin)) and 97-kDa (proMMP9, neutrophil type IV collagenase) gelatinases were observed in normal synovial tissue. The 97-kDa gelatinase was preferentially enhanced after IL-1. The same gelatinases were also found in extracts of isolated patellar cartilage, although in smaller quantities, and their expression was increased after IL-1. In the proteoglycan recovery phase that followed, the gelatinase expression returned to basal levels.

Hutchinson *et al.* (1992) examined the expression of stromelysin after huIL-1β administration in the rabbit and found it within both cartilage and synovia. However, whether stromelysin has a role in the cleavage and loss of proteoglycan is in question. Based on sequence data, the IL-1 induced cleavage of core protein appears not to be at the stromelysin site (Fosang *et al.*, 1991), but three residues further toward the C-terminal end between the glutamic acid and alanine residues (Sandy *et al.*, 1991). Thus it has been speculated that an as yet undefined enzyme called aggrecanase is induced by IL-1 to cleave proteoglycan core protein. Stromelysin could still play a role in cartilage breakdown; that is, cleaving link protein (Nguyen *et al.*, 1989), activating collagenase (Suzuki *et al.*, 1990) or even the undefined aggrecanase, or cleaving type IX and X collagen (Wu *et al.*, 1991). Thus stromelysin may play a significant role in cartilage breakdown, but that role remains to be defined.

Stromelysin has also been reported to be induced by i.a. IL-8 injection (Forrest *et al.*, 1992), and its presence is associated with the release of proteoglycan into the synovial fluid. However, IL-8 does not directly induce stromelysin; thus this would be a secondary effect.

Collagenase was also elevated in rabbit synovial fluid after 7 ng or more of huIL-1β given i.a., but collagenase did not show a clear dose response increase with IL-1 (McDonnell *et al.*, 1992). Hutchinson *et al.* (1992) reported (without showing data) that collagenase immunohistochemical staining was increased in the synovial lining, but not in the cartilage of the rabbit. As coculture of IL-1 and cartilage induces collagenase, leads to breakdown of collagen in long-term but not short-term culture, and collagenase inhibitors block collagen breakdown in such cultures, it is likely that collagenase is present in cartilage, but below the level of detection.

The role of the metalloproteinases is further complicated by the presence of a number of protease inhibitors. Thus α_2-macroglobulin, TIMP-1 and TIMP-2 all inhibit metalloproteinases. Under normal circumstances it is likely that the enzymes either are not activated or are bound up in complexes with inhibitor (Clark *et al.*, 1993). The role these inhibitors play in the induction and resolution of cytokine-induced arthritis is not defined. The reader is referred to Chapters 9 and 17, this volume, for further discussion of metalloproteinases in arthritis.

Other Enzymes

The effects of i.a. cytokines on the localization, activity, and release of other enzymes that may play a role in arthritis has not been determined. However, IL-1 has been shown to increase the level of cathepsin B in rabbit articular chondrocytes *in vitro* (Biaici and Lang, 1990). Inactivators of cysteine endopeptidases, especially the lipophylic Ep453, could almost completely prevent the IL-1 induced proteoglycan release from bovine nasal septum cartilage explants (Buttle and Saklatvala, 1992). Other inhibitors of cathepsin B, the fluoromethyl ketone derivatives, have been used successfully to treat antigen-induced arthritis in the rat (van Noorden *et al.*, 1988) and adjuvant-induced arthritis (Ahmed *et al.*, 1992), but has not been examined *in vivo* after IL-1 or TNF administration. Plasminogen activator is also increased (Campbell *et al.*, 1990b), as is the activity of aggrecanase suggesting multiple proteases in addition to the MMP are induced and could have a role in cytokine-induced arthritis.

PAIN

Prostaglandins

IL-1 induces the synthesis of prostaglandins in many cell types. After continuous release of muIL-1α in the rat from osmotic pumps, prostaglandins have been shown to be increased in plasma (Otterness *et al.*, 1991) but prostaglandins have not been detected in synovial lavage fluids after i.a. IL-1. However, indirect evidence suggests that they are present. Administration of non-steroidal anti-inflammatory drugs (NSAIDs) will block prostaglandin synthesis. In a variety of systems, prostaglandins enhance perception of pain, but do not cause pain themselves. Schweizer *et al.* (1988) have shown that induction of a pain reflex in the isolated rabbit ear was coincident with prostaglandin synthesis. We have found that NSAIDs improve mobility measured as daily running distance in the hamster suggesting that part of the inhibition of running by muIL-1α is prostaglandin dependent (Otterness *et al.*, unpublished). NSAIDs also decrease oedema and cell infiltration into the synovial lining. Van den Berg *et al.* (1992) have shown that NSAIDs do not reverse proteoglycan synthesis suppression or loss of proteoglycans in the mouse suggesting that these effects are not dependent on prostaglandins. We (unpublished) have confirmed the lack of reversal of proteoglycan synthesis inhibition and proteoglycan loss by NSAIDs in the hamster. In rabbits, treatment with indomethacin only reduced the external disease symptoms of antigen-induced arthritis, for example joint swelling, but had no effect or even aggravated inflammation and cartilage loss (Pettipher *et al.*, 1989).

Substance P

The role of substance P in inflammation and inflammatory pain has been extensively debated. Substance P has been considered a mediator of neurogenic inflammation because it induces vascular leakage when released by substances such as capsaicin. Neurokinin type 1 (NK$_1$) receptors in the dorsal horn of the spinal cord are thought to be responsible for transmitting pain impulses carried by afferent C-fibres using substance P as a neurotransmitter (Pernow, 1953). It has been speculated that substance P may play a role in inflammation by inducing the synthesis of IL-1 and TNF by macrophages (Lotz *et al.*, 1988), and releasing prostaglandin E$_2$ and collagenase from human synoviocytes (Lotz *et al.*, 1987).

O'Byrne *et al.* (1990) have shown that i.a. administration of huIL-1β or huTNF causes release of substance P into the synovial fluid. After lavage of the rabbit knee joint with 1 ml of fluid, the amount of substance P was measured by radioimmunoassay. A dose responsive increase in substance P, in leukocyte infiltrate, and in proteoglycan loss was observed from 10 to 100 ng of human IL-1α. The maximum substance P level was 500 fmol/joint. Although TNF does not induce cartilage degradation in the rabbit, it did induce comparable substance P suggesting that substance P does not contribute to cartilage degradation. Furthermore, there is a suggestion that substance P could have a beneficial effect on cartilage *in vitro*. The role of neuropeptides in RA joint pathology is reviewed in Chapter 16, this volume.

INHIBITORS OF CYTOKINES

IL-1 Antagonists

A natural IL-1 receptor antagonist (IL-1ra) has been cloned (Hannum *et al.*, 1990). It inhibits the activities of IL-1α and IL-β (Arend *et al.*, 1990) in a variety of systems. Henderson *et al.* (1991) examined the ability of i.v. IL-1ra to inhibit the effects of i.a. huIL-1β in the rabbit. IL-1ra was able to inhibit both the proteoglycan loss and the PMN infiltration that follows i.a. IL-1. If IL-1 plays a role in arthritis, this suggests that IL-1ra has suitable pharmacodynamics to inhibit the effects of IL-1 in the synovial cavity.

The multifunctional regulatory peptide, TGFβ, can counteract the effects of IL-1 on several cell types, including chondrocytes, possibly through reduction of IL-1 receptor expression or stimulation of IL-1ra release. *In vitro* TGFβ can suppress IL-1 induced proteoglycan degradation in monolayers of articular chondrocytes and in sliced cartilage (Chandrasekhar and Harvey, 1988; Andrews *et al.*, 1989). Van Beuning *et al.* (1993) investigated the muIL-1α counteractivities of TGFβ on murine patellar cartilage proteoglycan metabolism both *in vitro* and *in vivo*. Analogous to the *in vitro* effects, TGFβ injected i.a. 1 h prior to IL-1 suppressed IL-1 induced proteoglycan degradation. TGFβ also counteracted IL-1 induced suppression of chondrocyte proteoglycan synthesis to a great extent both *in vitro* and *in vivo*. Furthermore, TGFβ potentiated the *ex vivo* recovery of IL-1 induced suppression of proteoglycan synthesis in patellae. Repeated IL-1 injections in the murine knee joint resulted in cartilage depletion, but repeated injections of IL-1 in combination with TGFβ resulted in amelioration of the IL-1 induced cartilage pathology (van Beuning *et al.*, submitted). Further disucssions of cytokine antagonists is to be found in Chapters 12 and 13, this volume.

CELLULAR EFFECTS OF CYTOKINES

POLYMORPHONUCLEAR LEUKOCYTES (PMNs)

The extensive infiltration of PMNs suggests that these cells could be a source of the mediators that lead to cartilage loss and functional impairment during the IL-1 arthritis. Using a nitrogen mustard depletion of leukocytes, Pettipher *et al.* (1988, 1989) failed to find an inhibition of proteoglycan or keratan sulphate loss into synovial fluid caused by huIL-1β. Leukocyte infiltration was inhibited by greater than 95%.

CD18 is an adhesion molecule of the integrin family that is important in controlling infiltration of leukocytes in areas of inflammation. Its expression is induced by IL-1. McDonnell *et al.* (1992) utilized a monoclonal anti-human CD18 antibody to block PMN infiltration by greater than 98% at 12 and 24 h. Nonetheless, proteoglycan loss was unchanged (12 h) or enhanced (24 h). Neither IL-1 nor TNF are directly chemotactic for PMNs, but both are potent inducers of IL-8 (NAP-1) (Matsushima and Oppenheim, 1989; Schroder *et al.*, 1990), a potent chemotactic factor for PMNs (Yoshimura *et al.*, 1987; Colditz *et al.*, 1990). Rampart and Williams (1988) and Cybulsky *et al.* (1989) have shown that neutrophil influx to huIL-1β and TNF is dependent on protein synthesis (i.e. this is compatible with IL-8 as the major chemo-tactic factor) and suggests that neither C5a nor LTB$_4$ are important contributors to PMN infiltration. Sayers *et al.* (1988) found that neither inhibitors of prostaglandin formation nor leukotriene formation inhibited PMN influx to IL-1 or TNF. Pettipher *et al.* (1986) found that leukotriene inhibitors failed to block the influx of PMNs. The LTB$_4$ inhibitor MK-0591 was also without effect (Brideau, 1993). These results are all consistent with IL-8 as the primary mediator of IL-1 and TNF-induced PMN influx. Forrest *et al.* (1992) used anti-CD18 to block neutrophil influx to IL-8. Proteoglycan loss was unchanged.

In vitro studies show that IL-1 and TNF directly cause cartilage proteoglycan loss in appropriate species. The CD18 and nitrogen mustard experiments discussed above provide strong evidence that PMNs do not contribute significantly to IL-1 induced cartilage proteoglycan loss in the rabbit. This is also consistent with data from i.a. LPS (Pettipher *et al.*, 1986) or TNF (Henderson and Pettipher, 1989) injected rabbits where there is equivalent PMN infiltration, but no proteoglycan loss.

CHONDROCYTES

IL-1 is known to induce changes in the cell surface expression of class II MHC markers (Dingle *et al.*, 1990; Davies *et al.*, 1991b) and ICAM-1 (Davies *et al.*, 1991a) on chondrocytes. These changes have been both induced *in vitro* and detected in human arthritic patients (Davies *et al.*, 1991). The significance of expression of these cell surface markers while the cell is localized inside the chondron is not known, but it may be an expression of a generalized activation of the chondrocyte and indicative of the change in synthesis of many other proteins that are induced by IL-1. The response of articular chondrocytes to the pathological changes induced in arthritic joints is detailed in Chapter 9, this volume.

FUNCTIONAL CONSEQUENCES OF INTRA-ARTICULAR CYTOKINES

Relatively little work has been done on the physiological effects of i.a. cytokines. Stimpson *et al.* (1988a) found that 4–6 h after i.a. muIL-1α, the injected rats limped. After another 6 h, their movement returned to normal. In the rabbit, injection of IL-8 was associated with joint redness and limp without significant swelling (Endo *et al.*, 1991). In the hamster, we have examined the effect of i.a. muIL-1α on running (Otterness *et al.*, 1994a). Normally, a 3-month-old hamster will run about 10–12 km/night on a 30-cm diameter wheel. After 40 ng of IL-1, the running that night will fall to approximately half that distance, but running will be normal on the following night. If a second i.a. IL-1 injection is given, the running falls to a tenth of the normal distance. Again running is restored to normal the following night. Although systemic IL-1 can cause a decrease in motor activity (Otterness *et al.*, 1988), it seems unlikely that the effect was due to simple leakage of IL-1 from the joint into the systemic circulation because the amounts of administered IL-1 were too small to cause suppression of running when given intraperitoneally. The restoration of running in the face of continuing pathology (observed histologically as cellular infiltration, soft tissue swelling, and proteoglycan loss) suggests that it is not a local effect of tissue inflammation alone that leads to loss of running, but a systemic effect perhaps caused by movement of mediators from the joint to the systemic circulation. This is supported by our observations that the rise and fall of acute phase reactants synthesized in the liver correlates with running distance, not with local pathology (Otterness *et al.*, 1994c).

REVERSAL OF CYTOKINE-INDUCED CHANGES

Over time there is a replenishment of the proteoglycan lost from articular cartilage after cytokine injection. This has been studied in mice after muIL-1α induced proteoglycan depletion. The earliest change is restoration of the ability to synthesize proteoglycans. Synthesis is enhanced during the restoration phase and then returned to normal rates (van de Loo *et al.*, 1993). The elevated level of metalloproteases falls during the restoration phase (van de Loo *et al.*, 1993). Also, during the proteoglycan restoration phase, degradation of newly synthesized proteoglycan was impaired. Thus during the recovery phase, the two processes – enhancement of proteoglycan synthesis and decreased degradation – both occur over the same time scale and reinforce each other during replenishment of proteoglycan.

EFFECTS OF SYSTEMIC IL-1

IL-1 and TNF have been administered to animals by many routes besides intra-articular. Except in primed animals (see the next section), systemic administration (i.v., i.p., i.m., s.c.) of cytokine does not lead to arthritis. However, a number of general effects are observed (Dinarello, 1991).

Intravenous administration of IL-1 (endogenous pyrogen) leads to a fever. One of the paraventricular organs, the *ovum vasculorum lateral terminalis*, shows unusual sensitivity to induction of fever by prostaglandins and provides a site outside of the blood–brain barrier from which circulating IL-1 can induce prostaglandin production and fever (Stitt, 1991). These findings explain the high sensitivity of fever to inhibition by NSAIDs which do not cross the blood–brain barrier. In addition, systemic IL-1 causes NSAID-resistant appetite loss and decreased food consumption (Otterness *et al.*, 1988; Mrosovsky *et al.*, 1989). IL-1 also causes enhanced diuresis (Beasley *et al.*, 1988) and increased water consumption (Otterness *et al.*, 1991), both of which are NSAID sensitive. Leukocyte counts are elevated (NSAID resistant). Finally, acute phase reactant production is stimulated (Lewis *et al.*, 1992) (NSAID resistant). These effects (fever, decreased appetite, increased fluid consumption, increased leukocyte counts and acute phase reactants), mimic those observed in both acute inflammation and bacterial infection.

POTENTIATION OF ARTHRITIS

IL-1 and TNF may also play a role in potentiation of established arthritis. For example, muIL-1α causes a flare of low-grade streptococcal arthritis (Stimpson *et al.*, 1988a), and huIL-1β potentiates the induction of collagen arthritis in mice (Hom *et al.*, 1988; Killar and Dunn, 1989; Hom *et al.*, 1992). Although i.a. methylated bovine serum albumin (mBSA) alone does not cause arthritis in mice, subcutaneous huIL-1β along with i.a. mBSA will lead to an arthritis (Staite *et al.*, 1990). huIL-β administered i.a. during the immune development or within the first 2 days after induction/onset of antigen-induced arthritis in rats, reduced joint swelling and histopathology (Jacobs *et al.*, 1988). muIL-1α administered i.a. during the chronic phase of antigen-induced arthritis (AIA) in mice caused a flare of the arthritis (van de Loo *et al.*, 1992). Intra-articular injection of muTNFα but not muIL-6 (up to 1 μg) in the chronic phase of AIA, caused a short-lasting flare of the smouldering inflammation (van de Loo, in preparation). Potentiation by muIL-1α was also observed after inflammation induced by concanavalin A or zymosan in mice (van de Loo *et al.*, 1992). huTNF has been shown to potentiate collagen arthritis in rats (Cooper *et al.*, 1990; Brahn *et al.*, 1992). These results demonstrate a second possibility for cytokine involvement in arthritic disease: amplification of a nascent arthritis and flare-up of an established arthritis.

TRANSGENIC ANIMALS

Transgenic animals may prove to be a useful tool in understanding the pathogenesis of arthritic diseases by demonstrating the role of cytokines and growth factors (see chapter 27, this volume). *In vitro* studies often fail to mimic the full range of physiological and pathological effects these products have in the whole animal. In addition, administration of these products by single or multiple injection or by implantation of osmotic pumps for sustained release may fail to mimic the effects of *in vivo* local synthesis. Depending on the nature of the promoter, transgenic animals can be generated with specific localization and induction of the cytokine.

Transgenic mice of possible interest for arthritis have been made with over-expressing or deletion of genes for IL-4 (Tepper *et al.*, 1990), IL-6 (Turksen *et al.*, 1992; Woodroofe *et al.*, 1992), GM-CSF (Lang *et al.*, 1987), IFN-γ (Dalton *et al.*, 1993), TNF (Keffer *et al.*, 1991), TGFβ (Shull *et al.*, 1992) and collagenase (D'Armiento *et al.*, 1992). Since both TNF and IL-1 have been shown to play pathological roles in arthritis, insertion of a gene that causes unregulated production of these cytokines in an animal might be expected to give rise to an arthritis. A transgenic animal with over-expression of IL-1 has not yet been reported.

Transgenic mouse lines have been generated which express the human TNF gene (Keffer *et al.*, 1991). These transgenic mice show dysregulated patterns of TNF expression and also develop a chronic polyarthritis, which is demonstrated by a swelling of the ankles and impaired movement. Arthritis was the only noted pathology, despite widespread over-expression of TNFα. This macroscopic pathology was inherited with 100% frequency in transgenic progeny.

Histopathology showed hyperplasia of the synovial membrane. and PMN and lymphocytic inflammatory infiltrates of the synovial space by 3 weeks of age. In addition, pannus formation, articular cartilage destruction and massive production of fibrous tissue were observed in the advanced stages of the disease. However, serum levels of rheumatoid factor were not detectable at any disease stage.

Keffer *et al.* (1991) confirmed that the pathology observed is effected by the deregulated *in vivo* production of TNF. They completely suppressed arthritis development with monoclonal antibodies against human TNF. However, progeny of antibody-treated apparently normal transgenic mice developed arthritis within the usual time course. As yet, there are no reports of drug therapy to modify the disease development by *in vivo* blocking of a specific inflammatory cytokine in those mice with cytokine overexpression.

Transgenic mouse lines overexpressing IL-6 have been prepared using several different promoters. Those using a human keratin 14 promoter show abnormalities in the skin but no circulating elevated levels of IL-6 (Turksen *et al.*, 1992), whereas those using an immunoglobulin promoter/enhancer showed no apparent phenotype abnormalities in the skin but showed elevated plasma IL-6 levels, plasmacytosis, and mesangio-proliferative glomerulonephritis (Suematsu *et al.*, 1989). Putting mouse TNFα or TNFβ behind the insulin promoter leads to focal TNF production by the islet cells (Picarella *et al.*, 1993). These transgenics show elevated expression of leukocyte adhesion molecules VCAM-1 and ICAM-1 in islet endothelia, increased expression of MHC class I on islet cells and leukocyte infiltration. These results suggest that the promoter and the localization of site of TNF production could determine the nature of the disease.

'Knock out' mice (i.e. mice with a specific gene deletion) may provide another way to determine the biological function of individual cytokines. A cytokine 'knock out' mouse showing resistance to induction of arthritis could serve to further demonstrate a role for the cytokine in arthritis. Reinstatement of the susceptibility to arthritis induction by exogenous replacement of the deficient cytokine would solidify the need for the cytokine for induction of arthritis.

EVIDENCE FOR THE INVOLVEMENT OF CYTOKINES IN ANIMAL MODELS OF ARTHRITIS

IL-1 and TNF have been shown to play a significant pathological role in models of arthritis. Schwab *et al.* (1991, 1993) studied the flare-up reaction in streptococcal cell wall arthritis and showed that either the IL-1 receptor antagonist or anti-TNF antibody can block the arthritic flare. Van de Loo *et al.* (manuscript in preparation) studied the role of IL-1 in antigen reactivation of chronic antigen-induced arthritis in mice. Elevated levels of IL-1 and IL-6 were found in washouts of joint capsules taken 6 h after eliciting the flare-up. Blocking *de novo* synthesized IL-1 (α + β) by administering anti-IL-1 antibodies resulted in suppression of joint swelling, proteoglycan synthesis inhibition and the flare-up related cartilage pathology. Van de Loo *et al.* (1992) studied murine AIA and have shown with homologous blocking antibodies that anti-IL-1 (α + β) can prevent proteoglycan synthesis inhibition and can ameliorate the pathology of arthritis. In contrast to the flare-up reaction in AIA arthritis, anti-IL-1 treatment did not suppress the acute onset of joint inflammation. Anti-IL-1 antibodies also did not reverse the acceleration of proteoglycan degradation after IL-1 suggesting the proteoglycan degradation may be regulated differently than proteoglycan synthesis (van de Loo *et al.*, 1993).

Van Lent *et al.* (1992) studied an immune complex arthritis model (ICA) induced by passive immunization with rabbit anti-lysozyme antibodies followed by i.a. injection of poly-L-lysine coupled lysozyme. In contrast to AIA, ICA was less severe and less chronic. Anti-IL-1 antibodies in this model inhibited the onset of arthritis, joint swelling and inflammation, for example influx of PMNs (van Lent *et al.*, 1994). Possibly as a consequence of blocking inflammation, proteoglycan degradation in ICA was also largely prevented by anti-IL-1 treatment. Moreover, eliciting ICA in neutropenic mice resulted in an increased IL-1 bioactivity in the joint, yet proteoglycan degradation was absent indicating that degradation of cartilage in this arthritis was not a direct consequence of IL-1 but probably mediated through neutrophils (van Lent *et al.*, unpublished).

Schwab *et al.* (1991) found an ambiguous role for endogenous IL-1 in the onset of the flare reaction in streptococcal arthritis. Blocking IL-1 for the first 6 h of the flare enhances joint swelling. If the block was extended for more than 6 h by pretreatment with IL-1ra for 24 h before flare induction, joint swelling was suppressed by more than 50%. This indicates that IL-1 is pro-inflammatory, but also may initiate anti-inflammatory homeostatic responses. This is also shown in the study of Jacobs *et al.* (1988) where exogenous IL-1 injected i.a. before or directly after arthritis induction leads to reduced joint swelling, inflammation and cartilage destruction. Wooley *et al.* (1993) using huIL-1ra showed inhibition of the induction of collagen arthritis, but not therapeutic effects after disease onset. The study of Faherty *et al.* (1992) put further doubt on the usefulness of IL-1ra or monoclonal anti-IL-1 receptor antibodies as therapeutics as they could not block antigen-specific immune responses *in vivo*. Van den Berg *et al.* (submitted) demonstrated that anti-IL-1 antibodies were useful for the treatment of collagen-induced arthritis (CIA). Anti-IL-1 antibodies were effective both as prophylactic and therapeutic treatments, reducing joint swelling, inflammation, and cartilage pathology. Moreover, in the unilateral, zymosan-accelerated model of collagen induced arthritis in knee joints, it was demonstrated that anti-IL-1 antibodies prevented proteoglycan synthesis suppression. A novel IL-1 antagonist distinct from IL-1ra, M20 IL-1 inhibitor, was utilized in a prophylactic regimen in adjuvant arthritis and resulted in reduced pathological processes (Vivian *et al.*, 1992).

Issekeutz *et al.* (1994) found in rat adjuvant arthritis that anti-TNF, but not anti-IL-1, antibodies inhibited the chronic phase of the arthritis. Williams *et al.* (1991) using mu anti-TNF antibodies, and Piguet *et al.* (1992) using the hu p55 TNF receptor, found that prophylactic treatment can inhibit induction of murine collagen arthritis. Therapeutic administration was not effective. Van den Berg *et al.* (in preparation) compared both anti-IL-1 and anti-TNF treatments in collagen arthritis. Anti-TNF treatment resulted in arrest of the disease whereas anti-IL-1 treatment resulted in complete recovery. The applicability of inhibition of arthritis by anti-IL-1 and anti-TNF reagents to other animal models of arthritis and to human arthritis is currently an important area of research. Readers should refer to Chapter 13, this volume.

SUMMARY

The cytokines IL-1 and TNF cannot by themselves account for the pathology of RA or osteoarthritis. Nonetheless, their actions mimic in detail many processes observed in arthritic disease, and circumstances that could lead to continuous synthesis and release of IL-1 or TNF would be expected to lead to a chronic arthritis. Thus, both cytokines could play a significant role in the pathogenesis of arthritis. Moreover, the ability of the cytokines to cause a flare or increase the severity of an arthritis suggest that they would play a role even in arthritis lacking a cytokine etiology if they were induced by concurrent infection or other processes. These models of cytokine-induced arthritis then have value for studies into possible mechanisms of arthritic disease and as tools for design and development of cytokine-directed therapy.

REFERENCES

Ahmed NK, Martin LA, Watts LMHP, Thornberg L, Prior J & Esser ER (1992) Piptidyl fluoromethyl ketones as inhibitors of cathepsin B. Implication for treatment of rheumatoid arthritis. *Biochem Pharmacol* **44**: 1201–1207.

Andrews HH, Edwards TA, Crawston TE & Hazelman BL (1989) Transforming growth factor-beta causes partial inhibition of interleukin-1 stimulated cartilage degradation *in vitro*. *Biochem Biophys Res Comm* **162**: 144–150.

Arend WP, Welgus HG, Thompson RC & Eisenberg SP (1990) Biological properties of recombinant human monocyte-derived interleukin-1 receptor antagonist. *J Clin Invest* **85**: 1694–1697.

Arner EC, DiMeo TM, Ruhl DM & Pratta MA (1989). *In vivo* studies on the effects of human recombinant interleukin-1β on articular cartilage. *Agents Actions* **27**: 254–257.

Arner EC (1994) Effect of animal age and chronicity of interleukin-1 exposure on cartilage proteoglycan depletion *in vivo*. *J Orthop Res* **12**: 321–330.

Banks WA, Ortiz L, Plotkin SR & Kastin AJ (1992) Human interleukin (IL) 1α, murine IL-1α and murine IL-1β are transported from blood to brain in the mouse by a shared saturable mechanism. *J Pharm Exp Ther* **259**: 988–996.

Beasley D, Dinarello CA & Cannon JG (1988) Interleukin-1 induced naturesis in conscious rats: role of renal prostaglandins. *Kidney Int* **33**: 1059–1065.

Beutler BA, Milsark IW & Cerami A (1985) Cachectin/tumour necrosis factor: Production, distribution, and metabolic fate *in vivo*. *J Immunol* **135**: 3972–3977.

Biaci A & Lang A (1990) Effect of interleukin-1β on the production of cathepsin B by rabbit articular chondrocytes. *FEBS Lett* **277**: 93–96.

Brahn E, Peacock DJ, Banquerigo ML & Liu DY (1992) Effects of tumour necrosis factor α (TNFα) on collagen arthritis. *Lymphokine Cytokine Res* **11**: 253–256.

Bunning RAD & Russell RGG (1989) The effect of tumour necrosis factor α and γ-interferon on the resorption of human articular cartilage and on the production of prostaglandin E and of caseinase activity by human articular chondrocytes. *Arthritis Rheum* **32**: 780–784.

Brideau C, Chan C-C, Guevremont D, Hutchinson JH, McDonnell J & Moore V (1993) Inhibition of synovial LTB₄ production by a specific leukotriene biosynthesis inhibitor, MK-0591, in a rabbit model of joint inflammation. *Drug Dev Res* **29**: 188–194.

Buttle DJ & Saklatvala J (1992) Lysosomal cysteine endopeptidases mediate interleukin-1-stimulated cartilage proteoglycan degradation. *Biochem J* **287**: 657–661.

Campbell IK, Piccoli DS, Roberts MJ & Muriden KD (1990a). Effects of tumour necrosis factor α and β on resorption of human articular cartilage and production of plasminogen activator by human articular chondrocytes. *Arthritis Rheum* **33**: 542–552.

Campbell IK, Piccoli DS, Roberts MJ, Muriden KD & Hamilton JA (1990b). Regulation of plasminogen activator activity in arthritic joints. *J Rheumatol* **15**: 1129–1137.

Chandrasekhar S & Harvey AK (1988) Transforming growth factor-beta causes partial inhibition of interleukin-1-stimulated cartilage degradation *in vitro*. *Biochem Biophys Res Commun* **162**: 144–150.

Chandrasekhar S, Harvey AK, Hrubey PS & Bendele AM (1990). Arthritis induced by interleukin-1 is dependent on the site and frequency of intraarticular injection. *Clin Immunol Immunopathol* **55**: 382–400.

Chandrasekhar S, Harvey AK & Hrubey PS (1992) Intra-articular administration of interleukin-1 causes prolonged suppression of cartilage proteoglycan synthesis in rats. *Matrix* **11**: 1–10.

Clark IM, Powell LK, Ramsey S, Hazelman BL & Cawston TE (1993) The measurement of collagenase, tissue inhibitor of metalloproteinases (TIMP), and collagenase-TIMP complex in synovial fluids from patients with osteoarthritis and rheumatoid arthritis. *Arthritis Rheum* **36**: 372–379.

Colditz IG, Zwahlen RD & Baggiolini M (1990) Neutrophil accumulation and plasma leakage induced *in vivo* by neutrophil-activating peptide-1. *J Leukocyte Biol* **48**: 129–137.

Cooper WO, Fava RA, Gates CA & Townes AS (1990) Intra-articular injection of tumour necrosis factor-alpha (TNF) or transforming growth factor-beta (TGF-β) accelerates the onset and increases the incidence of collagen-induced arthritis. *Arthritis Rheum* **33**: S76.

Cybulsky MI, McComb DJ & Movat HZ (1989) Protein synthesis dependent and independent mechanisms of neutrophil emigration. Different mechanisms of inflammation in rabbits induced by interleukin-1, tumour necrosis factor alpha or endotoxin versus leukocyte chemoattractants. *Am J Pathol* **135**: 227–237.

D'Armiento J, Dalal SS, Okada Y, Berg RA & Chada K (1992) Collagenase expression in the lungs of transgenic mice causes pulmonary emphysema. *Cell* **71**: 955–961.

Dalton DK, Pitts-Meek S, Keshav S, Figari IS, Bradley A & Stewart TA (1993) Multiple defects of immune cell function in mice with disrupted interferon-γ genes. *Science* **259**: 1739–1742.

Da Silva JAP, Larbre JP, Spector TD, Scott DL & Willoughby DA (1992) Gender differences in cartilage response to interleukin-1. *Arthritis Rheum* **35**: S119.

Davies ME, Dingle JT & Pigott R (1991a) Expression of intercellular adhesion molecule 1 (ICAM-1) on human articular cartilage chondrocytes. *Connect Tiss Res* **26**: 207–216.

Davies ME, Horner A & Dingle JT (1991b) Immunorecognition of chondrocytes in articular cartilage activated by synovial chondrocytes. *Connect Tiss Res* **25**: 243–249.

Davies ME, Sharma H & Pigott R (1992) ICAM-1 expression on chondrocytes in rheumatoid arthritis: induction by synovial cytokines. *Mediators Inflam* **1**: 71–74.

DeMarco D & Kunkel SL (1991) IL-1 induced gene expression of neutrophil activating peptide (IL-8) and monocyte chemotactic peptide in human synovial cells. *Biochem Biophys Res Comm* **174**: 411–416.

Dinarello CA (1991) Interleukin 1 and interleukin-1 antagonism. *Blood* **77**: 1627–1652.

Dingle JT, Saklatvala J, Hembry RM, Tyler JA, Fell HB & Jubb R (1979) A cartilage catabolic factor, *Biochem J* **184**: 177–180.

Dingle JT, Thomas PD, King B & Bird DR (1987) *In vivo* studies of articular tissue damage mediated by catabolin/interleukin 1. *Ann Rheum Dis* **46**: 527–533.

Dingle JT, Davies ME, Mativi BY & Middleton HF (1990) Immunological identification of interleukin-1 activated chondrocytes. *Ann Rheum Dis* **49**: 889–892.

Dower SK, Kronheim SR, March CJ, Conlon PJ, Hopp TP, Gillis S et al. (1985) Detection and characterization of high affinity plasma membrane receptors for human interleukin-1. *J Exp Med* **162**: 501–515.

Elford PR & Cooper PH (1991) Induction of neutrophil-mediated cartilage degradation by interleukin-8. *Arthritis Rheum* **34**: 325–332.

Elford PR, Graeber M, Ohtsu H, Aeberhard M, Legendre B, Wishart WL et al. (1992) Induction of swelling, synovial hyperplasia and cartilage proteoglycan loss upon intra-articular injection of transforming growth factor β-2 in the rabbit. *Cytokine* **4**: 232–238.

Endo H, Akahoshi T, Takagishi K, Kashiwazaki S & Matsushima K (1991) Elevation of interleukin-8 (IL-8) levels in joint fluids of patients with rheumatoid arthritis and the induction by IL-8 of leukocyte infiltration and synovitis in rabbit joints. *Lymph Cytokine Res* **10**: 245–252.

Faherty DA, Claudy V, Plocinski JM, Kaffka K, Kilian P, Thompson RC & Benjamin WR (1992) Failure of IL-1 receptor antagonist and monoclonal anti-IL-1 receptor antibody to inhibit antigen-specific immune responses *in vivo*. *J Immunol* **148**: 766–771.

Feige U, Karbowski A, Rordorf-Adam C & Pataki A (1990) Arthritis induced by continuous infusion of hu-interleukin-1α into the rabbit knee-joint. *Int J Tissue Reac* **11**: 225–238.

Ferraiolo BL, Moore JA, Crase D, Gribling P, Wilking H & Baughman RA (1988) Pharmacokinetics and tissue distribution of recombinant human tumour necrosis factor α in mice. *Drug Metab Dist* **16**: 270–275.

Fibbe WE, Van Damme JBA Voogt PJ, Duinkerken N, Kluck PMC & Falkenburg JHF (1986) Interleukin-1 (22-K factor) induces release of granulocyte-macrophage colony-stimulating activity from human mononuclear phagocytes. *Blood* **68**: 1316–1321.

Forrest MJ, Eiermann GJ, Meurer R, Walakovits LA & MacIntyre DE (1992). The role of CD18 in IL-8 induced dermal and synovial inflammation. *Br J Pharmacol* **106**: 287–294.

Fosang AJ, Neame PJ, Hardingham TE, Murphy G & Hamilton JA (1991) Cleavage of cartilage proteoglycan between G1 and G2 domains by stromelysins. *J Biol Chem* **266**: 15579–15582.

Gilman SC, Hodge R & Chang J (1986) Articular synovitis in the rat knee joints induced by interleukin 1. *Arthritis Rheum* **29**: S29.

Hannum CH, Wilcox CJ, Arend WP, Joslin FG, Dripps DJ, Heimdal PL, Armes LG, Sommer A, Eisenberg SP & Thompson RC (1990) Interleukin-1 receptor antagonist activity of a human interleukin-1 inhibitor. *Nature* **343**: 336–340.

Hasty KA, Reife RA, Kang AH, & Stuart JM (1990) The role of stromelysin in the cartilage destruction that accompanies inflammatory arthritis. *Arthritis Rheum* **33**: 338–397.

Hay RV, Skinner RS, Newman OC, Kunkel SL, Lyle LR, Shapiro B & Gross MD (1993) Nuclear imaging of acute inflammatory lesions with recombinant interleukin-8. *J Nucl Med* **34**: 104.

Hayashida K, Ochi T, Fujimoto M, Owaki H, Shimaoka Y, Ono K et al. (1992) Bone marrow changes in adjuvant-induced and collagen-induced arthritis. Interleukin-1 and interleukin-6 activity and abnormal myelopoiesis. *Arthritis Rheum* **35**: 241–245.

Hechtman DH, Cybulsky MI, Fuchs HJ, Baker JB & Gimbrone Jr MA (1991) Intravascular IL-8 inhibitor of polymorphonuclear leukocyte accumulation at sites of acute inflammation. *J Immunol* **147**: 883–892.

Henderson B & Pettipher ER (1989) Arthritogenic actions of recombinant IL-1 and tumour necrosis factor α in the rabbit: evidence for synergistic interactions between cytokines *in vivo*. *Clin Exp Immunol* **75**: 306–310.

Henderson B, Thompson RC, Hardingham T & Lewthwaite J (1991) Inhibition of interleukin-1-induced synovitis and articular cartilage proteoglycan loss in the rabbit knee by recombinant human interleukin-1 receptor antagonist. *Cytokine* **3**: 246–249.

Hom JT, Bendele AM & Carlson DG (1988) *In vivo* administration with IL-1 accelerates the development of collagen-induced arthritis in mice. *J Immunol* **141**: 834–841.

Hom JT, Cole H, Estridge T & Gliszczynski VL (1992) Interleukin-1 enhances the development of type II collagen-induced arthritis only in susceptible and in resistant mice. *Clin Immunol Immunopathol* **62**: 56–65.

Hutchinson NI, Lark MW, MacNaul KL, Harper C, Hoerner LA, McDonnell J et al. (1992) *In vivo* expression of stromelysin in synovium and cartilage of rabbits injected intraarticularly with interleukin-1β. *Arthritis Rheum* **35**: 1227–1233.

Jacobs C, Young D, Tyler S, Callis G, Gillis S & Conlon PJ (1988). *In vivo* treatment with IL-1 reduces the severity and duration of antigen-induced arthritis in rats. *J Immunol* **141**: 2967–2974.

Kawatsu M, Takeo K, Kajikawa T, Funashashi I, Asaki T, Kakutani T, Yamashita T, Kawaharada H & Watanabe K (1990) The pharmacokinetic pattern of glycosylated human recombinant lymphotoxin in rats after intravenous administration. *J Pharmacobiodyn* **13**: 549–557.

Keffer J, Probert K, Cazlaris H, Georgopoulos S, Kaslaris E, Kiossis D et al. (1991) Transgenic mice expressing human tumour necrosis factor: a predictive genetic model of arthritis. *EMBO J* **10**: 4025–4031.

Killar LM & Dunn CJ (1989) Interleukin-1 potentiates the development of collagen-induced arthritis in mice. *Clin Sci* **76**: 535–538.

Klapproth J, Castell J, Geiger T, Andus T & Heinrich PC (1989) Fate and biological action of human recombinant interleukin 1β in the rat *in vivo*. *Eur J Immunol* **19**: 1485–1490.

Kudo S, Mizuno K, Hirai Y & Sjimzu T (1990) Clearance and tissue distribution of recombinant interleukin 1β in rats. *Cancer Res* **50**: 5751–5755.

Lang RA, Metcalf D, Cuthbertson RA, Lyons I, Stanley E, Kelso A et al. (1987) Transgenic mice expressing a hemopoietic growth factor gene (GM-CSF) develop accumulation of macrophages, blindness, and a fatal syndrome of tissue damage. *Cell* **51**: 675–686.

Lefebvre V, Peeters-Joris C & Vaes G (1990) Modulation by interleukin 1 and tumour necrosis factor of production of collagenase, tissue inhibitor of metalloproteinases and collagen types in differentiated and dedifferentiated articular chondrocytes. *Biochem Biophys Acta* **1052**: 366–378.

Lefebvre V, Peeters-Joris C & Vaes G (1991) Production of gelatin-degrading matrix metalloproteinases ('type IV collagenases') and inhibitors by articular chondrocytes during their dedifferentiation by serial subcultures and under stimulation by interleukin-1 and tumour necrosis factor α. *Biochem Biophys Acta* **1094**: 8–18.

Lewis EJ, Sedgwick AD & Hanahoe THP (1992) *In vivo* changes in plasma acute phase protein levels in the rat induced by slow release of IL-1, IL-6 and TNF. *Mediators Inflam* **1**: 39–44.

Libert C, Brouckaert P, Shaw A & Fiers W (1990) Induction of interleukin 6 by human and murine recombinant interleukin 1 in mice. *Eur J Immunol* **20**: 691–694.

Lisi PJ, Chu C-W, Koch GA, Endres S, Lonnermann G & Dinarello CA (1987) Development and use of radioimmunoassay for human interleukin 1β. *Lymphokine Res* **6**: 229–244.

Lotz M, Carson DA & Vaughan JH (1987) Substance P activation of rheumatoid synoviocytes: Neural pathway in pathogenesis of arthritis. *Science* **235**: 893–895.

Lotz M, Vaughan JH & Carson DA (1988) Effect of neuropeptides on production of inflammatory cytokines by human monocytes. *Science* **241**: 1218–1221.

Matsushima K & Oppenheim J (1989) Interleukin 8 and MCAF: novel inflammatory cytokines inducible by IL-1 and TNF. *Cytokine* **1**: 2–13.

McDonnell J, Hoerrner LA, Lark MW, Harper C, Dey T, Lobner J et al. (1992) Recombinant human interleukin-1β-induced increase in levels of proteoglycans, stromelysin, and leukocytes in rabbit synovial fluid. *Arthritis Rheum* **35**: 799–805.

McIntosh JDM, Mule JJ, Nordan RP, Rudikoff S, Lotze MT & Rosenberg SA (1989). *In vivo* induction of IL-6 by administration of exogenous cytokines and detection of *de novo* serum levels of IL-6 tumour-bearing mice. *J Immunol* **143**: 162–167.

Mizel SB, Dayer J-M, Krane SM & Mergenhagen SE (1981) Stimulation of rheumatoid cell collagenase and prostaglandin production by partially purified lymphocyte-activating factor (interleukin 1). *Proc Natl Acad Sci USA* **78**: 2474–2477.

Mrosovsky N, Molony LA, Conn CA & Kluger MJ (1989) Anorexic effects of interleukin 1 in the rat. *Am J Physiol* **254**: R1315–R1321.

Newton RC, Uhl J, Covington M & Black O (1988) The distribution and clearance of radiolabelled human interleukin-1β in mice. *Lymphokine Res* **7**: 207–215.

Nguyen Q, Murphy G, Roughly PJ & Mort JS (1989) Degradation of proteoglycan aggregate by a cartilage metalloproteinase. Evidence for the involvement of stromelysin in the generation of link protein hetero-geneity *in situ*. *Biochem J* **259**: 61–67.

O'Byrne EM, Blancuzzi V, Wilson DE, Wong M & Jeng AY (1990) Elevated substance P and accelerated cartilage degradation in rabbit knees injected with interleukin-1 and tumour necrosis factor. *Arthritis Rheum* **33**: 1023–1028.

Otterness IG, Seymour PA, Golden HW, Reynolds JA & Daumy GO (1988) The effects of continuous administration of murine interleukin-1α in the rat. *Physiol Behav* **43**: 787–804.

Otterness IG, Golden HW, Seymour PA, Eskra JD & Daumy GO (1991) Role of prostaglandins in the behavioural changes induced by murine interleukin 1α in the rat. *Cytokine* **3**: 333–338.

Otterness IG, Bliven ML & Micili AJ (1994a) Mobility changes in the golden hamster after induction of an IL-1-induced arthritis. *Med Inflam* **3**: 199–204.

Otterness IG, Bliven ML & Micili AJ (1994b) Comparison of mobility changes with histologic and bio-chemical changes during LPS-induced arthritis in the hamster. *Amer J Pathol* **144**: 1098–1108.

Otterness IG, Sipe JD, Sinohara H, Carraras I, Yamamoto K & Bliven ML (1994c) Serum amyloid A, but no other acute phase reactants, is a sensitive marker of mobility impairment in arthritic disease. *Amyloid Int J Clin Exp* **1**: in press.

Page-Thomas DP, King B, Stephens T & Dingle JT (1991) *In vivo* studies of cartilage regeneration after damage induced by catabolin/interleukin-1. *Ann Rheum Dis* **50**: 75–80.

Pernow, B (1953) Substance P. *Acta Physiol Scand* **29**: 1–90.

Pettipher ER, Higgs GA & Henderson B (1986) Interleukin 1 induces leukocyte infiltration and cartilage proteoglycan degradation in the synovial joint. *Proc Natl Acad Sci USA* **83**: 8749–8753.

Pettipher ER, Henderson B, Moncada S & Higgs GA (1988) Leucocyte infiltration and cartilage proteogly-can loss in immune arthritis in the rabbit. *Br J Pharmacol* **95**: 169–176.

Pettipher ER, Henderson B, Hardingham T & Ratcliffe A (1989) Cartilage proteoglycan depletion in acute and chronic antigen-induced arthritis. *Arthritis Rheum* **32**: 601–607.

Picarella DE, Kratz A, Li C-B, Ruddle NH & Flavell RA (1993) Transgenic tumour necrosis factor (TNF)-α production in pancreatic islets leads to insulitis, not diabetes. Distinct patterns of inflammation in TNF-α and TNF-β transgenic mice. *J Immunol* **150**: 4136–4150.

Piguet PF, Grau GE, Vesin C, Loetscher H, Gentz R & Lesslauer W (1992) Evolution of collagen arthritis in mice is arrested by treatment with antitumour necrosis factor (TNF) antibody or a recombinant soluble TNF receptor. *Immunology* **77**: 510–514.

Pratta MA, DiMeo TM, Ruhl DM & Arner EC (1989) Effects of IL-1β and tumour necrosis factor α on cartilage proteoglycan metabolism *in vitro*. *Agents Actions* **27**: 250–253.

Rampart M & Williams TJ (1988) Evidence that neutrophil accumulation induced by interleukin-1 requires both local protein biosynthesis and neutrophil CD18 antigen expression *in vivo*. *Br J Pharmacol* **94**: 1143–1148.

Reimers J, Wogensen LD, Welinder B, Hejnaes KF, Poulsen SS, Nilsson P & Nerup J (1991) The pharmacokinetics, distribution and degradation of human recombinant IL-1 beta in normal rats. *Scand J Immunol* **34**: 597–610.

Sandy JD, Boynton RE & Flannery CR (1991) Analysis of catabolism of aggrecan in cartilage explants by quantitation of peptides form the three gobular domains. *J Biol Chem* **266**: 8683–8685.

Sayers TJ, Wiltrout TA, Bull CA, Denn AC III, Pilaro AM & Lokesh B (1988) Effect of cytokines on polymorphonuclear neutrophil infiltration in the mouse. Prostaglandin- and leukotriene-independent induction of infiltration by IL-1 and tumour necrosis factor. *J Immunol* **141**: 1670–1677.

Schnyder JT & Dinarello CA (1987) Human monocyte or recombinant interleukin 1's are specific for the secretion of a metalloproteinase from chondrocytes. *J Immunol* **138**: 496–503.

Schroder JM, Sticherling M, Henneicke HH, Preissner WC & Christophers E (1990) IL-1α or tumour necrosis factor α stimulate release of three NAP-1/IL-8 related neutrophil chemotactic proteins in human dermal fibroblasts. *J Immunol* **144**: 2223–2232.

Schwab JH, Anderle SK, Brown RR, Dalldorf FG & Thompson RC (1991) Pro- and anti-inflammatory roles of interleukin-1 in recurrence of bacterial cell wall-induced arthritis. *Infect Immunit* **59**: 4436–4442.

Schwab JH, Brown RR, Anderle SK & Schlievert PM (1993) Superantigen can reactivate bacterial cell wall-induced arthritis. *J Immunol* **150**: 4151–4159.

Schweizer A, Feige U, Fontana A, Müller K & Dinarello CA (1988) Interleukin-1 enhances pain reflexes. Mediation through increased prostaglandin E2 levels. *Agents Actions* **25**: 248–251.

Sherry B, Jue D-M, Zentella A & Cerami A (1990) Characterization of high molecular weight glycosylated forms of murine tumour necrosis factor. *Biochem Biophys Res Comm* **173**: 1072–1078.

Shull MM, Ormsby I, Kier AB, Pawlowski S, Diebold RJ, Yin M, Allen R, Sidman C, Proetzel G, Calvin D, Annunziata N & Doetschman T (1992) Targeted disruption of the mouse transforming growth factor-β1 gene results in multifocal inflammatory disease. *Nature* **359**: 693–699.

Staite N, Richard KA, Aspar DG, Franz KA, Galinet LA & Dunn CJ (1990) Induction of an acute erosive monoarticular arthritis in mice with interleukin-1 and methylated bovine serum albumin. *Arthritis Rheum* **33**: 253–260.

Stimpson SA, Dalldorf FG, Otterness IG & Schwab JH (1988a) Exacerbation of arthritis by IL-1 in rat joints previously injured by peptidoglycan-polysaccharide. *J Immunol* **140**: 2964–2969.

Stimpson SA, Dalldorf FG, Otterness IG & Schwab JH (1988b) Pain and reactivation of arthritis induced by recombinant cytokines in rat ankles previously injured by peptidoglycan-polysaccharide. *Arthritis Rheum* **31**: S49.

Stimpson SA, Patterson DL, Eastin C & Noel LS (1990) Inflammation induced in rats by intraarticular injection of platelet-derived growth factor. *Prog Leuk Biol* **105**: 93–98.

Stitt JT (1991) Differential sensitivity in the sites of fever production by prostaglandin E1 within the hypothalamus of the rat. *J Physiol* **432**: 99–110.

Suematsu S, Matsuda T, Aozasa K, Akira S, Nakano N, Ohno S et al. (1989) IgG1 plasmacytosis in interleukin 6 transgenic mice. *Proc Natl Acad Sci USA* **86**: 7547–7551.

Suzuki K, Enghild JJ, Morodomi T, Salvesen G & Nagase H (1990) Mechanisms of activation of tissue procollagenase by matrix metalloproteinase 3 (stromelysin). *Biochemistry* **29**: 5783–5789.

Takai Y, Seki N, Senoh H, Yokota T, Lee F, Hamaoka T et al. (1989) Enhanced production of interleukin-6 in mice with type II collagen-induced arthritis. *Arthritis Rheum* **32**: 594–600.

Tartaglia LA, Weber RF, Figfari IS, Reynolds C, Palladino MA Jr & Goeddel DV (1991) The two different receptors for tumour necrosis factor mediate distinct cellular responses. *Proc Natl Acad Sci USA* **88**: 9292–9296.

Tepper RI, Levinson DA, Stanger BZ, Campos-Torres J, Abbas AK & Leder P (1990) IL-4 induces allergic-like inflammatory disease and alters T cell development in transgenic mice. *Cell* **62**: 457–467.

Turksen K, Kupper T, Degenstein L, Williams I & Fuchs E (1992) Interleukin 6: Insights to its function in skin by overexpression in transgenic mice. *Proc Natl Acad Sci USA* **89**: 5068–5072.

van Beuning HM, Arntz OJ & van den Berg WB (1991) *In vivo* effects of interleukin-1 on articular cartilage. Prolongation of proteoglycan metabolic disturbances in old mice. *Arthritis Rheum* **34**: 606–615.

van Beuning HM, van der Kraan PM, Arntz OJ & van den Berg WB (1993) Protection from interleukin-1-induced destruction of articular cartilage by transforming growth factor β: studies in anatomically intact cartilage *in vitro* and *in vivo*. *Ann Rheum Dis* **52**: 185–191.

van Beuning HM, van der Kraan PM, Arntz OJ & van den Berg WB (1993) Does TBGβ protect articular cartilage *in vivo*. In van den Berg WB (ed) *Joint Destruction in Osteoarthritis*, pp 127–131. Basel: Birkhauser Verlag.

van de Loo AAJ & van den Berg WB (1990) Effects of murine recombinant interleukin 1 on synovial joints in mice: measurement of patellar cartilage metabolism and joint inflammation. *Ann Rheum Dis* **49**: 238–245.

van de Loo AAJ, Arntz OJ & van den Berg WB (1992) Flare-up of experimental arthritis in mice with murine recombinant IL-1. *Clin Exp Immunol* **87**: 196–202.

van de Loo FAJ, Arntz OJ, Otterness IG & van den Berg WB (1992) Protection against cartilage proteoglycan synthesis inhibition by antileukin 1 antibodies in experimental arthritis. *J Rheumatol* **19**: 348–356.

van de Loo FAJ, Artnz OJ, Otterness IG & van den Berg WB (1993) Modulation of cartilage destruction in murine arthritis with anti-IL-1 antibodies. *Agents Actions* **39**: C211–C214.

van de Loo AAJ, Arntz OJ, Otterness IG & van den Berg WB (1994) Proteoglycan loss and subsequent replenishment of murine cartilage after a mild arthritic insult by IL-1 *in vivo*. *Agents Actions* **41**: 200–208.

van den Berg WB, Kruijsen MWM & van de Putte LBA (1982) The mouse patellae assay. An easy method of quantitating articular cartilage function *in vivo* and *in vitro*. *Rheumatol Int* **1**: 165–169.

van den Berg WB, van de Loo FAJ, Zwarts WA & Otterness IG (1988) Effects of murine recombinant interleukin 1 on intact homologous articular cartilage: a quantitative and autoradiographic study. *Ann Rheum Dis* **47**: 855–863.

van den Berg WB, van de Loo FAJ, van Lent PLEM & Joosten LAB (1993) Mechanisms of cartilage destruction in joint inflammation. In van den Berg WB (ed) *Joint Destruction in Osteoarthritis*, pp 49–60. Basel: Birkhauser Verlag.

van den Berg WB, Joosten LAB, Helsen M & van de Loo FAJ (1994) Amelioration of established murine collagen induced arthritis wth anti-IL-1 treatment. *Clin Exp Immunol* **95**: 237–243.

van Lent PLEM, van de Loo AAJ, van den Bersselaar LAM & van den Berg WB (1991) Chondrocyte nonresponsiveness of arthritic articular cartilage caused by short term immobilization. *J Rheumatol* **18**: 709–715.

van Lent PLEM, van den Bersselaar LAM, van den Hoek AEM, van de Loo AAJ, & van den Berg WB (1992) Cationic immune complex arthritis in mice, a new model: synergistic effect of complement and IL-1. *Am J Pathol* **140**: 1451–1461.

van Lent PL, van den Hoek AE, van den Bersselaar LA, van de Loo FAJ, Eykholt HE, Brouwer WF et al. (1994) Early cartilage degradation in cationic immune complex arthritis in mice: relative role of interleukin 1, the polymorphonclear cell (PMN) and PMN elastase. *J Rheumatol* **21**: 321–329.

van Noorden CJF, Smith RE & Rasnick D (1988) Cysteine proteinase activity in arthritic rat knee joints and the effects of a selective systemic inhibitor, Z-Phe-AlaCH$_2$F. *J Rheumatol* **15**: 1525–1535.

van Osch GJ, van der Kraan PM & van den Berg WB (1993) *In vivo* quantification of proteoglyan synthesis in articular cartilage of different topographical areas in murine knee joint. *J Orthop Res* **11**: 492–499.

Vivian B, David P, Iancu F, Yoau S, Elimelech O, Peter Y et al. (1992) The M20-IL-1 inhibitor prevents onset of adjuvant arthritis. *Biotherapy* **4**: 317–323.

Williams RO, Feldmann M & Maini RN (1991) Anti-tumour necrosis factor ameliorates joint disease in murine collagen-induced arthritis. *Proc Natl Acad Sci USA* **89**: 9784–9788.

Woessner JF (1991) Matrix metalloproteinases and their inhibitors in connective tissue remodelling. *FASEB J* **5**: 2145–2154.

Woodroffe C, Müller W & Rüther U (1992) Long-term consequences of interleukin-6 expression in transgenic mice. *DNA Cell Biol* **11**: 587–592.

Wooley PH, Whalen JD, Chapman DL, Berger AE, Richard KD, Aspar DG et al. (1993) The effect of an interleukin-1 receptor antagonist protein on type II collagen-induced arthritis and antigen-induced arthritis in mice. *Arthritis Rheum* **36**: 1305–1314.

Wu J, Lark MW, Chun LE & Eyre DR (1991) Sites of cleavage in collagen types II, IX, X and XI of cartilage. *J Biol Chem* **266**: 5625–5628.

Yoshimura T, Matsushima K, Tanaka S, Robinson EA, Appela E, Oppenheim JJ et al. (1987) Purification of a human monocyte-derived neutrophil chemotactic factor that has peptide sequence similarity to other host defense cytokines. *Proc Natl Acad Sci USA* **84**: 9233–9237.

27 Transgenic Animals in Rheumatoid Arthritis Research

Stephen Harris

INTRODUCTION

Since the mid-1980s several technologies have emerged that allow the production of transgenic animals – that is, organisms with a stable modification of genotype as a result of a defined genetic manipulation (Palmiter and Brinster, 1986; Jaenisch, 1988). This capability has provided the opportunity to investigate systematically the molecular mechanisms underlying a large number of fundamental biological processes in the context of the whole animal (Hanahan, 1989). In the past decade the widespread use of these technologies has resulted in significant advances being made in our understanding in areas such as gene structure and function, genome organization, mammalian development, immunobiology and the pathophysiology of many human diseases.

The complex nature of the immune system makes *ex vivo* study difficult. Transgenic animals can therefore contribute significantly to our present understanding of the development and functionality of the immune system specifically because the consequences of any genetic modification such as gene addition, deletion or subtle change can be evaluated within the context of the whole animal (Morahan, 1991; Fung-Leung and Mak, 1992; Mellor, 1992).

While the pathology associated with rheumatoid arthritis (RA) in man has been described in some detail, the factors that contribute to the initiation, establishment and progression of what many consider to be an autoimmune-based condition remain largely obscure (Harris, 1990; Mannik, 1992; Wordsworth, 1992; Sewell and Trentham, 1993). The generally accepted working hypothesis is that the progressive immune system dysfunction is triggered by exposure of immunologically susceptible individuals to antigenic stimuli. Currently, more is known about the immunogenetic component of RA than possible causative agents, whether endogenous or exogenous.

As documented elsewhere in this volume, there are several experimental animal models that exhibit some feature of the human condition RA. Many groups have also exploited established transgenic technologies to generate transgenic animals which either (a) exhibit a spontaneous autoimmunity in a particular organ, or (b) 'rescue' an established genetic susceptibility to develop autoimmunity (Hanahan, 1990; Lee and Sarvetnick, 1992). Some of these transgenic animals exhibit pathologies that resemble RA (see below; Hammer *et al.*, 1990; Iwakura *et al.*, 1991; Keffer *et al.*, 1991; Shiozawa *et al.*, 1992). These animals can therefore be employed to investigate the mechanism underlying the pathobiology of RA and thereby ultimately provide insights into novel forms of therapy.

An understanding of the relative strengths and weaknesses of the different

Mechanisms and Models in Rheumatoid Arthritis
ISBN 0–12–340440–1

approaches to generating transgenics is an essential prerequisite for their successful application to the understanding of complex biological questions. The main methodologies are therefore described before discussion of some specific examples of transgenic animals which provide insights into the pathobiology of RA.

PRODUCTION OF TRANSGENIC ANIMALS

The generation of transgenic animals requires the successful co-ordination of a series of mutually interdependent disciplines including embryology, animal husbandry and molecular biology skills (Hogan *et al.*, 1986). The methology chosen will depend on the nature of the biological question being addressed and the relative merits and limitations of the different techniques. The principal features of the dominant methods by which transgenic animals are currently produced are outlined below.

PRONUCLEAR DNA MICROINJECTION

The most widespread method by which transgenic animals are generated is by pronuclear DNA microinjection (Fig. 1; Gordon and Ruddle, 1981). This is technically the least demanding method that can be employed in a large number of different species, including commercially important animals such as the pig, goat, sheep and cattle. The efficiency with which transgenics are generated varies considerably between species; that is, from between 2–5% (eggs injected and transferred/transgenics identified) in mice to ≤1% in domestic animals. This probably reflects the various technical demands encountered in the different species (Clark *et al.*, 1992). While the precise behaviour of any particular transgene can never be predicted, a number of general principles have emerged from observing the organization and expression pattern of the many constructs employed to generate transgenics.

The size, complexity and species of origin of the DNA used in the production of transgene constructs can be varied considerably. However, very large DNA fragments, for example, YACS (Schedl *et al.*, 1992, 1993) and even chromosomal fragments (Richa and Lo, 1989), require careful manipulation if the physical integrity of transgene DNA is to be retained. While transgene copy number can vary significantly, most transgenics contain multiple copies of the transgene integrated at a single site within the genome, usually as a head-to-tail tandem array (Bishop and Smith, 1989). In general, a transgene array is transmitted in a stable Mendelian fashion to all subsequent generations; however, a proportion of founder animals are chimaeric and some of these never transmit the transgene (Whitelaw *et al.*, 1993).

The expression of a transgene can vary significantly between different transgenic lines due to variable transgene copy number and/or the genomic context at the integration site (i.e. the influence of flanking genomic sequences at different integration sites). The exceptions to these general observations have provided significant insights into how mammalian genomes are organized and gene expression is regulated. The first transgenes to exhibit copy number dependent expression, irrespective of integration site, led to the definition of a novel structural feature present within the genome – that is, the dominant locus control region (Grosveld *et al.*, 1987; Greaves *et al.*, 1989; Bonfier *et al.*, 1990). Similarly, transgenic lines that show variable patterns of transgene expression dependent on the mode of inheritance (i.e. on transmission

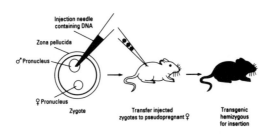

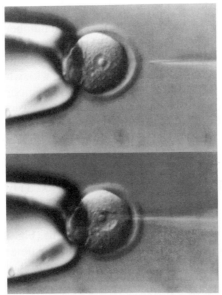

Figure 1. Generation of transgenic mice by microinjection. Top, zygotes isolated from donor females are microinjected with ≈100–200 copies of the transgene DNA fragment. Surviving zygotes are returned to the oviduct of a 0.5-day pseudopregnant female. Of the animals born, 10–30% should be transgenic. Bottom, the zygote (middle) is held in place by the holding pipette (left) ready for insertion of the injection pipette (right) into the pronucleus (top). Successful injection of the DNA containing solution into the pronucleus is indicated by a swelling of the nucleus (bottom). From Sedivy and Joyner (1992), with permission.

through the male or female gametes) are providing insights into how genomic imprinting is established and subsequently influences gene expression (DeChiara *et al.*, 1991; Reik, 1992).

In a significant proportion of cases, the transgene integration event results in an adverse recessive mutation that only becomes apparent when breeding experiments designed to generate animals homozygous for the transgene give rise to non-viable, often embryonic lethal, offspring. However, these insertional mutation events constitute a novel source of genetic variation that can be exploited to help define the role of endogenous genes in normal mouse development (Gridley *et al.*, 1987; Meisler, 1992).

Pronuclear DNA microinjection results in a genetic 'gain-of-function' (Merlino, 1991). This approach has been widely and successfully employed to explore the DNA sequences that determine the normal spatial, temporal and developmental regulation of many genes. Moreover, chimaeric transgenes (i.e. cDNA or a genomic coding region regulated by a heterologous promoter) have been extensively used to investigate the consequences of aberrant gene expression; either within the normal context of the gene or at ectopic sites (Cuthbertson and Klintworth, 1988). Other applications include either constitutive or conditional transgene specified cellular ablation (Breitmann and Bernstein, 1992) and the disruption or down-regulation of endogenous gene function using transgene encoded dominant negative (protein) or antisense RNA products (Sharp and Mullins, 1993). However, the ability to target a gene via homologous recombination in embryonic stem (ES) cells is in most instances likely to prove the more popular method for down-regulating gene function (see below).

A common problem encountered in the design phase of transgenic experiments involving pronuclear DNA microinjection is the limited number of fully characterized promoter/enhancer sequences available and, in particular, the absence of a tightly regulated conditional gene expression system. While the number of promoters is steadily increasing, this limitation restricts the precision with which a transgene can be targeted to a specific organ, tissue or cell type and the temporal control the investigator has over transgene expression. Another difficulty occasionally encountered is a transmission problem due to *in utero* lethality or impaired fertility as a consequence of transgene expression. At present, this can only be overcome using the binary transgenic approach (Ornitz *et al.*, 1991).

BLASTOCYST MICROINJECTION OF EMBRYONIC STEM (ES) CELLS

The other principal route by which transgenics are currently being generated involves gene targeting via homologous recombination in ES cells (Fig. 2; Kuehn *et al.*, 1987). This approach is critically dependent on the ability to isolate and manipulate *in vitro* pluripotent stem cells that retain the ability to contribute to the germline of a founder chimaeric animal after being returned to the embryonic environment. While pluripotent stem cells can readily be derived from the mouse; from either the inner cell mass of the blastocyst (ES cells; Evans and Kaufman, 1981; Martin, 1981) or the germinal ridge of the embryo (primordial germ cells or 'EG' cells; Matsui *et al.*, 1992; Resnick *et al.*, 1992), it is very important that the 'quality' of these cell lines be monitored. This is due to their tendency to lose the ability to contribute to the germline during extended periods of *in vitro* culture (see Bradley *et al.*, 1992).

The ability to culture pluripotent stem cells allows *in vitro* selection of those cells that have undergone a rare genetic manipulation of an endogenous gene (i.e. gene targeting via homologous recombination; Waldman, 1992). Two types of gene targeting construct are commonly employed: the sequence replacement or Ω-type; which results in sequence exchange, probably via a double cross-over event, and the sequence insertion or O-type; which results in a duplication of endogenous gene sequences, probably via a single crossover event (Fig. 3; Capecchi, 1989). Most gene-targeting experiments giving rise to 'knock-out' transgenic mice utilize sequence replacement protocols. However, sequence insertion type constructs are likely to become increasingly popular as these can be exploited to incorporate very subtle

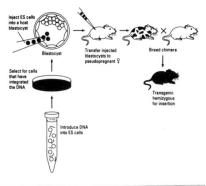

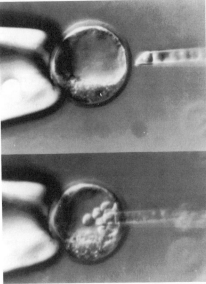

Figure 2. Generation of transgenic mice by gene targeting in ES cells. Top, DNA is introduced into ES cells by electroporation and those that incorporate and express the exogenous DNA are expanded on selective medium. Clones that have undergone gene targeting by homologous recombination are microinjected into recipient blastocysts which are then implanted into a 2.5-day pseudopregnant female. Chimaeric animals are bred to give rise to hemizygous transgenic offspring which are subsequently inbred to generate transgenic animals homozygous for the desired genetic modification. Bottom, the blastocyst (middle) is positioned on the holding pipette (left) ready for injection of ES cells (top). The inner cell mass can be seen at the base of the blastocyst. 15–20 ES cells are expelled from the microinjection pipette (right) into the blastocoel cavity (bottom). From Sedivy and Joyner (1992), with permission.

modifications into the endogenous target gene (Hasty *et al.*, 1991; Valencius and Smithies, 1991).

The generation of gene 'knock-out' transgenics is proving an increasingly popular method of gaining an insight into the *in vivo* significance of specific genes and/or their regulatory DNA sequences in areas such as oncology, neurobiology and immunology (e.g. Donehower *et al.*, 1992; Lee *et al.*, 1992; Mombaerts *et al.*, 1992; Shull *et al.*, 1992; Gruby *et al.*, 1993; Kopf *et al.*, 1993; Viville *et al.*, 1993). Investigators are also

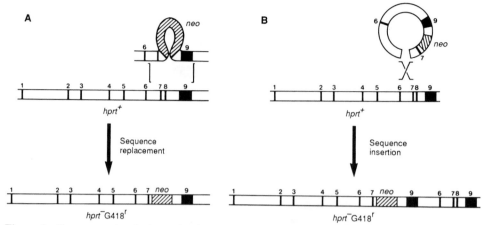

Figure 3. Gene targeting by homologous recombination. A schematic representation of the hypoxanthine phosphoribosyl transferase (*hprt*) gene is shown before (top) and after (bottom) being targeted by a sequence replacement (A) or sequence insertion (B) vector. Both targeting vectors contain sequences homologous to the *hprt* gene with the *neo* gene interrupting the homology in exon 8. Recombination results in either (A) replacement of endogenous sequences by those from the targeting vector, or (B) insertion of the vector sequences into the endogenous gene, resulting in a duplication of a portion of the gene. In this case, concomitant insertion of *neo* and disruption of *hprt* provides very effective enrichment for correctly targeted clones. For non-selectable target genes alternative enrichment or screening protocols have been developed. From Capecchi (1989), with permission.

exploiting gene targeting to validate or elucidate the role of specific genes during development (Joyner *et al.*, 1989, 1991) and to identify novel genes, using enhancer- or gene-trap based protocols (Friedrich and Soriano, 1991; Joyner, 1991; Beddington, 1992). Moreover, the validation of candidate genes implicated in human genetic disease by generating 'knock-out' transgenic models is providing the opportunity to perform preclinical testing of gene therapy protocols that could potentially have a major impact on the clinical treatment of many common human genetic disorders, for example Hyde *et al.* (1993).

The manipulation of an endogenous gene by homologous recombination in ES cells represents a genetic 'loss-' or 'modification-of-function'. However, 'gain-of-function' transgenics can also be generated using the ES cells route, as exemplified by the recent introduction of yeast artificial chromosome (YAC) clones into the mouse germline (Choi *et al.*, 1993; Jakobovits *et al.*, 1993; Strauss *et al.*, 1993). The outcome of a gene-targeting experiment, while always likely to be interesting and informative, may not always be straightforward to interpret (Davis and Bradley, 1993). Furthermore, one common criticism of gene-targeting experiments to generate 'knock-out' animals is: can the phenotype of an animal lacking a particular gene since conception be considered equivalent to an animal in which the gene has become functionally inactive since birth? In many cases this issue will only be resolved after extensive detailed analysis or once conditional gene inactivation protocols are available.

At present, the major limitation to gene targeting in a species other than the mouse is the absence of pluripotent ES-like cells. While several groups have described the isolation and culture of putative ES-like cells from other species (Handyside *et al.*,

1987; Doetschman *et al.*, 1988; Notarianni *et al.*, 1990; Piedrahita *et al.*, 1990; Saito *et al.*, 1992) germline transmission has yet to be formally demonstrated. In poultry, germline transmission of genetically modified primordial germ cells (PGCs) has been achieved (Vick *et al.*, 1993); however, gene-targeting experiments await successful *in vitro* culture of these PGCs.

OTHER APPROACHES

The first demonstration of germline transmission of an exogenously applied DNA sequence was achieved when mouse embryos were exposed to retrovirus (Jaenisch, 1976). While retroviruses are efficient delivery systems ideally suited for certain applications (e.g. transduction of dividing somatic cells) this approach has not been widely employed to generate mammalian transgenics. However, this is one of a number of approaches that has proved useful in poultry (see Clark *et al.*, 1992). An initial observation that a simple sperm-mediated DNA delivery protocol (Lavitrano *et al.*, 1989) could be employed to generated mouse transgenics caused a great deal of excitement; however, this observation has failed to be substantiated in a number of laboratories (Brinster *et al.*, 1989).

APPLICATION OF TRANSGENIC ANIMALS

The ability to manipulate the mammalian genome has provided exciting opportunities for basic and applied research in both academic and commercial environments. Some applications of the technology are described below.

GENE EXPRESSION AND GENOME ORGANIZATION

Transgenic animals have been used extensively to investigate the relationship between gene structure, expression and regulation (Palmiter and Brinster, 1986; Jaenisch, 1988). The *cis*-acting DNA sequences required to confer correct temporal, spatial and developmental patterns of expression have been identified for a variety of genes in many different tissues. The evidence for the *in vivo* importance of DNA sequence motifs such as enhancers, introns and locus control regions continues to grow as does our understanding of the mechanisms that underlie epigenetic phenomena such as genomic imprinting (Brinster *et al.*, 1988; Palmiter *et al.*, 1991; Reik, 1992; Sippel *et al.*, 1992).

DEVELOPMENTAL BIOLOGY

The ability to manipulate directly the mammalian genome provides tremendous opportunities for those interested in understanding the genetic and cellular basis of development and pattern formation. Access to an increasing number of novel developmental mutants in the mouse can be anticipated as a direct, or indirect, consequence of transgenic methodology. For example, transgene specified cell ablation (Palmiter *et al.*, 1987; Behringer *et al.*, 1988; Borelli *et al.*, 1989; Breitman *et al.*, 1990; Breitman and Bernstein, 1992) and the deletion (Le Mouellic *et al.*, 1992; Chisaka and

Capecchi, 1991; Chisaka *et al.*, 1992) or ectopic expression (Wolgemuth *et al.*, 1989; Kessel *et al.*, 1990) of candidate genes involved in pattern formation have been employed to investigate cell lineage relationships and the principles of positional information in the mouse, respectively. Random transgene insertional mutation events provide access to genes that exhibit novel phenotypes. More importantly, enhancer- or gene-trap protocols can be used to systematically identify novel genetic loci expressed at different stages of development and, ultimately, produce homozygous knock-out mice to identify and investigate the consequences of any *in vivo* mutant phenotype (Friedrich and Soriano, 1991; Joyner, 1991; Korn *et al.*, 1992; Beddington, 1992).

DISEASE MODELS

Many transgenics have resulted, either fortuitously or by design, in phenotypes in rodents that resemble a human disease state; for example, hypertension, atherosclerosis, inflammation, cancer, immune deficiencies, etc. Many of these models are the result of inappropriate expression of a 'normal' transgene product, either in the usual tissue or ectopically (e.g. Hanahan, 1988; Berns *et al.*, 1989). Dominant negative transgene products (i.e. those that disrupt normal function at the level of protein–protein interaction: Herskowitz, 1987; Stacey *et al.*, 1988); or antisense transgenes, that inhibit endogenous gene expression at the RNA level, can also be utilized to generate human disease models (Katsuki *et al.*, 1988; Munir *et al.*, 1990; Pepin *et al.*, 1992). Gene targeting via homologous recombination in ES cells is contributing significantly to the production of transgenic animal models, particularly human genetic disorders (e.g. Collins and Wilson, 1992; Silva *et al.*, 1992a, b; Tybulewicz *et al.*, 1992). These transgenic animal models provide tremendous opportunities to gain a better understanding of the mechanisms involved in the pathogenesis of a disease. They can also be used to validate novel therapeutic targets and to test both conventional pharmaceuticals and novel gene therapy protocols, for example, Hyde *et al.* (1993).

COMMERCIAL EXPLOITATION OF TRANSGENIC TECHNOLOGY

Unlike traditional animal breeding methods transgenic technology provides the opportunity to cross species barriers; that is, to sample and exploit traits outside the normal gene pool. Several groups have successfully utilized pronuclear DNA microinjection to attempt to manipulate the performance of commercially important species, including rabbit (Knight *et al.*, 1988; Riego *et al.*, 1993), pig (Hamer *et al.*, 1985), sheep (Wright *et al.*, 1991), goat (Ebert *et al.*, 1991), cattle (Krimpenfort *et al.*, 1991), poultry (Perry and Sang, 1993; Simkiss, 1993) and fish (Tewari *et al.*, 1992; Moav *et al.*, 1993). These include attempts to (a) improve the overall growth rate, by manipulating the hormones involved in growth; (b) improve meat quality, by increasing the lean meat/fat ratio; (c) enhance the commercial value of milk or wool by altering their composition; (d) increase feed efficiency on low-quality diets by altering intestinal metabolism; and (e) reduce susceptibility to disease by introduction of transgenes encoding disease resistance (for additional references and reviews, see Clark *et al.*, 1992).

ARTHRITIS IN TRANSGENIC RODENTS

RA is a relatively common chronic inflammatory disorder involving the progressive destruction of the cartilage and bone in the joints (Harris, 1990; Wordsworth, 1992; Chapters 1 and 2, this volume). While the aetiology of RA is largely unknown it is generally believed to be an autoimmune-based disease that occurs in genetically susceptible individuals following exposure to some exogenous or endogenous immunological challenge. As described elsewhere in this volume, significant insights into the biological mechanisms underlying autoimmunity and RA have been obtained from experimental animal models, though it has been argued that none of these reflects the full complexity of the human disease (Kaklamanis, 1992).

Many groups have exploited transgenic methodology to examine factors that may be involved in the initiation, progression or reversal of autoimmunity in a number of model organ systems (see Lee and Sarvetnick, 1992). Furthermore, some have generated transgenic animals that exhibit a spontaneous or predictable onset of a pathology of the joints that resembles RA. These transgenic animals may therefore provide useful models in which to further investigate the complex pathobiology of this disease. These examples are described below.

MHC MEDIATED ARTHRITIS

Several lines of genetic evidence have highlighted the probable involvement of genes within the MHC complex in the susceptibility of individuals to develop autoimmune disease. One such example is the significant association that exists between a cluster of interrelated rheumatic disorders, including reactive arthritis in the joints, and the class 1 MHC allele HLA-B27. All attempts to validate this association between human HLA-B27 and rheumatic disease in transgenic mice have so far been unsuccessful. However, Hammer *et al.* (1990) observe a spontaneous multi-organ chronic inflammation in transgenic rats co-expressing human β_2-microglobulin and this MHC allele which includes damage to peripheral and axial joints.

The spontaneous swelling, erythema and tenderness in the hindlimb joints of these animals lasts for several days or weeks and in some cases can be recurrent (Fig. 4a). On histological examination of the joints the synovium was found to be hyperplastic, oedematous and infiltrated by inflammatory cells. Pannus formation and destruction of articular cartilage and bone was also observed (Fig. 4b). Despite this extensive damage the mobility of the joint is retained on resolution of the inflammation. The lesions are similar to those observed in RA and more destructive than those seen in human B27-associated peripheral arthritis. The penetrance of the multi-organ inflammatory disease seen in these transgenic rats appears to correlate with the level of HLA-B27 expressed in the lymphoid tissue, though no further comment on joint associated disease has been presented (Taurog *et al.*, 1993). The failure to observe equivalent pathology in transgenic mice expressing HLA-B27 can be interpreted to reflect either (a) the failure to exceed the required threshold of HLA-B27 expression

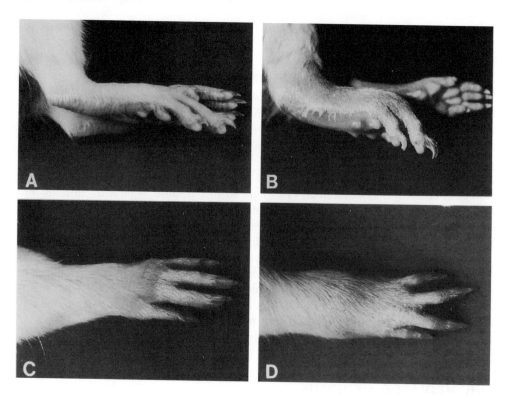

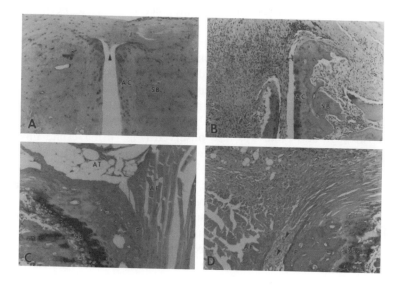

in the mice, or (b) species differences in the genetic susceptibility to HLA-B27 induced inflammation and autoimmunity.

VIRAL-MEDIATED DISEASE

Various exogenous aetiological agents have been implicated as possible mediators of RA in humans; including bacteria, mycoplasma and viruses (as described in Chapters 3 and 21, this volume). In support of this premise Iwakura *et al.* (1991) have described a chronic arthritis in transgenic mice containing a portion of the HTLV-1 genome.

In these animals transgene expression can be detected in a number of tissues although the only spontaneous pathology that develops involves the ankle joints. This occurs at age 2–3 and 5–10 months in females and males, respectively. Histological examination of the affected joints reveals extensive erosion of the bone and cartilage, pannus formation and an inflammatory infiltrate that occasionally extends into the tissue surrounding the joint. All of these changes resemble RA in humans. The incidence of the joint lesions correlates with transgene specific mRNA levels some 5–10 times higher in affected compared to unaffected transgenic animals. In a smaller number of transgenic animals they also detect rheumatoid factor, antibodies directed against both ss and dsDNA and, more recently, an increase in the proportion of the agalactosylated form of serum IgG (Endo *et al.*, 1993). While the authors propose several explanations for this phenotype, a more detailed analysis of the pathobiology of the joints and the associated immunological changes is required before the mechanism by which this HTLV-1 transgene mediates arthritis can be determined.

CYTOKINE-MEDIATED ARTHRITIS

As reagents have become available to investigate the inflammatory infiltrate in the joints of RA patients it has become increasingly apparent that aberrant expression of the cytokines that mediate immune and inflammatory function may, at least in part, contribute to the pathology of RA (Brennan and Feldman, 1992; also Chapter 2, this volume). Significant evidence for a direct causative involvement of a cytokine in RA is presented by Keffer *et al.* (1991).

Figure 4. Gross pathology and histopathology in peripheral and axial joints of B27/hβ_2m transgenic rats. Top, swelling and erythrema observed in distal hindlimb (B) and distal forelimb (D) of male transgenic rats at 6 and 4 months old, respectively. Normal distal hindlimb (A) and forelimb (C) from non-transgenic LEW rats, 3–6 months old. Bottom, peripheral and axial joint histopathology. Normal tarsal joint (A) and tail intervertebral joint (C) from nontransgenic LEW rats, 3–6 months old. Synovium (arrowhead), articular cartilage (AC), subchrondral bone (SB), joint capsule (J), annulus fibrosus (AF), vertebral endplate (P), ossification centre of subchondral bone (SB), and periarticular adipose tissue (AT) are labelled. (B) Tarsal joint from transgenic male (shown Top, D) showing chronic arthritis. There is a marked inflammatory infiltrate in the joint capsule and synovium, with pannus (asterisks) eroding articular cartilage and subchondral bone. (D) Tail intervertebral joint from transgenic male (shown Top, D), orientated as mirror image of (C), showing expansion of periarticular connective tissue by mononuclear inflammation and fibrosis (asterisks), invading and disrupting the attachment of the outer layers of the annulus to the vertebral end plate (arrowhead). From Hammer *et al.* (1990), with permission.

This group have generated several lines of transgenic mice containing the human tumour necrosis factor-α (hTNFα) gene with a modified 3′ non-translated region. Swelling of the ankles, impaired movement and chronic inflammatory polyarthritis are the principal abnormalities observed in the animals that express this transgene. Histological examination of affected joints reveals progressive, age related, evidence for synovial hyperplasia; inflammatory cell infiltration, pannus formation and the erosion of cartilage and bone. *In situ* hybridization reveals that the synovial cells of the joint constitute a major source of hTNFα production, suggesting a possible paracrine or autocrine mode of action.

Strong evidence for a central causative role of this cytokine in the pathogenesis of the disease in these animals is that the predictable onset of arthritis, which occurs at 3–4 weeks of age, can be blocked by the *in vivo* administration of monoclonal antibody to hTNFα (Fig. 5). However, it is likely that other local immunological factors are involved as TNFα expression does not elicit an autoimmune response in other organs; for example, Picarella *et al.* (1993) failed to observe any autoimmune destruction of pancreatic islets, even in the presence of an inflammatory infiltrate, in transgenic animals expressing murine TNFα from the insulin-promoter. Moreover, while Probert *et al.* (1993) observe wasting, ischaemia and lymphoid abnormalities in mice expressing hTNFα transgenes systemically (in their T-cell compartment) they report no joint pathology, again suggesting that localized ectopic production of hTNFα is the critical trigger of the joint pathology observed in these animals.

While the precise mechanism by which the deregulated expression of the hTNFα transgene mediates arthritis remains to be established the transgenic animals described by Keffer *et al.* (1991) represent the first predictive genetic model of RA in which novel therapeutic agents with a specific modality (i.e. functional antagonism of hTNFα action) could be tested (see Brennan *et al.*, 1992). This model is particularly important given the reported clinical benefit of neutralizing TNFα in RA patients reported in Chapter 2, this volume, by Maini and coworkers.

DESTRUCTIVE ARTHRITIS IN THE APPARENT ABSENCE OF AN INFLAMMATORY INFILTRATE

Evidence that localized destruction of cartilage and bone may occur in the absence of an inflammatory infiltration has been obtained by Shiozawa *et al.* (1992). They have established transgenic animals that display widespread constitutive expression of the murine c-fos gene from a MHC class I promoter (H-2K^b). These c-fos[+] trangenics are essentially normal except that they fail to raise antigen-specific IgG antibodies when challenged. They also do not develop any spontaneous arthritic abnormalities. In order to establish any role for antigen-specific IgG antibodies in the pathogenesis of arthritis Shiozawa *et al.* (1992) proceeded to generate an experimentally induced

Figure 5. Suppression of arthritis in monoclonal antibody treated Tg197 mice. Sections through the knee joints of normal (top), monoclonal antibody treated Tg197 progeny (middle) and non-treated Tg197 progeny (bottom). Thickening of the synovial layer (arrowheads) is effectively suppressed in the antibody treated transgenic mice. From Keffer *et al.* (1991), with permission.

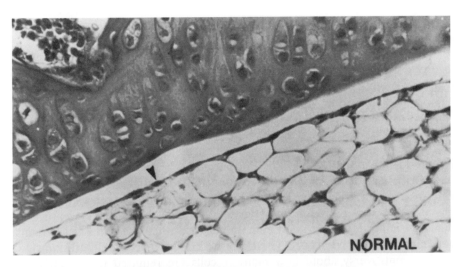

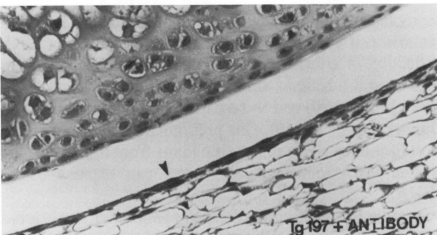

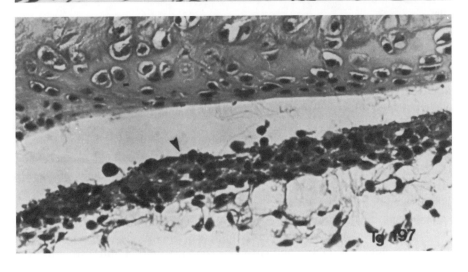

arthritis by intra-articular injection of ovalbumin into hyperimmunized transgenic (c-fos$^+$) and non-transgenic (c-fos$^-$) animals.

They observe a similar degree of destructive arthritis in both experimental groups. However, the damage in the transgenic c-fos$^+$ animals occurs in the apparent absence of a lymphocyte infiltrate. *In vitro* evidence is presented that the damage in the joint *in vivo* may, in part at least, be due to an alteration in the cartilage invasiveness of c-fos$^+$ cells derived from the activated synovium. They conclude that the experimentally induced arthritis in these transgenic animals is capable of being mediated by a localized, c-fos$^+$ expressing, antigen-activated, mesenchymal-derived population of cells normally resident within the synovium. Furthermore, they propose the normal role of antigen-specific IgG antibodies is to facilitate the recruitment of the lymphocyte infiltrate to an arthritic joint, at least in this experimental transgenic model. These animals may therefore represent an opportunity to investigate the very earliest pre-inflammatory infiltrate phase of autoimmune disease when the initial tissue damage and autoimmune dysfunction becomes established. This model is of interest in view of the current controversy about how many T cells are required to perpetuate RA (discussed in Chapters 2, 3 and 4, this volume).

While studying the involvement of deregulated expression of MHC molecules in a model of central nervous system (CNS) demyelination, Yoshioka *et al.* (1991) also observed physical tissue damage reminiscent of autoimmune disease in the apparent absence of any inflammatory infiltrate. In this case, ectopic expression of a syngeneic MHC class-I molecule was targeted specifically to the oligodendrocytes of the CNS using the myelin basic protein promoter. Expression of the transgene in the first few weeks after birth results in physical tremors, tonic seizures and death, in up to 50% of animals, due to an active demyelination. Those animals that survive this stage display evidence of hypomyelination. Due to the time of onset of the pathology they dismiss any significant autoimmune involvement in these animals; however, they also suggest the failure to observe any subsequent immune infiltrate could be due to the C57BL/6 genetic background. While the mechanism responsible for this phenotype remains to be elucidated they propose this model may closely resemble the initial events in virally induced CNS demyelination, prior to a secondary inflammatory response to auto-antigens.

GENE TARGETING AND RA

To date no gene-targeting experiments have been performed to address specifically questions relating to the pathogenesis of RA. However, many of the knock-out mutants being generated involve specific components and/or cell types of the immune system (see Fung-Leung and Mak, 1992). These animals therefore provide exciting opportunities for those interested in autoimmunity to evaluate how their transgenic or experimentally induced autoimmune models behave in the context of these novel genetic backgrounds. For example, Koh *et al.* (1992) have examined the pathogenesis of experimental allergic encephalomyelitis (EAE) in transgenic mice that are deficient for CD8$^+$ T lymphocytes. In this murine model of human multiple sclerosis, disease onset and susceptibility in mutant transgenic animals is similar to that in wild type controls. However, the mutant mice have a mild acute phase EAE with fewer deaths but a higher frequency of relapse and chronic EAE. It would be interesting to examine the progression of the RA-like pathology observed in some of the transgenic models described in this and other 'immune compromised' genetic backgrounds.

PERSPECTIVES

The ability to manipulate the mammalian genome provides exciting opportunities to investigate systematically specific aspects of the pathophysiology of complex human diseases. Immunobiology is ideally suited to this approach as many of the mutants that can be generated are likely to be viable when maintained in suitable conditions. Several interesting transgenic models have already been generated; however, there remains tremendous scope for further endeavour in this area.

As well as the primary pathology observed in any transgenic model, the power of mouse genetics, through interbreeding to different inbred strains and between transgenic lines, provides a unique opportunity to evaluate the progression of any disease in different genetic backgrounds. A challenge for the future will be to apply the techniques used in the experimental induction of an RA-like state to the range of transgenic animals likely to be generated in the near future. This powerful combination should provide significant insights into the aetiopathobiology of RA disease in humans. In turn this will aid the identification of novel disease targets and thereby enhance the prospects of discovering new therapeutic approaches to the prevention and relief of autoimmune diseases and RA in particular.

REFERENCES

Beddington RSP (1992) Transgenic strategies in mouse embryology and development. In Grosveld F & Kollias G (eds) *Transgenic Animals*, pp 47–78. London: Academic Press.

Behringer R, Mathews LS, Palmiter RD & Brinster RL (1988) Dwarf mice produced by genetic ablation of growth hormone-expressing cell. *Genes Dev* **2**: 453–461.

Berns A, Breuer M, Verbeek S & van Lohuizen M (1989) Transgenic mice as a means to study synergism between oncogenes. *Int J Cancer* (**Supplement 4**): 22–25.

Bishop JO & Smith P (1989) Mechanism of chromosomal integration of microinjected DNA. *Mol Biol Med* **6**: 283–298.

Bonifer C, Vidal M, Grosveld F & Sippel AE (1990) Tissue specific and position independent expression of the complete gene domain for chicken lysozyme in transgenic mice. *EMBO J* **9**: 2843–2848.

Borelli E, Heyman R, Arias C, Sawchenko PE & Evans RM (1989) Transgenic mice with inducible dwarfism. *Nature* **339**: 538–541.

Bradley A, Hasty P, Davis A & Ramirez-Solis R (1992) Modifying the mouse: design and desire. *Biol technology* **10**: 534–539.

Breitman ML & Bernstein A (1992) Engineering cellular deficits in transgenic mice by cellular ablation. In Grosveld F & Kollias G (eds) *Transgenic Animals*, pp 127–146. London: Academic Press.

Breitman ML, Rombola H, Maxwell IH, Klintworth GKK & Bernstein A (1990) Genetic ablation in transgenic mice with an attenuated diphtheria toxin A gene. *Mol Cell Biol* **10**: 474–479.

Brennan FM & Feldmann M (1992) Cytokines in autoimmunity. *Curr Opin Immunol* **4**: 754–759.

Brennan FM, Mainin RN & Feldmann M (1992). TNFα-A pivotal role in rheumatoid arthritis. *Brit J Rheumatol* **31**: 293–298.

Brinster, RL, Allen JM, Behringer RR, Gelinas RE & Palmiter RD (1988) Introns increase transcriptional efficiency in transgenic mice. *Proc Natl Acad Sci* **88**: 836–840.

Brinster RL, Sandgren EP, Behringer RR & Palmiter RD (1989) No simple solution for making transgenic mice. *Cell* **59**: 239–241.

Capecchi MR (1989) Altering the genome by homologous recombination. *Science* **244**: 1288–1292.

Chisaka O & Capecchi MR (1991) Regionally restricted developmental defects resulting from targeted disruption of the mouse homeobox gene Hox-1.5. *Nature* **350**: 473–479.

Chisaka C, Musci TS & Capecchi MR (1992) Developmental defects of the ear, cranial nerves and hindbrain resulting from targeted disruption of the mouse homeobox gene Hox-1.6. *Nature* **355**: 516–520.

Choi TK, Hollenbach PW, Pearson BE, Ueda RM, Weddell GN, Kurahara CG, Woodhouse CS, Kay RM & Loring JF (1993) Transgenic mice containing a human heavy chain immunoglobulin gene fragment cloned in a yeast artificial chromosome. *Nature Genetics* **4**: 117–123.

Clark AJ, Simons JP & Wilmut I (1992) Germline manipulation: applications in agriculture and biotechnology. In Grosveld F & Kollias G (eds) *Transgenic Animals*, pp 247–270. London: Academic Press.

Collins JM & Wilson FS (1992) More from the modellers. *Nature* **359**: 195–196.

Cuthbertson RA & Klintworth GK (1988) Transgenic mice – a gold mine for furthering knowledge in pathobiology. *Laboratory Investigation* **58**: 484–502.

Davis A & Bradley A (1993) Mutation of N-myc in mice: what does the phenotype tell us? *Bioessays* **15**: 273–275.

DeChiara TM, Roberton EJ & Efstratiadis A (1991) Parental imprinting of the mouse insulin-like growth factor II gene. *Cell* **64**: 849–859.

Doetschman T, Williams P & Maeda N (1988) Establishment of hamster blastocyst-derived embryonic stem (ES) cells. *Dev Biol* **127**: 224–227.

Donehower LA, Harvey M, Slagle BL, McArthur MJ, Montgomery Jr CA, Butel JS et al. (1992) Mice deficient for p53 are developmentally normal but susceptible to spontaneous tumours. *Nature* **254**: 215–221.

Ebert KM, Selgrath P, DiTullio P, Denman J, Smith TE, Memon MA et al. (1991) Transgenic production of a variant of human tissue-type plasminogen activator in goat milk: generation of transgenic goats and analysis of expression. *Bio/technology* **9**: 835–838.

Endo T, Iwakura Y & Kobata A (1993) Structural changes in the N-linked sugar chains of serum immunoglobulin G of HTLV-1 transgenic mice. *Biochem Biophy Res Comm* **192**: 1004–1010.

Evans MJ & Kaufman MH (1981) Establishment in culture of pluripotential cells from mouse embryos. *Nature* **292**: 154–156.

Friedrich G & Soriano P (1991) Promoter traps in embryonic stem cells: a genetic screen to identify and mutate developmental genes in mice. *Genes and Dev* **5**: 1513–1523.

Fung-Leung W-P & Mak TW (1992) Embryonic stem cells and homologous recombination. *Curr Opin Immunol* **4**: 189–194.

Gordon JW & Ruddle FH (1981) Integration and stable germ line transmission of genes injected into mouse pronuclei. *Science* **214**: 1244–1246.

Greaves DR, Wilson FD, Lang G & Kioussis D (1989) Human CD2 3′ flanking sequences confer high-level, T-cell specific, position-independent gene expression in transgenic mice. *Cell* **56**: 979–986.

Gridley T, Soriano P & Jaenisch R (1987) Insertional mutagensis in mice. *Trends in Genetics* **3**: 162–166.

Grosveld, F, Blom van Assendelft G, Greaves DR & Kollias G (1987) Position-independent, high-level expression of the human β-globin gene in transgenic mice. *Cell* **51**: 975–985.

Gruby MJ, Auchincloss H Jr, Lee R, Johnson RS, Spencer JP, Zulstra M et al. (1993) Mice lacking major histocompatibility complex class I and class II molecules. *Proc Natl Acad Sci* **90**: 3913–3917.

Hammer RE, Pursell VG, Rexroad CE, Wall RJ, Bolt DJ, Ebert KM et al. (1985) Production of transgenic rabbits, sheep and pigs by microinjection. *Nature* **315**: 680–683.

Hammer RE, Maika SD, Richardson JA, Tang J-P & Taurog JD (1990) Spontaneous inflammatory disease in transgenic rats expressing HLA-B27 and human β2m: an animal model of HLA-B27-associated human disorders. *Cell* **63**: 1099–1112.

Hanahan D (1988) Dissecting multistep tumorigenesis in transgenic mice. *Annu Rev Genet* **22**: 479–519.

Hanahan D (1989) Transgenic mice as probes into complex systems. *Science* **246**: 1265–1275.

Hanahan D (1990) Transgenic mouse models of self-tolerance and autoreactivity by the immune system. *Annu Rev Cell Biol* **6**: 493–537.

Handyside A, Hooper ML, Kaufman MH & Wilmut I (1987) Towards the isolation of embryonal stem cells in sheep. *Roux's Arch Dev Biol* **196**: 185–190.

Harris ED (1990) Rheumatoid arthritis. *New Eng J Med* **322**: 1277–1289.

Hasty P, Ramirez-Solis R, Krumlauf R & Bradley A (1991) Introduction of a subtle mutation into the Kox-2.6 locus in embryonic stem cells. *Nature* **350**: 243–246.

Herskowitz L (1987) Functional inactivation of genes by dominant negative mutations. *Nature* **329**: 219–222.

Hogan B, Costantini F & Lacy E (1986) *Manipulating the Mouse Embryo: a Laboratory Manual*. Cold Spring Harbor Lab.

Hyde SC, Gill DR, Higgins CF, Trezise AEO, MacVinish LJ, Cuthbert AW et al. (1993). Correction of the ion transport defect in cystic fibrosis transgenic mice by gene therapy. *Nature* **362**: 250–255.

Iwakura Y, Tosu M, Yoshida E, Takiguchi M, Sato K, Kitajma I et al. (1991) Induction of inflammatory arthropathy resembling rheumatoid arthritis in mice transgenic for HTLV-1. *Science* **253**: 1026–1028.

Jaenisch R (1976) Germline integration and mendelian transmission of the exogenous Moloney leukemia virus. *Proc Natl Acad Sci* **73**: 1260–1264.

Jaenisch R (1988) Transgenic animals. *Science* **240**: 1468–1474.

Jakobovits A, Moore AL, Green LL, Vergara GJ, Maynard-Currie CE, Austin HA et al. (1993) Germ-line transmission and expression of a human-derived yeast artificial chromosome. *Nature* **362**: 255–258.

Joyner AL (1991) Gene targeting and gene trap screens using embryonic stem cells: new approaches to mammalian development. *Bioassays* **13**: 649–656.

Joyner AL, Skarnes WC & Rossant J (1989) Production of a mutation in mouse En-2 gene by homologous recombination in embryonic stem cells. *Nature* **338**: 153–156.

Joyner AL, Auerbach BA, Davis CA, Herrup K & Rossant J (1991) Subtle cerebellar phenotype in mice homozygous for a targeted deletion of the En2 homodomain. *Science* **251**: 1239–1243.

Kaklamanis PHM (1992) Experimental animal models resembling rheumatoid arthritis. *Clin Rheumatol* **11**: 41–47.

Katsuki M, Sato M, Kimura M, Yokoyama M, Kobayashi K & Nomura T (1988) Conversion of normal behaviour to shiverer by myelin basic protein antisense cDNA in transgenic mice. *Science* **241**: 593–595.

Keffer J, Probert L, Cazlaris H, Georgopoulos S, Kaslaris E, Kioussis D & Kollias G (1991) Transgenic mice expressing human tumour necrosis factor: a predictive genetic model of arthritis. *EMBO J* **10**: 4025–4031.

Kessel M, Balling R & Gruss P (1990) Variations of cervical vertebrate after expression of a Hox1.1 transgene in mice. *Cell* **61**: 301–308.

Knight KL, Spieker-Polet H, Kazdin DS & Oi VT (1988) Transgenic rabbits with lymphocyte leukemia induced by the c-myc oncogene fused with the immunoglobulin heavy chain enhancer. *Proc Natl Acad Sci* **85**: 3130–3134.

Koh D-R, Fung-Leung W-P, Ho A, Gray D, Acha-Orbea H & Mak T-W (1992) Less mortality but more relapses in experimental allergic encephalomyelitis in $CD8^{-/-}$ mice. *Science* **256**: 1210–1213.

Korn R, Schoor M, Neuhaus H, Henseling U, Soininen R, Zachgo J et al. (1992) Enhancer trap integrations in mouse embryonic stem cells give rise to staining patterns in chimaeric embryos with a high frequency and detect endogenous gene. *Mechanisms of Development* **39**: 95–109.

Kopf M, Le Gros G, Bachmann M, Lamers MC, Bluethmann H & Kohler G (1993) Disruption of the murine IL-4 gene blocks Th2 cytokine responses. *Nature* **362**: 245–247.

Krimpenfort P, Rademakers A, Eyestone W, van der Schans A, van den Broek S, Kooiman P et al. (1991) Generation of transgenic dairy cattle using 'in vitro' embryo production. *Bio/technology* **9**: 844–847.

Kuehn MR, Bradley A, Robertson EJ & Evans MD (1987) A potential animal model for Lesch–Nyhan syndrome through introductions of hprt mutations into mice. *Nature* **326**: 285–298.

Lavitrano M, Camaioni A, Fazio VM, Dolci S, Farace MG & Spadafora C (1989) Sperm cells as vectors for introducing foreign DNA into eggs: genetic transformation of mice. *Cell* **57**: 717–723.

Lee K-F, Li E, Huber J, Landis SC, Sharpe AH, Chao MV et al. (1992) Targeted mutation of the gene encoding the low affinity NGF receptor p75 leads to deficits in the peripheral sensory nervous system. *Cell* **69**: 737–749.

Lee M-S & Sarvetnick N (1992) Transgenes and autoimmunity. *Curr Opin Immunol* **4**: 723–727.

Le Mouellic H, Lallemand Y & Brulet P (1992) Homeosis in the mouse induced by a null mutation in the Hox-3.1 gene. *Cell* **69**: 251–264.

Mannik M (1992) Rheumatoid factors in the pathogenesis of rheumatoid arthritis. *J Rheumatol* **19** (**supplement 32**): 46–49.

Martin GR (1981) Isolation of a pluripotent cell line from early mouse embryos cultured in medium conditioned by teratocarcinoma stem cells. *Proc Natl Acad Sci* **78**: 7634–7638.

Matsui Y, Zsebo K & Hogan BLM (1992) Derivation of pluripotential embryonic stem cells from murine primordial germ cells in culture. *Cell* **70**: 841–847.

Meisler MH (1992) Insertional mutation of 'classical' and novel genes in transgenic mice. *Trends in Genetics* **8**: 341–344.

Mellor AL (1992) Transgenic mice in immunology. In Grosveld F & Kollias G (eds) *Animals*, pp 147–168. London: Academic Press.

Merlino G (1991) Transgenic animals in biomedical research. *FASEB J* **5**: 2996–3001.

Moav B, Liu ZJ, Caldovic LD, Gross ML, Faras AJ & Hackett PB (1993) Regulation of expression of transgenes in developing fish. *Transgenic Research* **2**: 153–161.

Mombaerts P, Clarke AR, Rudnicki MA, Iacomini J, Itohara S, Lafaille JJ et al. (1992) Mutations in T-cell antigen receptor gene α and β block thymocytes development at different stages. *Nature* **360**: 225–231.

Morahan G (1991) Transgenic mice as immune system models. *Curr Opin Immunol* **3**: 219–223.

Munir MI, Rossiter BJ & Caskey CT (1990) Antisense RNA production in transgenic mice. *Somat Cell Mol Genet* **16**: 383–394.

Notarianni E, Laurie S, Moor RM & Evans MJ (1990) Maintenance and differentiation in cultures of pluripotential embryonic cell lines from pig blastocysts. *J Reprod Fert* **41** (**supplement**): 51–56.

Ornitz DM, Moreadith RW & Leder P (1991) Binary system for regulating transgene expression in mice:

targeting *int*-2 gene expression with yeast GAL4/UAS control elements. *Proc Natl Acad Sci* **88**: 698–702.

Palmiter RD & Brinster RL (1986) Germline transformation of mice. *Ann Rev Genet* **20**: 465–499.

Palmiter RD, Behringer RR, Quaife CJ, Maxwell F, Maxwell IH & Brinster RL (1987) Cell lineage ablation in transgenic mice by cell-specific expression of a toxin gene. *Cell* **50**: 435–443.

Palmiter RD, Sandgren EP, Averbock MR, Allen DD & Brinster RL (1991) Heterologous introns can enhance expression of transgenes in mice. *Proc Natl Acad Sci* **88**: 478–482.

Pepin MC, Pothier F & Barden N (1992) Impaired type II glucocorticoid-receptor function in mice bearing antisense RNA transgene. *Nature* **355**: 725–728.

Perry MM & Sang HM (1993) Transgenesis in chickens. *Transgenic Research* **2**: 125–133.

Picarella DE, Kratz A, Li C-B, Ruddle NH & Flavell RA (1993) Transgenic tumour necrosis factor (TNF)-α production in pancreatic islets leads to insulitis, not diabetes. Distinct patterns of inflammation in TNF-α and TNF-β transgenic mice. *J Immunol* **150**: 4136–4150.

Piedrahita JA, Anderson GB & BonDurant RH (1990) On the isolation of embryonic stem cells: Comparative behaviour of murine, porcine and ovine embryos. *Theriogenology* **34**: 865–878.

Probert L, Keffer J, Corbella P, Cazlaris H, Patsavoudi E, Stephens S et al. (1993) Wasting, ischaemia and lymphoid abnormalities in mice expressing T cell-targeted human tumour necrosis factor transgenes. *J Immunol* **151**: 1894–1906.

Reik W (1992) Genome imprinting. In Grosveld F & Kollias G (eds) *Transgenic Animals*, pp 99–126. London: Academic Press.

Resnick JL, Bixler LS, Cheng L & Donovan PJ (1992) Long-term proliferation of mouse primordial germ cells in culture. *Nature* **259**: 550–551.

Richa J & Lo CW (1989) Introduction of human DNA into mouse eggs by injection of dissected chromosome fragments. *Science* **245**: 176–177.

Riego E, Limonta J, Aguilar A, Perez A, Dearmas R, Solano R et al. (1993) Production of transgenic mice and rabbits that carry and express the human tissue plasminogen activator cDNA under the control of a bovine alpha-S1 casein promoter. *Theriogenology* **39**: 1173–1185.

Saito S, Strelchenko N & Niemann H (1992) Bovine embryonic stem cell-like cell lines cultured over several passages. *Roux's Arch Dev Biol* **201**: 134–141.

Schedl A, Beermann F, Thies E, Montoliu L, Kelsey G & Schutz G (1992) Transgenic mice generated by pronuclear injection of a yeast artificial chromosome. *Nucl Acids Res* **20**: 3073–3077.

Schedl A, Montoliu L, Kelsey G & Schutz G (1993) A yeast artificial chromosome covering the tyrosinase gene confers copy number-dependent expression in transgenic mice. *Nature* **362**: 258–261.

Sedivy JM & Joyner AL (1992) *Gene Targeting*. New York: WH Freeman.

Sewell KL & Trentham DE (1993) Pathogenesis of rheumatoid arthritis. *Lancet* **341**: 283–286.

Sharp MGF & Mullins JJ (1993) Loss of gene function methodology. *J Hypertension* **11**: 399–343.

Shull MM, Ormsby I, Kier AB, Pawlowski S, Diebold RJ, Yin M et al. (1992) Targeted disruption of the mouse transforming growth factor-β1 gene results in multifocal inflammatory disease. *Nature* **359**: 693–699.

Shiozawa S, Tanaka T, Fujita T & Tokuhisa T (1992) Destructive arthritis without lymphocyte infiltration in H2-fos transgenic mice. *J Immunol* **148**: 3100–3104.

Silva AJ, Stevens CF, Tonegawa S & Wang Y (1992a) Deficient hippocampal long-term potentiation in α-calcium-calmodulin kinase II mutant mice. *Science* **257**: 201–206.

Silva AJ, Paylor R, Wehner JM & Tonegawa S (1992b) Impaired spatial learning in α-calcium-calmodulin kinase II mutant mice. *Science* **257**: 206–211.

Simkiss K (1993) Surrogate eggs, chimaeric embryos and transgenic birds. *Comp Biochem Physiol* **104A**: 411–417.

Sippel AE, Saueressig H, Winter D, Grewal T, Faust N, Hecht A & Bonifer C (1992) The regulatory domain organization of eukaryotic genomes: implications for stable gene transfer. In Grosveld F & Kollias G (eds) *Transgenic Animals*, pp 1–26. London: Academic Press.

Stacey A, Bateman J, Choi T, Mascara T, Cole W & Jaenisch R (1988) Perinatal lethal osteogenesis imperfecta in transgenic mice bearing an engineered mutant pro-α1(I) collagen gene. *Nature* **332**: 131–136.

Strauss WM, Dausman J, Beard C, Johnson C, Lawrence JB & Jaenisch R (1993) Germ line transmission of yeast artificial chromosome spanning the murine α$_1$(I) collagen locus. *Science* **259**: 1904–1907.

Taurog JD, Maika SD, Simmons WA, Breban M & Hammer RE (1993) Susceptibility to inflammatory disease in HLA-B27 transgenic rat lines correlates with the level of B27 expression. *J Immunol* **150**: 4168–4178.

Tewari R, Michard-Vanhee C, Perrot E & Chourrout D (1992) Mendelian transmission, structure and expression of transgenes following their injection into the cytoplasm of trout eggs. *Transgenic Res* **1**: 250–260.

Tybulewicz VLJ, Tremblay ML, LaMarca ME, Willemsen R, Stubblefield BK, Winfield S et al. (1992)

Animal model of Gaucher's disease from targeted disruption of the mouse glucocerebrosidase gene. *Nature* **357**: 407–410.

Valancius V & Smithies O (1991) Testing an 'In–Out' targeting procedure for making subtle genomic modifications in mouse embryonic stem cell. *Mol Cell Biol* **11**: 1402–1408.

Vick L, Li Y & Simkiss K (1993) Trangenic birds from transformed primordial germ cells. *Proc R Soc Lond B* **251**: 179–182.

Viville S, Neefjes J, Lotteau V, Dierich A, Lemeur M, Ploegh H et al. (1993) Mice lacking the MHC Class II-associated invariant chain. *Cell* **72**: 635–648.

Waldman SA (1992) Targeted homologous recombination in mammalian cells. *Crit Rev in Oncol/Hematology* **12**: 49–64.

Whitelaw CBA, Springbett AJ, Webster J & Clark AJ (1993) The majority of G_0 transgenic mice are derived from mosaic embryos. *Transgenic Res* **2**: 29–32.

Wolgemuth DJ, Behringer RR, Mostoller MP, Brinster RL & Palmiter RD (1989) Transgenic mice overexpressing the mouse homeobox-containing gene Hox 1.4 exhibit abnormal gut development. *Nature* **337**: 464–467.

Wordsworth P (1992) Rheumatoid arthritis. *Curr Opin Immunol* **4**: 766–769.

Wright G, Carver A, Cottom D, Reeves D, Scott A, Simons P et al. (1991) High level expression of active human alpha-1-antitrypsin in the milk of transgenic sheep. *Bio/Technology* **9**: 830–834.

Yoshioka T, Feigenbaum L & Jay G (1991) Transgenic mouse model for central nervous system demyelination. *Mol Cell Biol* **21**: 5479–5486.

28 The Use of Animals in the Search for Anti-inflammatory Drugs

Richard J. Griffiths

INTRODUCTION

The use of animals in anti-inflammatory drug testing was until recently restricted to a selection of tests that were empirically found to be sensitive to the actions of one particular class of drug, cyclooxygenase inhibitors, which inhibit the enzyme that converts arachidonic acid to prostaglandins (see Chapter 14, this volume). These models, which include carrageenan-induced paw oedema, adjuvant arthritis and phenylbenzoquinine-induced writhing, and their use in the discovery of anti-inflammatory drugs have been extensively reviewed elsewhere (Otterness and Bliven, 1985). While cyclooxygenase inhibitors are not the only drugs with activity in these models, their profile in these tests is sufficiently characteristic to enable compounds with this pharmacological activity to be identified reliably. Although this class are generally referred to as non-steroidal anti-inflammatory drugs (NSAIDs) the use of this term will be avoided since it conveys little meaning with regard to pharmacological activity. The introduction of new types of drug, with a different pharmacological mechanism of action, into clinical trials will soon make the term confusing and outdated. Cyclooxygnase inhibitors are extensively used in the treatment of rheumatoid arthritis (RA), probably reflecting their analgesic activity more than anything else. They do not have any significant effect on the disease progression and there is a desperate need for pharmacological agents with increased efficacy (Brooks, 1993; Panayi, Chapter 4, this volume). The other major class of drug used in the treatment of RA are the so-called 'slow acting anti-rheumatic drugs' (SAARDs). These drugs, which include gold salts, D-penicillamine, chloroquine, methotrexate and sulphasalazine, can be considered as a class, not from any unifying basis for their mechanism of action, but rather because they share a slow onset of action and the lack of a defined mechanism of action. Animal studies were not an important feature of the development of any of these drugs. Since they are uniformly inactive in most models of arthritis they will not be discussed further here. Their clinical use and mechanism of action are discussed in Chapter 4, this volume.

In this review I concentrate on the recent changes in the way in which pharmacological testing of potential new anti-inflammatory agents is conducted, using representative examples of mechanism-based approaches. These approaches are still experimental for the most part, because they have not been proven in the clinic. The emphasis of *in vivo* studies in these examples is on demonstrating pharmacological/biochemical efficacy in a facile model at an early stage of drug discovery. This application of *in vivo* models complements the mechanism-based approach to drug design currently in vogue within the pharmaceutical industry. This strategy has been propelled by the explosive growth over the last decade in our knowledge of the molecular mechanisms of the inflammatory response which has identified a variety of enzymes and receptors as targets for drug discovery. The availability of these enzymes and receptors, preferably of human origin, and simple assays for measuring their function has enabled *in vitro* assays largely to replace whole animals as the first step in the discovery of new drugs. Although identification of active molecules in such mechanism based screens is still largely an empirical process, there is an ever-increasing contribution of rational drug design based on structure/function studies and molecular modelling techniques. Inhibitors of specific enzymes or receptors are taken through a hierarchy of *in vitro* tests to establish their intrinsic potency and specificity. Once a reasonable level of potency is reached, activity in a whole animal is determined using assays which do not attempt to model human disease but specifically evaluate the pharmacodynamics of the compound against the pharmacological target of interest. Even potent inhibitors may fail at this stage for a variety of reasons, for example, high plasma protein binding, lack of oral bioavailability, poor pharmacokinetics, etc. but at least these problems can be defined and addressed systematically. In contrast, if an animal is used as the first test system, the process of improving potency will be entirely empirical since the reason for any such increase will be very difficult to determine.

THE USE OF BIOCHEMICAL ENDPOINT ASSAYS IN ANIMALS TO DETERMINE BIOAVAILABILITY

EVALUATION OF ENZYME INHIBITORS

The Discovery of 5-Lipoxygenase Inhibitors

The first example of this mechanism-based approach is the discovery of orally active 5-lipoxygenase inhibitors. The enzyme 5-lipoxygenase transforms arachidonic acid to leukotrienes which are capable of producing symptoms of inflammation when injected into experimental animals and man (see Chapter 14, this volume). The availability of a source of the enzyme for *in vitro* studies was essential for initial screening purposes, and most work has been done on the enzyme from the rat basophil leukaemia cell. Isolated human neutrophils can be used as a secondary screen to ensure that activity is maintained in a whole cell and that there are not major interspecies differences in sensitivity to a particular inhibitor. Compounds active in the whole cell system can then be tested as inhibitors of leukotriene production in blood, to ensure that a high degree of protein binding does not reduce the free concentration of drug to a point where it is not pharmacologically active. However, the next step, activity in an animal, proved problematical for some time.

Two main approaches to demonstrating *in vivo* activity were tried. The first was to identify a model of inflammation which was sensitive to 5-lipoxygenase inhibitors; an equivalent of the carrageenan paw oedema assay used in the development of cyclo-oxygenase inhibitors. The second was to use a biochemical endpoint as the *in vivo* marker of activity. The turning point in the development of compounds with *in vivo* activity was, without doubt, the success of the second approach. The most widely used 'model' has been, in fact, a method that involves no manipulation of the animal other than dosing it with drug. Blood is withdrawn at appropriate times after dosing, and leukotriene production is stimulated by the addition of the calcium ionophore A23187. The drug is therefore tested for activity in a physiological milieu. This assay originally reported in 1985 has the additional advantage of being directly applicable to early pharmacology studies in man (Carey and Forder, 1985). The numerous orally active lipoxygenase inhibitors in clinical development have without exception all been examined in this assay at some point in their development (Carter *et al.*. 1991; McMillan *et al.*, 1992; McMillan *et al.*, Chapter 14, this volume).

If a drug is intended for use in arthritis, it is obviously desirable to show that it exhibits biochemical efficacy in an inflamed joint. Injection of zymosan into the rat (Griffiths *et al.*, 1991) or rabbit (McMillan *et al.*, 1992) knee joint stimulates LTB_4 production which is maximal within 3–4 h and can be inhibited by 5-lipoxygenase inhibitors. Prostaglandin production is also stimulated so the selectivity of a drug for the two major pathways of arachidonic acid metabolism can also be assessed. This test demonstrates efficacy in the compartment of interest and allows the detection of drugs with fundamental distributional problems that would preclude their use in arthritis.

The search for an inflammation model which can be reliably used to demonstrate *in vivo* efficacy of 5-lipoxygenase inhibitors has continued. The major problem with this approach of course is that one needs to have a selective 5-lipoxygenase inhibitor to validate the model. Thus the biochemical endpoint model is required to generate an inhibitor with sufficient potency and selectivity that it can be used to define the role of leukotrienes in a particular inflammatory model. Several models exist that are sensitive to the effects of 5-lipoxygenase inhibitors, but their role in the discovery of such drugs has been limited. Application of arachidonic acid to the skin of mice (Opas *et al.*, 1985) or rabbits (Aked and Foster, 1987) causes plasma protein extravasation which is partially dependent on leukotriene production. Intraperitoneal injection of zymosan in the rat also leads to leukotriene-dependent plasma protein extravasation (Griffiths *et al.*, 1991). Additionally, leukotriene production can be measured directly in these models, confirming 5-lipoxygenase inhibition as the mechanism of action of an active test agent and identifying false positives. For example, in the arachidonic acid induced inflammation model in the rabbit, glucocorticoids inhibit the oedema response without affecting leukotriene production (Griffiths and Blackham, 1988).

The Discovery of Collagenase Inhibitors

A major hindrance to the testing of enzyme inhibitors *in vivo* is if the process being measured is slow. This is exemplified by the search for *in vivo* efficacy of collagenase inhibitors. The enzyme collagenase is believed to be the rate-limiting enzyme that initiates the cleavage of collagen in its native, triple helical form (Werb, 1989). Collagen fibrils then become susceptible to the action of a variety of other enzymes. Since collagen is a major constituent of cartilage, many pharmaceutical companies have programmes designed to produce inhibitors of this enzyme which will hopefully prevent the loss of structural integrity of cartilage that occurs in arthritis. Collagen degradation *in vivo* is a relatively slow process (see Chapters 9 and 17, this volume). Quantifying collagen loss from cartilage is also not easy, which makes testing of drugs very difficult. The main approach to testing inhibitors of collagenase *in vivo* has been to rely on the production and activation of collagenase by an experimental animal and to measure a parameter that hopefully reflects the activity of the enzyme.

Collagenase inhibitors have been tested in two types of model. Adjuvant arthritis is a severe polyarthritis (see Chapter 20, this volume) which results in massive changes in bone turnover. Collagenase inhibitors have been tested in this model and are claimed to show efficacy using radiography and histology as endpoints (DiMartino *et al.*, 1991). However, these are at best semi-quantitative measures, and no measurement of enzyme inhibition in the tissue can be made. In a second model collagenase inhibitors have been tested as inhibitors of granuloma-induced cartilage degradation. This involves implanting xenogeneic cartilage in a material capable of inducing a chronic inflammatory response, such as cotton. Collagen degradation can be measured as the difference between the content of hydroxyproline (an amino acid unique to collagen) in implanted and non-implanted cartilage (Bottomley *et al.*, 1988). This model has the advantage of directly measuring collagen loss from a defined tissue, but as with the adjuvant model it suffers from a major drawback. This is that the endpoints are measured after a period of several days or weeks which raises the problem of ensuring sufficient exposure to the drug over a protracted period of time to give a reasonable chance of detecting an effect. In the early stages of drug discovery it is not uncommon for lead compounds to have short plasma half-lives and a less than optimum degree of potency. However it is important to be able to demonstrate activity *in vivo* at this stage. A primary *in vivo* assay that takes days or weeks is a severe liability to any project. There has clearly been a great contrast in the development of methods for assessing *in vivo* activity of inhibitors of 5-lipoxygenase compared to collagenase inhibitors, and this is reflected in the relative success achieved in these two areas. While in both areas compounds with potent *in vitro* activity have been produced, a number of 5-lipoxygenase inhibitors are now in clinical trials. In contrast there are no published reports of any collagenase inhibitor in clinical trials for arthritis. One of the major reasons for this difference has been the ability to detect *in vivo* activity easily and rapidly in one case but not the other. This information can be extremely valuable in guiding the work of medicinal chemists and avoiding pursuit of a chemical series that is not bioavailable. The ability to detect collagen damage reliably at a much earlier stage, prior to hydroxyproline loss (Dodge & Poole, 1989) or a more rapid way of inducing collagen breakdown would be a great step forward and enhance the chances of success in this field enormously. See Chapter 9, this volume for a review of the methods available for measuring cartilage breakdown.

EVALUATION OF RECEPTOR ANTAGONISTS

In contrast to the problems associated with testing enzyme inhibitors, developing a facile assay for initial *in vivo* efficacy studies of a receptor antagonist is generally much more straightforward. The primary reason for this is that a biological response mediated by a specific receptor can be elicited by administration of either the naturally occurring agonist, or a synthetic analogue, at an appropriate site. This approach has been employed successfully in the development of drugs in a number of therapeutic areas, for example, adrenoceptor antagonists and histamine H_2 antagonists, but has only recently been employed in the inflammation area. This type of assay can give a great deal of valuable information about bioavailability, potency and pharmacodynamics of a compound.

The Discovery of LTB₄ Receptor Antagonists

The development of potent, selective LTB_4 receptor antagonists is a good example of this. Receptor binding assays and functional responses such as a chemotaxis of intact cells can be used for the initial evaluation of such compounds. The *in vivo* efficacy of potent antagonists identified in such *in vitro* assays can be easily assessed by injecting LTB_4 into the skin of a suitable species, for example the guinea pig, and measuring the accumulation of neutrophils using either readiolabelled cells or a neutrophil marker enzyme such as myeloperoxidase (Bradley *et al.*, 1982). Inhibition of neutrophil accumulation in such a model system is an indicator that the drug is an LTB_4 antagonist. Specificity controls using other exogenously administered chemoattractants can be included in the assay to rule out the possibility that the drug has effects unrelated to LTB_4 antagonism. A number of potent and selective LTB_4 antagonists have been identified using such an approach (Fretland *et al.*, 1989; Huang *et al.*, 1992; Kishikawa *et al.*, 1992).

The Discovery of Non-peptide NK₁ Receptor Antagonists

Substance P and other neuropeptides have a variety of biological activities suggesting they may be important in the production of inflammatory responses and pain (Chapter 16, this volume). A variety of peptide analogues that antagonize the action of substance P have been described but their usefulness for *in vivo* studies is limited by lack of oral bioavailability and metabolic instability. The recent description of CP-96 345 (Snider *et al.*, 1991), a non-peptide antagonist of the NK_1 receptor, one subtype of the tachykinin family of receptors, is another illustration of how receptor antagonists can be easily characterized *in vivo*. Injection of tachykinins into the skin of experimental animals causes a rapid increase in vascular permeability to plasma proteins. CP-96 345 inhibits tachykinin-induced plasma protein extravasation in guinea pig skin, but not that induced by a variety of other inflammatory mediators, demonstrating the selectivity of the drug (Nagahisa *et al.*, 1992). CP-96 345 is orally bioavailable and is active in a variety of species (Lembeck *et al.*, 1992; Nagahisa *et al.*, 1992).

LTB_4 and NK_1 receptor antagonists are the prototypes of drugs that selectively inhibit the effects of inflammatory mediators at a particular receptor. While receptor antagonists are common in other therapeutic areas, for example anti-hypertensives, they are new to the inflammation area. The ease with which such drugs can be progressed from *in vitro* testing to *in vivo* testing, as exemplified by the two examples given, should ensure that these are the first of many such agents available for clinical testing.

THE CONTRIBUTION OF BIOLOGICAL REAGENTS TO THE STUDY OF DRUGS IN ANIMAL MODELS OF ARTHRITIS

The introduction of molecular biology into modern drug discovery has had two important impacts. The most obvious is the potential use of monoclonal antibodies and recombinant proteins as therapeutic agents in their own right. However, they have had a secondary use which has been beneficial to those interested in developing orally active agents for use in arthritis. This has been the ability to validate a model with a highly specific reagent such as a monoclonal antibody or recombinant protein. This is particularly important in areas where there is no simple way of ensuring that the mechanism of interest is involved in the biological response being measured. One area that illustrates this is the search for inhibitors of adhesion molecule function. A variety of molecules on the surface of leukocytes and endothelial cells can mediate the interaction of these two cell types. These molecules are involved in the initial attachment of cells to the endothelium (L, E and P selectin) and their subsequent transmigration into the tissues (members of the integrin and immunoglobulin superfamily of cell adhesion molecules, see Chapter 11, this volume). These systems are really receptor–ligand interactions but the ligand is membrane bound and not soluble. It is therefore not possible to induce leukocyte migration with these molecules in the same way that it can be induced with exogenous LTB_4 as described above (in fact, soluble versions of these molecules may in fact compete for the receptor and act as antagonists (Watson et al., 1991)). The contribution of each molecule to leukocyte migration can, however, be determined with suitable monoclonal antibodies that block the function of the targeted molecule. The relative importance of each of these molecules may vary from one type of response to another or even, in the same type of response, at different sites in the body. For example, neutrophil emigration from the circulation into sites of inflammation in the peritoneal cavity and subcutaneous tissues induced by a bacterial stimulus is dependent on the integrin CD18. However, in the pulmonary circulation this adhesion molecule complex does not contribute to neutrophil emigration in response to the same stimulus (Doerschuk et al., 1990). Similarly, the migration of different populations of lymphocytes to the joints of animals with adjuvant arthritis shows a differential dependency on the use of the integrin VLA-4 (Issekutz and Issekutz, 1991). The use of such antibodies is an invaluable tool for ensuring that low molecular weight inhibitors are tested in suitable, mechanistically validated models when initial studies are performed to determine bioavailability.

The use of the recombinant form of a naturally occurring IL-1 receptor antagonist (IL-1ra) is another example that illustrates the values of this approach (Arend et al., 1990). Injection of IL-1 into experimental animals causes a variety of biological effects such as neutrophil infiltration, proteoglycan depletion from cartilage and leukocytosis. Administration of IL-1ra selectively inhibits these responses to IL-1 (Henderson et al., 1991; McIntyre et al., 1991; Ulich et al., 1991). Having established efficacy and pharmacodynamics versus exogenous IL-1, IL-1ra has been used to investigate the role of IL-1 in models of inflammation. LPS-induced neutrophil recruitment (McIntyre et al., 1991; Ulich et al., 1991), septic shock (Ohlsson et al., 1990), and bacterial cell wall induced arthritis are all inhibited by IL-1 receptor antagonists (Schwab et al., 1991). These models can therefore be used to test novel IL-1ra against the endogenously produced cytokine (having first established efficacy against the exogenously administered cytokine as described for IL-1ra). The antagonism of cytokines is reviewed by Firestein in Chapter 13, this volume.

THE USE OF ANIMAL MODELS OF ARTHRITIS

The next step in the development of a drug once biochemical/pharmacological efficacy has been established is usually to ask the question 'what does the drug do in an animal model of disease?' The many different models available are described in detail in earlier chapters of this book (see overview in Chapter 18). They differ from the biochemical endpoint assays described above in that the pathology produced, and the endpoints against which drugs are tested, more closely resemble RA. The decision as to which is the most suitable model should be made (but frequently is not!) after consideration of a number of factors, related to both the model and the drug. It should be clear from the examples given in previous sections that every effort should be made to avoid testing the drug and the model at the same time. By this I mean that a drug with a defined pharmacological activity *in vitro* should not be taken straight into a model of arthritis in the hope that it will demonstrate efficacy. Lack of activity could either mean that the drug has poor bioavailability/pharmacokinetics or that the mechanism by which the drug acts is not important in that particular model. To avoid this pitfall, there are three considerations that need to be evaluated prior to testing the drug.

The first consideration is that the drug should be efficacious in the species chosen for study. The intrinsic potency of receptor antagonists (Ming Fong *et al.*, 1992; Sutherland *et al.*, 1992) and enzyme inhibitors (McMillan *et al.*, 1992) can vary dramatically between species. For example, certain LTB_4 receptor antagonists appear to have a very weak affinity for the receptor in the rabbit despite being potent antagonists in other species (Sutherland *et al.*, 1992). It is obviously pointless testing a drug in a particular model if it does not interact with the molecular target in the species in question.

If this factor is not a problem, the next hurdle is the question of pharmacokinetics of the drug in animals. Animal models of arthritis are usually of several weeks' duration. To optimize the chances of success, it is necessary to ensure that exposure of the animal to pharmacologically relevant concentrations of the drug is maintained for 24 h a day. This can be a considerable problem. For example, the plasma half-life of most cyclooxygenase inhibitors in the mouse is extremely short, for example, piroxicam has a plasma half-life of less than 2 h which is typical of this class of drug (Milne and Twomey, 1980). To maintain pharmacologically relevant concentrations of piroxicam by oral dosing would require multiple doses per day (it should be noted that in man the drug has a plasma half-life of approximately 2 days and is administered once a day (Hobbs and Twomey, 1979). This may be one factor that has contributed to the widely held belief that mouse models of arthritis are less susceptible to the effects of cyclooxygenase inhibitors than similar models in the rat. There are numerous studies in which cyclooxygenase inhibitors have been tested in collagen-induced arthritis in the mouse. This model is induced by immunizing a susceptible strain of rat (Trentham *et al.*, 1977) or mouse (Courtenay *et al.*, 1980) with heterologous type II collagen. This leads to the production of an immune response, which crossreacts with the collagen in joints, and leads to a severe destructive arthritis (reviewed in Chapter 23, this volume). Drugs have generally been dosed p.o. once daily in these studies, and the effects on disease symptoms are generally modest (Phadke *et al.*, 1985; Griswold *et al.*, 1988; Cannon *et al.*, 1990; Hom *et al.*, 1991). However, if piroxicam and other cyclooxygenase inhibitors are administered to mice in the diet, so that the plasma levels achieved approach those used clinically in man, complete inhibition of the disease is achieved along with pronounced suppression of antibody levels to type II collagen (Griffiths and Pettipher, unpublished observations). Removal of the drug from the diet results in an increase in antibody titres to collagen and clinical signs of disease. This is a clear exmaple of a situation in which failure to ensure adequate exposure to the drug would lead to an underestimate of efficacy. In the case of piroxicam this is also a good example of pharmacokinetics in a mouse not being predictive of man.

The third consideration is whether or not biological reagents have been used to establish the role of the mechanism in question in the model. Antibodies against IL-1 have been shown to be inhibitory in antigen-induced arthritis (van de Loo *et al.*, 1992) and collagen-induced arthritis in the mouse (Joosten *et al.*, 1992) so any drug that inhibits the production or action of this cytokine should be active in this model (subject to fulfilling the previous two criteria). This approach, if used judiciously, has the benefit of always producing a positive result!

If one had to choose an animal model on which to base a decision for developing a drug candidate, the one that has proved the most reliable for predicting activity in man is antigen-induced arthritis in rabbits (Dumonde and Glynn, 1962). It is unfortunately time consuming and requires large amounts of drug. However, it can give valuable information about drug effects on both the inflammatory and connective tissue changes that occur in disease. This is important since the effect of a drug on the inflammatory changes may not necessarily parallel the effects on the tissue damage (Blackham *et al.*, 1974; Blackham and Radzowonik, 1977; Pettipher *et al.*, 1988, 1989). This model was also the first to be used to compare biochemical efficacy of an anti-inflammatory drug with its effects on arthritis. Indomethacin was shown to inhibit completely the production of prostaglandins in the joint but only to partially inhibit joint swelling and to have no effect on histological changes (Blackham *et al.*, 1974).

In practice, activity of a drug in a chronic model of arthritis is greeted with enthusiasm by the investigators involved. A negative result, however, usually results in the conclusion that 'these models are not predictive for man anyway'! A strong case can be made for abandoning this step in the process if instead a drug candidate can be chosen on the basis of the type of mechanism-based studies described earlier. This is because if a potent, bioavailable drug has been developed to act on a particular mechanism, does lack of activity in a model such as adjuvant arthritis mean that development of such a drug should stop? In the case of prototypic agents the predictive value of any model is unknown. Once a particular mechanism is validated in the clinic, demonstrating activity in a model of arthritis is unnecessary, providing the relevant pharmacological activity can be shown *in vivo*.

SUMMARY

Animals continue to play a vital role in the discovery of new drugs for the treatment of arthritis. Demonstration of pharmacological activity in an animal is an absolute requirement for the justification of testing the drug in man. However, the nature of the role of *in vivo* models is evolving. The criteria for taking a compound forward for testing in man are changing from a situation in which activity in an animal model of disease is paramount, to the one where inhibition of a defined mechanism, which is believed to be important in human disease, is the major objective. The reasons for this are complex but probably relate to our lack of understanding of the aetiology of RA and how to mimic it in animals, not to any great physiological differences between man and animal. For example, there is no known mediator of the inflammatory response that is produced in humans but not in animals. However, the relative importance of each of these mediators may be different in human RA compared to the artificially induced 'diseases' produced in animals. The perfect model of the disease would be a transgenic animal containing all the genes that lead to susceptibility to RA, combined with a knowledge of the environmental conditions that cause expression of the disease. In the absence of such a model we have to make do with what we have! Valuable information on potential mechanisms that may lead to disease can be obtained from animal studies, since similar studies in man may be impossible to perform. However, the relative importance of these processes in human disease is difficult to predict. In the future we can therefore expect to see the entry into clinical trials of drugs with a defined mechanism of action which hopefully will prove of therapeutic benefit. From these studies we should learn which mechanisms are indeed important in the pathogenesis of RA.

REFERENCES

Aked DM & Foster SJ (1987) Leukotriene B_4 and prostaglandin E_2 mediate the inflammatory response of rabbit skin to intradermal arachidonic acid. *Br J Pharmacol* **93**: 545–552.

Arend WP, Welgus HG, Thompson RC & Eisenberg SP (1990) Biological properties of recombinant human monocyte-derived interleukin 1 receptor antagonist. *J Clin Invest* **85**: 1694–1697.

Blackham A & Radziwonik H (1977) The effect of drugs in established rabbit monoarticular arthritis. *Agents Actions* **7**: 473–480.

Blackham A, Farmer JB, Radziwonik H & Westwick J (1974) The role of prostaglandins in rabbit monoarticular arthritis. *Br J Pharmacol* **51**: 35–44.

Bottomley KMK, Griffiths RJ, Rising TJ & Steward A (1988) A modified air pouch model for evaluating the effects of compounds on granuloma induced cartilage degradation. *Br J Pharmacol* **93**: 627–635.

Bradley PB, Priebat DA, Christensen RD & Rothstein G (1982) Measurement of cutaneous inflammation: Estimation of neutrophil content with an enzyme marker. *J Invest Dermatol* **78**: 206–209.

Brooks P (1993) Clinical management of rheumatoid arthritis. *Lancet* **341**: 286–290.

Cannon, GW, McCall S, Cole BC, Griffiths MM & Radov LA (1990) Effects of indomethacin, cyclophosphamide and placebo on collagen-induced arthritis of mice. *Agents Actions* **29**: 315–323.

Carey F & Forder R (1985) Radioimmunossay of LTB_4 and 6-trans LTB_4: analytical and pharmacological characterization of immunoreactive LTB_4 in ionophore stimulated human blood. *Prostaglandins Leukot Med* **22**: 57–70.

Carter GW, Young PR, Albert DH, Bouska J, Dyer R, Bell, RL et al. (1991) 5-lipoxygenase inhibitory activity of zileuton. *J Pharmac Exp Ther* **256**: 929–937.

Courtenay JS, Dallman MJ, Dayan AD, Martin A & Mosedale I (1980) Immunization against heterologous type II collagen induces arthritis in mice. *Nature* **283**: 666–668.

DiMartino MJ, Wolff CE, High W, Crimmin MJ & Galloway WA (1991) Anti-inflammatory and chondroprotective activities of a potent metalloproteinase inhibitor. *J Cell Biol* **15E**: 179.

Dodge GR & Poole AR (1989) Immunohistochemical detection and immunochemical analysis of type II collagen degradation in human normal, rheumatoid and osteoarthritic articular cartilages and in explants of bovine articular cartilage cultured with interleukin 1. *J Clin Invest* **83**: 647–661.

Doerschuk CM, Winn RK, Coxson HO & Harlan JM (1990) CD18-dependent and independent mechanisms of neutrophil emigration in the pulmonary and systemic microcirculation of rabbits. *J Immunol* **144**: 2327–2333.

Dumonde DC & Glynn LE (1962) The production of arthritis in rabbits by an immunological reaction to fibrin. *Br J Exp Path* **43**: 373–383.

Fretland DJ, Widomski DL, Zemaitis JM, Djuric SW & Shone RL (1989) Effect of a leukotriene B_4 receptor antagonist on LTB_4-induced neutrophil chemotaxis in cavine dermis. *Inflammation* **13**: 601–605.

Griffiths RJ & Blackham A (1988) The effect of dexamethasone on inflammatory responses in rabbit skin. *Br J Pharmacol* **95**: 535P.

Griffiths RJ, Li SW, Wood BE & Blackham A (1991) A comparison of the anti-inflammatory activity of selective 5-lipoxygenase inhibitors with dexamethasone and colchicine in a model of zymosan induced inflammation in the rat knee joint and peritoneal cavity. *Agents Actions* **32**: 312–320.

Griswold DE, Hillegass LM, Meunier PC, DiMartino MJ & Hanna N (1988) Effects of inhibitors of eicosanoid metabolism in murine collagen-induced arthritis. *Arthritis Rheum* **31**: 1406–1412.

Henderson B, Thompson RC, Hardingham T & Lewthwaite J (1991) Inhibition of interleukin-1 induced synovitis and articular cartilage proteoglycan loss in the rabbit knee by recombinant human interleukin-1 receptor antagonist. *Cytokine* **3**: 246–249.

Hobbs DC & Twomey TM (1979) Piroxicam pharmacokinetics in man: Aspirin and antacid interaction studies. *J Clin Pharmacol* **19**: 270–281.

Hom, JT, Gliszczynski VL, Cole HW & Bendele AM (1991) Interleukin 1 mediated acceleration of type II collagen-induced arthritis: Effects of anti-inflammatory or anti-arthritic drugs. *Agents Actions* **33**: 300–309.

Huang F, Chan, W, Warus JD, Morrissette MM, Moriarty KJ, Chang MN, Travis JT, Mitchell LS, Nuss GW & Sutherland CA (1992) 4-[2-[methyl(2-phenethyl)amino-2-oxoethyl]-8-(phenylmethoxy)-2-naphthalenecarboxylic acid: A high affinity, competitive, orally active leukotriene B_4 receptor antagonist. *J Med Chem* **35**: 4253–4255.

Issekutz TB & Issekutz AC (1991) T lymphocyte migration to arthritic joints and dermal inflammation in the rat: Differing migration patterns and the involvement of VLA-4. *Clin Immunol Immunopath* **61**: 436–447.

Kishikawa K, Tateishi N, Maruyama T, Sco R, Toda M & Miyamoto T (1992) ONO-4057, A novel, orally active leukotriene B_4 antagonist: Effects on LTB_4-induced neutrophil functions. *Prostaglandins* **44**: 261–275.

Lemback F, Donnerer J, Tsuchiya M & Nagahisa A (1992) The non-peptide tachykinin antagonist CP-96,345 is a potent inhibitor of neurogenic inflammation. *Br J Pharmacol* **105**: 527–530.

McIntyre KW, Stepan GJ, Kolinsky KD, Benjamin WR, Plocinski JM, Kaffka KL et al. (1991) Inhibition of interleukin 1 (IL-1) binding and bioactivity *in vitro* and modulation of acute inflammation *in vivo* by IL-1 receptor antagonist and anti-IL-1 receptor monoclonal antibody. *J Exp Med* **173**: 931–939.

McMillan RM, Spruce KE, Crawley GC, Walker ERH & Foster SJ (1992) Pre-clinical pharmacology of ICI D2138, a potent orally-active non-redox inhibitor of 5-lipoxygenase. *Br J Pharmacol* **107**: 1042–1047.

Milne GM & Twomey TM (1980) The analgetic properties of piroxicam in animals and correlation with experimentally determined plasma levels. *Agents Actions* **10**: 31–37.

Ming Fong T, Yu H & Strader CD (1992) Molecular basis for the species selectivity of the neurokinin-1 receptor antagonists CP-96,345 and RP67580. *J Biol Chem* **267**: 25668–25671.

Nagahisa A, Kanai Y, Suga O, Taniguchi K, Tsuchiya M, Lowe JA et al. (1992) Anti-inflammatory and analgesic activity of a non-peptide substance P receptor antagonist. *Eur J Pharmacol* **217**: 191–195.

Ohlsson K, Bjork P, Bergenfeldt M, Hageman R & Thompson RC (1990) Interleukin-1 receptor antagonist reduces mortality from endotoxic shock. *Nature* **348**: 550–552.

Opas EE, Bonney RJ & Humes JL (1985) Prostaglandin and leukotriene synthesis in mouse ears inflamed by arachidonic acid. *J Invest Dermatol* **84**: 253–256.

Otterness IG & Bliven ML (1985) Laboratory models for testing nonsteroidal anti-inflammatory drugs. In Lombardino JG (ed) *Nonsteroidal Antiinflammatory Drugs*, pp 112–152. New York: Wiley.

Pettipher EH, Henderson B, Moncada S & Higgs GA (1988) Leukocyte infiltration and cartilage proteoglycan loss in immune arthritis in the rabbit. *Br J Pharmacol* **95**: 169–176.

Pettipher EH, Henderson B, Edwards JCW & Higgs GA (1989) Effect of indomethacin on swelling, lymphocyte influx and cartilage proteoglycan depletion in experimental arthritis. *Ann Rheum Dis* **48**: 623–627.

Phadke K, Fouts RL, Parrish JE & Butler LD (1985) Evaluation of the effects of various anti-arthritic drugs on type II collagen-induced mouse arthritis model. *Immunopharmacology* **10**: 51–60.

Schwab JH, Anderle SK, Brown RR, Dalldorf FG & Thompson RC (1991) Pro- and anti-inflammatory roles of interleukin-1 in recurrence of bacterial cell wall-induced arthritis in rats. *Infect Immun* **59**: 4436–4442.

Snider RM, Constantine JW, Lowe JA, Longo KP, Lebel W, Woodey HA et al. (1991) A potent nonpeptide antagonist of the substance P (NK1) receptor. *Science* **251**: 435–437.

Sutherland C, Mitchell L, Galemmo R, Treavis J, Sweeney D, Beale L et al. (1992) Evidence for species specific variation in high affinity leukotriene B_4 receptor conformation: relative activities of structurally diverse LTB_4 antagonists in several LTB_4 receptor binding assays. *6th International Conference of the Inflammation Research Association*, p 123. White Haven, PA.

Trentham DE, Townes AS & Kang AH (1977) Autoimmunity to type II collagen: an experimental model of arthritis. *J Exp Med* **146**: 857–868.

Ulich TR, Yin S, Guo K, del Castillo J, Eisenberg SP & Thompson RC (1991) The intratracheal administration of endotoxin and cytokines III. The interleukin-1 receptor antagonist inhibits endotoxin- and IL-induced acute inflammation. *Am J Pathol* **138**: 521–524.

van de Loo FAJ, Arntz OJ, Otterness IG & van den Berg WB (1992) Protection against cartilage proteoglycan synthesis inhibition by anti-interleukin 1 antibodies in experimental arthritis. *J Rheumatol* **19**: 348–356.

van den Berg WB, Joosten LAB, Helsen M & van de Loo FAJ (1994) Suppression of established CIA with anti-IL-1. *Clin Exp Rheum* **95**: 237–243.

Watson SR, Fennie C & Lasky LA (1991) Neutrophil influx into an inflammatory site inhibited by a soluble homing receptor-IgG chimaera. *Nature* **349**: 164–167.

Werb Z (1989) Proteinases and matrix degradation. In Kelley WN, Harris ED Jr, Ruddy S & Sledge CB (eds) *Textbook of Rheumatology*, pp 341–365. Philadelphia: WB Saunders.

Index